Amyotrophic Lateral Sclerosis

Second Edition

Amyotrophic Lateral Sclerosis

Second Edition

Edited by

Robert H Brown Jr MD DPhil
Day Laboratory for Neuromuscular Research
Massachusetts General Hospital East
Charlestown, Massachusetts, USA

Michael Swash MD FRCP FRCPath
Department of Neurology
St Bartholomew's and the Royal London School of Medicine and Dentistry
The Royal London Hospital, London, UK

Piera Pasinelli PhD
Day Laboratory for Neuromuscular Research
Massachusetts General Hospital
Charlestown, Massachusetts, USA

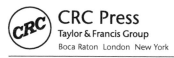

CRC Press
Taylor & Francis Group
Boca Raton London New York

CRC Press is an imprint of the
Taylor & Francis Group, an **informa** business

CRC Press
Taylor & Francis Group
6000 Broken Sound Parkway NW, Suite 300
Boca Raton, FL 33487-2742

First issued in paperback 2019

ISBN-13: 978-1-84184-463-3 (hbk)
ISBN-13: 978-0-367-39063-1 (pbk)

Visit the Taylor & Francis Web site at
http://www.taylorandfrancis.com

and the CRC Press Web site at
http://www.crcpress.com

Contents

Contributors

Ammar Al-Chalabi PhD FRCP
Senior Lecturer in Neurology
MRC Centre for Neurodegeneration Research
King's College London
Institute of Psychiatry
London
UK

Peter M Andersen MD DMSc
Department of Neurology
Umea University Hospital
Umea
Sweden

M Flint Beal MD
Chairman/Neurologist-in-Chief
Department of Neurology and Neuroscience
Weill Medical College of Cornell University
New York Presbyterian Hospital
New York, NY
USA

Camilla Blain MA MB BS MRCP
Department of Clinical Neuroscience
MRC Centre for Neurodegeneration Research
King's College London
Institute of Psychiatry
London
UK

Gian Domenico Borasio MD DipPallMed
Professor and Acting Chairman
Interdisciplinary Center for Palliative Medicine
Head, Motor Neuron Disease Research Group
Department of Neurology
Munich University Hospital – Grosshadern
Munich
Germany

Alice Brockington MB BS MRCP
Brain Research Fellow in Neurology
University of Sheffield
Sheffield
UK

Robert H Brown Jr MD DPhil
Director, Day Neuromuscular Research
  Laboratory
MassGeneral Institute for Neurodegenerative
  Disease
Massachusetts General Hospital East
Charlestown, MA
USA

Robin Conwit MD
Program Director
NINDS
Bethesda, MD
USA

Merit Cudkowicz MD
Neurology Clinical Trial Unit
Massachusetts General Hospital
Harvard Medical School
Boston, MA
USA

Mamede de Carvalho MD PhD
Professor, Department of Neurology
Neuromuscular Unit
Hospital de Santa Maria
Laboratory of EMG/EP
Institute of Molecular Medicine
Faculty of Medicine
Lisbon
Portugal

Andy Grierson
Academic Unit of Neurology
University of Sheffield
Sheffield
UK

Bradley T Hyman MD PhD
Harvard Medical School
Massachusetts General Hospital
MassGeneral Institute for Neurodegeneration
Charlestown, MA
USA

Devanand Jillapalli MD
Assistant Professor of Neurology
Department of Neurology
Upstate Medical University
Syracuse, NY
USA

Derek Jones MSc PhD Dip IPSM
Department of Clinical Neuroscience
MRC Centre for Neurodegeneration Research
King's College London
Institute of Psychiatry
London
UK

Blaz Koritnik MD MSc
Department of Clinical Neuroscience
MRC Centre for Neurodegeneration Research
King's College London
Institute of Psychiatry
London
UK

Jacqueline Lau
Neurology Clinical Trial Unit
Massachusetts General Hospital
Harvard Medical School
Boston, MA
USA

P Nigel Leigh PhD FRCP FMedSci
Professor, Department of Clinical Neuroscience
MRC Centre for Neurodegeneration Research
King's College London
Institute of Psychiatry
London
UK

Catherine Lomen-Hoerth MD PhD
Department of Neurology
University of California, San Francisco
San Francisco, CA
USA

Giovanni Manfredi
Department of Neurology and Neuroscience
Weill Medical College of Cornell University
New York, NY
USA

Valerie McGuire PhD MPH
Senior Research Scientist
Department of Health Research and Policy
Stanford University School of Medicine
Stanford, CA
USA

Chris Miller
Professor of Molecular Neuroscience
MRC Centre for Neurodegeneration Research
The Institute of Psychiatry
King's College London
Denmark Hill
London
UK

Robert Miller MD
California Pacific Medical Center
San Francisco, CA
USA

Hiroshi Mitsumoto MD DSc
Wesley J Howe Professor
Department of Neurology
Columbia University College of Physicians and
  Surgeons
and
Director, The Eleanor and Lou Gehrig
  MDA/ALS Research Center
Head, Neuromuscular Diseases Divisions
Columbia-Presbyterian Hospitals
Neurological Institutes
New York, NY
USA

Jennifer Murphy PhD
Department of Neurology
University of California, San Francisco
San Francisco, CA
USA

Brian Murray MB MSc
Consultant Neurologist
Blackrock Clinic
Blackrock, Co. Dublin
Ireland

Lorene M Nelson PhD MS
Associate Professor and Chief
Division of Epidemiology
Department of Health Research and Policy
Stanford University School of Medicine
Stanford, CA
USA

David Oliver FRCGP
Consultant in Palliative Medicine
Wisdom Hospice, Rochester
and
Honorary Senior Lecturer in Palliative Care
Kent Institute of Medicine and Health Sciences
University of Kent
UK

Piera Pasinelli PhD
Instructor in Neurology
Day Laboratory for Neuromuscular Research
Massachusetts General Hospital
Charlestown, MA
USA

Wim Robberecht MD PhD
Laboratory for Neurobiology
UZ Gasthuisberg
Leuven
Belgium

Michael Sendtner Prof Dr
Institute for Clinical Neurobiology
University of Würzburg
Würzburg
Germany

Pamela J Shaw MB BS MD FRCP
Professor of Neurology
and Director, Sheffield Care and Research Centre
  for Motor Neuron Disorders
Sheffield
UK

Jeremy M Shefner MD PhD
Professor of Neurology
Department of Neurology
Upstate Medical University
Syracuse, NY
USA

Claire L Simpson BSc PhD
MRC Centre for Neurodegeneration Research
King's College London
Institute of Psychiatry
London
UK

William H Stoothoff PhD
Harvard Medical School
Massachusetts General Hospital
MassGeneral Institute for Neurodegeneration
Charlestown, MA
USA

Michael Swash MD FRCP FRCPath
Professor, Department of Neurology
St Bartholomew's and the Royal London School
  of Medicine and Dentistry
Royal London Hospital
London
UK

Martin R Turner PhD MRCP
Department of Clinical Neuroscience
MRC Centre for Neurodegeneration Research
King's College London
Institute of Psychiatry
London
UK

Ludo Van Den Bosch PhD
Laboratory for Neurobiology
Campus Gasthuisberg
Leuven
Belgium

Markus Weber MD
Consultant, Department of Neurology
Kantonsspital St Gallen
St Gallen
and University of Basel
Switzerland

Victoria Williams MA PhD MRCP
Department of Clinical Neuroscience
MRC Centre for Neurodegeneration Research
King's College London
Institute of Psychiatry
London
UK

Anne-Marie A Wills MD
Schumann Fellow
MassGeneral Institute for Neurodegenarative
  Diseases
Charlestown, MA
USA

Preface

In this new edition of *Amyotrophic Lateral Sclerosis* we have set out to introduce new topics, and to bring forward new concepts in relation to older ideas. Research and understanding of ALS are evolving at a rapid rate, but there have been no commensurate rapid advances in the availability of definitive therapy. Thus, although there is a much greater understanding of the disease, the magnitude of the task of finding a means of prevention of the disease, and a cure for those afflicted, has become apparent. A sudden and complete resolution of the problem of ALS as a neurodegenerative disease seems unlikely. Consequently, it is important to tackle the disease on a number of fronts. Accordingly, this new edition is arranged in five sections: Clinical data, Functional studies, Genetics of ALS and related disorders, Pathogenic mechanisms, and Therapy of ALS and related disorders. Material from the first edition, in general, is not replicated in the new edition, and the new book should therefore be read with the first edition as a background. We hope that the information and discussion in this second edition will stimulate researchers and clinicians alike to further their efforts to understand the disease, in all its protean forms. Some of the material may be thought not directly in the mainstream of ALS research, but we believe that researchers and clinicians need to look outside their immediate understanding and to widen their approach to the disease; we hope we have encouraged this process. New advances depend on innovative ideas.

A multi-author book is as good as its editors can make it, but ultimately depends on the hard work of the contributors. We thank all our contributors for the effort they have made to follow our aims, and for the timely delivery of their manuscripts; it is no easy thing to undertake a comprehensive review of a difficult field while conducting a busy professional life, and we are most grateful. We also thank our publisher, and especially Martin Lister, our editorial manager, and Nick Dunton and his staff for their help and encouragement in keeping us to schedule. We hope our readers find the effort worthwhile.

Robert H Brown Jr MD
Michael Swash MD
Piera Pasinelli PhD

Foreword

Books about amyotrophic lateral sclerosis (ALS) continue to proliferate. The reasons are many, including the tragic nature of the lethal human disease. For an uncommon condition, it has captured the public mind and, surely, it is prominent in discussions of end-of-life issues and palliative care. More than that, the pathogenesis of the underlying motor neuron death is a challenge for neurobiologists, and the lack of effective therapy is a challenge for patients, their families and clinical investigators.

But, to my mind, the need for new books is good news because it results from the increasing number of molecular biologists, geneticists, clinicians, pathologists, neuropsychologists and ethicists who have been attracted to the field and have written an increasing number of papers, so documenting the increasing vigor of ALS research. The key to this burst of research was the discovery of the *SOD1* mutation in familial ALS, which was made in 1993 by one group of investigators led by Robert H Brown and another led by Teepu Siddique. The next year Mark Gurney described the transgenic mouse model of ALS, a transgenic murine disease created by inserting a human mutant *SOD1* gene that leads to a paralytic disease in mice, which displays the essential features of human ALS. At last, the methods of molecular biology could be applied to problems of pathogenesis of motor neuron diseases.

The first edition of this book was published in 2000. This, the second edition, has a new editor (Piera Pasinelli) who joined the two renowned and admired editors and investigators, Robert H Brown and Michael Swash. The current edition is not merely an update of the first one; new authors have been recruited and chapter titles reflect changing concepts of pathogenesis. The onrush of research makes it mandatory to summarize progress periodically.

The chapter authors are all recognized international authorities and the specific subjects cover the field. Among the authors, Drs Mitsumoto, Leigh and Shaw have edited ALS books themselves.

Clinical issues are covered thoroughly – from diagnosis to epidemiology, clinical trials and palliative care. Neurophysiology includes motor unit counting, functional aspects of the upper motor neuron, clinical neurophysiology and imaging. Genetics is detailed, with chapters on familial motor neuron diseases other than ALS, genotype and phenotype, modifying genes and molecular pathogenesis.

Pathogenesis is the theme for six chapters: animal models, cell death, aging and neurodegeneration, neurotrophins, axonal transport and mitochondrial dysfunction. All of this new information depends on research in the mutant SOD1 mouse.

It is difficult to think of any important topics that have been omitted. Clinicians working with patients, the patients and their families, and investigators will appreciate this new, up-to-date, thorough and handsomely produced volume.

Lewis P Rowland MD
Professor of Neurology
Eleanor and Lou Gehrig MDA/ALS Center
Neurological Institute
Columbia University Medical Center
New York, NY, USA

Color section

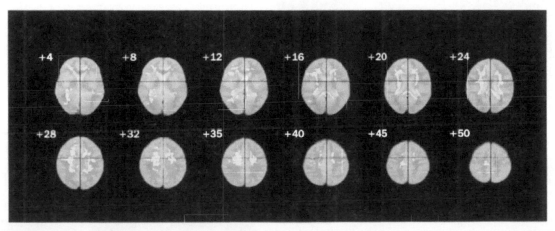

Plate 1 (Figure 3.2) Voxel-based morphometry (VBM). Axial slices through brain. Yellow areas represent statistically significant loss of cerebral white matter in amyotrophic lateral sclerosis patients who were impaired on a standardized test of verbal fluency (VF). VBM changes in patients who did not show impairments of VF were less obvious and were restricted mainly to frontal white matter (not shown). (Reproduced from reference 18 (Chapter 3), with permission)

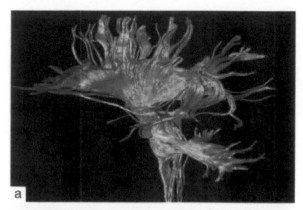

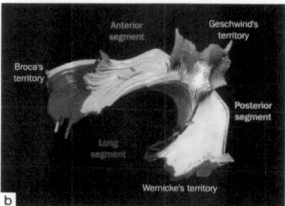

Plate 2 (Figure 3.3)   (a) Diffusion tensor magnetic resonance imaging tractography. *In vivo* dissection of subcortical fiber tracts. (b) Tractography reconstruction of the arcuate fasciculus using the two regions of interest approach. Broca's and Wernicke's territories are connected through direct and indirect pathways in the average brain. The direct pathway (long segment shown in red) runs medially and corresponds to classical descriptions of the arcuate fasciculus. The indirect pathway runs laterally and is composed of an anterior segment (green) connecting the inferior parietal cortex (Geschwind's territory) and Broca's territory and a posterior segment (yellow) connecting Geschwind's and Wernicke's territories. (Reproduced from reference 36 (Chapter 3), with permission of the authors and the editor of *Annals of Neurology*)

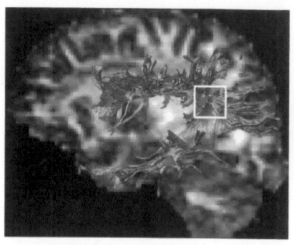

Plate 3 (Figure 3.4)   H-MRS and diffusion tensor magnetic resonance imaging (DT-MRI) tractography combined to derive measures of tissue damage in specific pathways. Tractography demonstrating parietotemporal fibers, and location (white square) of voxel from which NAA and creatine H-MRS measures were derived. (Repoduced with permission from reference 46 (Chapter 3))

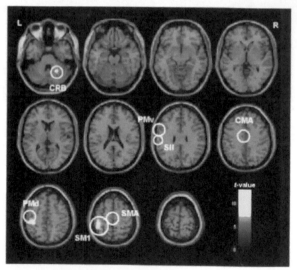

Plate 4 (Figure 3.5)   Functional magnetic resonance imaging can be used to visualize brain activation during a simple right-hand grip task. Normal subject. CMA, cingulate motor area, CRB, cerebellum; PMd, dorsal lateral premotor cortex; PMv, ventral lateral premotor cortex; SII, secondary somatosensory cortex; SM1, primary sensorimotor cortex; SMA, supplementary motor area; L, left; R, right. (Courtesy of Dr B Koritnik and Professor S Williams, King's College London, Centre for Neuroimaging Sciences)

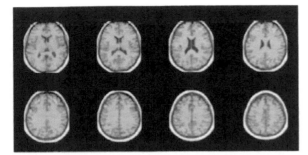

Plate 5 (Figure 3.6) Functional magnetic resonance imaging. Axial images showing (yellow/red) significantly decreased areas of activation, predominantly in dorsolateral prefrontal and temporal areas, in amyotrophic lateral sclerosis subjects compared to controls while performing a verbal fluency task. (Reproduced from reference 53 (Chapter 3), with permission)

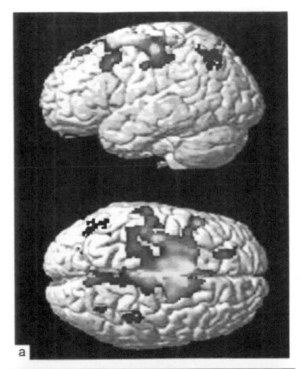

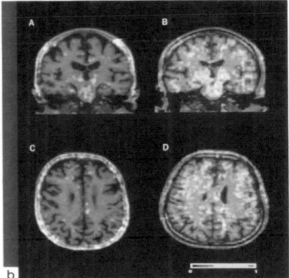

Plate 6 (Figure 3.7) (a) [11C]flumazenil positron emission tomography (PET) showing areas of significantly decreased ligand binding in amyotrophic lateral sclerosis (ALS) subjects compared to controls. (Reproduced from reference 83 (Chapter 3) with permission of the authors and by courtesy of the publishers and editor of *Brain*.) (b) [11C]PK11195 PET. Coronal (A,D) and axial (B,D) slices showing markedly increased ligand binding in anterior cortical areas and along corticospinal tracts in ALS subjects (B,D) compared to controls (A,D). (Reproduced with permission from reference 82 (Chapter 3))

a

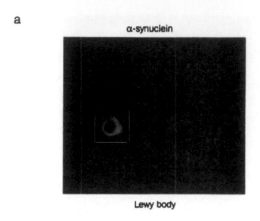

α-synuclein

Lewy body

Plate 7 (Figure 11.1)   (a) Confocal microscope image showing a Lewy body from a Parkinsons's disease (PD)-affected patient's brain that was stained with anti-α-synuclein antibody. (b) Schematic diagram of α-synuclein illustrating the major identified protein domains. The three mutations that have been found in familial PD are identified with arrows in the N-terminus of the protein

b

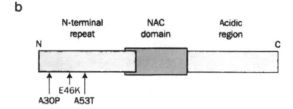

N-terminal repeat   NAC domain   Acidic region

N   C

E46K
A30P   A53T

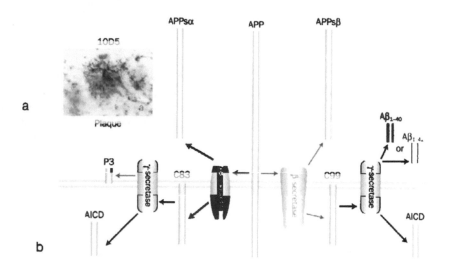

Plate 8 Figure 11.2   (a) Light microscope image of a plaque from an Alzheimer's disease (AD) brain section stained with 10D5 antibody, which recognizes the Aβ protein. Section was developed with HRP and DAB to visualize staining. (b) Diagram illustrating the different cleavage events that occur during amyloid precursor protein (APP) processing to yield the various end products. When APP is cleaved by α-secretase, the soluble APPsα is released into the extracellular space and the C83 fragment remains associated with the membrane. C83 is then cleaved by γ-secretase to yield the P3 and AICD fragment. Similarly, β-secretase cleaves APP to produce the soluble APPsβ and the membrane-associated C99 fragment. For reasons that are not understood, γ-secretase then cleaves the C99 fragment to produce either the Aβ1-40 or the more fibrillogenic Aβ1-42 peptide, along with the AICD fragment that is released into the intracellular space

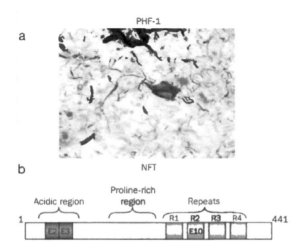

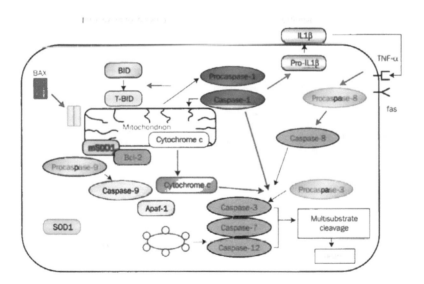

Plate 9 (Figure 11.3) (a) Light microscope image of Alzheimer's disease (AD) affected brain section stained with PHF-1 antibody, which recognizes abnormally phosphorylated tau in neurofibrillary tangles (NFTs) in AD brain. Section was developed with DAB and HRP to visualize staining, and figure shows a plaque present in AD brain (b) Schematic diagram of tau protein showing the longest human isoform found in adult brain. The longest isoform is characterized by the presence of two amino-terminal inserts (exons 2 and 3) and a fourth microtubule-binding domain (exon 10), which are all alternatively spliced to give rise to the six isoforms of tau found in adult human brain

Plate 10 (Figure 13.1) Cell death pathways in amyotrophic lateral sclerosis (ALS). This summarizes the major extrinsic and intrinsic pathways provoking apoptotic cell death. Both pathways have been implicated in mutant SOD1-related neuronal death. As indicated, in the intrinsic pathway (left) a toxic stimulus (such as mutant SOD1 protein) alters permeability of the mitochondrial membrane, release of cytochrome c, and activation of caspase-9, which is upstream of the executioner caspases 3, 7 and 12. Mitochondrial permeability changes may be triggered by multiple stimuli including caspase 1, cleavage of BID to T-BID, BAX translocation and binding of mutant SOD1 to Bcl-2 in the outer mitochondrial membrane. In the extrinsic pathway (right), stimuli exogenous to the cell (e.g. tumor necrosis factor-α or FAS ligand) bind surface receptors and thereby activate caspase-8, which is upstream of the executioner caspases. In SOD1-mediated ALS, the earliest changes are mitochondrial disruption and caspase-1 activation. This, in turn, may activate both the intrinsic pathway and, through the release of interleukin-1β, the extrinsic pathway. Death ultimately reflects both mitochondrial demise and cleavage of multiple substrates

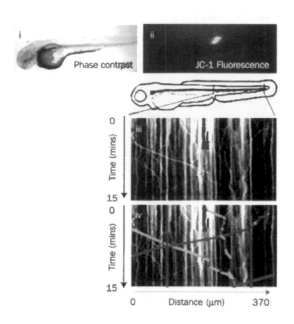

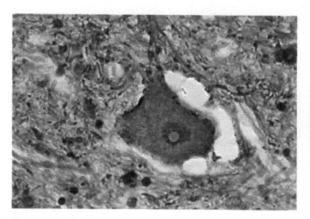

Plate 12 (Figure 16.3) Accumulation of phosphorylated neurofilament proteins in a spinal motor neuron from a sporadic amyotrophic lateral sclerosis patient. Immunocytochemistry using the SMI31 antibody to detect phosphorylated neurofilaments

Plate 11 (Figure 16.2c) Quantifying axonal transport *in vivo* in a live zebrafish embryo. (i and ii) Low-magnification phase contrast and fluorescent images of JC-1-injected 48-h zebrafish embryo. (iii and iv) High-power magnification kymograph of the annotated region of the same zebrafish. To create the kymograph the frames constituting the original time-lapse sequence were converted into a single montage with successive frames beneath one another. Along the *x*-axis of the montage is distance along the peripheral lateral line nerve; along the *y*-axis is time. The montage was then compressed along the *y*-axis so each individual frame was represented as a 1-pixel high line. In this way, the position of individual mitochondria can be shown on a two-dimensional image. Mitochondria that move towards the cell body (retrograde, shown in red) or growth cone (anterograde, shown in green) and stationary mitochondria (shown in blue) can be distinguished. Examples of mitochondria with anterograde, retrograde, or no net displacement are shown in (iv)

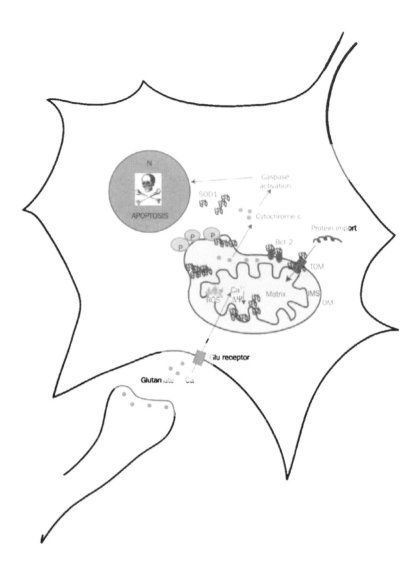

Plate 13 (Figure 17.1) Diagram of potential pathways of mitochondrial involvement in SOD1-related amyotrophic lateral sclerosis. Mutant SOD1 has been proposed to affect mitochondrial functions in several ways. All these mechanisms of mitochondrial involvement are not mutually exclusive and may interact and co-operate in establishing a vicious cycle, ultimately resulting in mitochondrial dysfunction and cell death. Mutant SOD1 may affect mitochondria directly within the organelles or indirectly from the cytoplasm in a yet undisclosed manner. Within mitochondria, mutant SOD1 may interfere with the anti-apoptotic function of Bcl-2, affect mitochondrial import by interfering with the translocation machinery (TOM/TIM), generate toxic reactive oxygen species (ROS) via aberrant superoxide chemistry, accumulate and aggregate in the intermembrane space (IMS) and in the matrix, promote outer membrane (OM) expansion and mitochondrial vacuolization. These changes may then result in abnormal mitochondrial energy metabolism, Ca^{2+} handling and release of pro-apoptotic factors

Section 1

Clinical data

1

The spectrum of motor neuron disorders

Brian Murray, Hiroshi Mitsumoto

INTRODUCTION

In its original sense, as proposed by Brain and Walton in 1969, the term motor neuron *disease* (MND) specifically refers to the single disease entity that is characterized by progressive weakness and muscle wasting usually leading to death within a few years of clinical onset[1]. However, it is now clear that there is a large family of motor neuron *diseases* that encompasses several entities including idiopathic sporadic degenerative conditions of the upper and/or lower motor neuron (UMN/LMN) pools such as amyotrophic lateral sclerosis (ALS); various familial disorders such as familial ALS (fALS), spinal muscular atrophy (SMA) and hereditary spastic paraparesis (HSP); and sporadic conditions caused by neoplasm, environmental toxins, or viral infections. In this chapter we provide a brief outline of the full clinical spectrum of motor neuron diseases each with different etiologies, presentations, prognoses and pathologies. Detailed discussions of etiology and treatment are found in later sections of this book. It is useful to consider the motor neuron disorders as overlapping conditions, some of which are purely motor in nature and others that, to a lesser or greater extent, encompass non-motor features such as dementia, supranuclear gaze palsy or parkinsonism (ALS-plus syndromes) (Figure 1.1).

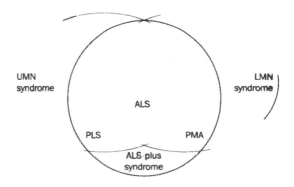

Figure 1.1 The spectrum of motor neuron diseases encompasses several different clinical and pathologic entities. Whether sporadic or familial, amyotrophic lateral sclerosis/ motor neuron disease (ALS/MND) is almost entirely limited to the motor system and involves both the upper and the lower motor neurons. Variants of this condition include forms with clinical features that are limited either to the upper motor neurons (primary lateral sclerosis: PLS) or the lower motor neurons (progressive muscular atrophy: PMA). Other disorders that are pathologically distinct from ALS/MND include those that involve upper motor neurons (UMN) as a significant part of their clinicopathologic presentation such as infection with human T lymphtropic virus types 1 and 2 (HTLV 1 and 2), lathyrism and the hereditary spastic paraplegias/parapareses (HSP). Similarly, there are several disorders that have a predilection for involvement of the lower motor neuron (LMN) system such as poliomyelitis, West Nile virus poliomyelitis, and the spinal muscular atrophies (SMA). Finally, while some conditions may feature clinical signs of upper and/or lower motor neuron involvement, they are associated with quite prominent non-motor features as can be seen in the frontotemporal dementias, spinocerebellar ataxias, Kennedy's disease, hexosaminidase A deficiency and Allgrove's syndrome

SPORADIC DISORDERS OF THE MOTOR NEURON SYSTEM IN ADULTS

- Amyotrophic lateral sclerosis (ALS)
- Primary lateral sclerosis (PLS)
- Progressive muscular atrophy (PMA)
- ALS with frontotemporal dementia (ALS/FTD)
- Western Pacific ALS
- Benign focal amyotrophy

Amyotrophic lateral sclerosis

As first fully described by Jean Martin Charcot in 1874, ALS is an idiopathic progressive neuro-degenerative disorder characterized by progressive muscle weakness and wasting with both clinical and pathologic evidence of combined upper and lower motor neuron loss[2]. It affects a broad age range but the peak incidence is in the 55–65-year-old age group with an overall male predominance (1.2:1) for all but the bulbar-onset form. There is evidence of a preclinical phase in ALS where the rate of motor neuron cellular loss is offset by the process of collateral reinnervation from unaffected motor units. This pattern of silent motor neuron cell attrition eventually becomes eloquent once motor neuron reserves can no longer keep pace with the rate of disease progression[3]. The classic clinical presentation is that of combined upper and lower motor neuron weakness in the extremities and/or bulbar innervated musculature (Table 1.1). Onset is most often restricted to regional weakness in one extremity (monomelic onset) with spread to other regions over time. In some instances, the initial appearance is difficult to distinguish from a mononeuropathy (pseudoneuritic onset) but progression into other nerve and root territories reveals the true nature of the underlying disease. Approximately 25% of all cases present in the bulbar-onset form: the initial problems are dysarthria and/or dysphagia. Rare cases present in overt respiratory failure from fulminant early involvement of the cervical and thoracic cord. The pattern of progression for monomelic onset disease is fairly predictable with initial spread within the same region of the neuraxis (e.g. if onset is in the lower cervical cord segment, then spread occurs in that segment first) before there is spread to other regions. If onset were in the left upper

---

Table 1.1 Clinical features in amyotrophic lateral sclerosis

UMN features	LMN features	Atypical features
Clumsiness (loss of dexterity)	Weakness (moderate–severe)	Sensory loss (objective)
Weakness (mild–moderate)	Muscle atrophy	Dysautonomia
Spasticity	Hyporeflexia–areflexia	Bladder or bowel involvement
Hyperreflexia (deep tendon and myotactic reflexes)	Hypotonicity or flaccidity	Parkinsonism
Pathologic reflexes (e.g. Babinski, Hoffmann's)	Muscle cramps	Cognitive dysfunction (usually frontotemporal in type)
Readily elicited reflexes in an atrophic limb	Fasciculations	Dysfunction of eye movements (saccades, gaze, pursuits)
Pseudobulbar palsy (spastic dysarthria, dysphagia, labile affect)	Bulbar palsy (flaccid dysarthria, dysphagia, no labile affect)	Pressure sores

UMN, upper motor neuron; LMN, lower motor neuron

extremity, one would see spread first to the contralateral side followed by involvement of thoracic and lumbar cord segments (as manifested by ventilatory and lower extremity involvement)[4]. Bulbar-onset ALS also follows a pattern of spread into the upper extremities and thence into the thoracic and lumbosacral segments. The hallmark of ALS is the coexistence of UMN and LMN signs in the same myotome with spread to other myotomes with the passage of time. Thus the clinician finds a combination of spasticity, muscle wasting, atrophy and hyperreflexia (or relative hyperreflexia) with often widespread fasciculations and/or cramps. Spread to the bulbar region may cause dysarthria, dysphagia, dysphonia and pseudobulbar affect. Weight loss, joint pains (secondary to severe muscle atrophy with altered mechanical stress on articular surfaces), depression and anxiety are also common features. Involvement of the muscles of ventilation may precipitate fulminant type II respiratory failure but more commonly presents as an insidiously progressive pattern of dyspnea on exertion, orthopnea and disturbed sleep. While it is fair to say that classic spinal type ALS is a disorder of combined UMN and LMN features, it is important to stress that these features may not become clinically evident simultaneously and it behoves the clinician to follow up on all suspected cases to ascertain any evidence of spread.

Certain symptoms and signs are considered relatively rare in the natural history of ALS. These include overt dementia at onset (< 5%, and usually of the frontotemporal type), Parkinsonism (5% and usually postural instability[5,6]), sphincter disturbance (occasionally seen as urinary frequency and urgency) and oculomotor dysfunction (not a clinical feature in the natural evolution of ALS).

Diagnostic and research criteria have been formulated for both the sporadic and the familial forms of ALS. A patient is defined as having 'definite ALS' if three or more regions of the neuraxis exhibit a combination of UMN and LMN signs. 'Probable ALS' refers to cases with UMN and LMN involvement in two regions, whereas 'possible ALS' refers to those with UMN and LMN signs in one region alone or cases with LMN in more than two regions lying rostral to any evidence of UMN disease in another region. Pure LMN disease does not satisfy the criteria for even possible ALS (www.wfnals.org). Cases with a family history are referred to as having familial ALS. These criteria include the use of ancillary tests, most important among them being electrodiagnostic studies. Indeed, those cases that meet the criteria for possible ALS but who also have additional laboratory evidence of involvement of other regions (e.g. electromyography evidence of LMN involvement) are classified as 'laboratory supported probable ALS'. However, none of these additional investigations are disease specific and a single, objective 'ALS test' remains elusive. The mean disease duration for spinal ALS is approximately 33 months with estimated 5- and 10-year survival rates of 21% and 9%, respectively[7]. The pathogenesis and treatment of this complex disorder are discussed at length in later chapters of this textbook.

Primary lateral sclerosis

First named by Erb in 1875, PLS is an uncommon disorder primarily of the upper motor neuron cellular pool whose clinical features are restricted to UMN symptoms and signs throughout the vast majority of the natural history[8]. The original diagnostic criteria that had been proposed for PLS stipulated that disease must have been present for more than 3 years, that disease be slowly progressive in nature and that there must be no alterative cause for symmetrical symptoms and signs of UMN disease[9]. The age at onset is somewhat younger than that of sporadic ALS: the mean ages at onset in three of the largest studies were 50.4 years[9], 53.4 years[10] and 44 years[11]. The most common presentation is with clumsiness and stiffness in muscles of the extremities with probably over half of all cases manifesting with a slowly ascending pattern of lower limb spasticity and weakness[11]. Bulbar presentations also occur, and are characterized by a strained vocal quality and often prominent pseudobulbar affect lability. A rare presentation is with slowly ascending or descending spastic hemiplegia, which is sometimes referred to as Mills' hemiplegic syndrome[12]. As would be expected from a disorder of UMNs, the degree of weakness in PLS is relatively mild. Examination reveals increased muscle tone, clasp-knife spasticity and spastic catches with poor manual dexterity leading to significant difficulties using utensils, buttoning clothes and writing. Reflexes are hyperactive, eventually becoming clonic, and pathological reflexes appear including frontal release signs, Hoffmann's sign and upgoing plantar responses. Non-habituating myotatic reflexes are also evident. A few patients may complain of urgency of micturition and there may be subtle evidence of frontal executive-type cognitive dysfunction. Standard investigations classically do not reveal clinical or electrodiagnostic evidence of LMN involvement until the latest stages although recent studies have reported both clinical and neurophysiologic features of LMN involvement throughout the course of the disease (thus posing the question as to whether PLS really exists)[10,13]. The bulk of disease burden is borne by the motor neuron cellular pool in the motor cortex, premotor cortex and corticospinal tracts with additional involvement of neuronal projection fibers to non-motor regions. Magnetic resonance imaging (MRI) of the brain may reveal quite striking focal atrophy in the motor cortex with degeneration of the corticospinal tracts, and novel imaging modalities, especially diffusion tensor MRI, may become especially useful in the early detection of UMN involvement in suspected cases of PLS[14,15]. Perhaps due to the general absence of clinical lower motor neuron involvement, PLS harbors a relatively favorable prognosis, with a mean disease duration of 224 months in the 26 cases studied by Norris *et al.* a median duration of 19 years in Pringle's series and, in LeForestier's study, a mean duration at the time of first presentation of 8.5 years[16]. The first International Conference of PLS held at San Jose, California in

2004 questioned the utility of the Pringle criteria and new recommendations were proposed such as the necessity for pure UMN involvement even 4 years after onset, normal somatosensory evoked potentials (SSEP) studies and electrodiagnostic confirmation of absent LMN involvement (personal communication, Ben Brooks MD, University of Wisconsin, 2004).

Progressive muscular atrophy

First described by Francois Aran in 1850, PMA is clinically characterized by pure lower motor neuron symptoms and signs throughout the course of its natural history. The initial presentation is most characteristically an asymmetric, distal predominant weakness of the upper limb. Compared to ALS, the rate of progression is slow, with a mean survival of 159 months (range 43–407) in Norris's study of 17 cases and a 3-year survival of 61.3% in Chio's series of 155 cases[16,17]. The mean age at presentation is approximately a decade younger than that for sporadic ALS (47 years[16] and 48.4 years[17]). While bulbar features may be an early feature of PMA it is more common that bulbar and/or respiratory features develop in later stages of disease[18]. The fact that PMA lacks clinical features of UMN involvement has led some to doubt its nosological relationship to ALS, but several pieces of evidence indicate otherwise. Autopsy studies of both sporadic and familial PMA have identified typical ALS pathology not only in spinal motor neurons but also in the motor cortex and corticospinal tracts[19,20]. Indeed, there may be a subset of more rapidly progressive PMA that develops pathologic evidence of UMN involvement but where UMN signs are clinically masked by severe degrees of terminal amyotrophy[18]. Furthermore, a recent study of 164 patients with MND included 30 cases with pure LMN disease (who were diagnosed as having PMA) in whom there was clear evidence of UMN involvement in 63% as detected by single-voxel magnetic resonance spectroscopy (MRS), in 63% by transcranial magnetic stimulation (TMS) and in 46% when both ancillary investigations were used together[21].

Amyotrophic lateral sclerosis with frontotemporal dementia

Frontotemporal dementia is not a single entity but a heterogeneous group of neurodegenerative disorders where the cognitive domains most affected are those concerning behavior, personality, executive control and language. Included within this family are cases that develop additional symptoms and signs of motor neuron disease. It has previously been estimated that less than 5% of all patients who present with features of motor neuron disease (be it bulbar- or limb-onset) also have readily apparent frontotemporal-type cognitive deficits. However, with adequate neuropsychological screening, up to 50% of all patients with MND display deficits in the frontotemporal domain[22,23]. In some instances, bulbar dysarthria or anarthria masks these important clinical features: the affect lability of pseudobulbar palsy may readily be confused or coexist with the disinhibition that so characterizes orbitofrontal degeneration in FTD. Just as FTD features may develop after onset of motor neuron disease, so too does the reverse occur; thus, motor neuron disease may evolve many months or even years after changes in personality, behavior and/or language[24]. This type of presentation harbors a particularly grim prognosis, with mean disease duration of about 2 years from onset to death[25]. In light of the knowledge that there is such a degree of clinical overlap between FTD and MND, it is important that formal neuropsychology testing be performed in all persons who might be undergoing recruitment in clinical research trials. The current diagnostic pathologic criteria for FTD include cases with motor neuron-type intraneuronal inclusions in the absence of tau-positive inclusions[26]. However, the recent discovery of distinct aggregated tau phosphoproteins in patients with sporadic ALS has raised the possibility for a role of tau protein in the pathogenesis of ALS/MND[27]. Neurofilament inclusion body disease (also referred to as neuronal intermediate filament inclusion disease, NIFID) is another apparently sporadic overlap disorder between FTD, PLS and corticobasal syndrome, with onset as early as the third decade of life. The underlying pathology is uniquely associated with intracytoplasmic neuronal and proximal axonal inclusion bodies strongly positive for neurofilaments, a major component of which is α-internexin protein[28].

Western Pacific amyotrophic lateral sclerosis

Western Pacific ALS was first described in Chamorro patients native to the island of Guam and other Mariana islands, where it occurred with an unusually high incidence (50–100 times higher than the rest of the world). A similar high incidence of ALS was later described in the Kii peninsula of Japan and southwest New Guinea. The disease is itself a spectrum disorder and may manifest in a number of ways, from a pure ALS-type disorder to a combined parkinsonism/dementia complex (PDC) or a combination of all three[29]. There appears to be an increased risk of developing this disorder in first-degree relatives, but the mode of transmission suggests a strong influence of exogenous/environmental factors that may be acting in concert with genetic susceptibility factors. The underlying pathology is most notable for neuronal loss in the setting of widespread tau-positive neurofibrillary tangles within the cerebral cortex and spinal cord, thus establishing this disorder as one of the tauopathies. Similar but less widespread tau tangles are found in the entorhinal cortex and hippocampi of normal individuals from the region, which suggests that a large tau burden is required before preclinical disease becomes clinically apparent[30]. The peak incidence of ALS and PDC appeared to occur between 1950 and 1960, but since then a number of clinical and epidemiologic changes have been observed. Where once this was more common in males, the disorder is now equally prevalent in both sexes and there has been a gradual increase in the age at onset[31,32]. More striking, however, has been a steady decline in the incidence of Western Pacific ALS over the past 40 years with a similar decline of PDC (up until 15 years ago when the incidence actually increased before recently leveling off). It is unlikely that there has been a significant change in genetic risk factors over such a short time frame, so this decline in ALS incidence may mirror a simultaneous decline in the influence of exogenous factors (PDC being relatively more vulnerable). Chief among the candidate environmental factors is β-methylamino-L-alanine (BMAA), an amino acid cyanobacterial neurotoxin that may act alone or in concert with other toxins including cycasin and/or toxic sterol glucosides. These toxins are present in cycad seed flour that is used to make traditional Chamorro tortillas, but it is now evident that massive amounts would need to be consumed to cause neurotoxicity. A more recent theory proposes that the Chamorros ingest sufficiently large amounts of cycad neurotoxin through a process of biomagnification: BMAA is produced by cyanobacteria in the cycad seeds which are then ingested and concentrated in the tissues of flying foxes, which in turn are eaten by the Chamorros at traditional feasts[33]. Since the 1960s, the flying fox population has dwindled, but this fact alone does not explain the decline in ALS[34]. Social factors are likely to be important: Chamorro women, for example, are working outside the home and are no longer as involved in the preparation of traditional meals, and there has been a general migration from the southern areas of highest incidence to northern regions with low incidence[31]. The higher than average incidence of ALS/PDC in non-Chamorro peoples in the Western Pacific has yet to be explained.

Benign monomelic amyotrophy/benign calf amyotrophy/wasted limb syndrome

Benign monomelic amyotrophy is known by many names in the English-language literature including Hirayama's juvenile SMA of the upper limbs and benign focal amyotrophy. The presentation is one of striking regional atrophy in one part of one limb with no UMN features. The most common pattern is unilateral atrophy in C7-T1 innervated musculature, sometimes with sparing of brachioradialis (oblique amyotrophy). Males aged between 15 and 25 years are most often affected and there is typically a pattern of deterioration for up to 5 years after which progression appears to halt. This condition is very benign and may even go unnoticed by the patient. A peculiar variant known as benign calf amyotrophy or 'wasted limb syndrome' (depending on the distribution of muscle atrophy) involves only one part of one lower extremity and also portends a very favorable prognosis with no actual disability. Whether upper or lower limb in type, there may be subtle electrophysiological evidence of involvement in other parts of the neuraxis. Muscle histopathology typically reveals chronic neurogenic atrophy with fibre-type grouping and secondary myopathic change. The cause of these conditions remains the subject of debate: some believe that the upper limb variant is due to flexion-induced spinal cord impingement against an aberrant posterior dura, whereas others propose that this is in fact a very limited/arrested form of sporadic spinal muscular atrophy or PMA[35-38].

As can be readily appreciated from what has been said before, it may be difficult to categorize patients who present with otherwise unexplained pure sporadic lower motor neuron disorders; are they a rare form of SMA, PMA or a benign monomelic amyotrophy? Indeed, a Dutch research group have approached this problem by dividing the clinical presentations into four distinct types: slowly progressive SMA, distal SMA, segmental distal SMA and segmental proximal SMA[39].

FAMILIAL MOTOR NEURON DISORDERS

- Familial ALS
    Autosomal dominant and recessive *SOD1* mutation-associated fALS
    Alsin, senataxin, p150 subunit of dynactin

Novel ALS loci
Chromosome 9-linked ALS/FTD
FTD-17 and fALS overlap

- Spinal muscular atrophies
- Kennedy's disease
- Hereditary spastic paraplegia

Familial amyotrophic lateral sclerosis

A clear family history is present in approximately 5% to 10% of all cases of ALS/MND. The most common mode of transmission appears to be autosomal dominant, but both autosomal recessive and X-linked forms also occur. Of the familial cases, about 20% of families have a mutation in the copper/zinc superoxide dismutase 1 (*SOD1*) gene located on chromosome 21 (ALS1) (see Chapter 9)[40]. Very rare mutations in other known genes account for just a few families clustered in different parts of the world, but several novel chromosomal loci have been linked to ALS families that may reveal other ALS genes in the near future[41].

A positive family history apart, there are few clinical clues to reliably distinguish familial autosomal dominant or recessive *SOD1* ALS from sporadic ALS. Onset is on average a decade earlier in the *SOD1*-associated disorders and there appears to be a predilection for lower-extremity onset as opposed to bulbar onset. Furthermore, there may be atypical features in fALS such as abnormal bladder control, cognitive abnormalities (rare), or sensory phenomena, but these are by no means hard and fast rules and there is considerable inter- and intrafamilial genetic heterogeneity[42,43]. The A4V mutation, for example, causes a LMN-predominant condition with rapid progression and a mean disease duration of approximately 1 year, whereas the H46R mutation, another cause of a LMN-predominant disorder, may last anywhere from 3 to 47 years[44-46]. The V148G mutation phenotype depends to a certain degree on the *CNTF* genotype; those with a null mutation in the latter gene have an early-onset disorder with rapid progression, whereas those with at least one copy of *CNTF* have late-onset disease[47].

Several mutations disrupt intracellular transport, traffic and/or regulation of the cytoskeleton, but there is no shared clinical phenotype. Mutations in the *alsin*/ALS2 gene on chromosome 2q33 lead to a rare form of juvenile-onset, autosomal recessive motor neuron disorder with one of two MND phenotypes, the first being a young-onset ALS disorder in a Tunisian family, and the second a PLS-like condition found in families in Kuwait and Saudi Arabia. It is noteworthy that certain mutations in this gene may also give rise to an infantile-onset ascending spastic paralysis, thus providing a genetic link between the known ALS and HSP phenotypes[48-50]. The alsin protein is a guanine exchange factor for Rab5 and Rac1, and loss of function may thus interfere with endosomal trafficking and cytoskeleton remodeling within the motor neuron cell population[51,52]. Other rare mutations with a possible important role for disturbed intracellular transport have been described in the gene encoding the p150 subunit of the dynactin transport protein; they cause a slowly progressive pure lower motor neuron disorder that has been described in only a single family to date[53]. The ALS8 mutation occurs in the vesicle trafficking protein *VAPB* gene (vesicle-associated membrane protein/synaptobrevin-associated membrane protein B) on chromosome 20, yet again suggesting a problem with intracellular transport. This time, however, the phenotype shows even more heterogeneity: patients may develop a slowly progressive form of ALS with young onset (31–45 years), a late-onset SMA phenotype, or a severe rapidly progressive ALS phenotype[54]. Thus, there are several non-*SOD1*-associated forms of fALS (see Chapter 8 for further discussion of these disorders as well as details on peripherin and neurofilament gene mutations in fALS) that also fail to conform to any clinical pattern, even when the putative pathogenetic mechanisms share certain similarities such as disturbed intracellular transport/traffic and regulation of the cytoskeleton.

ALS4 is a juvenile autosomal dominant very slowly progressive distal predominant atrophy with UMN signs but sparing of bulbar and respiratory muscles, and is caused by gain of function mutations in the senataxin gene on chromosome 9q34. As this gene contains a DNA/RNA helicase domain, the putative mechanisms in ALS4 include altered RNA processing or defective DNA repair, replication, or recombination[55]. Autosomal dominant familial ALS disorders have also been linked to sites on chromosomes 16q12 and 20ptel. The clinical syndromes are similar to sporadic ALS but both site and age at onset are more variable, with some cases beginning in the fourth decade. In the first of the two large European kindreds with linkages mapped to an overlapping site on chromosome 16q12, onset was in limbs with a mean survival of 13 months. In the other family, bulbar onset occurred in four affected family members while a further two cases had apparent evidence of frontotemporal cognitive deficits with hallucinations. The mean age of onset in this family was 61 years with mean disease duration of 35.5 months. Together, the families that are linked to chromosome 16q12 have been assigned to the ALS6 category whereas the family with linkage to chromosome 20ptel have been designated ALS7[56–58].

Hosler *et al.* have described a family with an autosomal dominant form of ALS linked to a site on chromosome 9q21–22. The motor neuron disorder first occurs in mid-life and may include features of FTD such as disinhibition and apathy[59]. Features of motor neuron involvement may also be detected clinically and pathologically in rare cases with tau mutation-associated frontotemporal dementia such as the amyotrophy described in a case with disinhibition–dementia–parkinsonism and amyotrophy complex (DDPAC) and the pyramidal features in several cases with pallidopontonigral degeneration (PPND)[60,61]. Another overlap disorder with features of FTD, parkinsonism and motor neuron

disease has recently been described in a Californian family. The pathology of this 17q-linked disorder includes tau and alpha synuclein inclusions, but no mutations in the tau gene have been identified[62].

Spinal muscular atrophy

The spinal muscular atrophies are a group of disorders characterized by progressive degeneration of the anterior horn cell population in the spinal cord. SMA has been categorized into four types based upon age at presentation; infantile (Werdnig–Hoffmann, birth to 6 months), intermediate (6–18 months), juvenile (Kugelberg–Welander, after 18 months) and adult (> 20 years). The pattern of inheritance is most often autosomal recessive, but both autosomal dominant and X-linked forms have been described. For almost all of the recessively inherited cases, the causative mutations (usually deletions) affect the survival motor neuron 1 gene (*SMN1*) located on chromosome 5. SMN1 protein appears to have many functions including pre-mRNA splicing and the synthesis of small nuclear ribonucleoproteins. The inversely homologous *SMN2* gene is located centromerically to *SMN1* on the same chromosome and encodes an unstable protein that is identical save for a skipped exon 7 that leaves the protein only partially capable of carrying out the functions of *SMN1*. It is now apparent that the degree of disease severity is dictated by the amount of functioning *SMN2* gene product: the more copies present, the less severe the disease[63].

The infantile form of SMA (Werdnig–Hoffmann) is particularly severe and is characterized by early onset of muscle weakness with severe atrophy, loss of tone (with the frog-legged posture), areflexia, diffuse fasciculations and a characteristic alert facial expression. These infants are unable to sit up and have great difficulty feeding. Although intercostal muscles are severely affected, the diaphragm may be spared, thus causing a bell-shaped chest deformity. The prognosis is grim with the vast majority not surviving beyond the first 2 years. Rare forms of infantile SMA may present with particularly severe respiratory distress or with cardiomyopathy and lactic acidosis[64,65].

Intermediate-type SMA is a milder version of Werdnig–Hoffmann syndrome: the children do manage to sit up and roll over, but usually do not develop sufficient power to walk. Minipolymyoclonus may be seen in the fingers, and severe contractures and skeletal deformities develop over the years. The juvenile form of SMA, Kugelberg–Welander disease, usually first occurs in young children and is characterized by slow progression of weakness, atrophy and fasciculations more prominent in proximal than distal muscles. In general, the later the onset, the more sedate the rate of progression and, although orthopedic issues abound, some cases remain ambulatory for up to three decades from the time of onset. About 10% of all SMA occurs in adults over the age of 20, the mode of inheritance most commonly being autosomal recessive (with mutations in the *SMN1* gene and variable copies of the *SMN2* gene). In about 30% of adult-onset SMA, however, the mode of inheritance appears to be autosomal dominant and others appear to occur sporadically. The disease usually manifests with weakness and wasting of the shoulder and hip girdles that progresses at a stately pace often marked by prolonged plateaus of arrested progression. Fasciculations are evident in three-quarters of patients, bulbar involvement is rare and muscles of ventilation are not involved. A useful clinical clue is greater weakness in triceps than biceps together with weakness in the quadriceps that is out of proportion to other lower extremity muscles. The creatinine kinase may be quite markedly elevated and electrodiagnostic studies are consistent with a chronic neurogenic disorder. Muscle biopsy is sometimes necessary to help distinguish adult-onset SMA from some of the limb-girdle muscular dystrophies and may reveal the grouped fascicular atrophy of chronic neurogenic disease, albeit sometimes with some secondary myopathic changes.

Kennedy's disease

Special mention must be made about a very slowly progressive adult-onset SMA-plus disorder known as Kennedy's disease or X-linked spinobulbar neuronopathy. As the latter name suggests, this disease primarily manifests in males in the third decade of life with an evolving SMA-pattern proximal limb weakness and wasting with markedly coarse or large limb fasciculations, calf muscle pseudohypertrophy, hand tremor and lower motor neuron bulbar signs. A deep central tongue furrow and perioral fasciculations are distinctive features that may or may not be present early in the disease course. The underlying genetic defect has been well characterized: individuals have an unstable trinucleotide (CAG, polyglutamine-repeat) repeat expansion mutation on the androgen receptor gene located on the X chromosome. This contributes to two additional distinguishing features in these patients, namely gynecomastia (up to 90% of cases) and testicular atrophy/infertility (40% of cases)[66,67]. Investigations in suspected cases hinge around the gene test result but clinicians should also determine the hormonal profile of their patients. The latter is usually consistent with a partial androgen resistance that tends to develop several years after disease onset[68]. Diabetes/glucose intolerance may also occur in 10–20% of cases. Up to 50% of cases may have clinical sensory impairment such as distal symmetrical hypesthesia, and between 80% and 95% may have electrophysiologic evidence of sensory dysfunction[66,69]. Characteristic motor system findings are consistent with a widespread mostly chronic disorder of the anterior horn cells and bulbar motor neurons. Skewed inactivation of the X chromosome in female carriers may cause prominent cramps and mild late-onset weakness in bulbar innervated musculature.

Hereditary spastic paraplegia

Hereditary (or familial) spastic paraplegia is a heterogeneous family of inherited disorders that cause progressive worsening of lower limb spasticity and weakness. The most common mode of inheritance is autosomal dominant, but autosomal recessive and X-linked types also occur and both inter- and intrafamilial heterogeneity is typical. HSP can be broadly divided into two types: 'pure HSP' and 'complicated HSP'[70]. The former is almost entirely a disorder of spastic paraparesis and reflects axonal degeneration in the longest descending and ascending tracts (corticospinal and funiculus gracilis) of the spinal cord. Symptoms such as clumsiness and tripping may begin at any time from childhood to old age. Those cases that begin in early childhood may have little progression in later life, whereas adolescent-onset disease tends to progress steadily[71]. Just as may be the case in ALS, some forms of HSP have normal plantar responses despite prominent lower extremity spasticity/hyperreflexia. Urinary urgency and mildly impaired vibratory sensation are quite common features in pure HSP, but involvement of the upper extremities and bulbar region is not characteristic[72]. Complicated HSP may include degeneration of other tissues and therefore may present with additional clinical features such as seizures, mental retardation, optic atrophy, retinopathy, deafness, dementia, hematologic dysfunction, autoimmune disease, extrapyramidal dysfunction, icthyosis, pigmentary skin changes, ataxia, amyotrophy, posterior column dysfunction and neurogenic bladder. Several HSP genes have been described and linkages to 23 chromosomal loci have thus far been made. The most common HSP mutations are in the *spastin* gene on chromosome 2p22 (with up to 50% of all HSP accounted for by the SPG3A and SPG4 *spastin* gene mutations). *Spastin* is a member of the AAA protein family (*A*TPase *a*ssociated with diverse cellular *a*ctivities). Aberrant interactions between mutant spastin and microtubules may cause disordered intracellular transport of organelles, which may explain why this disorder preferentially causes degeneration of the longest corticospinal tract[73]. Some of the other known HSP mutations appear to exert their pathogenetic mechanisms in

a variety of ways including altered myelin composition (proteolipid protein), abnormal mitochondrial oxidative phosphorylation (paraplegin), disturbed axonal transport (kinesin heavy chain gene, *KIF5A*) and impaired embryonic corticospinal tract development (L1 cell adhesion molecule, X-linked, Xq28)[71]. As mentioned previously in this chapter, *alsin* mutations on chromosome 2 may cause a PLS-like disorder, an ALS-like disorder or an HSP-like presentation, but there is no evidence for a role of any of the other HSP genes in the cause of sporadic or familial amyotrophic lateral sclerosis[74].

MOTOR NEURON INVOLVEMENT IN OTHER DISORDERS

- Motor neuron diseases of presumed immune origin
     Lymphoproliferative disorders
     Paraneoplastic motor neuron disease
     Multifocal motor neuropathy with conduction block (MMNCB)

- Spinocerebellar ataxia types 2 and 3

- Adult hexosaminidase A deficiency

- Adult adrenomyeloneuropathy

- Allgrove's syndrome

- Adult polyglucosan body disease

- Post-irradiation motor neuronopathy

Motor neuron diseases of presumed immune origin

A subacute, painless and predominantly lower motor neuron disorder may occur as part of the presentation of several lymphoproliferative disorders including Hodgkin's lymphoma and non-Hodgkin's lymphoma (with or without myeloma or macroglobulinemia)[75]. The most common site of onset is in the lower extremities but the distribution is typically rather patchy. In some patients, treatment of the underlying disorder may halt the progression of the lower motor neuron disorder, but in those with combined UMN and LMN features the outlook is less favorable. Pathology includes inflammation and neuronal loss in the anterior horns of the spinal cord and inflammation in the ventral roots. A lumbar puncture may reveal elevated protein levels and/or oligoclonal bands.

A paraneoplastic motor neuron disorder has been described in association with several tumor types, the most common being small cell lung cancer. The onset and progression of this combined UMN/LMN condition may be quite rapid and precede the diagnosis of the underlying tumor. Unfortunately, treatment of the cancer usually does not lead to resolution of the motor neuron disorder. Several solid cancers have been associated with the development of motor neuron disorders including lung, colon, renal, ovarian, uterine and breast (a PLS-like presentation). Features such as sensory loss, sphincter disturbance, encephalopathy (in the form of limbic encephalitis) and Lambert–Eaton-type neuromuscular junction disease occur in many of these presumed paraneoplastic disorders (especially in association with small cell cancer) and should guide the clinician to search for an underlying tumor[76]. Unequivocal evidence supports the role of anti-Hu antibody in causing a motor neuron disorder and there is reason to assume a causative role for other antibodies (anti-ampiphysin, anti-Yo, anti-beta IV spectrin) in some rare cases of breast cancer[77,78]. However, the rarity of other solid cancer-associated cases suggests a coincidental relationship[79].

Although not strictly a motor neuronopathy but rather an immune-mediated motor neuropathy, MMNCB is an important part of the differential diagnosis of the pure lower motor neuron disorders because it responds to treatment with intravenous immunoglobulin (IVIG) therapy. This rare disorder is most commonly encountered in males under the age of 45. The clinical picture

is that of slowly evolving weakness more often in an upper extremity and in the distribution of one or more peripheral motor nerves with no objective sensory involvement and no upper motor neuron signs. Wristdrop, grip paresis and footdrop are common presentations but rare variants presenting as a slowly evolving proximal lower extremity paresis may also be encountered. Cranial nerve and/or bulbar involvement is not a feature of MMNCB. As befits a disorder that is largely demyelinating in its initial stages, there is usually little or no atrophy until late in the disease course. Fasciculations and muscle cramps are frequent and reflexes are diminished only in areas of muscle weakness. As the disorder evolves, individual peripheral nerve distributions may merge into what appear to be monomelic patterns of weakness with later development of wasting. About 50% of patients have high anti-GM1 antibody titers in serum; this ganglioside autoantigen is abundant in adaxonal membranes at the nodes of Ranvier of motor nerves. Electrodiagnostic studies are key in the evaluation; the electrical sine qua non of MMNCB is the demonstration of conduction blocks in two or more motor nerves at sites that are not common entrapment points and in the presence of normal sensory responses[80]. The underlying pathology is likely to be that of initial conduction block with secondary axonal degeneration, thus helping to explain the lack of muscle wasting despite profound weakness early in the course of disease[81]. Those with high titers of GM1 autoantibodies, definite conduction blocks, higher compound muscle action potential amplitudes, and younger age at onset appear to respond most favorably to IVIG therapy[82].

Spinocerebellar ataxias

The spinocerebellar ataxias (SCA) are an ever-expanding family of neurodegenerative disorders that are characterized by loss of neurons and support cells within the spinocerebellar system. Most cases present with features of gait and limb ataxia but many also feature peripheral nerve involvement, extrapyramidal disease and disordered eye movements. Symptoms such as cramps, fasciculations, muscle weakness, hypo/areflexia and muscle wasting have been described in several forms of SCA including SCA 1, 6 and 7, but the most common association between motor neuron features and the SCA family is with SCA 3 and, to a lesser extent, SCA 2. SCA 3, also known as Machado Joseph disease, is an autosomal dominant inherited CAG trinucleotide repeat expansion disorder with onset usually in the third decade. The mutation produces mutant ataxin-3 protein that results in the aggregation of harmful intracellular polyglutamine-containing proteins[83]. Some of the key clinical characteristics are dystonia, parkinsonism, eye movement abnormalities and ataxia, but some patients also develop motor neuron features both of the limbs and of the bulbar region. Electrodiagnostic studies may reveal changes consistent with a motor neuropathy in these cases[84,85]. SCA 2, another CAG trinucleotide repeat expansion disease, may present in a similar fashion to SCA 3 with parkinsonism, ataxia, tremor and motor neuron disease including facial fasciculations[86–88]. While Friedreich's ataxia usually includes both upper and lower motor neuron signs, the co-existent cardiomyopathy and sensory features make it hard to mistake it for MND.

Radiation-induced lower motor neuron syndrome

Many case reports have described a syndrome of progressive weakness and wasting of the lower extremities in individuals who have previously undergone retroperitoneal and/or para-aortic region radiotherapy treatment for testicular or lymphoid cancers. The pattern of involvement is usually asymmetrical and is accompanied by fasciculations and areflexia. There is usually a latency of months to years between the time of the radiotherapy and the onset of the flaccid paraparesis and, while most cases eventually stabilize, some appear to deteriorate slowly over many years.

Myokymic potentials and non-resolving conduction blocks are important electrodiagnostic features. There is considerable debate as to the exact cause of this disorder and in particular whether this is a direct effect of radiation-induced injury to motor neurons or to motor anterior primary rami. A recent meta-analysis of the 47 cases that have been reported in the English literature to date suggests that there is insufficient evidence to support a direct effect of radiation therapy on motor neurons/nerves; the authors even speculate that the pattern is more suggestive of a predisposing viral etiology[89].

Adult polyglucosan body disease

Adult polyglusocan body disease is a very rare autosomal recessive disorder characterized by progressive UMN and LMN degeneration beginning in the fifth or sixth decade of life with early symptoms of poor bladder control (neurogenic pattern) and, in approximately two-thirds of cases, with cognitive dysfunction. Patients may develop extrapyramidal and cerebellar features, and additional sensory loss may also occur with electrodiagnostic evidence of an axon-loss sensorimotor polyneuropathy. MRI may reveal non-enhancing, symmetrical white matter signal changes in the periventricular regions along with spinal cord atrophy. The disorder gains its name from the presence of abundant periodic acid Schiff (PAS)-positive polyglucosan bodies in affected tissues and is associated with reduced activity of the glycogen branching enzyme (GBE). A number of mutations in the *GBE* gene have been described but the disease may occur in the absence of a *GBE* mutation[90,91].

Adrenomyeloneuropathy

Loss of function mutations in the *ABCD1* (adenosine triphosphate binding cassette, subfamily D) peroxisomal transporter gene on the X chromosome result in two phenotypes, the more severe being adrenoleukodystrophy, a childhood-onset disorder characterized by seizures, cognitive decline, spasticity, blindness and deafness. The milder adult-onset version, adrenomyeloneuropathy, presents as a slowly progressive spastic paraparesis with relatively abrupt onset, central demyelination (that may be seen as white matter signal change on MRI of the spinal cord), additional sensorimotor peripheral neuropathy and a neurogenic bladder. Laboratory tests may reveal mild adrenal deficiency, and sural nerve biopsy may show curvilinear empty lipid clefts within Schwann cells. The gene defect results in high intracellular levels of very-long-chain fatty acids (VLCFAs); demonstration of raised VLCFAs in plasma or cultured skin fibroblasts is the most useful diagnostic test. There is no specific therapy but recent animal research has identified a potential role for the upregulation of a closely related transporter gene in the treatment of both the severe childhood- and milder adult-onset disorders[92].

Allgrove's syndrome

Allgrove's syndrome is a rare autosomal recessive disorder caused by mutations in the *aladin* gene on chromosome 12q13. There can be considerable clinical heterogeneity both within and between families: a combination of *a*chalasia, *a*lacrima and *a*drenocorticotropic deficiency have defined this condition (indeed it is most commonly called triple A syndrome), but recently described features such as mental retardation, dysautonomia and bulbospinal amyotrophy have broadened the phenotype[93,94].

Hexosaminidase A deficiency

Adult hexosaminidase (Hex) A is a rare autosomal recessive GM2-gangliosidosis caused by mutations in the *Hex A* gene on chromosome 15q23–24. In infants, a complete absence of *Hex A* activity causes Tay Sachs syndrome, but juveniles and adults with Hex A deficiency are compound heterozygotes and thus have some residual enzyme activity[95,96]. The clinical presentation is that of slowly progressive proximal muscle-predominant weakness in the upper and lower extremities with frequent cramps. In some cases with additional features of spasticity and/or bulbar dysfunction it can be extremely difficult to distinguish between Hex A and ALS. That being said, atypical features usually develop in Hex A and include sphincter impairments, cognitive changes, psychiatric complaints, cerebellar signs, extrapyramidal features, and sensory loss. Widespread complex repetitive discharges are an important sign to watch out for during electrodiagnostic studies.

MOTOR NEURON DISORDERS DUE TO VIRAL INFECTION AND TOXIC AGENTS

- Viral infections
    Poliomyelitis
    Postpolio syndrome
    West Nile virus
    Tropical spastic paraparesis/HTLV-associated myelopathy
    Human immunodeficiency virus

- Lathyrism

- Konzo

- Heavy metals

- Shellfish poisoning

Viral infections

Neurotropic viruses are adept at gaining entry to the central nervous system where they take up residence in both neurons and glial cells. Potentially important viruses with respect to involvement of the motor neuron cell population are the retroviruses (HIV, HTLV1 and HTLV2), enteroviruses (including polio virus) and the flaviviruses (including West Nile virus), many of which have yet to be fully characterized. The more common virus-induced motor neuron disorders are discussed below.

Poliovirus is a single-stranded RNA virus of the enterovirus group of picornaviruses and is spread via the feco-oral route. Prior to the introduction of an effective vaccination program, acute poliomyelitis was a relatively common disorder that occurred in epidemics during the summer months, and primarily affected children and teenagers. Acute poliomyelitis (acute anterior poliomyelitis) is now a rare disorder in the western world but is still encountered in certain regions where immunization programmes have yet to take full effect[97]. Only a minority of cases (0.1–1%) actually develop acute paralytic poliomyelitis, onset of which is characterized by frequent localized or generalized fasciculations with myalgias and hyperesthesia. Soon afterwards, there is rapid development of muscle weakness that may remain localized or appear in a fairly generalized pattern including involvement of the muscles of ventilation. Bulbar muscle involvement is rare and reflects the relative rarity of involvement by the virus of brainstem motor nuclei. Clinical examination reveals a pattern of lower motor neuron weakness that is soon followed by focal or regional muscle atrophy. Recovery from the acute illness is often prolonged and sometimes incomplete.

Post polio syndrome is a disorder of new weakness and fatigue in muscles that were affected by polio more than 10 years previously. It occurs in up to 60% of patients who have recovered from the acute paralytic illness. Additional clinical features include chronic generalized fatigue, fasciculations, joint pains, cramps, myalgias and reduced endurance. The underlying cause has yet to be determined; the leading hypothesis that there is a new-onset peripheral disintegration of motor units that were previously affected by acute polio supports the notion that metabolically exhausted motor units undergo a process of premature aging. Investigation of this syndrome serves only to support what is largely a clinical diagnosis[98].

West Nile virus is an arthropod-borne flavivirus that first rose to the attention of neurologists in the USA in 1999, when it caused an outbreak of meningitis and encephalitis. It has subsequently spread from its original eastern seaboard location across the Midwest and into the western United States[99]. One of the most dramatic presentations of West Nile virus infection is an irreversible, acute flaccid paralysis (AFP) that may occur in any number of limbs and in a typically asymmetrical pattern with or without other clinical features such as meningitis, encephalitis and cranial mononeuropathies. Additional aching pains may be present in affected limbs, but actual loss of sensation is not a characteristic feature. Involvement of respiratory muscles may precipitate acute respiratory failure, and bladder and bowel dysfunction may occur in up to a third of all cases. Investigations usually reveal a fever and cerebrospinal fluid pleocytosis[100]. Cerebral imaging is usually normal but MRI of the spinal cord may show increased signal in the cauda equina, in the conus medullaris, or in the anterior horns. Electrodiagnostic studies typically reveal normal SNAPs with low-amplitude CMAPs: motor conduction velocities are within the realm of motor axon loss rather than demyelination. Needle electrode examination characteristically reveals changes consistent with acute loss of motor units including fibrillation potentials, positive sharp waves and a neurogenic recruitment pattern of motor unit action potentials. On occasion, electrodiagnostic studies and neuroimaging findings are most consistent with an acute polyradiculitis pattern rather than with involvement of the anterior horn cells themselves[101].

Human T lymphotropic viruses (HTLV) types 1 and 2 are the retroviruses responsible for tropical spastic paraparesis (TSP) that is endemic to the Caribbean, Central/South America, southern United States, Melanesia, equatorial Africa and South Africa. The same disorder is also found in temperate parts of southwestern Japan where it is known as HTLV-associated myelopathy (HAM). Mode of transmission is via breastfeeding, transplacental transfer, sexual contact, intravenous drug abuse and blood transfusions; the vast majority of infected persons are asymptomatic, although capable of transmitting the virus. Patients with very high proviral loads appear prone to developing an intense T cell-mediated inflammatory response to tax and env viral proteins that is centered in the thoracic cord but also involves subcortical tissues (leading to white matter MRI signal change). The characteristic clinical picture is that of a slowly evolving spastic paraparesis in the third and fourth decades of life with sphincter disturbance but without symptoms in the upper limbs (apart from brisk reflexes) or the bulbar region. Patients may complain of distal paresthesiae and may have ataxia from posterior column dysfunction. On occasion, the clinical presentation may more closely resemble that of ALS but the presence of atypical features such as urgency of micturition or sensory disturbance and/or being resident in an endemic area warrants serological testing for HTLV1.

Although phylogenetically related to HTLV1, HTLV2 is an antigenically distinct virus that has recently come to the fore as a potential cause of a slowly evolving spastic paraparesis spread via sexual contact and/or contaminated needles. It was originally endemic among Amerindian tribal members but has now spread to the general population and is particularly prevalent in intravenous drug abusers. The clinical condition is no different from that caused by HTLV1, but it is difficult to ascertain the true extent of neurologic disease due to HTLV2, because of frequent coincident infection with HIV[102]. Because of the high incidence of asymptomatic carrier status in the population, it can be difficult to establish a diagnosis of these disorders without first excluding other possibilities such as multiple sclerosis and HIV-related neurologic disease. There is no specific treatment for either HTLV1 or HTLV2.

Acquired immune deficiency syndrome caused by HIV infection type 1 (and in one case report in HIV2) can cause a progressive disorder of weakness and wasting that is similar to ALS but with a subacute presentation with rapid deterioration and young onset. White-matter lesions may be identified in the subcortical regions and/or brainstem and additional evaluation may reveal generalized adenopathy, progressive dementia, elevated proteins in cerebrospinal fluid, low white cell counts and, of course, low CD4 counts[103,104]. These additional features are the main means to distinguish true ALS from this HIV-associated ALS mimic disease. Treatment with highly active anti-retroviral therapy can halt or reverse the deleterious changes and may be reflected in disappearance of MRI signal change.

Shellfish poisoning/domoic acid

In the winter of 1987, an outbreak of serious illness occurred in 107 individuals who had consumed cultivated mussels from Prince Edward Island in Canada. The initial gastrointestinal upset was followed within 48 hours by seizures, myoclonus, profound amnesia, confusion and, in a few elderly individuals, by coma and death. A detailed study of 14 cases with neurologic involvement described generalized weakness in all cases and an alternating hemiparesis/ophthalmoplegia in two. Electrodiagnostic studies revealed changes consistent with either a motor neuronopathy or a motor axonopathy, but pathological confirmation of motor neuron involvement was not achieved[105]. The causative toxin was domoic acid that had been bioconcentrated in mussels that had filtered toxin-producing phytoplankton diatoms (*Pseudo-nitzschia pungens*)[106]. Domoic acid is a potent stimulator of kainate-type glutamate receptors and there is evidence that this interaction leads to a large calcium influx into the cell and results in disturbed intracellular homeostasis. The particular abundance of this receptor in the CA3 region of the human hippocampus may explain the vulnerability of this region to domoic acid toxicity and the resulting amnestic syndrome (amnestic shellfish poisoning, ASP) that was described in several cases[107]. Domoic acid may be found in the tissues of several shellfish species, crabs and even fish (mackerel and anchovies) and hence many countries are monitoring domoic acid levels in their fishery stocks with the Canadian authorities having imposed a limit of 20 µg domoic acid/g shellfish tissue.

Lathyrism and Konzo

Lathyrism is a toxic nutritional disorder that occurs in epidemic form in famine- and drought-prone regions including India, Ethiopia and Bangladesh (but also described in China and Europe). It is caused by ingestion of foodstuffs made from *Lathyrus sativus*. This drought-resistant chickling pea contains an excitotoxic amino acid, β-*N*-oxalylamino-L-alanine (BOAA) that can excessively stimulate glutamate receptors. Onset may be acute or insidious; young men seem particularly prone and typically present with cramps and spasms in the lower extremities followed by an evolving spastic paraparesis with neurogenic bladder and lower-extremity sensory disturbances including formications[108]. Konzo (meaning 'tied legs') is clinically similar to lathyrism: it also has a predilection for males and occurs in epidemics in certain African populations that are prone to protein–calorie deficiency. The neurotoxin is derived from flour made from short-soaked cassava roots. These roots liberate cyanohydrins that generate thiocyanates that, in turn, may excessively stimulate glutamate receptor subtypes[109]. Both lathyrism and Konzo exhibit striking loss of Betz cells and, though both disorders are self-limiting, the outcome may be that of permanent disability.

CONCLUSION

Whether sporadic or familial, motor neuron disease may be defined as a progressive disorder that affects the upper and/or lower motor neurons and manifests as motor weakness in the extremities, the bulbar muscles and/or the respiratory muscles (Table 1.2). The adult form of MND, which is familial in less than 10% of instances, can exist in several motor-predominant forms including ALS, PLS and PMA, and is characterized pathologically by loss of motor neurons with the presence of ubiquitinated intraneuronal inclusion bodies within the motor system. Frontotemporal dementia and aphasia, although usually subtle, may accompany the motor disorder and indicate the additional presence of non-motor system disease. Several different fALS-associated mutations have been identified in genes encoding proteins involved in cell transport, trafficking, free radical regulation and DNA repair, but no distinct fALS phenotype has emerged and the individual rarity of these mutations has yet to explain the much more common sporadic form of MND.

There are a host of neurologic disorders that include features of MND such as the spinal muscular atrophies, Kennedy's disease and the HSP family, most of which include atypical features such as sensory loss, cognitive changes, endocrine changes and sphincter disturbances. Yet again, despite considerable knowledge of the underlying etiology of most of these conditions, no clear-cut unifying link between these disorders and ALS/MND has been identified. The fact that ALS/MND overlaps clinically with so many disorders illustrates how difficult it may be to confirm the diagnosis quickly and also highlights the need for a reliable biologic disease marker to help make an accurate diagnosis and track disease progression.

Table 1.2 The motor neuron disorders. Summary of the main clinical features that are encountered in the various motor neuron diseases discussed in the chapter. As may be appreciated, there are many features that overlap between the different disease entities, but in many instances there are clinical clues that may guide the clinician to an early and accurate diagnosis

Disorder	Inheritance/gene	UMN	LMN	Atypical
ALS	Sporadic	Yes	Yes	No
PLS	Sporadic	Yes	No	No
PMA	Sporadic	No	Yes	No
ALS/FTD	Sporadic	Yes	Yes	FTD
Western Pacific ALS	Complex: genetic and environmental	Yes	Yes	Dementia, parkinsonism, high incidence in region
ALS/FTD Chr 9	AD	Yes	Yes	FTD
ALS 1	AD or AR; SOD1	Yes	Yes	Young onset
ALS 2	AR, alsin	Yes	Yes	Young onset; ALS or PLS and overlap with HSP phenotype
ALS 3	AD, other	Variable	Variable	Variable
ALS 4	AD, senataxin	Yes	Yes	Young onset, can be CMT-like or ALS-like, slow progression, normal life expectancy, sparing of bulbar and respiratory muscles
ALS 5	AR	Yes	Yes	Young onset
ALS 6	AD	Yes	Yes	Young onset; variable site of onset, rare
ALS 7	AD	Yes	Yes	FTD with/without hallucinations
ALS 8	AD, VAPB	Yes	Yes	Young onset
Progressive LMN disease	AD, DCTN1	No	Yes	Slow progression, early adult onset, early facial paralysis, vocal cord paralysis
SMA	AR, rare AD, rare X-linked, rare 'sporadic'. Adult: 30% AD	No	Yes	Very slow progression; no UMN signs at any time; rare forms in newborns with cardiomyopathy, lactic acidosis
Kennedy's disease	X-linked recessive	Yes	Yes	Gynecomastia, infertility, glucose intolerance
HSP	AD, AR, X-linked	Yes	No	Variable: can be 'complicated' by ataxia, sensory signs, optic atrophy, seizures, mental retardation
SCA 3	AD	Yes	Yes	Ataxia, 'protuberant eyes', gaze palsy, dementia, extrapyramidal features
Hex A	AR, Hex A gene	Yes	Yes	Severe cramps, sensory loss, cerebellar signs, dementia, psychosis, extrapyramidal signs
DDPAC/PPND	AD, tau gene	Yes	Yes	Early onset, FTD, parkinsonism
AAA syndrome	AR, aladin gene	No	Yes	Alacrima, achalasia, ACTH deficiency, MR, seizures, optic atrophy, autonomic dysfunction

Continued...

Table 1.2   Continued...

Disorder	Inheritance/gene	UMN	LMN	Atypical
Adrenomyeloneuropathy	AR, ABC reporter gene mutation	Yes		Young onset, mild adrenal insufficiency, sensory impairments, neurogenic bladder
Polyglucosan disease	AR, GBE gene	Yes	Yes	Sensory loss, dementia, sphincter disturbance
Paraneoplastic ALS	Sporadic	Yes	Yes	Sensory symptoms/signs, encephalopathy, anti-Hu antibody, subacute course
Polio	Sporadic	No	Yes	Pains and paresthesiae at onset, fulminant onset, co-existent meningism, raised enteroviral titers
West Nile	Sporadic	No	Yes	Seizures, mononeuropathies, raised CSF protein and cells, and/or West Nile virus titers, co-existent meningitis/encephalitis, neuropathies, fulminant onset
HTLV-1	Sporadic	Yes	No	Neurogenic bladder, sensory ataxia, sensory involvement
HTLV-2	Sporadic	Yes	No	Neurogenic bladder, sensory ataxia, sensory involvement, ± HIV-positive
HIV	Sporadic	Yes	Yes	Dementia, sensory loss, associated AIDS-defining disease
Lathyrism	Sporadic	Yes	No	Self-limiting, leg formications
Konzo	Sporadic	Yes	No	Self-limiting
Domoic acid	Sporadic	No evidence	Possible	Acute seizures, GI upset, encephalopathy, coma Chronic amnestic syndrome
Benign focal amyotrophy	Usually sporadic	No	Yes	Very limited region of LMN involvement; prolonged stability

AD, autosomal dominant; AR, autosomal recessive; SOD1, Cu/Zn superoxide dismutase 1; VAPB, vesicle-associated membrane protein/synaptobrevin-associated membrane protein B; GBE, glycogen branching enzyme; CMT, Charcot–Marie–Tooth; FTD, frontotemporal dementia; DCTN1, Dynactin 1; ABC, adenosine triphosphate binding cassette

REFERENCES

1. Brain WR, Walton JN. Brain's Diseases of the Nervous System. London: Oxford University Press, 1969: 595–606

2. Charcot JM. De la sclérose latérale amyotrophique. Prog Med 1874; 23: 235–7, 24: 341–2, 29: 453–5

3. Swash M, Ingram D. Preclinical and subclinical events in motor neuron disease. J Neurol Neurosurg Psychiatry 1988; 51: 165–8.

4. Brooks BR, Sufit RL, DePaul R, et al. Design of clinical therapeutic trials in amyotrophic lateral sclerosis. Adv Neurol 1991; 56: 521–46

5. Eisen A, Calne D. Amyotrophic lateral sclerosis, Parkinson's disease and Alzheimer's disease: phylogenetic characteristics. Can J Neurol Sci 1992; 19: 117–23

6. Desai J, Swash M. Extrapyramidal involvement in amyotrophic lateral sclerosis; backward falls and

retropulsion. J Neurol Neurosurg Psychiatry 1999; 67: 214–16

7. Murray B. Natural history and prognosis of amyotrophic lateral sclerosis. In: Mitsumoto HM, Przedborski S, Gordon P, eds. Amyotrophic Lateral Sclerosis. New York: Taylor & Francis Group, 2006: 227–55

8. Erb WH. Über einen wenig bekannten spinalen symptomen-complex. Berl Klin Wochenschr 1875; 12: 357–9

9. Pringle CE, Hudson AJ, Munoz DG, et al. Primary lateral sclerosis. Clinical features, neuropathology and diagnostic criteria. Brain 1992; 115: 495–520

10. Le Forestier N, Maisonabe T, Piquard A, et al. Does primary lateral sclerosis exist? A study of 20 patients and a review of the literature. Brain 2001; 124: 1989–99

11. Zhai P, Pagan F, Statland J, et al. Primary lateral sclerosis: A heterogeneous disorder composed of different subtypes? Neurology 2003; 60: 1258–65

12. Mills CK. A case of unilateral progressive ascending paralysis, probably representing a new form of degenerative disease. J Nerv Ment Dis 1900; 27: 195–200

13. Kuipers-Upmeijer J, de Jager AEJ, Hew JM, et al. Primary lateral sclerosis: clinical, neurophysiological, and magnetic resonance findings. J Neurol Neurosurg Psychiatry 2001; 71: 615–20

14. Ulug AM, Grunewald T, Lin MT, et al. Diffusion tensor imaging in the diagnosis of primary lateral sclerosis. J Magn Reson Imaging 2004; 19: 34–9

15. Toosy AT, Werring DJ, Orrell RW, et al. Diffusion tensor imaging detects corticospinal tract involvement at multiple levels in amyotrophic lateral sclerosis. J Neurol Neurosurg Psychiatry 2003; 74: 1250–7

16. Norris F, Shepherd R, Denys E, et al. Onset, natural history and outcome in idiopathic adult motor neuron disease. J Neurol Sci 1993; 118: 48–55

17. Chio A, Brignolio F, Leone M, et al. A survival analysis of 155 cases of progressive muscular atrophy. Acta Neurol Scand 1985; 72: 407–13

18. Ince PG, Evans J, Knopp M, et al. Corticospinal tract degeneration in the progressive muscular atrophy variant of ALS. Neurology 2003; 60: 1252–8

19. Tsuchiya K, Sano M, Shiotsu H, et al. Sporadic amyotrophic lateral sclerosis of long duration mimicking spinal progressive muscular atrophy exists: additional autopsy evidence with a clinical course of 19 years. Neuropathology 2004; 24: 228–35

20. Cervenakova L, Protas II, Hirano A, et al. Progressive muscular atrophy variant of familial amyotrophic lateral sclerosis (PMA/ALS). J Neurol Sci 2000; 177: 124–30

21. Kaufmann P, Pullman SL, Shunga DC, et al. Objective tests for upper motor neuron involvement in amyotrophic lateral sclerosis (ALS). Neurology 2004; 62: 1753–7

22. Wilson CM, Grace GM, Munoz DG, et al. Cognitive impairment in sporadic ALS: a pathologic continuum underlying a multisystem disorder. Neurology 2001; 57: 651–7

23. Lomen-Hoerth C, Murphy J, Langmore S, et al. Are amyotrophic lateral sclerosis patients cognitively normal? Neurology 2003; 60: 1094–7

24. Lomen-Hoerth C. Characterization of amyotrophic lateral sclerosis and frontotemporal dementia. Dement Geriatr Cogn Disord 2004; 17: 337–41

25. Hodges JR, Davies R, Xuareb J, et al. Survival in frontotemporal dementia. Neurology 2003; 61: 349–54

26. Yoshida M. Amyotrophic lateral sclerosis with dementia: the clinicopathologic spectrum. Neuropathology 2004; 24: 87–102

27. Yang W, Sopper MM, Leystra-Lantz C, Strong MJ. Microtubule-associated tau protein positive neuronal and glial inclusions in ALS. Neurology 2003; 61: 1766–73

28. Mackenzie IR, Feldman H. Neurofilament inclusion body disease with early onset frontotemporal dementia and primary lateral sclerosis. Clin Neuropathol 2004; 23: 183–93

29. Plato CC, Galasko D, Garruto RM, et al. ALS and PDC of Guam: Forty-year follow-up. Neurology 2002; 58: 765–73

30. Perl DP, Hof PR, Purohit DP, et al. Hippocampal and entorhinal cortex neurofibrillary tangle formation in Guamanian Chamorros free of overt neurologic dysfunction. J Neuropathol Exp Neurol 2003; 62: 381–8

31. Plato CC, Garruto RM, Galasko D, et al. Amyotrophic lateral sclerosis and parkinsonism dementia complex of Guam: Changing incidence rates during the past 60 years. Am J Epidemiol 2003; 157: 149–57

32. Galasko D, Salmon DP, Craig UK, et al. Clinical features and changing patterns of neurodegenerative disorders on Guam, 1997-2000. Neurology 2002; 58: 90–7

33. Cox PA, Sachs OW. Cycad neurotoxins, consumption of flying foxes, and ALS/PDC disease in Guam. Neurology 2002; 58: 956–9

34. Cox PA, Banack SA, Murch SJ. Biomagnification of cyanobacterial neurotoxins and neurodegenerative

disease among the Chamorro people of Guam. Proc Natl Acad Sci USA 2003; 100: 13380–3

35. Schroder R, Keller E, Flacke S, et al. MRI findings in Hirayama's disease; flexion-induced cervical myelopathy or intrinsic motor neuron disease? J Neurol 1999; 246: 1069–74

36. Restuccia D, Rubino M, Valeriani M, et al. Cervical cord dysfunction during neck flexion in Hirayama's disease. Neurology 2003; 60: 1980–3

37. Felice KJ, Whitaker CH, Grunnet ML. Benign calf amyotrophy. Clinicopathologic study of 8 patients. Arch Neurol 2003; 60: 1415–20

38. Gourie-Devi M, Nalini A. Long-term follow-up of 44 patients with brachial monomelic amyotrophy. Acta Neurol Scand 2003; 107: 215–20

39. Van den Berg-Vos RM, Visser J, Franssen H, et al. Sporadic lower motor neuron disease with adult onset: Classification of subtypes. Brain 2003; 126: 1036–47

40. Rosen DR, Siddique T, Patterson D, et al. Mutations in Cu/Zn superoxide dismutase gene are associated with familial amyotrophic lateral sclerosis. Nature 1993; 362: 59–62

41. Kunst CB. Complex genetics of amyotrophic lateral sclerosis. Am J Hum Genet 2004; 75: 933–47

42. Mase G, Ros S, Gemma A, et al. ALS with variable phenotypes in a six-generation family caused by leu144phe mutation in the SOD1 gene. J Neurol Sci 2001; 191: 11–18

43. Prudlo J, Alber B, Kalscheur VM, et al. Chromosomal translocation t (18;21)(q23;22.1) indicates novel susceptibility loci for frontotemporal dementia with ALS. Ann Neurol 2004; 55: 134–8

44. Juneja T, Pericak-Vance MA, Laing NG, et al. Prognosis in familial amyotrophic lateral sclerosis: progression and survival in patients with glu100gly and ala4val mutations in Cu, Zn superoxide dismutase. Neurology 1997; 48: 55–7

45. Ohi T, Saita K, Takechi S, et al. Clinical features and neuropathological findings of familial amyotrophic lateral sclerosis with a His46Arg mutation in Cu/Zn superoxide dismutase. J Neurol Sci 2002; 197: 73–8

46. Cudkowicz ME, McKenna-Yasek D, Sapp PE, et al. Epidemiology of mutations in superoxide dismutase in amyotrophic lateral sclerosis. Ann Neurol 1997; 41: 210–21

47. Giess R, Holtmann B, Braga M, et al. Early onset of severe familial amyotrophic lateral sclerosis with SOD-1 mutation: Potential impact of CNTF as a candidate modifier gene. Am J Hum Genet 2002; 70: 1277–86

48. Devon RS, Helm JR, Rouleau GA, et al. The first nonsense mutation in alsin results in a homogeneous phenotype of infantile-onset ascending spastic paralysis with bulbar involvement in two siblings. Clin Genet 2003; 64: 210–15

49. Hadano S, Hand CK, Osuga H, et al. A gene encoding a putative GTPase regulator is mutated in familial amyotrophic lateral sclerosis 2. Nat Genet 2001; 29: 166–73

50. Yang Y, Hentati A, Deng HX, et al. The gene encoding alsin, a protein with three guanine-nucleotide exchange factor domains, is mutated in a form of recessive amyotrophic lateral sclerosis. Nat Genet 2001; 29: 160–5

51. Topp JD, Gray NW, Gerard RD, Horaxdovsky BF. Alsin is a Rab5 and Rac1 guanine nucleotide exchange factor. J Biol Chem 2004; 279: 24612–23

52. Kunita R, Otomo A, Mizumura H, et al. Homo-oligomerization of ALS2 through its unique carboxyl-terminal regions is essential for the ALS2-associated Rab5 guanine nucleotide exchange activity and its regulatory function in endosomal trafficking. J Biol Chem 2004; 279: 38626–35

53. Puls I, Jonnakuty C, LaMonte BH, et al. Mutant dynactin in motor neuron disease. Nat Genet 2003; 33: 455–6

54. Nishimura AL, Mitne-Neto M, Silva HC, et al. A mutation in the vesicle trafficking protein VAPB causes late onset spinal muscular atrophy and amyotrophic lateral sclerosis. Am J Hum Genet 2004; 75: 822–31

55. Chen Y-Z, Bennett CL, Huynh HM, et al. DNA/RNA helicase gene mutations in a form of juvenile amyotrophic lateral sclerosis. Am J Hum Genet 2004; 74: 1128–35

56. Sapp PC, Hosler BA, McKenna-Yasek D, et al. Identification of two novel loci for dominantly inherited familial amyotrophic lateral sclerosis. Am J Hum Genet 2003; 73: 397–493

57. Ruddy DM, Parton MJ, Al-Chalabi A, et al. Two families with familial amyotrophic lateral sclerosis are linked to a novel locus on chromosome 16q. Am J Hum Genet 2003; 73: 390–6

58. Abalkhail H, Mitchell J, Habgood J, et al. A new familial amyotrophic lateral sclerosis locus on chromosome 16q12.1-16q12.2. Am J Hum Genet 2003; 73: 383–9

59. Hosler BA, Siddique T, Sapp PC, et al. Linkage of familial amyotrophic lateral sclerosis with frontotemporal dementia to chromosome 9q21-q22. JAMA 2000; 284: 1664–9

60. Lynch T, Sano M, Marder KS, et al. Clinical characteristics of a family with chromosome 17-linked disinhibition–dementia–parkinsonism–amyotrophy complex. Neurology 1994; 44: 1878–84

61. Tsuboi Y, Uitti RJ, Delisle MB, et al. Clinical features and disease haplotypes of individuals with the N279K tau gene mutation: a comparison of the pallidopontonigral degeneration kindred and a French family. Arch Neurol 2002; 59: 943–50

62. Wilhelmsen KC, Forman MS, Rosen HJ, et al. 17q-linked frontotemporal dementia–amyotrophic lateral sclerosis without tau mutations with tau and alpha-synuclein inclusions. Arch Neurol 2004; 61: 398–406

63. Iannaconne ST, Burghes A. Spinal muscular atrophies. Adv Neurol 2002; 88: 83–98

64. Grohmann K, Varon R, Stolz P, et al. Infantile spinal muscular atrophy with respiratory distress type 1 (SMARD1). Ann Neurol 2003; 54: 719–24

65. Tarnopolsky MA, Bourgeois JM, Fu MH, et al. Novel SCO2 mutation (G1521A) presenting as a spinal muscular atrophy type 1 phenotype. Am J Med Genet 2004; 125A: 310–14

66. Sperfeld AD, Karitzky J, Brummer D, et al. X-linked bulbospinal neuronopathy: Kennedy disease. Arch Neurol 2002; 59: 1921–6

67. Paparounas K. Kennedy disease: Insights and questions. Arch Neurol 2004; 61: 603–4

68. Dejager S, Bry-Gauillard E, Bruckert E, et al. A comprehensive endocrine description of Kennedy's disease revealing androgen insensitivity linked to CAG repeat length. J Clin Endocrinol Metab 2002; 87: 3893–901

69. Ferrante MA, Wilbourn AJ. The characteristic electrodiagnostic features of Kennedy's disease. Muscle Nerve 1997; 20: 323–9

70. Harding AE. Classification of the hereditary ataxias and paraplegias. Lancet 1983; 1: 1151–5

71. Fink JK. Advances in the hereditary spastic paraplegias. Exp Neurol 2003; 184: S106–10

72. Online Mendelian Inheritance in Man; OMIM 182600

73. McDermott CJ, Grierson AJ, Wood JD, et al. Hereditary spastic paraparesis: disrupted intracellular transport associated with spastin mutation. Ann Neurol 2003; 54: 748–59

74. McDermott CJ, Roberts D, Tomkins J, et al. Spastin and paraplegin gene analysis in selected cases of motor neurone disease (MND). Amyotroph Lateral Scler Other Motor Neuron Disord 2003; 4: 96–9

75. Rudnicki SA, Dalmau J. Paraneoplastic syndromes of the spinal cord, nerve and muscle. Muscle Nerve 2000; 23: 1800–18

76. Rosenfeld MR, Posner JB. Paraneoplastic motor neuron disease. Adv Neurol 1991; 56: 445–59

77. Berghs S, Ferracci F, Maksimova E, et al. Autoimmunity to beta IV spectrin in paraneoplastic lower motor neuron syndrome. Proc Nat Acad Sci 2001; 98: 6945–50

78. Ogawa M, Nishie M, Kurahashi K, et al. Anti-Hu associated paraneoplastic sensory neuronopathy with motor neuron involvement. J Neurol Neurosurg Psychiatry 2004; 75: 1051–3

79. Forsyth PA, Dalmau J, Graus F, et al. Motor neuron syndromes in cancer patients. Ann Neurol 1997; 41: 722–30

80. Olney RK, Lewis RA, Putnam TD, Campellone JV Jr. Consensus criteria for the diagnosis of multifocal motor neuropathy. American Association of Electrodiagnostic Medicine. Muscle Nerve 2003; 27: 117–21

81. Taylor BV, Dyck PJ, Engelstad J, et al. Multifocal motor neuropathy: Pathologic alterations at the site of conduction block. J Neuropathol Exp Neurol 2004; 63: 129–37

82. Vucic S, Black KR, Chong PS, Cros D. Multifocal motor neuropathy: decrease in conduction blocks and reinnervation with long-term IVIg. Neurology 2004; 63: 1264–9

83. Goti D, Katzen SM, Mez J, et al. A mutant ataxin-3 putative-cleavage fragment in brains of Machado–Joseph disease patients and transgenic mice is cytotoxic above a critical concentration. J Neurosci 2004; 24: 10266–79

84. Durr A, Stevanin G, Cancel G, et al. Spinocerebellar ataxia 3 and Machado–Joseph disease: Clinical, molecular, and neuropathological features. Ann Neurol 1996; 39: 490–9

85. ven de Warrenburg BP, Notermans NC, Schelhaas HJ, et al. Peripheral nerve involvement in spinocerebellar ataxia. Arch Neurol 2004; 61: 257–61

86. Geschwind DH, Periman S, Figueroa CP, et al. The prevalence and wide clinical spectrum of the spinocerebellar ataxia type 2 repeat in patients with autosomal dominant ataxia. Am J Hum Genet 1997; 60: 842–50

87. Furtado S, Payami H, Lockhart PJ, et al. Profile of families with parkinsonism-predominant spinocerebellar ataxia type 2 (SCA2). Mov Disord 2004; 19: 622–9

88. Infante J, Berciano J, Volpini V, et al. Spinocerebellar ataxia type 2 with levodopa-responsive parkinsonism culminating in motor neuron disease. Mov Disord 2004; 19: 848–52

89. Esik O, Vonoczky K, Lengyel Z, et al. Characteristics of radiogenic lower motor neuron disease, a possible link with a preceding viral infection. Spinal Cord 2004; 42: 99–105

90. Sindern E, Ziemssen F, Ziemssen T, et al. Adult polyglucosan body disease: A post-mortem study. Neurology 2003; 61: 263–5

91. Klein CJ, Boes CJ, Chapin JE, et al. Adult polyglucosan body disease: Case description of an expanding genetic and clinical syndrome. Muscle Nerve 2004; 29: 323–8

92. Pujol A, Ferrer I, Camps C, et al. Functional overlap between ABCD1 (ALD) and ABCD2 (ALD2) transporters: A therapeutic target for X-adrenoleukodystrophy. Hum Mol Genet 2004; 13: 2997–3006

93. Goizet C, Catargi B, Tison F, et al. Progressive bulbospinal amyotrophy in triple A syndrome with AAAS mutation. Neurology 2002; 58: 962–5

94. Barat P, Goizet C, Tullio-Pelet A, et al. Phenotypic heterogeneity in AAAS gene mutation. Acta Paediatr 2004; 93: 1257–9

95. Mitsumoto H, Sliman RJ, Schafer IA, et al. Motor neuron disease and adult hexosaminidase A deficiency in two families: evidence for multisystem degeneration. Ann Neurol 1985; 17: 378–85

96. Drory VE, Birnbaum M, Peleg L, et al. Hexosaminidase A deficiency is an uncommon cause of a syndrome mimicking amyotrophic lateral sclerosis. Muscle Nerve 2003; 28: 109–12

97. Minor PD. Polio eradication, cessation of vaccination and re-emergence of disease. Nat Rev Microbiol 2004; 2: 473–82

98. Trojan DA, Cashman NR. Post-poliomyelitis syndrome. Muscle Nerve 2005; 31: 6–19

99. Tyler KL. West Nile Virus infection in the United States. Arch Neurol 2004; 61: 1190–5.

100. Leis AA, Stokic DS, Webb RM, et al. The spectrum of muscle weakness in human West Nile Virus. Muscle Nerve 2003; 28: 302–8

101. Park M, Hui JS, Bartt RE. Acute anterior radiculitis associated with West Nile Virus infection. J Neurol Neurosurg Psychiatry 2003; 74: 823–5

102. Araujo A, Hall WW. Human T-lymphotropic virus type II and neurological disease. Ann Neurol 2004; 56: 10–19

103. Moulignier A, Moulonguet A, Pialoux G, Rozenbaum W. Reversible ALS-like disorder in HIV infection. Neurology 2001; 57: 995–1001

104. MacGowan DJL, Scelsa SN, Waldron M. An ALS-like syndrome with new HIV infection and complete response to antiretroviral therapy. Neurology 2001; 57: 1094–7

105. Teitelbaum JS, Zatorre R, Carpenter S, et al. Neurologic sequelae of domoic acid intoxication due to the ingestion of contaminated mussels. N Engl J Med 1990; 322: 1781–7

106. Perl TM, Bedard L, Kosatsky T, et al. An outbreak of toxic encephalopathy caused by eating mussels contaminated with domoic acid. N Engl J Med 1990; 322: 1775–80

107. Jeffery B, Barlow T, Moizer K, et al. Amnesic shellfish poisoning. Food Chem Toxicol 2004; 42: 545–57

108. Getahun H, Lambein F, Vanhoorne M, Van der Stuyft P. Pattern and associated features of the neurolathyrism epidemic in Ethiopia. Trop Med Int Health 2002; 7: 118–24

109. Tor-Agbidye J, Palmer VS, Lasarev MR, et al. Bioactivation of cyanide to cyanate in sulphur amino acid deficiency: Relevance to neurological disease in humans subsisting on cassava. Tox Sci 1999; 50: 228–35

2

Epidemiology of amyotrophic lateral sclerosis

Lorene M Nelson, Valerie McGuire

Amyotrophic lateral sclerosis (ALS), also known as Lou Gehrig's disease, is the most common motor neuron disease. The pathologic hallmark of ALS is the selective death of motor neurons in the brain and spinal cord that innervate skeletal muscles, with symptoms of progressive weakness, muscle wasting and spasticity. ALS onset occurs most often in the fifth to seventh decades of life, although cases in young adults and elderly persons are well recognized. Median survival after clinical onset is 2–3 years. The causes of ALS are unknown and the apparent selectivity for motor neurons remains unexplained. If modifiable risk factors for ALS could be identified, strategies to prevent or delay the development of ALS could reduce the individual and societal burden of this serious disease.

Three major classifications of ALS are recognized. Familial (hereditary ALS) is the subject of the third section of this text and will be addressed only briefly in this chapter. The Western Pacific form of ALS that occurred beginning in the mid-20th century is the best-known geographic cluster of ALS and, unfortunately, its causes remain unknown. Sporadic ALS comprises the remainder of cases, and the goal of epidemiologic research has been to identify risk factors for this group of patients.

EPIDEMIOLOGY OF FAMILIAL AMYOTROPHIC LATERAL SCLEROSIS

Genetic susceptibility is an important determinant of the risk for ALS. In most case series or population-based studies, 5–10% of ALS cases report at least one affected first-degree relative[1-5]; however, a clear pattern of Mendelian inheritance is evident for only a small percentage of familial cases. When Mendelian inheritance is observed, the most common form is autosomal dominant[6-9]; autosomal recessive or X-linked recessive forms are more rarely observed[10]. A major breakthrough was achieved in 1993 with the discovery that mutations of the superoxide dismutase gene (*SOD1*) account for 20% of familial ALS cases[8]; over 100 mutations of the *SOD1* gene have been identified in total. Transgenic *in vitro* and *in vivo* models of SOD1-mediated motor neuron death have yielded insights into the pathogenic mechanisms of motor neuron disease. Eight additional loci have been associated with familial forms of ALS and motor neuron disease (ALS2–ALS8, ALS-frontotemporal dementia (FTD))[11]; however, together these loci explain only a very small percentage of ALS. Very little is known about susceptibility genes or other risk factors for sporadic ALS, which comprises more than 90% of ALS cases. (Please refer to Chapter 9 for an excellent summary of the role of genetics in familial and sporadic ALS.)

WESTERN PACIFIC ALS AND OTHER GEOGRAPHIC CLUSTERS OF AMYOTROPHIC LATERAL SCLEROSIS

Western Pacific amyotrophic lateral sclerosis

Western Pacific ALS was first described among the Chamorro people of Guam in the early 1950s, with incidence and mortality rates estimated to range from 50 to 100/100 000 per year[12,13], a rate that was 25–50 times higher than the incidence of ALS in the USA. Some ALS patients in this region acquired pathologic characteristics similar to Parkinson's disease and Alzheimer's disease, referred to as ALS parkinsonism–dementia complex (ALS-PDC) [14–16]. An excess incidence of ALS and ALS-PDC also has been recognized in two other indigenous populations, Irian Jaya (western New Guinea)[17] and the Kii Peninsula of Japan. In both males and females, the incidence of ALS on Guam peaked in 1950–1954, and started to decline thereafter (Figure 2.1). Over the next several decades, the incidence of ALS in both males and females declined steadily, and the annual incidence rates in 1980–1984 for males and females were 5/100 000 and 4/100 000, respectively[18]. Since the beginning of the Western Pacific epidemic of ALS, the average age at onset has increased by 16 years for ALS[19].

The rapid rise and subsequent fall of ALS incidence rates in the Western Pacific suggest that the cause may be an environmental agent that peaked after World War II and has declined, but not completely disappeared. Although many hypotheses have been proposed to explain the epidemic of ALS-PDC in the western Pacific, the hypothesis that has garnered the most attention has focused on a traditional food source, the seed of the *Cycas circinalis* cycad palm tree that was commonly used by native Chamorro people to prepare tortillas. A

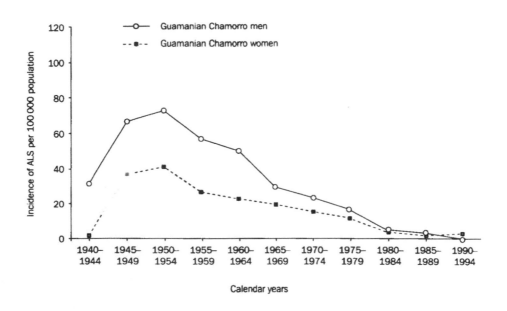

Figure 2.1   Average annual incidence rates (per 100 000 population) of amyotrophic lateral sclerosis for Guamanian Chamorro patients with amyotrophic lateral sclerosis, 1940–1994 (From reference 18)

glutamate analog found in the seed of the cycad palm, β-*N*-methylamino-L-alanine (BMAA), was initially suspected of causing ALS-PDC[20]; however, the concentration of BMAA in flour that has been washed is thought to be too low to induce disease[21]. Recently, Cox and Sacks[22] proposed that high concentrations of BMAA or its metabolites could have been ingested by the Chamorro people while consuming flying foxes (bats) that fed on the cycad nut. If biomagnification occurred, the flesh of the bats would contain high levels of BMAA. Although the flying fox species is extinct, Banack and Cox[23] obtained museum specimens of these bats and reported that consuming a single bat could contribute a high concentration of BMAA to the diet.

Environmental excitotoxins other than BMAA are well-recognized causes of neurodegeneration. The classic example of a neurodegenerative disorder caused by an environmental excitotoxin is lathyrism, a disease of upper motor neurons caused by excessive consumption of the chickling pea which contains an unusual amino acid (β-*N*-oxalylamino-L-alanine) that acts as a glutamate-like excitotoxin[24]. Limb weakness suggestive of motor neuron involvement was also observed among several individuals in Canada who ingested seaweed-contaminated mussels that contained domoic acid, an excitotoxin that acts similarly to kainic acid[25]. The observation that glutamate analogs in the diet can cause neurodegeneration supports the hypothesis that exposure to motor neuron-specific environmental toxicants or chemicals with excitotoxic properties may increase the risk of ALS. A later section of this chapter describes the evidence regarding the potential role of the neurotoxicants such as heavy metals, solvents and pesticides, in the etiology of ALS.

Other geographic clusters of amyotrophic lateral sclerosis

The reporting of geographic clusters of patients with ALS in US communities has been prompted by public concerns regarding possible exposure to toxic chemicals or other environmental agents. A certain number of areas with higher than expected ALS incidence are expected to arise on the basis of chance alone, and, once investigated, many apparent disease clusters do not turn out to be significant[26,27]. Many cluster investigations end with no resolution because what initially appears to be a statistical excess of cases is not borne out by more systematic investigation.

Although many reported clusters of ALS have not withstood scientific scrutiny, there are a few notable exceptions. The very high incidence of ALS-PDC observed in the Western Pacific left little doubt that an epidemic had occurred. More recently, two studies have been reported noting a higher incidence of ALS among young servicemen who were deployed to the first Persian Gulf War than servicemen who were not deployed[28,29]. Haley[28] utilized national mortality statistics to show a higher than expected estimate of the incidence of ALS among Gulf War veterans diagnosed before 45 years of age. In another study, Horner *et al.*[29] used both active and passive methods to identify all incident cases of ALS that occurred in the 10-year period following the first Persian Gulf War. The investigators reported a two-fold increased risk of developing ALS among veterans deployed to the Gulf arena compared with those who were not deployed (relative risk (RR) 1.9, 95% confidence interval (CI) 1.3–2.8)[29]. The risk of ALS was significant for military personnel who were members of the Air Force and the Army. Some concern was noted regarding the possible under-reporting of ALS cases. However, capture–recapture analysis suggested little under-reporting of ALS cases among deployed military personnel and only modest under-reporting of ALS cases among the non-deployed[30].

The observation that ALS incidence was higher among Persian Gulf War veterans raised the concern that environmental exposures, physiological or psychological stress was responsible for the excess, but as yet no explanation for the higher ALS incidence has been identified. Additional concern about an excess risk among men who served in the military was stimulated by the findings of a recent prospective cohort study of men who were participants in a study of the American Cancer Society[31]. Compared to men who had never been employed by the military, men who served in the military had a 1.6-fold increased risk of ALS mortality (95% CI 1.1–2.2). This finding was observed among several branches of service and was not restricted to a single time period[31]. Additional studies are needed to confirm these findings and to identify risk factors associated with the excess risk of ALS among US veterans. To this aim, the Department of Veteran Affairs (VA) recently established a National Registry of Veterans with ALS. The primary goals of the Registry are (1) to provide the VA with data on the current number and characteristics of veterans with ALS; (2) to provide a mechanism to inform veterans with ALS about research studies and clinical trials for which they may be eligible to participate; and (3) to establish a resource for the conduct of large-scale studies to identify epidemiologic and genetic factors that may be associated with ALS among US veterans.

DESCRIPTIVE EPIDEMIOLOGY OF AMYOTROPHIC LATERAL SCLEROSIS

When pursuing etiologic clues about what might cause ALS, epidemiologists adopt two general approaches: *descriptive study designs* to describe the frequency of ALS in a population, and *analytic study designs* to test specific hypotheses about risk factors for ALS. Early epidemiologic research focused on descriptive approaches, with estimation of incidence, prevalence and mortality rates of ALS from population-based studies. The first clues as to risk factors come from such studies where the frequency of ALS was examined in subgroups defined on the basis of age, gender, race/ethnicity and geographic location. Other studies have focused on analytic epidemiologic approaches, such as the case–control design, to identify risk factors for ALS.

Amyotrophic lateral sclerosis case definition for epidemiologic studies

Two major consensus conferences have been conducted to propose a uniform case definition of ALS for use in research studies. The first conference was convened by the World Federation of Neurology (WFN) ALS Research Subcommittee[32], where disease definitions were developed, and a subsequent conference where case definition criteria were further refined[33]. Table 2.1 summarizes the WFN 'El Escorial' criteria for the diagnosis of ALS which require the presence, evolution and progression of upper motor neuron (UMN) and lower motor neuron (LMN) findings at multiple levels. The diagnosis of ALS requires evidence of both UMN and LMN involvement; however, it often presents initially as either LMN involvement (PMA, with primary involvement of LMNs that innervate skeletal muscles) or UMN involvement (PBP, with primary involvement of bulbar motor neurons). However, most patients who present with either PMA or PBP ultimately develop signs that support the diagnosis of ALS. Patients with ALS may be classified as definite, probable, possible or suspected. Ross *et al.*[33] reported a method whereby, using a combination of clinical, electrodiagnostic and radiologic data, some patients who would be classified as having 'possible' ALS, according to the WFN El Escorial criteria, would be considered as having 'laboratory-supported, definite ALS.'

Incidence, prevalence and mortality of amyotrophic lateral sclerosis

Because ALS is a disease of short duration, most descriptive epidemiologic studies have focused on estimating the incidence of ALS (i.e. the frequency of newly diagnosed ALS patients in a population), or estimating the mortality of ALS (i.e. the frequency of ALS deaths in a population). The incidence of ALS in the USA and most European countries ranges from 1.5 to 2.5 ALS cases per 100 000 population members per year[2,34–37]. In countries outside the USA, ALS is often referred

---

Table 2.1 El Escorial World Federation of Neurology criteria for the diagnosis of amyotrophic lateral sclerosis (ALS). (From references 32 and 33)

The diagnosis of ALS requires the presence of the following:

* signs of lower motor neuron (LMN) degeneration by clinical, electrophysiologic or neuropathologic examination in one or more of four regions (bulbar, cervical, thoracic or lumbosacral)

* signs of upper motor neuron (UMN) degeneration by clinical examination, *and* progressive spread of signs within a region or other regions

Assessment of diagnostic certainty:

Definite ALS: UMN and LMN signs in bulbar region and at least two of the other spinal regions *or* UMN and LMN signs in three spinal regions *and* signs progress over a 12-month period following diagnosis

Probable ALS: UMN and LMN signs in at least two regions with UMN signs rostral to a region with LMN signs *and* signs progress over a 12-month period following diagnosis

Possible ALS: UNM and LMN signs in only one region *or* UNM signs in two or more regions (i.e. progressive bulbar palsy, primary lateral sclerosis)

Suspected ALS: LMN signs in two or three regions (i.e. primary muscular atrophy)

---

to as motor neuron disease (MND) and incidence rates range from 0.86 to 2.4/100 000 per year[38–44]. Since almost all patients with ALS die of their disease, mortality rates for ALS parallel incidence rates. However, because of under-reporting of ALS on death certificates, reported mortality rates for ALS in the USA are lower than incidence rates (approximately 1.5/100 000 per year for all ages combined compared to incidence rates of 2/100 000 per year). Fewer studies have focused on the prevalence of ALS, which is based on a count of all ALS cases within a population at a given point in time. With a median survival of 3 years, the prevalence of ALS is approximately 6/100 000, or nearly three times the incidence rate of 2/100 000 per year.

Gender and age distribution

Most epidemiologic studies report incidence rates among men that are 20–60% higher than incidence rates among women[37,40,43,45], although in the most recent studies, the differences in male and female incidence rates are less striking. The largest recent ALS incidence study in the USA was conducted in a three-county region of Western Washington State during the years 1990–1995. In this study and most other population-based studies, the incidence of ALS was shown to increase with age, peaking at ages 65–74 years for both men and women (Figure 2.2)[2,37,39]. In contrast, the age distribution of ALS peaked earlier, at 55–60 years, in referral-center-based studies[46,47], probably due to a form of selection bias where younger-onset patients with ALS are more likely than older-onset patients to seek the specialty care that ALS referral centers can provide.

Comparing age- and gender-specific rates among various studies often is not straightforward because of methodologic differences in how ALS cases were ascertained, how diagnostic criteria were applied, and different age distributions of the underlying populations. In order to make meaningful comparisons, the calendar years studied should be similar in all studies so that any differences in incidence rates are not due to changing rates over time. Chancellor and Warlow[48] compared the age- and gender-specific ALS incidence rates from eight surveys that were judged to have near-complete case ascertainment. Analyses were restricted to men and women aged 45–74

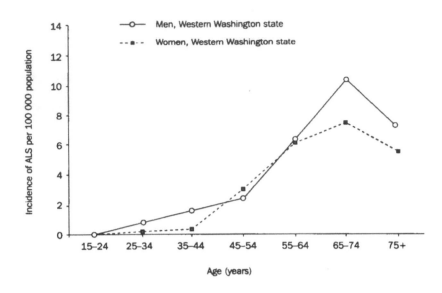

Figure 2.2 Average annual age- and sex-specific incidence rates (per 100 000 population) of amyotrophic lateral sclerosis (ALS) in western Washington State, 1990–1995 (From reference 37)

years[2,49–55] to provide comparable data across studies. Several more ALS incidence studies were subsequently incorporated, including studies from western Washington State[37], Texas[56], Scotland,[57] Ireland[40], Italy[43,58,59] and Sweden[60]. Table 2.2 shows the incidence of ALS in men and women from these 16 different studies, age-adjusted to the 1990 US population for those 45–74 years old. In the three US studies[2,37,56] and the Finnish study[54], the differences in rates are less striking between men and women than in the other surveys. Generally, rates tended to be higher for northern latitudes than for southern latitudes. Differences in incidence rates across regions may reflect differences in case definition or case ascertainment, or differences in the prevalence of risk factors in certain populations. The incidence and mortality rates for MND have been higher in recent decades than were previously reported in industrialized countries[36,41,42]. This increase may be accounted for by improved ascertainment, better reporting and loss of competing causes of mortality in a susceptible cohort[61–63].

Racial/ethnic distribution of amyotrophic lateral sclerosis

Previous studies have suggested that ALS incidence and mortality may be lower among African, Asian and Hispanic Americans than among non-Hispanic Caucasians. ALS mortality rates for Caucasians exceed those for non-Caucasians by 70%[47]. A study by Annegers et al.[56] in Texas reported that the incidence of ALS was lower for African-Americans and Hispanics than among non-Hispanic Caucasians. However, the degree of case ascertainment among African-Americans and Hispanics was less than complete and probably resulted in an underestimation of the incidence of ALS in these groups. In the study in western Washington State, the age-adjusted incidence rates were higher for non-Hispanic Caucasians than other groups; however, only ten patients were from groups other than non-Hispanic Caucasians[37]. Further research is needed to obtain estimates of the incidence of ALS in larger studies that can be conducted in multiracial populations with uniform access to medical care.

Table 2.2   Incidence of amyotrophic lateral sclerosis in men and women in recent studies, age-adjusted to the 1990 US population for those 45–74 years of age. (From references 37, 43 and 58)

Country	Year(s) of survey	Latitude	Incidence rates Men	Women	Combined	Male:female ratio
Middle Finland[54]	1976–1981	66°	8.9	8.3	8.5	1.1
Northern Sweden[51]	1969–1980	66°	8.6	4.5	6.4	1.9
Middle Sweden[52]	1970–1981	60°	5.6	3.5	4.5	1.6
Scotland[57]	1988	56°	6.7	3.8	5.2	1.8
Denmark[53]	1974–1986	56°	4.2	2.9	3.5	1.4
Ireland[40]	1995–1997	53°	6.7	5.3	6.0	1.3
Washington, USA[37]	1990–1995	47°	5.8	5.3	5.5	1.1
Minnesota, USA[2]	1925–1984	45°	7.4	6.4	6.9	1.2
Southern Sweden[60]	1961–1990	45°	7.5	4.8	6.1	1.6
Reggio Emilia, Italy [59]	1985–1992	44°	6.7	4.5	5.5	1.5
Piemonte, Italy[58]	1966–1986	44°	3.4	2.2	2.7	1.5
Piemonte, Italy[43]	1995-1996	44°	6.1	4.7	5.4	1.3
Ontario, Canada[55]	1978–1982	44°	5.4	3.7	4.5	1.5
Sardinia[50]	1965–1974	40°	3.7	1.4	2.5	2.6
Israel[49]	1959–1974	32°	2.7	1.5	2.0	1.8
Texas, USA[56]	1985–1988	29°	3.7	3.6	3.6	1.0

Risk factors for amyotrophic lateral sclerosis

ALS basic research has undergone exciting progress in recent years, with evidence accumulating that genetic susceptibility, impaired regulation of glutamate neurotransmission, oxidative stress, abnormal protein aggregation, and abnormalities of axonal transport may play important roles in the pathogenesis of ALS. Despite these insights into disease pathogenesis, there is little information regarding the causal factors that initiate these pathogenic mechanisms, and rigorous epidemiologic studies of genetic and environmental risk factors are vitally needed to provide insight about the upstream causal factors for ALS.

The epidemiologic study of ALS and motor neuron diseases has spanned several recent decades and has undergone evolution over this time period. Findings from many of the earlier epidemiologic studies did not produce consistent results, leading some to believe that the field of epidemiology could offer little insight into the etiology of ALS. Many of these studies held little promise of identifying risk factors for ALS because of methodologic deficiencies such as using convenience samples of ALS patients matched to ill-defined control groups, crude assessment of risk factors and very small sample sizes, resulting in poor statistical power to detect differences between risk subgroups. In recent years, there has been a resurgence of interest in conducting epidemiologic studies to identify environmental and life-style risk factors for ALS, and many studies are under way, but the number of published studies remains small.

The epidemiologic evidence regarding risk factors for ALS is summarized in Table 2.3. Findings from earlier epidemiologic studies emphasized the contribution of occupational exposures, excessive physical activity, electrical shock and skeletal fractures as potential risk factors for ALS. More

Table 2.3   Risk factors for amyotrophic lateral sclerosis (ALS): strength and certainty of associations

	Strength of association
Known or likely risk factors for ALS	
Age	↑↑↑
Disease-causing mutations, Mendelian inheritance (ALS1–ALS8)	↑↑↑
Geographic clusters (Persian Gulf War, Western Pacific ALS–PDC)	↑ RR 2.0–50+
Gender (male > female)	↑ RR 1.2–1.4
Family history of ALS	↑ RR 3.0–4.0
Cigarette smoking	↑ RR 1.7–3.5
Potential risk factors, more research needed	
Environmental and occupational exposures	
lead, mercury, or other heavy metal exposure	
pesticide exposure (insecticides, herbicides)	
industrial occupations, solvent exposure	
employment as an electrical worker or farmer	
Lifestyle factors	
diet (fat, fiber, glutamate, antioxidant intake)	
other sources of tobacco besides cigarettes	
vigorous physical activity, extreme athleticism	
Other factors	
anthropometric measures (weight, body mass index)	
severe electrical shock	
skeletal fracture	
infectious agents	
Factors not yet widely investigated	
Prescription and over-the-counter medication use	
Caffeine intake	
Recreational drug use	
Residential exposures (pesticides, hobby chemicals)	
Hormonal and reproductive factors (in women)	

recently, epidemiologic studies have begun to investigate the role of life-style factors such as diet and cigarette smoking as factors that might influence the risk of developing ALS.

Occupational exposures

A synthesis of the literature that has implicated occupational exposures prevents any firm conclusions regarding the role of metals, pesticides and solvents in the etiology of ALS. There are several limitations of using retrospective studies to identify environmental risk factors for ALS, including: (1) uncertainty about the timing and duration of exposure and their relation to disease onset; (2) inadequacies of using job title or industry as a surrogate measure for exposure to chemicals in the occupational setting; and (3) difficulty of comparing studies from different areas and different time periods since exposures may vary by geographic region and calendar period. It is unlikely that an entire class of chemicals such as metals or pesticides would cause ALS. Instead, motor neuron-specific toxicants with a particular chemical structure or toxic mechanism of action are more likely to be responsible for selective motor neuron death, particularly among individuals who have a genetic background that impairs their ability to detoxify such chemicals. Future population-based studies of occupational exposures, in combination with studies of environmental response genes, may help to elucidate the role of specific chemicals in the etiology of ALS. We present here a brief summary of evidence regarding the potential associations of ALS with metal, pesticide and solvent exposure.

Metals

Several lines of investigation have linked ALS to heavy metal exposure, including studies finding increased metal content in tissues of ALS patients[64,65] and epidemiologic studies that have reported associations of ALS with exposure to lead[66–70], mercury[68,71] or heavy metals as a class[71]. The relative risk estimates associated with exposure to lead, mercury or other heavy metals have ranged from 2.0 to 6.0 and were significant in all but two studies[72,73]. Only three studies assessed duration of exposure to lead in relation to the risk of ALS[66–67,70]. Armon *et al.*[67] reported an increased risk of ALS among men with more than 200 cumulative lifetime hours of exposure to lead (odds ratio (OR) 5.5, 95% CI 1.4–21.0). Similar results were found in a case–control study from Scotland among workers who were employed for more than 12 months in occupations involving lead exposures (OR 5.7, 95% CI 1.6–30.0)[66].

Kamel et al.[70] reported that among subjects who reported more than 2000 lifetime days of lead exposure, the risk estimate was 2.3 (95% CI 1.1–4.9), compared to subjects with no exposure to lead.

Physiologic measures of lead in bone have been obtained in two epidemiologic studies. A study in the early 1970s reported no association between bone lead and risk of ALS, following examination of lead concentration in bone from 25 ALS cases and from 17 autopsy controls[69]. More recently, blood lead and bone lead were measured in 107 cases and a subset of 41 population-based controls in a case–control study of ALS conducted in New England[70]. Blood lead levels were significantly higher in ALS cases than controls, and measures of lead concentration in tibia and patella were somewhat higher among ALS cases than controls. The evidence from this study of a possible association between physiologic measures of lead concentration and risk of ALS merits further investigation.

Specific occupations associated with metal exposures also have been investigated as risk factors for ALS. Welders were over-represented among ALS patients in three case–control studies[67,72,74], while a fourth study failed to observe any association with welding[72]. No significant associations have been observed between ALS and other metal-related industries, such as metal working and metal casting[46,75,76].

In summary, although no single study has provided definitive proof that exposure to lead or other heavy metals causes ALS, further investigation is warranted. When possible, information obtained from subjects by self-report should be supplemented with expert industrial hygiene review and measurements of lead in blood and bone.

Pesticides

The potential role of farming occupations or agricultural chemical exposure in the etiology of ALS has been the subject of several studies. Studies in Italy, Greece, and Sweden have identified weak associations of agricultural work and rural residence with the risk of developing motor neuron disease[60,77–80]. However, many other studies reported no association between farming or rural living and motor neuron disease[66,74,81–89]. Inconsistent findings also have been reported in case–control studies that have specifically investigated exposure to pesticide chemicals and risk of ALS. Two case–control studies in the USA and Italy reported an increase in risk of ALS associated with exposure to agricultural chemicals, but the risk estimates were imprecise and not statistically significant[72,90]. Still other studies have not observed an association between exposure to agricultural chemicals and the risk of ALS[66,74,85]; however, a population-based study in western Washington State found that men with occupational exposure to pesticides, in particular insecticides and fertilizers had a greater than two-fold increase in risk of ALS (OR 2.4, 95% CI 1.2–4.8)[91]. A significant exposure–response trend was observed when an expert panel of industrial hygienists grouped exposed individuals into low and high categories[91]. This study is the first to identify pesticide exposure as a possible risk factor for ALS, and the finding merits future investigation.

Solvents

Several case–control studies have examined the association of past exposure to solvents and other industrial chemicals with the risk of developing ALS; however, exposure to this class of toxicants is not easily quantified or validated. Three studies reported a two- to three-fold increase in risk with solvent exposure[66,85,90], while three other studies did not observe any association between exposure to solvents and risk of ALS[74,82,83]. Only one study collected detailed information regarding the past occupational exposure to specific classes of organic solvents rather than the broad category of solvents. The overall risk of ALS associated with self-reported exposure to solvents was 1.6 (95% CI 1.1–2.5)[91]. In the same study, when an expert industrial hygiene panel reviewed occupational histories, overall solvent exposure was not associated with the risk of developing ALS, but risk estimates were elevated for exposure to two classes of solvents: alcohols/ketones and degreasers/cleaning solvents[91]. Several epidemiologic studies have examined occupation as a surrogate for exposure to solvents or industrial chemicals, and have implicated solvent exposure in leather workers[87,92] and painters[76,79], but other studies have been negative in this respect[4,88,93,94].

Electrical work and electrical shock

Employment in electrical occupations has been the subject of several epidemiologic investigations of ALS[95-98]; these studies are summarized in a recent review[99]. Håkansson et al.[100] assessed a cohort of 538 221 engineering industry workers and found a greater than two-fold increase in risk for ALS in cases with the highest exposure to electromagnetic fields (EMF) (OR 2.2, 95% CI 1.0–4.7). However, other investigators have found no association between EMF exposure and risk of ALS[98,101]. More often, epidemiologic studies have identified associations between electrical work and ALS, with an approximately two-fold increased incidence of ALS among individuals with a history of work in electrical occupations[96,98,101]. In a cohort study, Savitz et al.[97] reported a three-fold increase in risk for ALS (RR 3.1, 95% CI 1.1–9.8) among men employed as electrical workers for 20 years or longer. Individuals in electrical occupations may have greater potential for electrical shocks, or may have exposure to solvents or other toxicants that may explain the increased risk. Past case–control studies have shown elevated risks associated with electrical shock[72,84,90,101-103], although many of the odds ratios were not statistically significant due to the rarity of the exposure.

Lifestyle risk factors

To date, very few studies have investigated the association of ALS with life-style factors such as diet, cigarette smoking and alcohol consumption, but the role of physical activity has attracted considerable interest.

Physical activity

Several early epidemiologic studies reported associations between measures of vigorous physical activity and the risk of ALS[50,52,104-107]; however, more recent population-based studies have failed to confirm these findings[86,108,109]. Early studies found an increased risk of ALS among workers who engaged in heavy physical labor[85,104] and among men who had a history of participating in athletic activities[110]. In a population-based case–control study of ALS conducted in western Washington State, the investigators collected detailed information regarding physical activity in the workplace and recreational settings[108]. The risk of developing ALS was not associated with overall physical activity or with vigorous activity either in workplace or recreational settings. The only association observed was among those who participated in organized sports in high school, whose risk of ALS was increased by 50% (OR 1.5, 95% CI 1.03–2.25). A recent case–control study in Amsterdam conducted with patients from an ALS referral center also reported no association between several overall measures of physical activity level and the occurrence of ALS[109].

Investigators from Italy examined mortality data for 24 000 Italian professional and semi-professional football (soccer) players who played between 1970 and 2001, and reported a nearly seven-fold increase in risk of developing ALS compared to the underlying population (standardized proportional mortality ratio (SMR) 6.5, 95% CI 2.1–15.1) with a significant dose–response result for years of play[111]. Based on these findings, a population-based case–control study is under way in Italy to evaluate the association of professional sports activities with the risk of ALS[12]. This study may add important new information to determine whether sustained vigorous physical activity is associated with ALS.

In summary, conflicting findings do not as yet allow the conclusion that vigorous physical activity is associated with an increased risk of ALS. However, it is possible that some aspect of physical activity itself (e.g. early life extensive recreational activity or sustained sports-related activity), or exposures that occur during physical activity (e.g. pesticides or fertilizers applied to playing fields) may be associated with the risk of developing ALS.

Cigarette smoking

Only recently have epidemiologic studies collected extensive information regarding the role of cigarette smoking in the etiology of ALS. Early studies reported no association with cigarette smoking, possibly due to small sample size, use of prevalent cases and hospital-based control subjects. Kamel et al.[78], in a case–control study conducted in New England, reported a 70% increased risk for ALS among ever smokers (OR 1.7, 95% CI 1.0–2.8). In a population-based case–control study in Washington State, a similar result was observed for subjects who had ever smoked cigarettes (adjusted OR 2.0, 95% CI 1.3–3.2), with a greater than three-fold increase in risk among current smokers compared to never smokers (adjusted OR 3.5, 95% CI 1.9–6.4)[113]. A dose–response trend with increasing pack years of smoking was significant. Weisskopf et al.[114] examined the association of tobacco use and ALS mortality among participants in the Cancer Prevention Study II cohort of the American Cancer Society. The authors reported a nearly 70% increase in ALS mortality among current smokers compared to never smokers (OR 1.7, 95% CI 1.2–2.2); however, this association was noted only among women.

The investigators from the western Washington State study proposed two mechanisms by which cigarette smoke could contribute to the risk of ALS[113]: direct toxic injury to motor neurons from one or more of the thousands of chemicals in cigarette smoke or oxidative stress caused by the formation of free radicals during the metabolism of the chemical constituents of cigarette smoke[115]. The hypothesis that tobacco exposure is associated with ALS warrants further investigation, ideally with studies that investigate the other sources of tobacco exposure such as pipes and cigars, dose and duration of tobacco exposure, and timing of smoking cessation.

Diet

Diet may play a role in the pathogenesis of ALS, but few studies have addressed this issue and early case–control studies examined differences in consumption of only a few food items[68,70,74,90]. Only one case–control study has utilized a food frequency questionnaire to obtain detailed information on nutrient intake[116]. The investigators reported that high dietary fat intake (> 93 g per day compared with < 42 g per day) increased the risk of ALS nearly three-fold (adjusted OR 2.7, 95% CI 0.9–8.0). Similar findings were observed for the intake of polyunsaturated fat, saturated fat and linoleic acid. The brain is particularly vulnerable to oxidative damage since it is rich in polyunsaturated fatty acids, especially linoleic acid, which come largely from dietary intake[117–119].

Fiber intake was evaluated in the study from western Washington State[116]. Dietary fiber intake (> 18 g per day compared with < 10 g per day) significantly decreased the risk of ALS (adjusted OR 0.3, 95% CI 0.1–0.7)[116], suggesting a possible protective effect against the development of ALS. Dietary fiber could potentially reduce absorption of a dietary toxin associated with ALS since fiber has been shown to cause luminal dilution of potential carcinogens[120,121]. Dietary fiber also shortens transit time in the large intestine[120] and could reduce the contact time and the absorption of dietary toxins.

In the western Washington State study, glutamate intake (> 15 g per day compared with < 8.6 g per day) was associated with an increased risk of ALS (OR 3.2, 95% CI 1.2–8.0)[116]. Glutamate is a neurotransmitter that has been implicated in excitotoxic cell death. Since glutamate is widely present in the food supply, high levels of glutamate in the diet in combination with a disordered glutamate metabolism in the brain could cause excitotoxic cell death of motor neurons.

Dietary antioxidants may confer a protective effect on the development of ALS given the postulated role of oxidative stress in the pathogenesis of the disease. A recent prospective study assessed the relationship between the use of vitamin E, vitamin C, vitamin A and multivitamin supplements and ALS mortality[122]. The study population included 957 740 subjects who participated in the American Cancer Society Prevention Study II. Information on vitamin supplements was obtained at baseline and on a subset of participants 10 years later. Subjects were classified as never users, occasional users (fewer than 15 times per month) and regular users (15 times or more per month). Regular users of vitamin E supplements were at decreased risk of death from ALS. The investigators reported a dose–response trend with a 62% reduction in risk of death from ALS among individuals who used vitamin E supplements for more than 10 years (age- and smoking-adjusted OR 0.38, 95% CI 0.16–0.92). The use of vitamin C, vitamin A and multivitamins had no apparent effect on the risk of ALS. This finding is of interest since animal studies have shown that transgenic mice over-expressing one of the *SOD1* genes have delayed onset of motor neuron disease when given vitamin E supplementation. Additional studies using comprehensive dietary assessment methods are needed before firm conclusions can be drawn regarding the role of specific macronutrients and micronutrients as risk or protective factors for ALS.

Fractures

Early case–control studies identified physical trauma and skeletal fractures as risk factors for ALS, with OR ranging from 1.3 to 10.0[72,77,79,81–83,101,123,124]. More recently conducted population-based studies have suggested that the overall excess of fractures may be due to subclinical weakness resulting in fractures that occur close in time before the diagnosis of ALS. In a population-based case–control study in Scotland, the investigators did not find an association with a lifetime history of fractures, but reported a 15-fold increase in risk for fractures that occurred 5 years prior to date of diagnosis (95% CI

2.3–654)[66]. Extensive information regarding a history of physical trauma was collected in a population-based study of incident ALS cases in western Washington State, but again, the only association found was with fractures that occurred within the 5-year period prior to date of diagnosis[84]. Together, these findings suggest that physical injuries may be a consequence rather than a cause of ALS.

FUTURE DIRECTIONS

Because of these methodologic limitations, case–control studies have yielded conflicting results and very few definitive conclusions about risk factors are possible. Compared to many other neurologic disorders, the epidemiologic study of ALS is still in its infancy, and further research is needed to identify genetic, life-style and environmental risk factors for motor neuron disease. Epidemiologic studies will yield more consistent findings regarding risk factors for ALS by making several methodologic improvements:

(1) Conducting studies in well-defined populations that allow the inclusion of a large number of ALS cases and control subjects;

(2) Recruiting incident rather than prevalent cases, to enable the identification of etiologic factors for the disease;

(3) Increasing the sample size of ALS cases and controls to improve the statistical power to detect associations;

(4) Including individuals from racial/ethnic groups other than solely Caucasians;

(5) Assessing exposures to environmental toxicants using the most rigorous and objective methods possible, including blinded exposure assessments and biomarkers of exposure when possible;

(6) Collecting and storing genomic DNA for the future evaluation of candidate susceptibility genes.

Future investigation of risk factors for ALS in existing large cohort studies also could yield important clues as to the etiology of ALS. The methodologic challenges of conducting ALS epidemiologic research have prompted some investigators to join forces in conducting multisite studies that include the collection of risk factor information and genomic DNA so that interesting hypotheses regarding gene–environment interaction can be addressed.

CONCLUSIONS

The past two decades have seen significant advances in understanding the molecular genetic basis of familial ALS. These advances hold great promise for identifying pathogenic mechanisms that may be involved in both familial and sporadic ALS. Within the next decade, it is within the reach of laboratory scientists to identify the biochemical chain of events by which highly penetrant genes cause Mendelian forms of ALS, and a major goal of the future is to identify the causes of ALS in the 90–95% of individuals for whom no cause is apparent. Insights regarding the biochemical pathways involved in disease pathogenesis may enable the identification of susceptibility genes for sporadic ALS, and may help to inform epidemiologic investigations of environmental and life-style factors that influence the risk of developing ALS. The field will benefit from molecular epidemiologic studies that are hypothesis driven and conducted in well-defined populations. Such epidemiologic studies hold great promise for advancing our understanding of the causes of ALS.

REFERENCES

1. Williams DB, Windebank AJ. Motor neuron disease (amyotrophic lateral sclerosis). Mayo Clin Proc 1991; 66: 54–82
2. Yoshida S, Mulder DW, Kurland LT, et al. Follow-up study on amyotrophic lateral sclerosis in Rochester, Minnesota, 1925-1984. Neuroepidemiology 1986; 5: 61–70
3. Mulder DW, Kurland LT, Offord KP, Beard CM. Familial adult motor neuron disease: amyotrophic lateral sclerosis. Neurology 1986; 36: 511–17
4. Li TM, Alberman E, Swash M. Comparison of sporadic and familial disease amongst 580 cases of motor neuron disease. J Neurol Neurosurg Psychiatry 1988; 51: 778–84
5. Williams DB, Floate DA, Leicester J. Familial motor neuron disease: Differing penetrance in large pedigrees. J Neurol Sci 1988; 86: 215–30
6. Majoor-Krakauer D, Willems PJ, Hofman A. Genetic epidemiology of amyotrophic lateral sclerosis. Clin Genet 2003; 63: 83–101
7. Harding AE. Inherited neuronal atrophy and degeneration predominantly of lower motor neurons. In: Dyck PJ, Thomas PK, eds. Peripheral Neuropathy. Philadelphia: WB Saunders, 1993: 1051–64
8. Siddique T, Figlewicz DA, Pericak-Vance MA, et al. Linkage of a gene causing familial amyotrophic lateral sclerosis to chromosome 21 and evidence of genetic-locus heterogeneity. N Engl J Med 1991; 324: 1381–4
9. Siddique T, Nijhawan D, Hentati A. Familial amyotrophic lateral sclerosis. J Neural Transm Suppl 1997; 49: 219–33
10. Al-Chalabi A, Andersen PM, Chioza B, et al. Recessive amyotrophic lateral sclerosis families with the D90A SOD1 mutation share a common founder: Evidence for a linked protective factor. Hum Mol Genet 1998; 7: 2045–50
11. Veldink JH, Van den Berg LH, Wokke JH. The future of motor neuron disease: The challenge is in the genes. J Neurol 2004; 251: 491–500
12. Kurland LT, Mulder DW. Epidemiologic investigations of amyotrophic lateral sclerosis: 1. Preliminary report on geographic distribution, with special reference to the Mariana Islands, including clinical and pathologic observations. Neurology 1954; 4: 355–78
13. Kurland LT, Mulder DW. Epidemiologic investigations of amyotrophic lateral sclerosis. 2. Familial aggregations indicative of dominant inheritance. Neurology 1955; 5: 182–96
14. Hirano A, Kurland LT, Krooth RS, Lessell S. Parkinsonism–dementia complex, an endemic disease on the island of Guam. I. Clinical features. Brain 1961; 84: 642-661
15. Hirano A, Malamud N, Kurland LT. Parkinsonism–dementia complex, an endemic disease on the

island of Guam. II. Pathological features. Brain 1961; 84: 662–79

16. Gajdusek DC, Salazar AM. Amyotrophic lateral sclerosis and parkinsonian syndromes in high incidence among the Auyu and Jakai people of West New Guinea. Neurology 1982; 32: 107–26

17. Shiraki H. The neuropathology of amyotrophic lateral sclerosis (ALS) in the Kii Peninsula and other areas of Japan. In: Norris FH Jr, Kurland LT, eds. Motor Neuron Diseases: Research on Amyotrophic Lateral Sclerosis and Related Disorders. New York: Grune & Stratton, 1969: 80–94

18. Plato CC, Garruto RM, Galasko D, et al. Amyotrophic lateral sclerosis and parkinsonism–dementia complex of Guam: Changing incidence rates during the past 60 years. Am J Epidemiol 2003; 157: 149–57

19. McGeer PL, Schwab C, McGeer EG, et al. Familial nature and continuing morbidity of the amyotrophic lateral sclerosis–parkinsonism dementia complex of Guam. Neurology 1997; 49: 400–9

20. Whiting MG. Toxicity of cycads. Econ Bot 1963; 17: 271–302

21. Duncan MW. beta-Methylamino-L-alanine (BMAA) and amyotrophic lateral sclerosis–parkinsonism dementia of the western Pacific. Ann NY Acad Sci 1992; 648: 161–8

22. Cox PA, Sacks OW. Cycad neurotoxins, consumption of flying foxes, and ALS-PDC disease in Guam. Neurology 2002; 58: 956–9

23. Banack SA, Cox PA. Biomagnification of cycad neurotoxins in flying foxes. Neurology 2003; 61: 387–9

24. Spencer PS, Nunn PB, Hugon J, et al. Guam amyotrophic lateral sclerosis–parkinsonism–dementia linked to a plant excitant neurotoxin. Science 1987; 237: 517–22

25. Teitelbaum JS, Zatorre RJ, Carpenter S, et al. Neurologic sequelae of domoic acid intoxication due to the ingestion of contaminated mussels. N Engl J Med 1990; 322: 1781–7

26. Armon C, Daube JR, O'Brien PC, et al. When is an apparent excess of neurologic cases epidemiologically significant? Neurology 1991; 41: 1713–18

27. Kurtzke JF. On statistical testing of prevalence studies. J Chron Dis 1966; 19:909–22

28. Haley RW. Excess incidence of ALS in young Gulf War veterans. Neurology 2003; 61: 750–6

29. Horner RD, Kamins KG, Feussner JR, et al. Occurrence of amyotrophic lateral sclerosis among Gulf War veterans. Neurology 2003; 61: 742-749. Erratum in: Neurology 2003; 61: 1320

30. Coffman CJ, Horner RD, Grambow SC, Lindquist J. Estimating the occurrence of amyotrophic lateral sclerosis among Gulf War (1990–1991) veterans using capture–recapture methods. Neuroepidemiology 2005; 24: 141–50

31. Weisskopf M, O'Reilly E, McCullough M, et al. Prospective study of military service and risk of amyotrophic lateral sclerosis. Neurology 2005; 64: 32–7

32. Brooks BR. El Escorial World Federation of Neurology criteria for the diagnosis of amyotrophic lateral sclerosis. Subcommittee on Motor Neuron Diseases/Amyotrophic Lateral Sclerosis of the World Federation of Neurology Research Group on Neuromuscular Diseases and the El Escorial 'Clinical limits of amyotrophic lateral sclerosis' workshop contributors. J Neurol Sci 1994; 124: 96–107

33. Ross MA, Miller RG, Berchert L, et al. Towards earlier diagnosis of amyotrophic lateral sclerosis: revised criteria. rhCNTF ALS Study Group. Neurology 1998; 50: 768–72

34. Sorenson EJ, Stalker AP, Kurland LT, Windebank AJ. Amyotrophic lateral sclerosis in Olmsted County, Minnesota, 1925 to 1998. Neurology 2002; 59: 280–2

35. Kurtzke JF. Which 'neurodegenerative diseases' are on the rise? Health Environ Digest 1989; 3: 3–8

36. Lilienfeld DE, Perl DP. Projected neurodegenerative disease mortality in the United States, 1990–2040. Neuroepidemiology 1993; 12: 219–28

37. McGuire V, Longstreth WT Jr, Koepsell TD, van Belle G. Incidence of amyotrophic lateral sclerosis in three counties in western Washington state. Neurology 1996; 47: 571–3

38. Armon C, Kurland LT. Classic and western Pacific amyotrophic lateral sclerosis: epidemiologic comparisons. In: Hudson AJ, ed. Amyotrophic Lateral Sclerosis: Concepts in Pathogenesis and Etiology. Toronto: University of Toronto Press, 1989: 144–65

39. Christensen PB, Hojer-Pedersen E, Jensen NB. Survival of patients with amyotrophic lateral sclerosis in two Danish counties. Neurology 1990; 40: 600–4

40. Traynor BJ, Codd MB, Corr B, et al. Incidence and prevalence of ALS in Ireland, 1995-1997: A population-based study. Neurology 1999; 52: 504–9

41. Seljeseth YM, Vollset SE, Tysnes OB. Increasing mortality from amyotrophic lateral sclerosis in Norway? Neurology 2000; 55: 1262–6

42. Maasilta P, Jokelainen M, Loytonen M, et al. Mortality from amyotrophic lateral sclerosis in Finland, 1986-1995. Acta Neurol Scand 2001; 104: 232–5

43. Piemonte and Valle d'Aosta Register for Amyotrophic Lateral Sclerosis (PARALS). Incidence of ALS in Italy: evidence for a uniform frequency in Western countries. Neurology 2001; 56: 239–44

44. Mandrioli J, Faglioni P, Merelli E, Sola P. The epidemiology of ALS in Modena, Italy. Neurology 2003; 60: 683–9

45. Armon C. Motor neuron disease. In Gorelick PB, Alter M, eds. Handbook of Neuroepidemiology. New York: Marcel Dekker, 1994: 407–56

46. Gunnarsson L-G, Lindberg G, Soderfeldt B, Axelson O. Amyotrophic lateral sclerosis in Sweden in relation to occupation. Acta Neurol Scand 1991; 83: 394–8

47. Kurtzke JF. Risk factors in amyotrophic lateral sclerosis. Adv Neurol 1991; 56: 245–70

48. Chancellor AM, Warlow CP. Adult onset motor neuron disease: Worldwide mortality, incidence and distribution since 1950. J Neurol Neurosurg Psychiatry 1992; 55: 1106–15

49. Kahana E, Zilber N. Changes in incidence of amyotrophic lateral sclerosis in Israel. Arch Neurol 1984; 41: 157–60

50. Rosati G, Pinna L, Granieri E, et al. Studies on epidemiological, clinical, and etiological aspects of ALS disease in Sardinia, Southern Italy. Acta Neurol Scand 1977; 55: 231–44

51. Forsgren L, Almay BG, Holmgren G, Wall S. Epidemiology of motor neuron disease in northern Sweden. Acta Neurol Scand 1983; 68: 20–9

52. Gunnarsson LG, Palm R. Motor neuron disease and heavy manual labor: an epidemiologic survey of Varmland County, Sweden. Neuroepidemiology 1984; 3: 195–206

53. Hojer-Pedersen E, Christensen PB, Jensen NB. Incidence and prevalence of motor neuron disease in two Danish counties. Neuroepidemiology 1989; 8: 151–9

54. Murros K, Fogelholm R. Amyotrophic lateral sclerosis in Middle-Finland: An epidemiological study. Acta Neurol Scand 1983; 67: 41–7

55. Hudson AJ, Davenport A, Hader WJ. The incidence of amyotrophic lateral sclerosis in southwestern Ontario, Canada. Neurology 1986; 36: 1524–8

56. Annegers JF, Appel S, Lee JR, Perkins P. Incidence and prevalence of amyotrophic lateral sclerosis in Harris County Texas, 1985–1988. Arch Neurol 1991; 48: 589–93

57. Scottish Motor Neuron Disease Research Group. The Scottish motor neuron disease register: A prospective study of adult onset motor neuron disease in Scotland. Methodology, demography and clinical features of incident cases in 1989. J Neurol Neurosurg Psychiatry 1992; 55: 536–41

58. Chiò A, Tribolo A, Oddenino E, Schiffer D. A cross-sectional and cohort study of motor neuron disease in Piedmont, Italy. In: Clifford Rose F, ed. New Evidence in MND/ALS Research. London: Smith-Gordon, 1991: 59–62

59. Guidetti D, Bondavalli M, Sabadini R, et al. Epidemiological survey of amyotrophic lateral sclerosis in the province of Reggio Emilia, Italy: Influence of environmental exposure to lead. Neuroepidemiology 1996; 15: 301–12

60. Gunnarsson LG, Lygner PE, Veiga-Cabo J, de Pedro-Cuesta J. An epidemic-like cluster of motor neuron disease in a Swedish county during the period 1973–1984. Neuroepidemiology 1996; 15: 142–52

61. Gompertz B. On the nature of the function expressive of the law of human mortality. Philos Trans R Soc London 1825; 115: 513–85

62. Riggs JE. Longitudinal Gompertzian analysis of amyotrophic lateral sclerosis mortality in the U.S., 1977–1986: Evidence for an inherently susceptible population subset. Mech Ageing Dev 1990; 55: 207–20

63. Nielson S, Robinson I, Hunter M. Longitudinal Gompertzian analysis of ALS mortality in England and Wales, 1963-1989: estimates of susceptibility in the general population. Mech Ageing Dev 1992; 64: 210–16

64. Kurlander HM, Patten BM. Metals in spinal cord tissue of patients dying of motor neuron disease. Ann Neurol 1979; 6: 21–4

65. Mitchell JD. Heavy metals and trace elements in amyotrophic lateral sclerosis. Neurol Clin 1987; 5: 43–60

66. Chancellor AM, Slattery JM, Fraser H, Warlow CP. Risk factors for motor neuron disease: A case–control study based on patients from the Scottish Motor Neuron Disease Register. J Neurol Neurosurg Psychiatry 1993; 56: 1200–6

67. Armon C, Kurland LT, O'Brien PC, Mulder DW. Antecedent medical diseases in patients with amyotrophic lateral sclerosis: A population-based case-controlled study in Rochester, Minnesota, 1925–1987. Arch Neurol 1991; 48: 283–6

68. Felmus MT, Patten BM, Swanke L. Antecedent events in amyotrophic lateral sclerosis. Neurology 1976; 26: 167–72

69. Campbell AMG, Williams ER, Barltrop D. Motor neuron disease and exposure to lead. J Neurol Neurosurg Psychiatry 1970; 33: 877–85

70. Kamel F, Umbach DM, Munsat TL, et al. Lead exposure and amyotrophic lateral sclerosis. Epidemiology 2002; 13: 311–19

71. Pierce-Ruhland R, Patten BM. Repeat study of antecedent events in motor neuron disease. Ann Clin Res 1981; 13: 102–7

72. Deapen DM, Henderson BE. A case–control study of amyotrophic lateral sclerosis. Am J Epidemiol 1986; 123: 790–9

73. Gresham LS, Molgaard CA, Golbeck AL, Smith R. Amyotrophic lateral sclerosis and occupational heavy metal exposure: A case–control study. Neuroepidemiology 1986; 5: 29–38

74. Gunnarsson LG, Bodin L, Soderfeldt B, Axelson O. A case–control study of motor neuron disease: Its relation to heritability, and occupational exposures, particularly to solvents. Br J Ind Med 1992; 49: 791–8

75. Schulte PA, Burnett CA, Boeniger MF, Johnson J. Neurodegenerative diseases: Occupational occurrence and potential risk factors, 1982 through 1991. Am J Public Health 1996; 86: 1281–8

76. Graham AJ, Macdonald AM, Hawkes CH. British motor neuron disease twin study. J Neurol Neurosurg Psychiatry 1997; 62: 562–9

77. Granieri E, Murgia SB, Rosati G, et al. The frequency of amyotrophic lateral sclerosis among workers in Sardinia. IRCS Med Sci 1983; 11: 898

78. Kamel F, Umbach DM, Munsat TL, et al. Association of cigarette smoking with amyotrophic lateral sclerosis. Neuroepidemiology 1999; 18: 194–202

79. Chiò A, Meineri P, Tribolo A, Schiffer D. Risk factors in motor neuron disease: a case-control study. Neuroepidemiology 1991; 10: 174–84

80. Holloway SM, Emery AE. The epidemiology of motor neuron disease in Scotland. Muscle Nerve 1982; 5: 131–3

81. Kurtzke JF, Beebe GW. Epidemiology of amyotrophic lateral sclerosis: 1. A case–control comparison based on ALS deaths. Neurology 1980; 30: 453–62

82. Kondo K, Tsubaki T. Case–control studies of motor neuron disease. Association with mechanical injuries. Arch Neurol 1981; 38: 220–6

83. Strickland D, Smith SA, Dolliff G, et al. Amyotrophic lateral sclerosis and occupational history: A pilot case–control study. Arch Neurol 1996; 53: 730–3

84. Cruz DC, Nelson LM, McGuire V, Longstreth WT Jr. Physical trauma and family history of neurodegenerative diseases in amyotrophic lateral sclerosis: A population-based case–control study. Neuroepidemiology 1999; 18: 101–10

85. Granieri E, Carreras M, Tola R, et al. Motor neuron disease in the province of Ferrara, Italy in 1964–1982. Neurology 1988; 38: 1604–8

86. Armon C, Kurland LT, Daube JR, O'Brien PC. Epidemiologic correlates of sporadic amyotrophic lateral sclerosis. Neurology 1991; 41: 1077–84

87. Buckley J, Warlow C, Smith P, et al. Motor neuron disease in England and Wales, 1959–1979. J Neurol Neurosurg Psychiatry 1983; 46: 197–205

88. Holloway SM, Mitchell JD. Motor neuron disease in the Lothian Region of Scotland 1961–81. J Epidemiol Community Health 1986; 40: 344–50

89. Provinciali L, Giovagnoli AR. Antecedent events in amyotrophic lateral sclerosis: Do they influence clinical onset and progression? Neuroepidemiology 1990; 9: 255–62

90. Savettieri G, Salemi G, Arcara A, et al. A case–control study of amyotrophic lateral sclerosis. Neuroepidemiology 1991;10:242–5

91. McGuire V, Longstreth WT Jr, Nelson LM, et al. Occupational exposures and amyotrophic lateral sclerosis. A population-based case–control study. Am J Epidemiol 1997; 145: 1076–88

92. Hawkes CH, Fox AJ. Motor neuron disease in leather workers. Lancet 1981; 1: 507

93. Martyn CN. Motor neuron disease and exposure to solvents. Lancet 1989; 1: 394

94. Gunnarsson LG, Lindberg G. Amyotrophic lateral sclerosis in Sweden 1970–83 and solvent exposure. Lancet 1989; 1: 958

95. Davanipour Z, Sobel E, Bowman JD, et al. Amyotrophic lateral sclerosis and occupational exposure to electromagnetic fields. Bioelectromagnetics 1997; 18: 28–35

96. Johansen C, Olsen JH. Mortality from amyotrophic lateral sclerosis, other chronic disorders, and electric shocks among utility workers. Am J Epidemiol 1998; 148: 362–8

97. Savitz DA, Checkoway H, Loomis DP. Magnetic field exposure and neurodegenerative disease mortality among electric utility workers. Epidemiology 1998; 9: 398–404

98. Noonan CW, Reif JS, Yost M, Touchstone J. Occupational exposure to magnetic fields in case-referent studies of neurodegenerative diseases. Scand J Work Environ Health 2002; 28: 42–8

99. Li C-Y, Sung F-C. Association between occupational exposure to power frequency electromagnetic fields and amyotrophic lateral sclerosis: A review. Am J Ind Med 2003; 43: 212–20

100. Håkansson N, Gustavsson P, Johansen C, Floderus B. Neurodegenerative diseases in welders and other workers exposed to high levels of magnetic fields. Epidemiology 2003; 14: 420–6; discussion 427–8

101. Feychting M, Jonsson F, Pedersen NL, Ahlbom A. Occupational magnetic field exposure and neurodegenerative disease. Epidemiology 2003; 14: 413–19; discussion 427–8

102. Gawel M, Zaiwalla Z, Rose FC. Antecedent events in motor neuron disease. J Neurol Neurosurg Psychiatry 1983; 46: 1041–3

103. Sienko DG, Davis JP, Taylor JA, Brooks BR. Amyotrophic lateral sclerosis. A case–control study following detection of a cluster in a small Wisconsin community. Arch Neurol 1990; 47: 38–41

104. Breland AE, Currier RD. Multiple sclerosis and amyotrophic lateral sclerosis in Mississippi. Neurology 1967; 17: 1011–16

105. Palo J, Jokelainen M. Geographic and social distribution of patients with amyotrophic lateral sclerosis. Arch Neurol 1977; 34: 724

106. Bracco L, Antuono P, Amaducci L. Study of epidemiological and etiological factors of amyotrophic lateral sclerosis in the province of Florence, Italy. Acta Neurol Scand 1979; 60: 112–24

107. Roelofs-Iverson RA, Mulder DW, Elveback LR, et al. ALS and heavy metals: A pilot case–control study. Neurology 1984; 34: 393–5

108. Longstreth WT, McGuire V, Koepsell TD, et al. Risk of amyotrophic lateral sclerosis and history of physical activity: A population-based case–control study. Arch Neurol 1998; 55: 201–6

109. Veldink JH, Kalmijn S, Groeneveld GJ, et al. Physical activity and the association with sporadic ALS. Neurology 2005; 64: 241–5

110. Kurtzke JF. Risk factors in amyotrophic lateral sclerosis. Ann Neurol 1991; 56: 245–70

111. Chiò A, Benzi G, Dossena M, et al. Severely increased risk for amyotrophic lateral sclerosis among Italian professional football players. Brain 2005; 128: 472–6

112. Beghi E, Chiò A, Hardiman O, et al. Amyotrophic lateral sclerosis and professional sports activities – a population-based case–control study. Neuroepidemiology 2004; 23: 155

113. Nelson LM, McGuire V, Longstreth WT, Matkin C. Population-based case–control study of amyotrophic lateral sclerosis in western Washington State. I. Cigarette smoking and alcohol consumption. Am J Epidemiol 2000; 151: 156–63

114. Weisskopf MG, McCullough ML, Calle EE, et al. Prospective study of cigarette smoking and amyotrophic lateral sclerosis. Am J Epidemiol 2004; 160: 26–33

115. Howard DJ, Ota RB, Briggs LA, et al. Environmental tobacco smoke in the workplace induces oxidative stress in employees, including increased production of 8-hydroxy-2'-deoxyguanosine. Cancer Epidemiol Biomarkers Prev 1998; 7: 141–6

116. Nelson LM, Matkin C, Longstreth WT, McGuire V. Population-based case–control study of amyotrophic lateral sclerosis in western Washington State. II. Diet. Am J Epidemiol 2000; 151: 164–73

117. Penzes L, Fischer HD, Noble RC. Some aspects on the relationship between lipids, neurotransmitters, and aging. Z Gerontol 1993; 26: 65–9

118. Bourre JM, Bonneil M, Clement M, et al. Function of dietary polyunsaturated fatty acids in the nervous system. Prostaglandins Leukot Essent Fatty Acids 1993; 48: 5–15

119. Liu D. The roles of free radicals in amyotrophic lateral sclerosis. J Mol Neurosci 1996; 7: 159–67

120. Hillemeier C. An overview of the effects of dietary fiber on gastrointestinal transit. Pediatrics 1995; 96: 997–9

121. Lupton JR, Turner ND. Potential protective mechanisms of wheat bran fiber. Am J Med 1999; 106: 24S–7S

122. Ascherio A, Weisskopf MG, O'Reilly E, et al. Vitamin E intake and risk of amyotrophic lateral sclerosis. Ann Neurol 2005; 57: 104–10

123. Angelini C, Armani M, Bresolin N. Incidence and risk factors in the Venice and Padua districts of Italy, 1972–1979. Neuroepidemiology 1983; 2: 236–42

124. Kurland LT, Radhakrishnan K, Smith GE, et al. Mechanical trauma as a risk factor in classic amyotrophic lateral sclerosis. Lack of epidemiologic evidence. J Neurol Sci 1992; 113: 133–43

Section 2

Functional studies

3

Neuroimaging in amyotrophic lateral sclerosis

Martin R Turner, Victoria Williams, Camilla Blain, Derek Jones, Blaz Koritnik, P Nigel Leigh

INTRODUCTION

Neuroimaging is central to the diagnostic process in amyotrophic lateral sclerosis (ALS). At present, however, it is central only in its capacity to exclude other conditions. Neuroimaging, particularly magnetic resonance imaging (MRI), is uniquely powerful in identifying tumors and other lesions of the brain, spinal cord, or nerve roots that can masquerade as ALS. High-quality MRI of these structures is widely available and most patients with suspected ALS have MRI scans of the brain and/or spinal cord, although this may not always be necessary. There are some instances where the clinical and electrophysiologic evidence rules out a focal lesion or other disease processes.

Unfortunately, there is no reliable neuroimaging 'hallmark' for ALS. In particular, early changes in the motor cortex and spinal cord cannot yet be detected by any standard, clinically applicable imaging technique. Nevertheless, the developments described in this review may lead to new diagnostic tests that will help in the early diagnosis of ALS.

Prior to the advent of neuroimaging, there was limited scope for understanding the nature and importance of the cerebral lesions in ALS. This has diagnostic significance, as well as implications for understanding pathophysiology, given that the detection of upper motor neuron (UMN) involvement is an important element of the El Escorial research diagnostic criteria[1]. The development of new technologies to investigate neurologic disease *in vivo* has opened up the possibility of developing surrogate markers of disease to improve diagnosis, to delineate phenotypes and genotypes, and to monitor therapy.

Whereas the degeneration of anterior horn motor neurons (AHMNs) characterizes the lower motor neuron (LMN) involvement in ALS, UMN involvement occurs through degeneration of the corticospinal tracts (CSTs) along its length, including its origins within the motor cortex[2]. Most obvious to the pathologist is loss of the giant Betz cells[3–5], but this is not always evident even in patients with well-documented UMN signs in life[6]. Betz cells, estimated to number about 30 000 in humans[7], make a relatively small contribution to the corticospinal tract overall[8]. Smaller pyramidal neurons must contribute the majority of fibers entering the CST. In keeping with the notion that cortical involvement in ALS is more diffuse than sometimes assumed, degenerating nerve fibers can be traced to areas outside the primary motor cortex including the prefrontal and temporal regions[2,6,9].

Forms of ALS that manifest only LMN signs (progressive muscular atrophy – PMA) show pathologic evidence of UMN involvement[10,11]. One of the pressing goals of clinical investigation

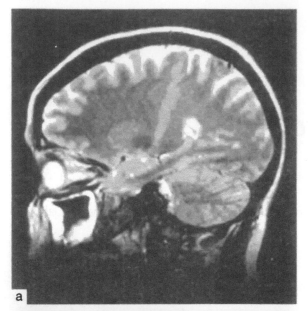

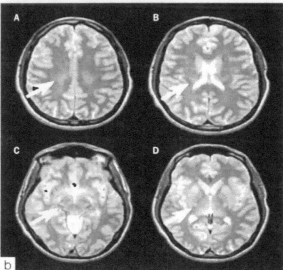

Figure 3.1 (a) Sagittal T2-weighted image of high signal in corticospinal tract in a patient with rapidly progressive amyotrophic lateral sclerosis with predominant upper motor neuron signs. (Reproduced from reference 14, with permission). (b) Signal hyperintensity in the intracranial corticospinal tract in a patient with amyotrophic lateral sclerosis (proton density-weighted images). (A) Centrum semiovale; (B) corona radiata; (C) posterior limb of the internal capsule; (D) cerebral peduncle. (Reproduced from reference 15 with permission of the editor of *Neurology* and the authors)

is to demonstrate subtle degrees of UMN damage early in the disease, so increasing the certainty of

diagnosis (by inclusion or exclusion) in patients with LMN syndromes.

Just as ALS is clinically[12] and genetically[13] heterogeneous, so the nature of damage to the CSTs is likely to differ between patients. In some cases, degeneration may involve the whole CST almost simultaneously, with Wallerian degeneration predominating. We speculated that this might be the case in a patient who had very rapidly progressive ALS with prominent UMN signs and in whom the MRI scan showed marked signal change along the course of the CST from the motor cortex through the subcortical white matter and into the internal capsule[14,15] (Figure 3.1). Using conventional myelin stains, loss of myelin in the CST is most obvious distally in the spinal cord, and may be difficult to detect in the brainstem, internal capsule and subcortical white matter[6]. More sensitive techniques, however, indicate that the CST is usually damaged, albeit to varying degrees from case to case, along its entire course[3] (see reference 16, for an authoritative review of the early pathologic literature). This argues against any simplistic concept of 'dying back' versus 'dying forward' processes.

Histopathology alone can never resolve these issues but, as we will see, more sensitive neuroimaging techniques have the potential to study cellular (even molecular) processes *in vivo* at an early stage of disease evolution. When such analyses can be combined with understanding of genotype–phenotype interactions, it may be possible to probe the mechanisms of cellular damage in life. Thus the challenge for neuroimaging is to evolve techniques that go beyond descriptions of structure to describing molecular events in the brain, spinal cord and even peripheral nerve and muscle.

NEUROIMAGING: STATE OF THE ART

The development of neuroimaging techniques in the past 30 years has permitted the detailed study of brain pathology *in vivo*, and has revolutionized the study of neurologic diseases more than any other single development. In particular, modern neuroimaging techniques can provide insight into dynamic processes that reflect a variety of brain functions.

Conventional magnetic resonance imaging techniques

Conventional techniques that can be applied in almost all modern neuroimaging units include T1- and T2-weighted images, proton density-weighted images and fluid attenuated inversion recovery (FLAIR)-weighted images. Diffusion-weighted imaging (DWI) is becoming more widely available. As mentioned, the role of imaging in ALS traditionally has been to aid in the exclusion of disease mimics. Numerous studies describing structural changes in the brains of subjects with ALS detected by MRI have been published. Cortical atrophy, T2 ribbon-like hypointensity of the motor cortex and T2-weighted high signal in the corticospinal tracts (Figure 3.1) have all been reported. In general, these observed abnormalities with standard imaging modalities are insufficiently sensitive or specific to provide useful diagnostic information or to allow accurate measurement of disease progression.

One study[15] looked at the diagnostic utility of several imaging modalities. Twenty-nine patients with ALS and 23 healthy volunteers were studied with conventional MRI (T1-weighted, T2-weighted and proton density-weighted) sequences as well as diffusion tensor imaging (see below). The scans were visually examined and regions within and outside the CSTs were classified as normal or abnormal by two neuroradiologists with a consensus rating scheme. A ribbon of T2-weighted hypointensity in the motor cortex was identified in five of 25 patients with UMN signs; proton density signal hyperintensity in the corona radiata was found in four of 16 patients with UMN signs. These changes were not seen in any of the healthy volunteers. There were no significant differences found between the two groups in the other CST regions or non-CST regions examined. No abnormalities were identified on T1-weighted images in either group, and no significant differences were found between the ALS patients and the controls using a FLAIR sequence. In conclusion, T2-weighted hypointensity in the motor cortex may be a helpful sign in ALS, but signal changes in the CST are nonspecific. However, systematic large-scale studies comparing these changes in ALS and other conditions involving the motor system are warranted.

Volumetric imaging

Few studies have been published of quantitative imaging measures of brain volume loss in patients with ALS. Ellis et al.[17] found no differences in total brain volume between 16 ALS patients and eight normal controls. There was a loss of frontal gray matter in the ALS group and of CST white matter volume in the eight bulbar-onset patients (Figure 3.2). Abrahams et al.[18] studied 11 cognitively impaired and 12 cognitively unimpaired ALS patients, compared to 12 controls. There were no significant differences in *gray* matter volume between the groups. The impaired group had a significant loss of white matter volume in extensive motor and non-motor regions. The unimpaired group had a significant reduction in frontal white matter compared to controls. A further study[19] of patients with ALS/frontotemporal dementia (FTD) and ALS patients without cognitive impairment demonstrated *gray*, but not white matter, atrophy in both groups in bilateral motor and pre-motor cortices as well as frontal and temporal regions and the left thalamus. Each of these studies suggests that the damage in ALS extends beyond motor regions, even in patients without frank cognitive impairment.

Diffusion imaging

Diffusion tensor magnetic resonance imaging (DT-MRI) is an exciting and relatively new imaging technique that has proved to be highly

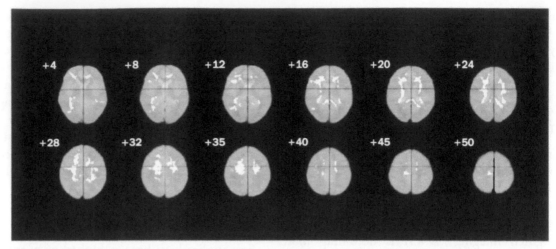

Figure 3.2 Voxel-based morphometry (VBM). Axial slices through brain. Yellow areas represent statistically significant loss of cerebral white matter in amyotrophic lateral sclerosis patients who were impaired on a standardized test of verbal fluency (VF). VBM changes in patients who did not show impairments of VF were less obvious and were restricted mainly to frontal white matter (not shown). (Reproduced from reference 18, with permission). See also Plate 1

valuable in the study of a wide variety of neurologic diseases. It provides insights into the state of the microstructure of tissue, which are not available through standard MR sequences.

DT-MRI capitalizes on the constant random thermal motion of water molecules within tissue. In an unbounded medium, such as the cerebrospinal fluid (CSF), water molecules are free to diffuse in any direction – and will tend to diffuse at the same rate in each direction. However, within parenchyma, cell membranes and cellular inclusions will hinder the molecular motion in one or more direction, leading to a reduction in the 'apparent diffusivity'. In gray matter, on the scale of typical voxel sizes, there is no particular order – and so the apparent diffusivity will be approximately the same in all directions, albeit reduced compared to that in the CSF. In highly ordered tissue such as the white matter, however, water molecules will diffuse more readily along the long axes (where they are relatively unhindered) than across them. The apparent diffusivity in white matter therefore has a natural directionality, which is termed diffusion anisotropy.

By far the most commonly used diffusion-weighted magnetic resonance (MR) sequence is the pulsed-gradient spin echo (PGSE) sequence. In this sequence, two large magnetic field gradients (matched in amplitude and duration) are placed either side of a 180° refocusing pulse. Stationary molecules will be equally dephased and rephased by the two pulsed gradients and thus there will be no reduction in the amplitude of the spin echo. However, for molecules that move during the measurement period (i.e. diffusing molecules), the phase change due to the first pulsed gradient will not be matched in amplitude by the phase change due to the second gradient. If the motion of the molecules in the voxel is not uniform, the result will be a distribution of phases within the voxel. This reduction in coherence will lead to a reduction in the amplitude of the spin echo signal. The amount of phase dispersion or 'diffusion weighting' will depend on the strength of the diffusion encoding gradient and also on the duration and temporal separation of the pulsed gradient pair.

One cannot fully describe diffusion characteristics by applying diffusion encoding gradients along just one axis. In diffusion tensor imaging, a number of measurements of the spin echo are made (at least six) with a different (non-collinear) direction of the diffusion gradient for each measurement. These measurements are subsequently used to estimate the diffusion tensor, which yields several important indices of water displacement. The mean diffusivity (MD) characterizes the total amount of diffusivity (irrespective of directionality). The more hindered the motion of water molecules, the lower the mean diffusivity. Thus, CSF has a much higher diffusivity than parenchyma. The most popular index of directionality is the fractional anisotropy (FA) which characterizes anisotropy on a scale from zero to one. If the apparent diffusivity is the same in all directions, then diffusion is isotropic and the FA is zero. Conversely, the more preferred the displacement is along one axis over others, the higher the FA. The extreme case is when molecules can move along only one axis, corresponding to an FA of one. Thus, in areas such as the CSF, the MD will be high and the FA will be low. Throughout parenchyma, the MD is lower (about four times less than that of free water) – but is roughly constant. The FA is higher in white matter and is highest in the most organized fiber pathways such as the corpus callosum and cerebral peduncles.

Clinical applications of diffusion tensor magnetic resonance imaging

DT-MRI has been used to investigate a number of neurologic diseases, in particular stroke and multiple sclerosis. From the foregoing discussion, it should be clear that any pathologic process that affects the tissue microstructure (cellular membranes, myelin layers, cellular inclusions) will result in differences in the hindrance to diffusion with an accompanying change in the mean diffusivity and/or diffusion anisotropy. For reviews of clinical applications to both normal and diseased populations see reviews by Neil et al.[20], Moseley[21], Sotak[22], Horsfield and Jones[23], and Lim and Helpern[24]. In this chapter, we restrict ourselves to reviewing key DT-MRI studies of ALS.

Using measures taken from diffusion-weighted images, Segawa et al.[25] found no differences

between the groups in diffusion characteristics in the posterior limb of the internal capsule, although, in a subsequent study, a reduction in anisotropy was found within periventricular white matter lesions in five ALS patients. In the first published study of DT-MRI in ALS, Ellis et al.[26] studied 20 patients. Six regions of interest (ROIs) were placed on coronal images along the CSTs within the posterior limb of the internal capsule bilaterally. The FA and MD values were each averaged to produce a single mean value for each individual. The FA was significantly reduced in the ALS patients overall compared to controls. The reduction in FA was significant between the ten bulbar-onset patients and controls, but not between the limb-onset group and controls. The FA correlated with measures of disease severity, but not with disease duration. The MD was significantly higher in both the limb- and bulbar-onset groups when compared to controls. The MD was correlated with disease duration but not with disease severity. Of six patients without definite UMN signs, five had a normal MD. Both MD and FA correlated with the threshold to motor conduction measured using transcranial magnetic stimulation, a marker of UMN damage.

Subsequently, a number of DT-MRI studies in ALS have been published (summarized in Table 3.1). Toosy et al.[27] studied 21 patients with El Escorial probable or definite ALS and 14 controls. Measurements were taken from ROIs placed along the CSTs at the internal capsule, cerebral peduncles, pons and pyramids. In normal controls, they identified a reduction in FA and an increase in MD caudally along the CSTs. The ALS patients had a lower FA along the CT than the control group. There was some evidence that the MD was higher in the ALS group at the level of the internal capsule, but this difference was not maintained lower in the CST. They found no correlation between diffusion indices and the ALS functional rating scale (ALSFRS) score, or a measure of the rate of disease progression. They did not comment on correlation with disease duration.

Table 3.1   Summary of diffusion tensor magnetic resonance studies in amyotrophic lateral sclerosis

Study	No. pts	Type	FA changes in CST	MD changes in CST	Clinical correlations
Segawa et al., 1994[25]	16	Diffusion-weighted images, ROI	Unchanged	Unchanged	N/A
Ellis et al., 1999[26]	20	ROI	Reduced	Increased	MD – duration FA – severity MD and FA – threshold to cortical magnetic stimulation
Toosy et al., 2003[27]	21	ROI	Reduced	Increased in IC	No correlation with severity or progression
Jacob et al., 2003[28]	3	Longitudinal ROI	Reduced over time in UMN pt	N/A	N/A
Sach et al., 2004[29]	12	VBM	Reduced in CSTs, extramotor regions and in patients with LMN disease only	N/A	FA – CMCT
Graham et al., 2004[15]	19	ROI	Reduced in PLIC	Unchanged	FA – MRC grading and disease severity scale
Karlsborg et al., 2004[30]	8	ROI	Reduced in pons	Increased in IC	N/A
Yin et al., 2004[31]	8	ROI	Reduced	Unchanged	N/A
Cossottini et al., 2005[32]	20	ROI	Reduced (unchanged in LMN)	Increased (unchanged in LMN)	N/A

CMCT, central motor conduction time; CP, cerebral peduncle; CST, corticospinal tract; FA, fractional anisotropy; IC, internal capsule; LMN, lower motor neuron; MD, mean diffusivity; PLIC, posterior limb of internal capsule; ROI, region of interest; UMN, upper motor neuron; VBM, voxel-based morphometry; MRC, Medical Research Council

Two further large studies deserve specific mention. Sach et al.[29] examined 12 controls and 15 patients with ALS, six of whom had no clinical signs of UMN involvement at the time of the study but went on to develop them later in their disease. Diffusion-weighted gradients were applied in six directions, and 20 contiguous coronal slices were obtained covering the pyramidal tract fibers from the cortex to the brainstem. FA maps were compared between patients and controls. A significant decrease in FA in the CSTs in subcortical white matter, posterior limb of the internal capsule and the brainstem was identified. In addition, reduced FA was found in extramotor areas in the ALS group – in the corpus callosum and the right thalamus. A negative correlation was found between FA and central motor conduction time (an electrophysiologic marker of UMN disease). The group with no UMN signs at the time of the study also had significant reductions in FA in the subcortical white matter, internal capsule and brainstem.

Finally, Graham et al.[15] studied 15 patients with UMN signs, four with PMA and 14 healthy volunteers. ROIs were positioned at three levels within the CST (subcortical white matter of the precentral gyrus, corona radiata and posterior limb of the internal capsule), subcortical white matter of the post-central gyrus and in three control brain regions (frontal white matter and corpus callosum). The only significant region of reduced FA was identified in the posterior limb of the internal capsule in patients with UMN signs. The FA correlated with muscle weakness as measured by MRC grading and with the ALS rating scale. There was a trend towards reduced FA in the subcortical white matter of the precentral gyrus. The MD did not differ between patients with UMN signs and healthy volunteers and did not correlate with any of their clinical measures. There was a trend towards reduced FA in the posterior limb of the internal capsule in the LMN patients compared to controls. The mean FA in the LMN group fell between the control and UMN groups, although it was not significantly different to either. The authors went on to consider whether the FA could be used to diagnose UMN damage. Setting an upper threshold of FA in the posterior limb of the internal capsule 1 SD above the mean FA of patients with UMN signs gave a positive predictive value for the diagnosis of ALS (with or without UMN signs) of 82%, a sensitivity of 95% and a specificity of 71%.

In normal controls and ALS patients, FA had a tendency to increase and MD to decrease from the internal capsules caudally. There was no difference between left and right sides (in contrast to previous studies). Only the mean of the FA and MD in all the ROIs were further considered. There was significant reduction in FA and increase in MD in the ALS group compared to the control group. There were no significant differences between the PMA and control groups. MD correlated with disease duration and FA with ALSFRS (although not with duration). The diffusivity along the tract was not significantly different between the control and ALS groups, although the diffusivities in the transverse direction were. The authors postulated that the reduction in FA was therefore due to increased diffusion across the nerve fibers, rather than reduced diffusion along them. This pattern of diffusion abnormality is thought to be a hallmark of Wallerian degeneration.

In summary, the published studies of DT-MRI in ALS have generally shown a reduction in FA and an increase in MD in the CSTs of patients with ALS. Where clinical correlations have been reported, FA has been inversely correlated with markers of disease progression and MD with disease duration. These two diffusion indices may therefore be reflecting different pathologic processes.

An exciting development yet to be applied extensively to ALS is DT-MRI tractography[33–35]. This is a technique that aims to elucidate the three-dimensional trajectories and origins/terminations of white matter fasciculi within the brain non-invasively, by 'stitching' together, in a piece-wise fashion, discrete estimates of fiber orientation.

Within the major fasciculi, it has been shown that fasciculus reconstructions from DT-MRI tractography are remarkably similar to those obtained by postmortem dissection (Figure 3.3). Applications of tractography to study diseased populations has, however, been limited. An immediately obvious application is to look for the effect of tumors on white matter tracts, which has implications for neuronavigation and surgery (for example, see reference 37). However, an emerging application is to use tractography as a method for obtaining tract-specific quantitative measurements. ROI-based approaches can not only be laborious, but also be problematic for tracts that follow a tortuous route in and out of the imaged plane or for tracts that run very close to other tracts. By using tractography to isolate the location of particular tracts, Jones et al.[38] were able to obtain tract-specific measurements of FA and MD in the cingulum, uncinate, inferior occipital frontal and superior longitudinal fasciculi of schizophrenic patients and controls, revealing fasciculus-specific group differences. This approach is an exciting prospect for the study of the CSTs in patients with ALS.

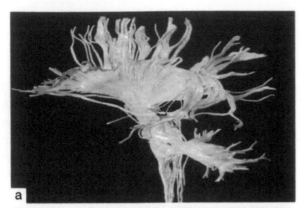

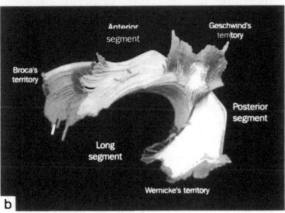

Figure 3.3 (a) Diffusion tensor magnetic resonance imaging tractography. *In vivo* dissection of subcortical fiber tracts. (b) Tractography reconstruction of the arcuate fasciculus using the two regions of interest approach. Broca's and Wernicke's territories are connected through direct and indirect pathways in the average brain. The direct pathway (long segment shown in red) runs medially and corresponds to classical descriptions of the arcuate fasciculus. The indirect pathway runs laterally and is composed of an anterior segment (green) connecting the inferior parietal cortex (Geschwind's territory) and Broca's territory and a posterior segment (yellow) connecting Geschwind's and Wernicke's territories. (Reproduced from reference 36, with permission of the authors and the editor of *Annals of Neurology*). See also Plate 2

Magnetic resonance spectroscopy

Proton magnetic resonance spectroscopy (H-MRS) allows non-invasive *in vivo* quantification of the metabolite composition of the brain. When the signal from water is suppressed, the characteristic proton spectra of several metabolites can be detected. The most prominent signal is due to *N*-acetylaspartate (NAA), a compound found only in neurons. NAA is often expressed as a ratio to creatine and phosphocreatine (P+Cr) or to choline (Cho), which are found throughout neurons and glia. A reduction in NAA/P+Cr or NAA/Cho is therefore held to be a marker of relative neuronal/axonal loss or dysfunction. Relative reductions in NAA have been found in a variety of neurodegenerative disorders such as Alzheimer's disease.

Several studies have reported a reduction in NAA concentration or NAA/Cho ratio in the motor cortex, brainstem and cerebellum of subjects with ALS (see Table 3.2 for references). Other studies have demonstrated that NAA is lowest in subjects with more signs of UMN damage and more normal in those with few UMN signs. Further reduction in NAA has been observed with worsening clinical status over time. There is significant overlap between the concentrations of NAA found in subjects with and without ALS, and currently this technique is insufficiently accurate to provide a diagnostic tool.

Sequences with shorter (40 ms or less) echo times can demonstrate the weaker proton spectra of a variety of substances including glutamate (Glu) and glutamine (Gln). Glu and Gln, grouped together as 'Glx' are of particular interest given the putative excitotoxic pathogenicity of Glu in ALS. Studies by different groups have shown unchanged or reduced concentrations of Glx in the motor cortex (Figure 3.4) and one group reported elevated Glx in the medulla, particularly in subjects with prominent bulbar symptoms. Levels of Glx may vary with the course of the disease; further studies will be required to clarify the role of spectroscopy in the investigation of disease pathogenesis.

Functional magnetic resonance imaging

Functional MRI (fMRI) is a non-invasive method of measuring cortical activity, allowing mapping of specific brain regions. Oxy- and deoxyhemoglobin

Table 3.2   Summary table of spectroscopy studies in amyotrophic lateral sclerosis (ALS)

Group	Subjects	Regions included	Metabolites measured	Results
Pioro et al., 1994[39] CSI	5 ALS 5 PUMS 2 SMA 6 NC	Centered on precentral gyrus postcentral, subparietal gyri included	(NAA/Cr+PCr)	ALS – ratio reduced in precentral, postcentral, superior parietal and posterior superior frontal gyri (in descending order) PUMS ratio reduced in precentral gyrus
Jones et al., 1995[40]	7 ALS 7 NC	Anterior to the central sulcus, contralateral to side with severe weakness	NAA/(Cr+PCr) NAA/Cho (Cr+PCr)/Cho	NAA/Crx and NAA/Cho reduced in ALS patients
Gredal et al., 1997[41]	7 ALS 7 PMA 8 NC	Motor cortex cerebellum (gray and white matter) avoiding CSF	[Cho] [NAA] [Cr+PCr]	[NAA] lower in cerebellum than cortex in controls [NAA] in cortex significantly reduced in ALS but not PMA compared with normal controls
Kalra et al., 1998[42] CSI	23 ALS	Centered on central sulcus Covering both precentral gyri	NAA/Cr	NAA/Cr ratio increased after 3 weeks of riluzole treatment. In untreated patients, the ratio fell
Block et al., 1998[43]	22 ALS 11 PUMS 4 MMN 20 NC	Anterior to central sulcus, adjacent white matter	NAA/Cho NAA/PCr Cho/PCr Ino/PCr (Glu+Gln)/PCr	NAA/Cho and NAA/PCr ratios reduced in ALS patients (continued reduction in NAA/Cho on follow-up scans) Cho/PCr and Ino/PCr ratios increased in ALS patients NAA/Cho ratio reduced in MMN patients
Ellis et al., 2000[44]	8 limb 8 bulbar 8 NC	4 in motor region 8 in parieto-occipital region anterior to central sulcus, predominantly white matter	NAA/(Cr+PCr), NAA/Cho, Cho/(Cr+PCr)	NAA/(Cr+PCr) correlated with El Escorial category, ALS severity scale and MRC score
Cwik et al., 1998[45]	12 ALS 5 NC	Centered in pons and upper medulla (upper edge aligned with upper end of fourth ventricle)	NAA/Cr	Brainstem NAA/Cr reduced in ALS subjects, most abnormal in patients with severe spasticity or prominent bulbar weakness

Cho, choline; Cr, creatinine; Gln, glutamine; Glu, glutamate; Glx, glutamine + glutamate; Ino, inositol; NAA, N-acetylaspartate; NC, normal control; P, phosphocreatine; PUMNs, patients with possible upper motor neuron signs; SMA, patients with spinal muscular atrophy; CSI, chemical shift imaging

have different magnetic susceptibility and therefore different MR characteristics. BOLD (blood oxygen level dependent) changes in signal result from a small but detectable difference in T2*-weighted signal intensity in regions of brain activation due to an increase in oxygenated blood in these areas[47–50]. Changes in signal are detected using rapid gradient echo sequences.

fMRI has been used to investigate motor cortex activity in ALS patients. MRI scanning typically takes place using BOLD imaging whilst subjects repeatedly perform a simple motor paradigm (for example, movement of a joystick or pressing a button). The data are acquired at rest and during the movement task; regions that show significant signal differences between the rest and motor task

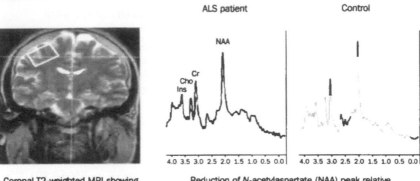

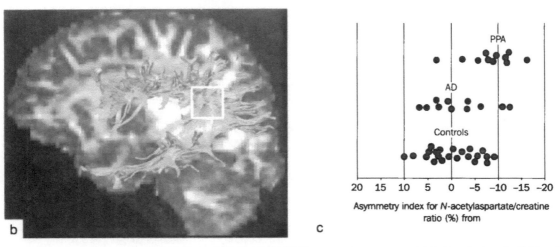

Figure 3.4 (a) Proton magnetic resonance spectroscopy (H-MRS) spectra from an amyotrophic lateral sclerosis (ALS) patient and control subject, showing a lower N-acetylaspartate (NAA) peak in the ALS motor cortex. (The white box in the left panel indicates the voxel analyzed for H-MRS.) (b) H-MRS and diffusion tensor magnetic resonance imaging (DT-MRI) tractography combined to derive measures of tissue damage in specific pathways. Tractography demonstrating parietotemporal fibers, and location (white square) of voxel from which NAA and creatine H-MRS measures were derived. (c) NAA and creatine measurements from voxel localized by DT-MRI tractography. PPA, primary progressive aphasia; AD, Alzheimer's disease. (Reproduced with permission from reference 46). See also Plate 3

epochs can be identified. As all other conditions remain the same during the task and rest period, those areas that show this signal difference are assumed to be areas activated by the task. These regions of activation may then be compared between study and control groups.

fMRI studies have, in keeping with positron emission tomography (PET) (see below), shown an increase in the volume of brain activation compared to that in normal controls when subjects with ALS carry out motor tasks (Figure 3.5). Konrad and colleagues[51] found activation more anteriorly in his ALS group than in the control group when they were performing a simple finger flexion task. Activation was seen within the motor region and included the premotor cortex in the ALS group. In addition, the supplementary motor area (SMA) activation was higher and more anterior, towards the pre-SMA.

Schoenfeld and colleagues[52] found more bilateral activity and difficulty-related cerebellar activity in their ALS group with a button-press task. When the groups were controlled for relative task difficulty, there were fewer differences. They

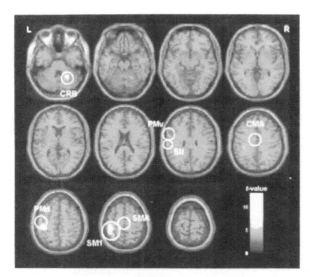

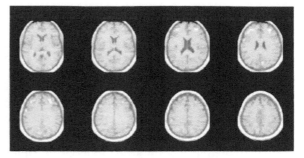

Figure 3.6   Functional magnetic resonance imaging. Axial images showing significantly decreased areas of activation, predominantly in dorsolateral prefrontal and temporal areas, in amyotrophic lateral sclerosis subjects compared to controls while performing a verbal fluency task. (Reproduced from reference 53, with permission of the editor of *Brain*). See also Plate 5

Figure 3.5   Functional magnetic resonance imaging can be used to visualize brain activation during a simple right-hand grip task. Normal subject. CMA, cingulate motor area; CRB, cerebellum; PMd, dorsal lateral premotor cortex; PMv, ventral lateral premotor cortex; SII, secondary somatosensory cortex; SM1, primary sensorimotor cortex; SMA, supplementary motor area; L, left; R, right. (Courtesy of Dr B Koritnik and Professor S Williams, King's College London, Centre for Neuroimaging Sciences). See also Plate 4

hypothesized that the abnormal activation in ALS patients was related to functional compensation rather than a direct result of disease.

Conversely, both in PET and unpublished fMRI studies, the abnormal spread of activation was not seen in subjects with LMN weakness only, suggesting that these changes may not be merely an adaptation to weakness. This 'boundary shift effect' may represent abnormal excitability or loss of inhibitory control, which allows spread of activation to the adjacent cortex. This may have particular significance in view of the postulated role of Glu excitotoxicity in disease pathogenesis.

Abrahams *et al.*[53], using a verbal fluency and confrontation naming fMRI task, identified significantly reduced activation in frontal and temporal regions despite matched performances between the patients and controls during the paradigm (Figure 3.6). This study adds to the increasing body of evidence for extramotor pathology and executive dysfunction in subjects with ALS.

Although fMRI is currently insufficiently sensitive to provide a diagnostic test for neuronal damage, it does provide further evidence of extramotor involvement in this condition and may have a role in defining pathogenic mechanisms. With improvements in imaging technology and increases in field strengths, the imaging modalities discussed above are likely to become increasingly important in the study of the disease.

Single photon emission tomography

Single photon emission computerized tomography (SPECT) involves scanning using a detector that rotates around the patient, in a manner similar to computerized tomography (CT), but which is sensitive to gamma radiation directly released by radionuclides introduced to the patient's body.

After crossing the intact blood–brain barrier the SPECT radionuclide *N*-isopropyl-[^{123}I]p-iodoamphetamine (IMP) binds to amphetamine receptors on neurons, and has been used to explore cerebral perfusion[54]. A study in ALS identified differences in the fixation of the tracer that correlated with disease severity[55]. Other studies have combined this technique with the detection of CST abnormalities on MRI[56,57]. SPECT also demonstrated potential in delineating patients with cognitive impairment by the study of frontal lobe uptake[58].

Positron emission tomography

PET has the advantage over SPECT in that it has higher image resolution and can more readily provide quantitative data on cerebral changes in ALS[59], based as it is on absolute levels of gamma radioactive emission (indirectly, via positronic decay and annihilation), from an identifiable volume of tissue[60], and furthermore is unrivalled in its sensitivity[61,62].

The PET tracer 2-[^{18}F]2-deoxy-D-glucose (FDG) is used to measure regional changes in cerebral metabolic rate for glucose (rCMRG). The tracers $^{15}O_2$ and $H_2^{15}O$ have been used to study regional cerebral blood flow (rCBF), and this has permitted so-called 'activation' studies. The development of radioligands has raised the possibility of identifying changes in specific neurochemical and cellular systems (Table 3.3).

Positron emission tomography studies of cerebral metabolism in amyotrophic lateral sclerosis

Dalakas and colleagues published the first PET study in ALS using FDG[63]. The authors concluded that subjects with UMN signs (i.e. classical ALS) showed significantly decreased uptake of FDG in most cortical areas, and in the brainstem and basal ganglia, compared to normal controls. Subjects with only LMN signs showed no significant changes. In a follow-up study of the same group, Hatazawa and colleagues found that the greatest reduction in FDG uptake was in the sensorimotor cortex and putamen, but that smaller decreases were present in other areas in ALS subjects[64]. Such changes were not apparent in subjects with LMN signs only, nor in subjects with the post-poliomyelitis syndrome. These observations suggested that cerebral dysfunction in ALS might be more widespread than previously thought.

A study by Ludolph and colleagues cemented the view of ALS as a multi-system cerebral disorder with extramotor involvement[65]. Using FDG,

Table 3.3 Positron emission tomography tracers that have been used particularly in the field of neurosciences (adapted from reference 60)

Parameter	Tracer/ligand
Blood flow	$H_2[^{15}O]$, $C[^{15}O]_2$
Blood volume	$[^{11}C]O$, $C[^{15}O]$
Oxygen extraction	Combination
Glucose metabolism	2-[^{18}F]2-deoxy-D-glucose
Tumor metabolism	[^{11}C]-amino acids, 2-[^{18}F]2-deoxy-D-glucose
Receptor measurements	[^{11}C]methylspiperon, [^{11}C]raclopride, [^{18}F]DOPA, [^{18}F]carazolol, [^{11}C]flumazenil, [^{11}C](R)PK11195, [^{11}C]WAY100635
Stimulus research	$H_2[^{15}O]$, 2-[^{18}F]2-deoxy-D-glucose

they studied 18 ALS subjects and 14 controls and found significantly reduced rCMRG throughout the entire cortex, more focally in frontal and occipital areas. Trends towards reduced rCMRG were also seen in the caudate nucleus and thalamus. They did not specifically detect reduced rCMRG in the motor cortex, but their ROI for the frontal area did not specifically include the motor cortex. In addition to PET, the group carried out detailed neuropsychological assessments in 17 ALS subjects as well as the 14 controls and noted marked deficits in tests of verbal and nonverbal fluency. There was positive correlation between reduced rCMRG in the whole cortex, thalamus and caudate nucleus, and errors in the verbal fluency test scores, supporting the view that the cognitive changes reflected frontal changes. The analytical approaches available were subject to several potential errors, including the effects of (unquantified) cerebral atrophy, multiple comparisons and inevitable assumptions about the kinetic modeling of FDG uptake in the diseased brain.

A later study examined rCBF and cerebral metabolic rate for oxygen (rCMRO$_2$) in ALS patients with and without dementia compared to controls, using $^{15}O_2$ and $C^{15}O_2$[66]. Both parameters were significantly decreased in those patients with progressive dementia compared to ALS patients without evidence of cognitive impairment.

Against these conclusions, Hoffman and colleagues noted reductions in rCMRG in several areas of their ALS subjects, but these were no longer significant after correction for multiple comparisons[67]. They noted positive correlations between UMN dysfunction and reduced rCMRG, but, paradoxically, in the SMAs there seemed to be an increase in rCMRG associated with deteriorating function. There was no overall correlation between duration or severity of disease and rCMRG. They concluded that there were no widespread changes of rCMRG in ALS, and pointed out that patient selection, nutritional status and severity of disease might account for the differences between their own and previous studies.

Positron emission tomography activation studies

Activation studies have the potential to explore the possibility that characteristic changes in brain function in disease might be more evident during brain activity than at rest. This approach has been widely applied to the study of cognitive function and to the study of brain plasticity following damage[68-73]. Although brain activation studies can in theory be performed using FDG, the use of $C^{15}O_2$ or better, $H_2^{15}O$, offers greater flexibility in designing experiments. Unlike FDG, these latter radiotracers enable one to measure rCBF repeatedly over a shorter time, which permits the repetition of specific motor or cognitive tasks.

Kew and colleagues used a simple motor paradigm (developed by Deiber, Playford and colleagues[72,74]), in which the ALS and control subjects were asked to move a joy-stick either in a specified direction (the 'stereotyped task'), or according to their own choice (the 'free selection task')[75,76]. The latter task is more effective in activating prefrontal regions. $C^{15}O_2$ was used as the tracer for rCBF measurements[77]. Data analysis methods dealt with many of the difficulties and

uncertainties of the initial PET studies[78-80], although co-registration with MRI was not available at that time. The process yielded statistical parametric maps representing ALS versus controls, rest versus activation, and stereotyped task versus free selection task. Mean adjusted change in rCBF (ml/100 g tissue/minute) was also measured in different brain areas in relation to stereotactic coordinates, to give z-scores for each location in order to estimate the magnitude as well as the significance of rCBF changes.

In the first study of 12 ALS subjects and six controls[75], the following changes were observed in ALS subjects compared to controls:

(1) Decreases in resting rCBF were present in premotor, motor, parietal and insular cortex.

(2) During activation with the stereotyped task, significant increases in rCBF were present in the 'face area' (but not the arm and hand area) of the contralateral motor cortex in ALS subjects compared to controls, and in several other areas including the contralateral ventral premotor cortex, the contralateral anterior insula and the ipsilateral anterior cingulate cortex.

(3) With the free selection task, overall increases in rCBF were greater in ALS subjects compared to controls, and focal increases were also more marked than with the stereotyped task.

(4) For the whole brain, the overall changes in rCBF comparing the stereotyped and free selection tasks were not significant between ALS and control subjects. However, impaired responses to activation were detected in three areas. These were the medial prefontal cortex (anterior cingulate area), the parahippocampal gyrus and retrosplenial cortex areas.

Subsequently, in a comparative study in patients with PMA, the link between the presence of UMN signs and cortical impairment was confirmed – the increased activation of the motor face area (the 'boundary shift effect') was not seen in patients with LMN syndromes and comparable weakness, suggesting that the change was not simply a consequence of limb weakness[81]. Subsequent neuroimaging studies using other techniques (see below) have also demonstrated that measures of UMN involvement clinically seem to correlate with cerebral changes[82–84]. The boundary shift effect is of potential interest in understanding mechanisms of cortical damage, as it might be related to increased excitatory or decreased inhibitory activity within the motor cortex.

Subsequent studies explored the relationship between impaired activation of prefrontal and limbic areas and cognitive changes, especially abnormal verbal fluency[75,85]. These showed that impaired activation of prefrontal regions was indeed associated with abnormal verbal fluency.

Positron emission tomography ligand studies

Early PET ligand studies detected abnormalities of dopamine systems in ALS using [^{18}F]6-fluorodopa[86,87], presumably reflecting the subtle loss of substantia nigra dopamine neurons that is known to occur in ALS[88,89]. Other ligands linked to this transmitter system, such as [^{11}C]raclopride, offer little prospect of providing a useful marker of neuronal degeneration, since nigro-striatal damage appears to be minimal in most cases of ALS, outside the bounds of the combined neurodegenerative 'ALS-plus' disease such as that found on Guam.

Flumazenil

Flumazenil binds to the benzodiazepine subunit of the γ-amino butyric acid (GABA)$_A$ receptor present on neurons throughout the cerebral cortex. [^{11}C]flumazenil PET therefore provides a marker for cortical neuronal loss or dysfunction. It may also reflect altered GABAergic inhibitory function.

A pilot study in sporadic ALS indicated significant and widespread motor and extramotor cortical [^{11}C]flumazenil binding decreases compared with healthy controls[90]. In a larger study, possibly with a more homogeneous group of 24 sporadic ALS patients, the decreases in [^{11}C]flumazenil

binding were more consistently localized to motor cortex, posterior motor association, and premotor regions[83] (Figure 3.7a). In this latter study, the degree of UMN involvement – measured using a clinical 'UMN score' – correlated with widespread and marked cortical decreases over the dominant hemisphere.

[^{11}C]PK11195

The ligand PK11195 (1-[2-chlorophenyl]-N-methyl-N-[1-methyl-propyl]-3-isoquinolone carboxamide) binds specifically to the 'peripheral benzodiazepine binding site' (PBBS). The PBBS is expressed by mitochondria in cells of the mononuclear phagocyte lineage and within the central nervous system is highly expressed by activated, though not resting, microglia – the brain's intrinsic population of tissue macrophages. The entantiomeric PET ligand [^{11}C](R)-PK11195 can therefore be used to measure microglial activation in acute and chronic inflammatory, and non-inflammatory, brain disease[91]. It has been used as a sensitive *in vivo* marker of active disease in a variety of acute and slowly progressive neurologic conditions, including stroke[92–94], herpes encephalitis[95], Rassmussen's encephalitis[96], Alzheimer's disease and frontotemporal dementia[97,98], multiple system atrophy[99], corticobasal degeneration[100] and in multiple sclerosis, where it correlated with disability and neuropathological findings[101].

Microglial cell activation has been implicated in the pathogenesis of several neurodegenerative disorders[102,103]. There is evidence that inflammatory mechanisms, in which microglial cells may play a central role, are important mediators of cell death or survival in neurodegenerative diseases[104], specifically in ALS[105–107]. Moreover, drugs aimed at inflammatory pathways have beneficial effects on survival of transgenic mouse models of ALS[108,109]. There are also a number of emerging hypotheses concerning selective motoneuronal cell death, in which microglia may have the central role[110–112].

In a study of ten sporadic ALS patients compared with controls, [^{11}C](R)-PK11195 demonstrated evidence of widespread microglial

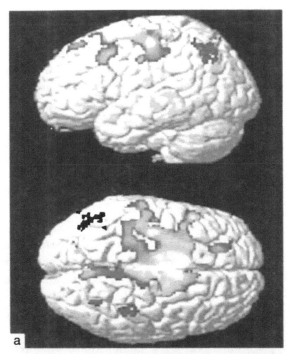

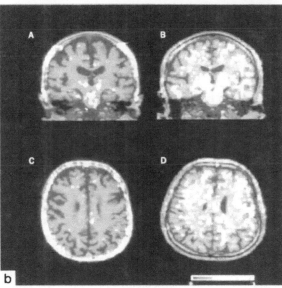

Figure 3.7 (a) [¹¹C]flumazenil positron emission tomography (PET) showing areas of significantly decreased ligand binding in amyotrophic lateral sclerosis (ALS) subjects compared to controls. (Reproduced from reference 83 with permission of the authors and by courtesy of the publishers and editor of *Brain*. (b) [¹¹C]PK11195 PET. Coronal (A,D) and axial (B,D) slices showing markedly increased ligand binding in anterior cortical areas and along corticospinal tracts in ALS subjects (B,D) compared to controls (A,D). (Reproduced with permission from reference 82). See also Plate 6

activation in both motor (pons and motor cortex) and extramotor (dorsolateral prefrontal cortex, thalamus) areas (Figure 3.7b). Overall the changes were surprisingly rather 'low grade' compared to other patient groups studied with this ligand. However, once again the UMN score clinically was highly correlated with the degree of cerebral change, strikingly within the motor cortex and thalamus using this ligand. In a study involving a single patient with definite primary lateral sclerosis and lateralized involvement clinically, there was a very striking uptake of [¹¹C](R)-PK11195 within the motor cortex contralateral to the clinical signs[113].

Regionally increased PK11195 binding does not necessarily imply the presence of ameboid or phagocytic microglia/brain macrophages, but may also indicate active tissue responses to disconnection, in retrograde, anterograde or trans-synaptic projection areas[101,114]. While in these areas, activated microglia do not herald overt destructive tissue pathology, they may render these regions susceptible to secondary recruitment of peripheral blood-borne inflammatory cells, as has been demonstrated in models of motoneuron injury[115,116]. Such remote activation of microglia may potentially be responsible for secondary progressive brain pathology extending beyond the initially affected neural system. One example of an area with secondary, remote activation of microglia might be in the thalamus. Although concerned with the integration of sensory information, its reciprocal connections with multiple cortical areas[117] may account for the significant microglial activation demonstrated in this study[82]. Indeed, neurodegeneration in the thalamus is noted to be amongst the earliest features of the wobbler mouse model of ALS[118]. The significant correlation between thalamic microglial activation and UMN burden clinically seen in the PET study may therefore reflect its connectivity with motor pathways.

[¹¹C]WAY100635

The localization of the serotonin (5-hydroxytryptamine) 5-HT$_{1A}$ receptor on pyramidal neurons[119], which are found throughout the neocortex, makes this receptor a potential marker of motor and extramotor cerebral involvement in ALS[120]. WAY100635, (N-[2-[4-(2-methoxyphenyl)-1-piperazinyl]ethyl]-N-(2-pyridinyl)-cyclohexane carboxamide), is a selective ligand for the serotonin 5-HT$_{1A}$ receptor[121], and [^{11}C]WAY100635 PET is a sensitive marker of *in vivo* 5-HT$_{1A}$ receptor binding[122].

In a study of 21 non-depressed sporadic ALS patients compared with controls, a marked reduction (21%) in both the global cortical and raphe binding of [^{11}C]WAY100635 in ALS patients was seen[84]. A ROI analysis including all cortical regions demonstrated reductions in binding ranging from 16 to 29% compared with the control group, and trends to greater reductions in those patients with bulbar involvement. Statistical Parametric Mapping (SPM, Wellcome Department of Cognitive Neurology) revealed that the greatest differences between sporadic ALS cases and controls lay in frontotemporal regions, cingulate and lateral precentral gyri. The reductions in binding were not related to depression or other drug use.

It is postulated that the reduction of cortical 5-HT$_{1A}$ receptor binding in sporadic ALS represents loss of, or damage to, neurons bearing these receptors, with the possibility that these reductions reflect alterations in receptor expression or function. In respect of the latter, this might relate to control of motorneuronal excitability, cognitive or neurotrophic functions.

THE INFLUENCE OF GENOTYPE ON THE CEREBRAL LESION

Of ALS cases, 5–10% are associated with mutations of the superoxide dismutase-1 (*SOD1*) gene on chromosome 21[123–125]. Most of the 109 known *SOD1* gene mutations are associated with variable phenotypes, a survival period typically in the order of 1–4 years (as for sporadic cases), and are inherited dominantly[124]. The D90A *SOD1* gene mutation is usually inherited as a recessive trait.

Homozygous patients (homD90A) show a characteristic and predictable phenotype beginning with lower limb spasticity and paresis prior to upper limb and bulbar involvement, with slow progression and long survival – averaging 14 years[126]. The disease has a high penetrance in homozygotes[127]. D90A patients worldwide have been shown to share a common founder some 18 000 years ago. To explain this paradox the existence of a linked disease-modifying factor has been postulated, although the D90A *SOD1* mutation may simply be less toxic than others[126–129].

The cerebral lesion has been studied in a group of homD90A ALS patients with a sporadic ALS group of similar disability, both compared with healthy controls. Whilst a comparative study using DT-MRI did not detect significant differences in CST involvement between the sporadic and homD90A patient groups[130], studies with [^{11}C]flumazenil PET demonstrated that reductions in cortical ligand binding compared with healthy controls appeared to be more frontally located in the homD90A group including the frontotemporal junction. Moreover, in a study of two 'at risk' healthy subjects, homozygous for the mutation but with no clinical signs, changes were detected in this latter area, raising the possibility (with the caveat of a small study) that cortical changes are among the first and might precede the 'clinical horizon'.

Transcranial magnetic stimulation studies in homD90A patients have demonstrated reduced cortical excitability providing evidence that intracortical inhibitory circuits may be selectively preserved compared to sporadic cases[131,132]. In an attempt to localize where there might be a relative preservation of inhibitory neurons, a direct comparison of homD90A and sporadic patients' [^{11}C] flumazenil binding was made. This revealed a relative preservation of binding in motor and motor-association areas in the homD90A group[132].

These studies comparing groups of patients of similar clinical features and functional disability, one sporadic and the other genetically homogeneous, have begun to unravel the effects of genotype on cerebral involvement in ALS. The limited nature of cortical change seen in the homD90A patients may be critical in determining the delayed progression of disease in this group, or certainly reflect it.

FUTURE DIRECTIONS

Developments in magnetic resonance imaging

MRI offers the hope of relatively cheap, ubiquitous neuroimaging, and recent developments have demonstrated its potential to illuminate cerebral pathogenesis in ALS. One of the most exciting advances lies in the use of so-called 'smart' contrast agents. An example is the ultra-small superparamagnetic iron oxide (USPIO) contrast agent which is taken up by macrophages, and used to visualize their activity after stroke[133]. The blood–brain barrier is thought to remain intact in ALS. Whilst this is an advantage, in that studies using such an agent to study macrophage activity in ALS would not be confounded by contrast 'leakage' rather than direct uptake, there are obvious hurdles to overcome in understanding the dynamics of contrast uptake and transport across this barrier as a result.

Through stronger field strengths and improved segmentation software, MRI offers the potential for improved understanding of cortical atrophy in ALS. The increasing availability of this type of imaging means that longitudinal studies can be more easily performed.

Developments in positron emission tomography

Where PET excels is in its ability to image the brain at the receptor level. Furthermore, the annihilation of positrons into three photons ('three-gamma annihilation') is postulated to be a potential future development in PET that holds the promise of improved resolution if the technical difficulties can be overcome[134]. PET cameras for small animals already exist and there is great potential to study transgenic models of ALS in this way.

The development of novel PET ligands with specificity for receptors that have relevance to pathogenic mechanisms arising from laboratory research can be a useful tool for testing hypotheses generated *in vitro* in the *in vivo* patient setting. A Glu receptor ligand would have potential use in exploring mechanisms of pathologic cortical hyperexcitability, or in studying the actions of the drug riluzole, for example. CNS 5161[135] is a use-dependent *N*-methyl-D-aspartate (NMDA) channel blocker, and [^{11}C]CNS 5161 is under active development as a PET ligand[136,137], with clear potential for study in ALS. Finally, the development of new PET ligands targeting microglial activation, e.g. CGP42112[138], may offer superior visualization of this important potential therapeutic target.

REFERENCES

1. Brooks BR, Miller RG, Swash M, Munsat TL. El Escorial revisited: revised criteria for the diagnosis of amyotrophic lateral sclerosis. Amyotroph Lateral Scler Other Motor Neuron Disord 2000; 1: 293–9
2. Smith MC. Nerve fiber degeneration in the brain in amyotrophic lateral sclerosis. J Neurol Neurosurg Psychiatry 1960; 23: 269–82
3. Charcot JM, Marie P. Deux nouveaux cas de la sclerose laterale amyotrophique suivis d'autopsie. Arch Neurol 1885; 10: 168–86
4. Lawyer T, Netsky MG. Amyotrophic lateral sclerosis. A clinicoanatomic study of 53 cases. Arch Neurol Psychiatry 1953; 69: 171–92
5. Piao YS, Wakabayashi K, Kakita A, et al. Neuropathology with clinical correlations of sporadic amyotrophic lateral sclerosis: 102 autopsy cases examined between 1962 and 2000. Brain Pathol 2003; 13: 10–22
6. Brownell B, Oppenheimer DR, Hughes JT. The central nervous system in motor neurone disease. J Neurol Neurosurg Psychiatry 1970; 33: 338–57

7. Lassek A. The pyramidal tract: Basic considerations of corticospinal neurons. Res Publ Assoc Nerv Ment Disord 1948; 27: 106–28

8. Meyer G. Forms and spatial arrangement of neurons in the primary motor cortex of man. J Comp Neurol 1987; 262: 402–28

9. Davison C. Amyotrophic lateral sclerosis. Origin and extent of the upper motor neuron lesion. Arch Neurol Psychiatry 1941; 46: 1036–56

10. Sasaki S, Iwata M. Immunocytochemical and ultrastructural study of the motor cortex in patients with lower motor neuron disease. Neurosci Lett 2000; 281: 45–8

11. Ince PG, Evans J, Knopp M, et al. Corticospinal tract degeneration in the progressive muscular atrophy variant of ALS. Neurology 2003; 60: 1252–8

12. Kato S, Shaw P, Wood-Allum C, et al. Amyotrophic lateral sclerosis. In: Dickson DW, ed. Neurodegeneration: The Molecular Pathology of Dementia and Movement Disorders. Basel: ISN Neuropath Press, 2003

13. Bruijn LI, Miller TM, Cleveland DW. Unraveling the mechanisms involved in motor neuron degeneration in ALS. Annu Rev Neurosci 2004; 27: 723–49

14. Ellis CM, Simmons A, Dawson J, et al. Distinct hyperintense MRI signal changes in the corticospinal tracts of a patient with motor neuron disease. ALS Other Motor Neuron Disord 1999; 1: 41–4

15. Graham JM, Papadakis N, Evans J, et al. Diffusion tensor imaging for the assessment of upper motor neuron integrity in ALS. Neurology 2004; 63: 2111–19

16. Chou SM. Pathology of motor system disorder. In: Leigh PN, Swash M, eds. Motor Neuron Disease: Biology and Management. London: Springer-Verlag, 1995: 53–118

17. Ellis CM, Suckling J, Amaro E Jr, et al. Volumetric analysis reveals corticospinal tract degeneration and extramotor involvement in ALS. Neurology 2001; 57: 1571–8

18. Abrahams S, Goldstein LH, Suckling J, et al. Frontotemporal white matter changes in amyotrophic lateral sclerosis. J Neurol 2005; 252: 321–31

19. Chang JL, Lomen-Hoerth C, Murphy J, et al. A voxel-based morphometry study of patterns of brain atrophy in ALS and ALS/FTLD. Neurology 2005; 65: 75–80

20. Neil J, Miller J, Mukherjee P, Huppi PS. Diffusion tensor imaging of normal and injured developing human brain – a technical review. NMR Biomed 2002; 15: 543–52

21. Moseley ME. Diffusion tensor imaging and aging – a review. NMR Biomed 2002; 15: 553–60

22. Sotak CH. Nuclear magnetic resonance (NMR) measurement of the apparent diffusion coefficient (ADC) of tissue water and its relationship to cell volume changes in pathological states. Neurochem Int 2004; 45: 569–82

23. Horsfield MA, Jones DK. Applications of diffusion tensor MRI to white matter diseases – a review. NMR Biomed 2002; 15: 570–7

24. Lim KO, Helpern JA. Neuropsychiatric applications of DTI – a review. NMR Biomed 2002; 15: 587–93

25. Segawa F, Kishibayashi J, Kamada K, et al. [MRI of paraventricular white matter lesions in amyotrophic lateral sclerosis – analysis by diffusion-weighted images]. In Japanese. No To Shinkei 1994; 46: 835–40

26. Ellis CM, Simmons A, Jones DK, et al. Diffusion tensor MRI assesses corticospinal tract damage in ALS. Neurology 1999; 53: 1051–8

27. Toosy AT, Werring DJ, Orrell RW, et al. Diffusion tensor imaging detects corticospinal tract involvement at multiple levels in amyotrophic lateral sclerosis. J Neurol Neurosurg Psychiatry 2003; 74: 1250–7

28. Jacob S, Finsterbusch J, Weishaupt JH, et al. Diffusion tensor imaging for long-term follow-up of corticospinal tract degeneration in amyotrophic lateral sclerosis. Neuroradiology 2003; 45: 598–600

29. Sach M, Winkler G, Glauche V, et al. Diffusion tensor MRI of early upper motor neuron involvement in amyotrophic lateral sclerosis. Brain 2004; 127: 340–50

30. Karlsborg M, Rosenbaum S, Wiegell M, et al. Corticospinal tract degeneration and possible pathogenesis in ALS evaluated by MR diffusion tensor imaging. Amyotroph Lateral Scler Other Motor Neuron Disord 2004; 5: 136–40

31. Yin H, Lim CC, Ma L, et al. Combined MR spectroscopic imaging and diffusion tensor MRI visualizes corticospinal tract degeneration in amyotrophic lateral sclerosis. J Neurol 2004; 251: 1249–54

32. Cosottini M, Giannelli M, Siciliano G, et al. Diffusion-tensor MR imaging of corticospinal tract in amyotrophic lateral sclerosis and progressive muscular atrophy. Radiology 2005; 237: 258–64

33. Mori S, Crain BJ, Chacko VP, van Zijl PC. Three dimensional tracking of axonal projections in the brain by magnetic resonance imaging. Ann Neurol 1999; 45: 265–9

34. Basser PJ, Pajevic S, Pierpaoli C, et al. In vivo trac-tography using DT-MRI data. Magn Reson Med 2000; 44: 625–32

35. Conturo TE, Lori NF, Cull TS, et al. Tracking neu-ronal fiber pathways in the living human brain. Proc Natl Acad Sci USA 1999; 96: 10422–7

36. Catani M, Jones DK, Ffytche DH. Perisylvian lan-guage networks of the human brain. Ann Neurol 2005; 57: 8–16

37. Nimsky C, Ganslandt O, Hastreiter P, et al. Preop-erative and intraoperative diffusion tensor imaging-based fiber tracking in glioma surgery. Neuro-surgery 2005; 56: 130–7

38. Jones DK, Catani M, Pierpaoli C, et al. A diffusion tensor magnetic resonance imaging study of frontal cortex connections in very-late-onset schizophrenia-like psychosis. Am J Geriatr Psychiatry 2005; 13: 1092–9

39. Pioro EP, Antel JP, Cashman NR, Arnold DL. Detection of cortical neuron loss in motor neuron disease by proton magnetic resonance spectroscopic imaging in vivo. Neurology 1994; 44: 1933–8

40. Jones AP, Gunawardena WJ, Coutinho CM, et al. Preliminary results of proton magnetic resonance spectroscopy in motor neurone disease (amy-otrophic lateral sclerosis). J Neurol Sci 1995; 129 (Suppl): 85–9

41. Gredal O, Rosenbaum S, Topp S, et al. Quantifica-tion of brain metabolites in amyotrophic lateral sclerosis by localized proton magnetic resonance spectroscopy. Neurology 1997; 48: 878–81

42. Kalra S, Cashman NR, Genge A, Arnold DL. Recovery of N-acetylaspartate in corticomotor neu-rons of patients with ALS after riluzole therapy. Neuroreport 1998; 9: 1757–61

43. Block W, Karitzky J, Traber F, et al. Proton mag-netic resonance spectroscopy of the primary motor cortex in patients with motor neuron disease: Sub-group analysis and follow-up measurements. Arch.Neurol 1998; 55: 931–6

44. Ellis CM, Simmons A, Glover A, et al. Quantitative proton magnetic resonance spectroscopy of the sub-cortical white matter in motor neuron disease. ALS Other Motor Neuron Disord 2000; 1: 123–9

45. Cwik VA, Hanstock CC, Allen PS, Martin WR. Estimation of brainstem neuronal loss in amy-otrophic lateral sclerosis with in vivo proton mag-netic resonance spectroscopy. Neurology 1998; 50: 72–7

46. Catani M, Piccirilli M, Cherubini A, et al. Axonal injury within language network in primary progres-sive aphasia. Ann Neurol 2003; 53: 242–7

47. Logothetis NK, Pfeuffer J. On the nature of the BOLD fMRI contrast mechanism. Magn Reson Imaging 2004; 22: 1517–31

48. Fink GR. Functional MR imaging: From the BOLD effect to higher motor cognition. Clin Neu-rophysiol 2004; 57 (Suppl): 458–68

49. Stephan KE, Harrison LM, Penny WD, Friston KJ. Biophysical models of fMRI responses. Curr Opin Neurobiol 2004; 14: 629–35

50. Nair DG. About being BOLD. Brain Res Brain Res Rev 2005; 50: 229–43

51. Konrad C, Henningsen H, Bremer J, et al. Pattern of cortical reorganization in amyotrophic lateral sclerosis: A functional magnetic resonance imaging study. Exp Brain Res 2002; 143: 51–6

52. Schoenfeld MA, Tempelmann C, Gaul C, et al. Functional motor compensation in amyotrophic lateral sclerosis. J Neurol 2005; 252: 944–52

53. Abrahams S, Goldstein LH, Simmons A, et al. Word retrieval in amyotrophic lateral sclerosis: a functional magnetic resonance imaging study. Brain 2004; 127: 1507–17

54. Nishizawa S, Tanada S, Yonekura Y, et al. Regional dynamics of N-isopropyl-(123I)p-iodoampheta-mine in human brain. J Nucl Med 1989; 30: 150–6

55. Ludolph AC, Elger CE, Bottger IW, et al. N-iso-propyl-p-123I-amphetamine single photon emis-sion computer tomography in motor neuron dis-ease. Eur Neurol 1989; 29: 255–60

56. Udaka F, Sawada H, Seriu N, et al. MRI and SPECT findings in amyotrophic lateral sclerosis. Demonstration of upper motor neurone involve-ment by clinical neuroimaging. Neuroradiology 1992; 34: 389–93

57. Waragai M, Takaya Y, Hayashi M. Serial MRI and SPECT in amyotrophic lateral sclerosis: A case report. J Neurol Sci 1997; 148: 117–20

58. Abe K, Fujimura H, Toyooka K, et al. Single-pho-ton emission computed tomographic investigation of patients with motor neuron disease. Neurology 1993; 43: 1569–73

59. Turner MR, Leigh PN. Positron emission tomogra-phy (PET) – its potential to provide surrogate markers in ALS. Amyotroph Lateral Scler Other Motor Neuron Disord 2000; 1 (Suppl 2): S17–22

60. Paans AM. Positron emission tomography: Back-ground, possibilities and perspectives in neuro-science. Acta Neurol Belg 1997; 97: 150–3

61. Jones T. The role of positron emission tomography within the spectrum of medical imaging. Eur J Nucl Med 1996; 23: 207–11

62. Herholz K, Heiss WD. Positron emission tomography in clinical neurology. Mol Imag Biol 2004; 6; 239–69

63. Dalakas MC, Hatazawa J, Brooks RA, Di Chiro G. Lowered cerebral glucose utilization in amyotrophic lateral sclerosis. Ann Neurol 1987; 22: 580–6

64. Hatazawa J, Brooks RA, Dalakas MC, et al. Cortical motor–sensory hypometabolism in amyotrophic lateral sclerosis: A PET study. J Comput Assist Tomogr 1988; 12: 630–6

65. Ludolph AC, Langen KJ, Regard M, et al. Frontal lobe function in amyotrophic lateral sclerosis: A neuropsychologic and positron emission tomography study. Acta Neurol Scand 1992; 85: 81–9

66. Tanaka M, Kondo S, Hirai S, et al. Cerebral blood flow and oxygen metabolism in progressive dementia associated with amyotrophic lateral sclerosis. J Neurol Sci 1993; 120: 22–8

67. Hoffman JM, Mazziotta JC, Hawk TC, Sumida R. Cerebral glucose utilization in motor neuron disease. Arch Neurol 1992; 49: 849–54

68. Colebatch JG, Deiber MP, Passingham RE, et al. Regional cerebral blood flow during voluntary arm and hand movements in human subjects. J Neurophysiol 1991; 65: 1392–401

69. Chollet F, DiPiero V, Wise RJ, et al. The functional anatomy of motor recovery after stroke in humans: A study with positron emission tomography. Ann Neurol 1991; 29: 63–71

70. Frith CD, Friston KJ, Liddle PF, Frackowiak RS. PET imaging and cognition in schizophrenia. J R Soc Med 1992; 85: 222–4

71. Liddle PF, Friston KJ, Frith CD, Frackowiak RS. Cerebral blood flow and mental processes in schizophrenia. J R Soc Med 1992; 85: 224–7

72. Playford ED, Jenkins IH, Passingham RE, et al. Impaired activation of frontal areas during movement in Parkinson's disease: A PET study. Adv Neurol 1993; 60: 506–10

73. Weiller C, Chollet F, Friston KJ, et al. Functional reorganization of the brain in recovery from striatocapsular infarction in man. Ann Neurol 1992; 31: 463–72

74. Deiber MP, Passingham RE, Colebatch JG, et al. Cortical areas and the selection of movement: a study with positron emission tomography. Exp Brain Res 1991; 84: 393–402

75. Kew JJ, Goldstein LH, Leigh PN, et al. The relationship between abnormalities of cognitive function and cerebral activation in amyotrophic lateral sclerosis. A neuropsychological and posi-

tron emission tomography study. Brain 1993; 116: 1399–423

76. Kew JJ, Leigh PN, Playford ED, et al. Cortical function in amyotrophic lateral sclerosis. A positron emission tomography study. Brain 1993; 116: 655–80

77. Lammertsma AA, Cunningham VJ, Deiber MP, et al. Combination of dynamic and integral methods for generating reproducible functional CBF images. J Cereb Blood Flow Metab 1990; 10: 675–86

78. Friston KJ, Passingham RE, Nutt JG, et al. Localisation in PET images: Direct fitting of the intercommissural (AC-PC) line. J Cereb Blood Flow Metab 1989; 9: 690–5

79. Friston KJ, Frith CD, Liddle PF, Frackowiak RS. Plastic transformation of PET images. J Comput Assist Tomogr 1991; 15: 634–9

80. Friston KJ, Frith CD, Liddle PF, Frackowiak RS. Comparing functional (PET) images: The assessment of significant change. J Cereb Blood Flow Metab 1991; 11: 690–9

81. Kew JJ, Brooks DJ, Passingham RE, et al. Cortical function in progressive lower motor neuron disorders and amyotrophic lateral sclerosis: A comparative PET study. Neurology 1994; 44: 1101–10

82. Turner MR, Cagnin A, Turkheimer FE, et al. Evidence of widespread cerebral microglial activation in amyotrophic lateral sclerosis: An [(11)C](R)-PK11195 positron emission tomography study. Neurobiol Dis 2004; 15: 601–9

83. Turner MR, Hammers A, Al Chalabi A, et al. Distinct cerebral lesions in sporadic and 'D90A' SOD1 ALS: Studies with [11C]flumazenil PET. Brain 2005; 128: 1323–9

84. Turner MR, Rabiner EA, Hammers A, et al. [11C]-WAY100635 PET demonstrates marked 5-HT1A receptor changes in sporadic ALS. Brain 2005; 128: 896–905

85. Abrahams S, Goldstein LH, Kew JJ, et al. Frontal lobe dysfunction in amyotrophic lateral sclerosis. A PET study. Brain 1996; 119: 2105–20

86. Snow BJ, Peppard RF, Guttman M, et al. Positron emission tomographic scanning demonstrates a presynaptic dopaminergic lesion in Lytico-Bodig. The amyotrophic lateral sclerosis–parkinsonism–dementia complex of Guam. Arch Neurol 1990; 47: 870–4

87. Takahashi H, Snow BJ, Bhatt MH, et al. Evidence for a dopaminergic deficit in sporadic amyotrophic lateral sclerosis on positron emission scanning. Lancet 1993; 342: 1016–18

88. Burrow JN, Blumbergs PC. Substantia nigra degeneration in motor neurone disease: A quantitative study. Aust NZ J Med 1992; 22: 469–72

89. Kato S, Oda M, Tanabe H. Diminution of dopaminergic neurons in the substantia nigra of sporadic amyotrophic lateral sclerosis. Neuropathol Appl Neurobiol 1993; 19: 300–4

90. Lloyd CM, Richardson MP, Brooks DJ, et al. Extramotor involvement in ALS: PET studies with the GABA(A) ligand [(11)C]flumazenil. Brain 2000; 12: 2289–96

91. Banati RB. Visualising microglial activation in vivo. Glia 2002; 40: 206–17

92. Pappata S, Levassseur M, Gunn RN, et al. Thalamic microglial activation in ischaemic stroke patients detected in vivo by PET and [11C]PK11195. Neurology 2000; 55: 1052–4

93. Gerhard A, Neumaier B, Elitok E, et al. In vivo imaging of activated microglia using [11C]PK11195 and positron emission tomography in patients after ischemic stroke. Neuroreport 2000; 11: 2957–60

94. Gerhard A, Schwarz J, Myers R, et al. Evolution of microglial activation in patients after ischemic stroke: a [(11)C](R)-PK11195 PET study. Neuroimage 2005; 24: 591–5

95. Cagnin A, Myers R, Gunn RN, et al. In vivo visualization of activated glia by [11C] (R)-PK11195-PET following herpes encephalitis reveals projected neuronal damage beyond the primary focal lesion. Brain 2001; 124: 2014–27

96. Banati RB, Goerres GW, Myers R, et al. [11C](R)-PK11195 positron emission tomography imaging of activated microglia in vivo in Rasmussen's encephalitis. Neurology 1999; 53: 2199–203

97. Cagnin A, Brooks DJ, Kennedy AM, et al. In-vivo measurement of activated microglia in dementia. Lancet 2001; 358: 461–7

98. Cagnin A, Rossor M, Sampson EL, et al. In vivo detection of microglial activation in frontotemporal dementia. Ann Neurol 2004; 56: 894–7

99. Gerhard A, Banati RB, Goerres GB, et al. [11C](R)-PK11195 PET imaging of microglial activation in multiple system atrophy. Neurology 2003; 61: 686–9

100. Gerhard A, Watts J, Trender-Gerhard I, et al. In vivo imaging of microglial activation with [(11)C](R)-PK11195 PET in corticobasal degeneration. Mov Disord 2004; 19: 1221–6

101. Banati RB, Newcombe J, Gunn RN, et al. The peripheral benzodiazepine binding site in the brain in multiple sclerosis: Quantitative in vivo imaging of microglia as a measure of disease activity. Brain 2000; 123: 2321–37

102. McGeer PL, Kawamata T, Walker DG, et al. Microglia in degenerative neurological disease. Glia 1993; 7: 84–92

103. McGeer PL, McGeer, EG. Glial cell reactions in neurodegenerative diseases: pathophysiology and therapeutic interventions. Alzheimer Dis Assoc Disord 1998; 12 (Suppl 2): S1–6

104. Perry VH. The influence of systemic inflammation on inflammation in the brain: Implications for chronic neurodegenerative disease. Brain Behav Immun 2004; 18: 407–13

105. McGeer PL, McGeer EG. Inflammatory processes in amyotrophic lateral sclerosis. Muscle Nerve 2002; 26: 459–70

106. Kriz J, Nguyen M, Julien J. Minocycline slows disease progression in a mouse model of amyotrophic lateral sclerosis. Neurobiol Dis 2002; 10: 268

107. Ferri A, Nencini M, Casciati A, et al. Cell death in amyotrophic lateral sclerosis: Interplay between neuronal and glial cells. FASEB J 2004; 18: 1261–3

108. Zhu S, Stavrovskaya IG, Drozda M, et al. Minocycline inhibits cytochrome c release and delays progression of amyotrophic lateral sclerosis in mice. Nature 2002; 417: 74–8

109. Drachman DB, Frank K, Dykes-Hoberg M, et al. Cyclooxygenase 2 inhibition protects motor neurons and prolongs survival in a transgenic mouse model of ALS. Ann Neurol 2002; 52: 771–8

110. Ciesielski-Treska J, Ulrich G, Chasserot-Golaz S, et al. Mechanisms underlying neuronal death induced by chromogranin A-activated microglia. J Biol Chem 2001; 276: 13113–20

111. Raoul C, Estevez AG, Nishimune H, et al. Motoneuron death triggered by a specific pathway downstream of Fas. potentiation by ALS-linked SOD1 mutations. Neuron 2002; 35: 1067–83

112. Tortarolo M, Veglianese P, Calvaresi N, et al. Persistent activation of p38 mitogen-activated protein kinase in a mouse model of familial amyotrophic lateral sclerosis correlates with disease progression. Mol Cell Neurosci 2003; 23: 180–92

113. Turner MR, Gerhard A, Al-Chalabi A, et al. Mills' and other isolated upper motor neuron syndromes: In vivo study with [11C]-PK11195 PET. J Neurol Neurosurg Psychiatry 2005; 76: 871–4

114. Banati RB. Brain plasticity and microglia: Is transsynaptic glial activation in the thalamus after limb denervation linked to cortical plasticity and

central sensitisation? J Physiol Paris 2002; 96: 289–99

115. Flugel A, Bradl M, Kreutzberg GW, Graeber MB. Transformation of donor-derived bone marrow precursors into host microglia during autoimmune CNS inflammation and during the retrograde response to axotomy. J Neurosci Res 2001; 66: 74–82

116. Raivich G, Jones LL, Kloss CU, et al. Immune surveillance in the injured nervous system: T-lymphocytes invade the axotomized mouse facial motor nucleus and aggregate around sites of neuronal degeneration. J Neurosci 1998; 18: 5804–16

117. Behrens TE, Johansen-Berg H, Woolrich MW, et al. Non-invasive mapping of connections between human thalamus and cortex using diffusion imaging. Nat Neurosci 2003; 6: 750–7

118. Rathke-Hartlieb S, Schmidt VC, Jockusch H, et al. Spatiotemporal progression of neurodegeneration and glia activation in the wobbler neuropathy of the mouse. Neuroreport 1999; 10: 3411–16

119. Azmitia EC, Gannon PJ, Kheck NM, Whitaker-Azmitia PM. Cellular localization of the 5-HT1A receptor in primate brain neurons and glial cells. Neuropsychopharmacology 1996; 14: 35–46

120. Azmitia EC. Modern views on an ancient chemical: serotonin effects on cell proliferation, maturation, and apoptosis. Brain Res Bull 2001; 56: 413–24

121. Forster EA, Cliffe IA, Bill DJ, et al. A pharmacological profile of the selective silent 5-HT1A receptor antagonist, WAY-100635. Eur J Pharmacol 1995; 281: 81–8

122. Rabiner EA, Messa C, Sargent PA, et al. A database of [(11)C]WAY-100635 binding to 5-HT(1A) receptors in normal male volunteers: normative data and relationship to methodological, demographic, physiological, and behavioral variables. Neuroimage 2002; 15: 620–32

123. Rosen DR, Siddique T, Patterson D, et al. Mutations in Cu/Zn superoxide dismutase gene are associated with familial amyotrophic lateral sclerosis. Nature 1993; 362: 59–62

124. Andersen PM, Sims KB, Xin WW, et al. Sixteen novel mutations in the Cu/Zn superoxide dismutase gene in amyotrophic lateral sclerosis: A decade of discoveries, defects and disputes. Amyotroph Lateral Scler Other Motor Neuron Disord 2003; 4: 62–73

125. Andersen PM. Genetic aspects of amyotrophic lateral sclerosis/motor neuron disease. In: Shaw PJ, Strong MJ, eds. Motor Neuron Disease. Oxford: Butterworth Heinemann, 2003: 207–36

126. Andersen PM, Forsgren L, Binzer M, et al. Autosomal recessive adult-onset amyotrophic lateral sclerosis associated with homozygosity for Asp90Ala CuZn-superoxide dismutase mutation. A clinical and genealogical study of 36 patients. Brain 1996; 119: 1153–72

127. Andersen PM, Nilsson P, Keranen ML, et al. Phenotypic heterogeneity in motor neuron disease patients with CuZn-superoxide dismutase mutations in Scandinavia. Brain 1997; 120: 1723–37

128. Al-Chalabi A, Andersen PM, Chioza B, et al. Recessive amyotrophic lateral sclerosis families with the D90A SOD1 mutation share a common founder: evidence for a linked protective factor. Hum Mol Genet 1998; 7: 2045–50

129. Parton MJ, Broom W, Andersen PM, et al. D90A-SOD1 mediated amyotrophic lateral sclerosis: A single founder for all cases with evidence for a Cis-acting disease modifier in the recessive haplotype. Hum Mutat 2002; 20: 473

130. Blain CRV, Williams VC, Turner MR, et al. Corticospinal tract damage in patients homozygous for the D90A SOD1 gene mutation compared to sporadic ALS: a diffusion tensor imaging study. Neurology 2005; 64 (6 Suppl 1): A293

131. Weber M, Eisen A, Stewart HG, Andersen PM. Preserved slow conducting corticomotoneuronal projections in amyotrophic lateral sclerosis with autosomal recessive D90A CuZn-superoxide dismutase mutation. Brain 2000; 123: 1505–15

132. Turner MR, Osei-Lah A, Hammers A, et al. Abnormal cortical excitability in sporadic but not homozygous D90A SOD1 ALS. J Neurol Neurosurg Psychiatry 2005; 76: 1279–85

133. Saleh A, Schroeter M, Jonkmanns C, et al. In vivo MRI of brain inflammation in human ischaemic stroke. Brain 2004; 127: 1670–7

134. Kacperski K, Spyrou NM, Smith FA. Three-gamma annihilation imaging in positron emission tomography. IEEE Trans Med Imag 2004; 23: 525–9

135. Hu LY, Guo J, Magar SS, et al. Synthesis and pharmacological evaluation of N-(2,5-disubstituted phenyl)-N'-(3-substituted phenyl)-N'-methyl-guanidines as N-methyl-D-aspartate receptor ion-channel blockers. J Med Chem 1997; 40: 4281–9

136. Hammers A, Asselin MC, Brooks DJ, et al. Correlation of memory function with binding of [11C]CNS 5161, a novel putative NMDA ion

channel PET ligand. Neuroimage 2004; 22 (Suppl 2): T54

137. Asselin MC, Hammers A, Turton DR, et al. Initial kinetic analyzes of the in vivo binding of the putative NMDA receptor ligand [11C]CNS 5161 in humans. Neuroimage 2004; 22 (Suppl 2): T137

138. Roulston CL, Lawrence AJ, Jarrott B, Widdop RE. Non-angiotensin II [(125)I] CGP42112 binding is a sensitive marker of neuronal injury in brainstem following unilateral nodose ganglionectomy: Comparison with markers for activated microglia. Neuroscience 2004; 127: 753–67

4

Motor unit number estimation in amyotrophic lateral sclerosis

Devanand Jillapalli, Jeremy M Shefner

INTRODUCTION

Progressive loss of motor units over time is a defining characteristic of amyotrophic lateral sclerosis (ALS). Documentation of this progressive loss through a non-invasive, potentially repeatable measure is desirable for many reasons. Such a measure could provide information about disease severity at the time of patient presentation, and could be used to follow disease progression either as a routine clinical tool or in the context of an experimental trial. Although clinical neurophysiologic techniques have played a critical role in the diagnosis of ALS, they have had limited success in assessing disease progression. Results of routine nerve conduction studies and needle electromyography do reflect the number of functioning motor units, but are rendered relatively insensitive by the physiologic compensatory mechanisms of peripheral reinnervation. Motor unit number estimation (MUNE) techniques attempt to measure the number of motor units in a muscle. To the extent that MUNE provides a valid measure of the number of functioning motor units and can be performed reliably and reproducibly it is a valuable tool for prognosis and disease assessment, both in the clinic and in the experimental setting.

MUNE was first performed in 1965, when McPhedran *et al.* measured the twitch tension of single motor units and the maximal tension in the soleus muscle of the cat[1]. MUNE was first performed in human subjects in 1971[2], but it was not until 20 years later that neurophysiologists showed serious interest in its potential to follow the course of diseases where motor units are lost over time. In the past 15 years, MUNE has provided a wealth of information regarding the properties of single motor units in health, normal aging and neurogenic disease. In addition to providing a metric for the average number of motor units and the average surface-recorded single motor unit potential (SMUP) size in a muscle, MUNE has enabled quantitative serial assessment of motor unit decline and concomitant SMUP size increase in aging and in the progression of diseases where there is motor unit loss over time. It has furthered the understanding of physiologic and mechanical properties of motor units in health and disease states characterized by motor unit loss. In addition, MUNE is increasingly used as an outcome measure in clinical trials designed to halt or slow the loss of motor units.

This chapter examines the different methods of MUNE, their advantages and limitations. In addition, the utility of MUNE in understanding the electrophysiologic characteristics of motor units, assessing the various clinical aspects of ALS including severity and progression, and the role of MUNE as an outcome measure in clinical trials is discussed.

METHODS OF MOTOR UNIT NUMBER ESTIMATION AND COMPARISION OF DIFFERENT METHODS

The concept of obtaining a motor unit number estimate is remarkably simple. First, a maximal response is evoked from the muscle that is being studied. Most MUNE techniques employ electrical stimulation; less commonly, force measurements are used to obtain a maximal response. Second, the average size of the constituent motor units in that muscle is obtained. MUNE techniques differ in the way the single motor units are sampled to calculate the average size of a single motor unit. Last, the maximal response is divided by the average size of the single motor unit to yield the functioning number of motor units in that muscle. Each MUNE technique is associated with important theoretical assumptions and practical limitations. Several methods have been developed, but of these, the incremental technique, multiple point stimulation technique (MPS), F-wave technique (F-MUNE), spike-triggered averaging technique (STA) and the statistical method of MUNE are the most widely used. All techniques continue to evolve to address perceived limitations. Since the incremental technique, MPS, F-MUNE and statistical MUNE methods use electrical stimulation delivered percutaneously to excite motor units, they are classified as 'stimulation MUNE techniques'. In contrast, motor units in STA are activated volitionally and therefore the STA method is classified as a 'voluntary MUNE technique'.

Methods of motor unit number estimation

The incremental technique

This technique is the originally described MUNE method, and is applicable to the study of small muscles in either the hands or the feet[2]. A maximum compound motor action potential (CMAP) is recorded in response to supramaximal stimulation of the nerve innervating the muscle being recorded. Starting from a subthreshold value, stimulus strength is then gradually increased until an initial all-or-none potential is recorded. This potential is taken to be the response of the single lowest threshold motor unit; with gradual increases in stimulus intensity, 11 successive incremental responses are obtained. Each increment is taken to represent the addition of another single motor unit. The number (11) of component quantal increments is divided into submaximal CMAP to derive the average motor unit size. The average motor unit size is then divided into the supramaximal CMAP to yield the MUNE.

A crucial assumption of the incremental method is that each response increment resulting from graded stimulation represents the addition of a single motor unit. However, the threshold for a given motor unit is probabilistic rather than absolute[3-5]. Thus, even at lower levels of motor unit threshold, an incremental step could represent either the difference between the amplitudes of the alternation of two or more motor units or the summation of two or more motor units with similar threshold always activated simultaneously, rather than a single motor unit. The net effect is an erroneous estimate of motor units. Another assumption is that the motor units used in the calculation of the average motor unit size are representative of the total population of motor units in the entire muscle. However, several studies have suggested the possibility of a systematic bias in excluding larger motor units with higher threshold, which could overestimate MUNE[3,4,6]. Another potential source of variability in the incremental method, which extends to most of the other methods to be discussed below, is the fact that single motor units in patients with ALS show increased motor unit variability as compared to normal subjects, when subjected to repeated constant electrical stimulation[7]. For the incremental method, this could result in amplitude variation, which is attributed to the addition of single motor units but which in fact could be the result of variable amplitude within individual units.

Modifications of the incremental technique have been made since its original description. Ballantyne and Hansen introduced digital subtraction to evaluate single motor units and eliminate the confounding effect of phase cancellation[8]. Others have used a variety of methods to account for alternation; these methods reduced the MUNE as expected, but in general did not reduce the variability of measurement[4,9].

Multiple point stimulation technique

The multiple point stimulation technique was developed to avoid the problem of alternation associated with the incremental technique. Brown and Milner-Brown in 1976 suggested stimulation at multiple locations along the nerve to obtain a more representative sample of motor units and more importantly to avoid the problem of alternation[3]. In the first description of this technique, Kadrie and colleagues stimulated the median or ulnar nerves at 10–20 different sites from the level of the wrist to the upper arm in normal subjects[10]. At each site, using threshold intensities, a single motor unit was evoked without subresponses. Thus 10–20 single motor units were collected over the length of the nerve. These units were then averaged and divided into the CMAP obtained with supramaximal stimulation to yield an estimate of the motor units.

Like the incremental technique, MPS assumes that the motor potentials evoked with threshold stimulation are single motor units and that the sample of motor units collected is representative of the population of motor units within that muscle. Although prior studies have suggested a relationship between graded electrical stimulation and fiber size[2,9-12], it now appears that the primary determinant of activation to electrical stimulation is the position of the axon in the nerve bundle, with axons close to the stimulus more likely to be activated than those far away[13-16]. That MPS probably provides an unbiased sample is based on observations that there is a wide range of motor unit sizes and latencies, both from individual trials and across subjects; the size distribution of

motor units for individual trials is similar to that for pooled subjects[17,18]. Doherty et al. refined this technique further by developing special software that allowed template subtraction of any stimulus or artifact contained within the null response from single motor units to accurately define these single units[19]. In an attempt to combine the speed of the incremental technique with the advantage of MPS in reducing alternation, Wang and Delwaide developed the 'adapted MPS' technique[20]. They used incremental stimulation at several points along the median nerve but, unlike the original incremental technique, collected 2–3 evoked potentials at any one point. In all they collected about ten single motor units after stimulating at 4–10 sites along the nerve.

F-wave technique

Stashuk et al. described a method of MUNE based on automated analysis of F-waves[21]. The F-wave is a late response due to the re-excitation of a small percentage of motor neurons in the spinal cord in response to antidromic impulses[22]. In the original description of this method[21], F-responses were acquired at stimulus intensities adjusted to evoke M-potentials 10–50% of the supramaximal CMAP by delivering a succession of 300 stimuli at a rate of 2 Hz. Using a computer algorithm, the F-waves were extracted free of the positively displaced baseline. From among these F-waves, a sample of F-waves representing single motor units was automatically selected using the criterion that, for a particular F-wave to be considered as a single motor unit, the F-response must repeat with identical morphology and latency two or more times in 300 stimuli. MUNE was obtained by dividing the supramaximal CMAP by this average motor unit potential size.

An important assumption of this technique is that a sample of single motor units can be identified from a group of F-responses at submaximal stimulus intensities and that this sample is representative of the motor unit population under study. Doherty et al. found that the distribution of single motor units obtained using this method varied widely in size and were similar to those collected from the same subjects using other methods[15,19]. Another potential source of error could be the increased variability of motor units in patients with ALS as compared to normal subjects[7]. This increase in variability can change the morphology of the same F-wave, so that even though it is the same single motor unit occurring twice, it can be erroneously excluded from the computer-generated sample.

Spike-triggered averaging technique

Brown and colleagues described this technique in 1988[23,24]. The fundamental difference of this technique as compared to other MUNE techniques is that the single motor units are evoked by low levels of voluntary contraction and are identified using needle electromyography rather than surface recording. Since motor units are activated by voluntary contraction rather than electrical stimulation, alternation is avoided. In the original description of this technique, two channels were used: one, to record the intramuscular recording of electrical activity; and the other for surface recording of electrical potentials in the biceps-brachialis muscle[23,24]. Low levels of isometric contractions were used to activate a single motor unit. The intramuscular needle electrode was then adjusted to isolate this activated motor unit such that the negative rise time gradient was the steepest and then captured. This captured single motor unit was used as a trigger to time lock the surface-recorded motor unit potentials which then were averaged. This process is repeated in other locations in the muscle to record additional motor units. The mean of at least ten surface-recorded motor potentials is calculated and divided into the supramaximal CMAP to yield an estimate of the number of motor units.

An important assumption is that there is no bias in selection of motor units and that the sample is representative of the population of motor units. Since low levels of voluntary contraction are used to activate motor units, there is the possibility of a systematic bias favoring small motor

units[25]. Using decomposition-enhanced STA applied to the vastus medialis muscle, Conwit et al. showed that average surface-recorded single motor units increased in size as the force level increased from 5% of maximum voluntary contraction to 30%, suggesting that STA performed only at low levels of contraction may result in biased sampling of small motor units[26]. Motor unit decomposition is an evolving technique based on the identification of multiple single motor units in an interference pattern, and has the potential to resolve the issue of sampling bias[27–29]. Yet another important limitation is the increased variability of single motor units in patients with ALS which can cause the same motor unit spike to vary in morphology, making it difficult for triggering[7].

Statistical method

Daube first reported the statistical method of MUNE in an abstract in 1988[30]. Since then several papers have been published improving or utilizing this technique[31–36]. In contrast to other methods of MUNE, the statistical method relies on alternation to estimate single motor unit size and makes no attempt to identify individual motor units. It assumes that multiple submaximal responses to a constant stimulus follow a Poisson distribution. In such a distribution, the variance of the responses directly estimates the size of the motor units firing at this intensity[31,37]. As currently employed, response variability to four different levels of stimulus intensity are measured, then averaged to yield a mean SMUP amplitude[32,35,36]. This value is then divided into the supramaximal CMAP to yield MUNE, to which the number of large motor units separately identified is added to give the MUNE for trial one. The entire procedure is repeated and MUNE values averaged to increase the reproducibility[38,39].

An important assumption of the statistical method is that, in order for the Poisson distribution to apply, motor units with a similar threshold must be the same size, and each unit must have a small probability of being activated by a single stimulus. Neither of these assumptions is likely to be met; however, modeling studies have shown that the technique is relatively robust to both problems. A more significant problem may be that, in patients with ALS, single motor units are much more variable in their individual response amplitudes than are units from normal subjects[7]. For a method that estimates motor unit size based on variable motor unit recruitment, variability in individual motor unit size could constitute a significant confounding factor. A variety of ways to deal with this issue have been proposed[40]; it is not yet certain how successful they will be. However, the statistical method has advantages as well as disadvantages. It estimates motor unit sizes over a wider range of thresholds than any other method of MUNE, reducing the potential for any systematic bias in the selection of motor units with a particular threshold range. With careful training, statistical MUNE is highly reliable with respect to both inter- and intrarater comparisons[40].

Comparisons of individual methods of motor unit number estimation

The best MUNE method is obviously the one that most closely estimates the true number of motor units in a given muscle. Unfortunately, however, such a gold standard has proved elusive. Anatomical counts have been attempted, but are not without assumptions and limitations. The results of several such studies carried out in animals and human subjects reported in the literature are summarized in Table 4.1[2,41–45]. As can be seen, in general, MUNE values obtained by physiologic methods closely match anatomical counts. Average MUNE values for thenar muscles in normal subjects less than age 60 years, pooling data from published sources, were: 270.4 for the incremental method, 151 for STA, 266 for F-wave and 251 for the MPS method[13]. The fact that there is such a close concordance of MUNE values generated by various MUNE methods suggest that, despite the assumptions and limitations discussed above, these methods represent the true number of motor

units in a muscle to a fairly reasonable degree. Since there is no clear gold standard against which the various physiologic methods can be compared, reproducibility of a method becomes very important in evaluating the various methods of MUNE. Studies show higher reproducibility if a second estimate is performed and the two are averaged[34,38,46]. Reproducibility can be increased by enlarging the number of motor units sampled[47]. There are few studies comparing one method of MUNE against another[33,48]. Stein and Yang compared spike-triggered averaging, intramuscular microstimulation of motor nerve branches and graded whole nerve stimulation and two other techniques using average force generated by single units, and concluded that the estimates by the different methods were not statistically different from one another[48].

There is no clear evidence that any one method is far superior to the others. Therefore, practical considerations predominate in the selection of the method to be used in a clinical or experimental situation[13]. The incremental, MPS and STA techniques do not require any special software, unless modifications with template matching are desired. STA requires needle insertion; however, it is a preferred method for proximal muscles[49]. Statistical and automated F-MUNE requires special software that limits the availability of these methods. The statistical method is an automated technique that does not require the degree of operator skill of some of the other methods. Finally, the shortest time to perform MUNE is the incremental method, while the longest is the statistical[13].

MOTOR UNIT NUMBER ESTIMATION STUDIES IN AMYOTROPHIC LATERAL SCLEROSIS PATIENTS AND MODELS

Motor unit loss in amyotrophic lateral sclerosis

A fundamental observation of MUNE studies in ALS is that there is motor unit loss over time[50–54].

Table 4.1 Comparison of anatomical and physiologic estimates of motor units

Study	Subjects	Nerve or spinal cord used in anatomical count	Anatomical count	Physiologic method	Physiologic count
McComas et al. (1971)[2]	Human	Lateral terminal branch of the deep peroneal nerve	323*	Incremental method on EDB	199
Eisen et al. (1974)[43]	Animal	Nerve to rat soleus	30	Incremental method on soleus	33
Lee et al. (1975)[41]	Human	Recurrent motor branch of the median nerve	203	STA on thenar muscles	167
Peyronnard et al. (1977)[44]	Animal	Deep peroneal nerve	153	Incremental method	120
Law et al. (1975)[42]	Animal	Sciatic nerve to soleus	52†	Incremental method Twitch tension	22 22
Arasaki et al. (1997)[45]	Animal	Alpha motor unit in the spinal cord identified by retrograde transport of cholera toxin	103	MPS equivalent	93

EDB, extensor digitorum brevis; STA, spike-triggered averaging; MPS, multiple point stimulation

*One factor for the anatomical estimate to exceed the physiologic estimate is the existence of a nerve branch, which does not terminate in the EDB but runs on to supply the dorsal interosseous muscles

†The axon diameter of these fibers was $\geq 3\,\mu m$, arbitrarily chosen to show the involvement of fibers of all sizes

Though consistent with known pathophysiology, such an observation is not particularly insightful. Muscle atrophy and weakness reflects motor unit loss; however, physiologic compensation in early disease makes clinical assessment insensitive[55]. Classical electrophysiologic methods have been successfully employed to document the presence of disease, but are poor markers of progression. CMAP amplitude may remain normal until up to 50% of motor units are lost due to physiologic compensation[55,56]. Analysis of the recruitment pattern in needle electromyography provides a sensitive but subjective estimate of the number of functioning motor units in a muscle[57]. Fibrillation potentials are a sensitive marker for ongoing denervation, but have not been successfully quantified. In contrast, MUNE assesses the number of functioning motor units in muscle. Because of its quantitative nature, MUNE can be used to follow motor unit loss serially over time. Unlike other physiologic methods, MUNE is not affected by compensatory reinnervation of surviving motor units. Thus, MUNE may allow meaningful assessment of motor unit loss even in the very early stages and over time.

Brown and Jaatoul applied the incremental technique of MUNE at intervals in patients with ALS and controls[50]. They calculated rates of decay of motor units in patients and found a high rate of decay of 175 times the fallout rate of controls, in the initial stages, but that this motor unit fallout slowed once the motor unit count was very low in late stages. Dantes and McComas examined the relationship between MUNE and time interval from the onset of disease using MUNE (incremental method) in 123 patients with ALS[53]. Based on their data, they concluded that, once the disease affects a muscle, the rate of motor unit loss is greatest early in the disease course and diminishes more slowly thereafter (Figure 4.1). Motor unit losses were as frequent in the younger (< 60 years) group of subjects as that of the older. Motor unit losses in ALS are not only seen in the early phases of the disease as described above, but are well documented even in the preclinical or asymptomatic phase of the disease. Aggarwal and Nicholson used the statistical method of MUNE in a longitudinal study of 19 asymptomatic carriers of cytosolic copper/zinc superoxide dismutase (*SOD1*) gene mutation over a 3-year period[54]. At

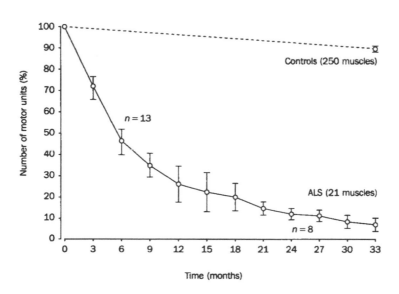

Figure 4.1   Rate of loss of motor units in amyotrophic lateral sclerosis (ALS) patients using incremental motor unit number estimation. (From reference 53, with permission)

the beginning of the study, motor unit numbers in all carriers were not statistically different from those in the *SOD1*-negative family controls[58]. However, in their 3-year follow up, two of these 19 carriers developed motor unit loss (51% in one and 37% in the other) before the onset of symptoms. The fact that motor unit decline occurs well before the onset of symptoms suggests that early treatment may have a significant impact on slowing or even halting motor unit loss.

The transgenic mouse model of ALS has also proved amenable to MUNE. Feeney *et al* investigated the progression of motor unit loss in *SOD1* G93A mice with protracted course of the disease and control mice[59]. No motor unit loss was seen at 70 days of age. The onset of symptoms in these animals began at 196 days of age. They found a biphasic loss of motor neurons: an initial loss occurring at 126 days (in the presymptomatic stage of the disease) followed by a period of stabilization, and a gradual loss during which symptoms began. Shefner *et al* investigated the effect of neurophilin ligands on *SOD1* G93A mice[60]. MUNE dropped by 31% before behavioral abnormalities appeared.

Utility of motor unit number estimation techniques in the study of motor units in amyotrophic lateral sclerosis

Since all MUNE techniques originate with an estimate of an average of individual SMUP size, they are potentially useful in the study of other aspects of ALS progression besides progressive motor unit loss. MUNE studies clearly show a progressive increase in SMUP size as motor unit numbers decline, in both animal models and human disease[50,52,60]. Late in the disease, it is often possible to study giant single motor units in detail. Brown and colleagues followed giant motor units in small hand muscles of ALS patients, and pointed out evidence suggesting incipient neuromuscular junction failure[51,52]. A tendency toward reduction in motor unit size in the very late stages of disease also supports the view that motor unit innervation

is reduced when the motor neuron is close to death[51,59]. Changes in motor unit size may also be a therapeutic target. Shefner *et al* studied transgenic *SOD1* mice treated with a neurophilin ligand, and showed a dose-dependent increase in motor unit size late in disease. This change was not associated with a survival effect, but points to the potential of MUNE to detect changes beyond motor unit numbers[60].

The MPS MUNE technique has also been adapted to the study of individual motor units over time[61]. Gooch and Harati tracked individual motor units in ALS patients with rapidly progressive disease over an 8–12-week period[62]. The amplitudes of each unit remained relatively constant with less than 30% variation between the highest and lowest values. Any trend during that time was toward decreasing motor unit size. Chan *et al* followed two motor units in an ALS patient over a 2-year period and found stable physiologic properties over the 2-year period for one unit while the other unit rapidly declined over a 5-month period[63]. Such longitudinal studies may further our understanding of single motor unit properties including what happens to large motor units prior to death.

Mechanical properties of motor units in amyotrophic lateral sclerosis

Motor unit estimation studies using twitch tensions of single motor units have contributed to the understanding of the mechanical properties of single motor units. Motor unit twitch tension correlates well with voltage recorded on the surface of the muscle for first dorsal interosseous[64,65] and hypothenar[10]. As motor units drop out with ALS disease progression, physiologic compensation by collateral innervation increases both single motor unit size and twitch tensions of single motor units; however, in later stages of ALS, reinnervated motor units become functionally incompetent[65]. It appears that reinnervated motor units with significant fiber grouping are less efficient in force generation than are normally ordered units. Other similar observations of twitch properties of motor units in late stages of ALS confirm that units with large electrical potentials do not necessarily exert the expected increase in force[5]. Very large motor units were observed to have normal twitch tension instead of increased tension and in surviving motor units in later stages there is a decline of twitch tension[5,66]. These observations suggest that, in later stages of the disease process, large motor units become less efficient contractile units and this factor is likely to contribute to clinical muscle weakness.

APPLICATION OF MOTOR UNIT NUMBER ESTIMATION IN CLINICAL TRIALS AND CLINICAL MANAGEMENT OF PATIENTS

Application of motor unit number estimation in clinical trials

To the extent that MUNE accurately assesses the number of functioning motor units, it would seem to be an excellent candidate for a surrogate outcome measure in clinical trials. Felice obtained serial data on 21 patients with ALS using the following variables: MUNE (MPS method), mean thenar SMUP, thenar maximal CMAP, isometric hand grip strength, total Medical Research Council manual muscle testing score, Appel ALS rating scale and forced vital capacity[67]. MUNE showed a significantly higher rate of change than other measures and, in addition, was the most sensitive index for documenting changes in disease progression over time. Bromberg et al., in a cross-sectional study of 31 patients with ALS, compared MUNE with several other measures and showed that MUNE measures were better suited to provide information on the natural history of the disease process and were clinically useful to follow disease progression[68]. In another single-site study, fiber density, CMAP amplitude, MUNE (incremental method) of abductor digiti minimi and grip strength were examined longitudinally in ten patients over a 6-month interval[69]. MUNE and fiber density were more sensitive measures of the

rate of ALS progression than the other measures tested.

To be useful in clinical trials, reproducibility and reliability of MUNE in ALS must be maximized. Using the statistical method, Olney et al. found excellent reproducibility at all levels of disease[34]. Using MPS MUNE, Felice found excellent test–retest reproducibility in ALS patients ($r = 0.99$)[70]. MUNE using STA was more variable than other methods; however, reproducibility increased as patients became weaker[71]. These data suggest that MUNE is a sensitive endpoint measure of disease progression in ALS, highly reproducible and reliable – all attributes quite useful as outcome measures for a clinical trial.

MUNE has been used as an outcome measure in several clinical trials, although most often at single sites[40,49,72-74]. Smith et al. measured MUNE at multiple sites in a trial of recombinant human ciliary neurotrophic factor or placebo[74]. No standardized training, monitoring, or quality assurance methods were put in place; not surprisingly, intersite and intrasite variability was too large to detect even a modest clinical effect (the trial was negative, so that other measures also showed no differences between groups). In contrast, rigorous evaluator training, standards for test–retest reliability and stringent data monitoring were all employed in a recent multicenter clinical trial assessing the safety and efficacy of creatine, for which statistical MUNE was a secondary outcome measure[40]. Evaluator training led to test–retest variability of less than 20% at all 15 participating sites. MUNE dropped by 24% in 6 months, consistent with the rate of decline of other outcome measures. Interpatient variability and the sensitivity of MUNE to detect a small treatment difference were similar to other outcome measures.

Motor unit number estimation in clinical management of amyotrophic lateral sclerosis patients

In addition to its potential utility as an outcome measure in clinical trials, MUNE can be used to assess prognosis in patients with ALS. In a longitudinal study of patients with ALS, Yuen and Olney showed that a greater decline in MUNE identified a group with a worse prognosis[69]. Armon and Brandstater derived linear estimates of rates of disease progression using single MUNE evaluations in predicting patient survival, enabling them to stratify patients into groups based on rate of progression[75,76]. Predictions regarding prognosis can be made even in an individual patient. In one study, the rate of decline in MUNE over a 3-month interval for an individual patient was a significant prognostic factor that was quantitative and measurable[77]. These findings have potential implications in clinical management of patients with ALS.

SUMMARY

Motor unit number estimation is a physiologic method of assessing the number of functioning motor units in a muscle. Several methods have been developed, each with its advantages, assumptions and limitations. Since there is no standard reference method against which these methods can be compared for accuracy, each method is evaluated for reproducibility and compared against one another. Application of MUNE in assessing the physiologic and mechanical properties of motor units in human and animal models of ALS has led to understanding of the rate of motor unit loss, the reinnervation of surviving motor units, increase in motor unit variability and their adaptation in the terminal stages of the disease. Studies have shown that the rate of decline in MUNE can be used for prognosis with implication in the clinical management of patients with ALS. Since MUNE is the most sensitive measure of motor unit loss in the early stages of ALS, long before other clinical and electrophysiologic measures, it is increasingly being used as an endpoint measure in clinical trials.

REFERENCES

1. McPhedran AM, Wuerker RB, Henneman E. Properties of motor units in a homogenous red muscle (soleus) of the cat. J Neurophysiol 1965; 28: 71–84
2. McComas AJ, Fawcett PR, Campbell MJ, Sica RE. Electrophysiological estimation of the number of motor units within a human muscle. J Neurol Neurosurg Psychiatry 1971; 34: 121–31
3. Brown WF, Milner-Brown HS. Some electrical properties of motor units and their effects on the methods of estimating motor unit numbers. J Neurol Neurosurg Psychiatry 1976; 39: 249–57
4. Milner-Brown HS, Brown WF. New methods of estimating the number of motor units in a muscle. J Neurol Neurosurg Psychiatry 1976; 39: 258–65
5. Milner-Brown HS, Stein RB, Lee RG. Contractile and electrical properties of human motor units in neuropathies and motor neuron disease. J Neurol Neurosurg Psychiatry 1974; 37: 670–6
6. Sica RE, McComas AJ, Upton AR, Longmire D. Motor unit estimations in small muscles of the hand. J Neurol Neurosurg Psychiatry 1974; 37: 55–67
7. Jillapalli D, Shefner J. Single motor unit variability with threshold stimulation in patients with amyotrophic lateral sclerosis and normal subjects. Muscle Nerve 2004; 30: 578–84
8. Ballantyne JP, Hansen S. New method for the estimation of the number of motor units in a muscle. 2. Duchenne, limb-girdle and facioscapulohumeral, and myotonic muscular dystrophies. J Neurol Neurosurg Psychiatry 1974; 37: 1195–201
9. Galea V, de Bruin H, Cavasin R, McComas AJ. The numbers and relative sizes of motor units estimated by computer. Muscle Nerve 1991; 14: 1123–30
10. Kadrie HA, Yates SK, Milner-Brown HS, Brown WF. Multiple point electrical stimulation of ulnar and median nerves. J Neurol Neurosurg Psychiatry 1976; 39: 973–85
11. Erlanger J, Gasser H. Electrical Signs of Nervous Activity. Philadelphia, PA: University of Pennsylvania Press, 1937
12. Tasaki I. Electric stimulation and the excitatory process in the nerve fiber. Am J Physiol 1939; 125: 380–95
13. Shefner JM. Motor unit number estimation in human neurological diseases and animal models. Clin Neurophysiol 2001; 112: 955–64
14. Chan KM, Doherty TJ, Andres LP, et al. Longitudinal study of the contractile and electrical properties

of single human thenar motor units. Muscle Nerve 1998; 21: 839–49

15. Doherty TJ, Komori T, Stashuk DW, et al. Physiological properties of single thenar motor units in the F-response of younger and older adults. Muscle Nerve 1994; 17: 860–72

16. McComas AJ. Invited review: motor unit estimation: methods, results, and present status. Muscle Nerve 1991; 14: 585–97

17. Doherty TJ, Brown WF. The estimated numbers and relative sizes of thenar motor units as selected by multiple point stimulation in young and older adults. Muscle Nerve 1993; 16: 355–66

18. Doherty TJ, Stashuk DW, Brown WF. Determinants of mean motor unit size: impact on estimates of motor unit number. Muscle Nerve 1993; 16: 1326–31

19. Doherty T, Stashuk D, Brown W. Multiple point stimulation and F-response MUNE technique. Clin Neurophysiol Suppl 2003; 55: 31–40

20. Wang FC, Delwaide PJ. Number and relative size of thenar motor units estimated by an adapted multiple point stimulation method. Muscle Nerve 1995; 18: 969–79

21. Stashuk DW, Doherty TJ, Kassam A, Brown WF. Motor unit number estimates based on the automated analysis of F-responses. Muscle Nerve 1994; 17: 881–90

22. Fisher MA. AAEM Minimonograph no.13: H reflexes and F waves: physiology and clinical indications. Muscle Nerve 1992; 15: 1223–33

23. Brown WF, Strong MJ, Snow R. Methods for estimating numbers of motor units in biceps-brachialis muscles and losses of motor units with aging. Muscle Nerve 1988; 11: 423–32

24. Strong MJ, Brown WF, Hudson AJ Snow R. Motor unit estimates in the biceps-brachialis in amyotrophic lateral sclerosis. Muscle Nerve 1988; 11: 415–22

25. Henneman E, Somjen G, Carpenter D. Functional significance of cell size in spinal motoneurons. J Neurophysiol 1965; 28: 560–80

26. Conwit RA, Tracy B, Jamison C, et al. Decomposition-enhanced spike-triggered averaging: contraction level effects. Muscle Nerve 1997; 20: 976–82

27. Doherty TJ, Stashuk DW. Decomposition-based quantitative electromyography: methods and initial normative data in five muscles. Muscle Nerve 2003; 28: 204–11

28. Boe SG, Stashuk DW, Doherty TJ. Motor unit number estimation by decomposition-enhanced spike-triggered averaging: Control data, test–retest reliability,

and contractile level effects. Muscle Nerve 2004; 29: 693–9

29. Bromberg M. Spike triggered averaging MUNE technique. Clin Neurophysiol Suppl 2003; 55: 99–107

30. Daube JR. Statistical estimates of number of motor units in thenar and foot muscles in patients with amyotrophic lateral sclerosis or the residual of poliomyelitis. Muscle Nerve 1988; 11: 957–8 (abstr)

31. Daube JR. Estimating the number of motor units in a muscle. J Clin Neurophysiol 1995; 12: 585–94

32. Shefner JM, Jillapalli D, Bradshaw DY. Reducing intersubject variability in motor unit number estimation. Muscle Nerve 1999; 22: 1457–60

33. Lomen-Hoerth C, Olney RK. Comparison of multiple point and statistical motor unit number estimation. Muscle Nerve 2000; 23: 1525–33

34. Olney RK, Yuen EC, Engstrom JW. Statistical motor unit number estimation: Reproducibility and sources of error in patients with amyotrophic lateral sclerosis. Muscle Nerve 2000; 23: 193–7

35. Lomen-Hoerth C, Olney RK. Effect of recording window and stimulation variables on the statistical technique of motor unit number estimation. Muscle Nerve 2001; 24: 1659–64

36. Daube J. MUNE by statistical analysis. Clin Neurophysiol Suppl 2003; 55: 51–71

37. Lomen-Hoerth C, Slawnych MP. Statistical motor unit number estimation: From theory to practice. Muscle Nerve 2003; 28: 263–72

38. Simmons Z, Epstein DK, Borg B, et al. Reproducibility of motor unit number estimation in individual subjects. Muscle Nerve 2001; 24: 467–73

39. Olney RK. Motor Unit Number Estimation (MUNE). Proc Amyotroph Lateral Scler Other Motor Neuron Disord 2002; 3 (Suppl 1): S91-2(abstr)

40. Shefner JM, Cudkowicz ME, Zhang H, et al. and the Northeast ALS Consortium. The use of statistical MUNE in a multicenter clinical trial. Muscle Nerve 2004; 30: 463–9

41. Lee RG, Ashby P, White DG, Aguayo AJ. Analysis of motor conduction velocity in the human median nerve by computer simulation of compound muscle action potentials. Electroencephalogr Clin Neurophysiol 1975; 39: 225–37

42. Law PK, Caccia MR. Physiological estimates of the sizes and the numbers of motor units in soleus muscles of dystrophic mice. J Neurol Sci 1975; 24: 251–6

43. Eisen A, Karpati G, Carpenter S, Danon J. The motor unit profile of the rat soleus in experimental myopathy and reinnervation. Neurology 1974; 24: 878–84

44. Peyronnard JM, Lamarre Y. Electrophysiological and anatomical estimation of the number of motor units in the monkey extensor digitorum brevis muscle. J Neurol Neurosurg Psychiatry 1977; 40: 756–64

45. Arasaki K, Tamaki M, Hosoya Y, Kudo N. Validity of electromyograms and tension as a means of motor unit number estimation. Muscle Nerve 1997; 20: 552–60

46. Galea V, Fehlings D, Kirsch S, McComas A. Depletion and sizes of motor units in spinal muscular atrophy. Muscle Nerve 2001; 24: 1168–72

47. Slawnych M, Laszlo C, Hershler C. Motor unit number estimation: Sample size considerations. Muscle Nerve 1997; 20: 22–8

48. Stein RB, Yang JF. Methods for estimating the number of motor units in human muscles. Ann Neurol 1990; 28: 487–95

49. Bromberg MB. Electrodiagnostic studies in clinical trials for motor neuron disease. J Clin Neurophysiol 1998; 15: 117–28

50. Brown WF, Jaatoul N. Amyotrophic lateral sclerosis. Electrophysiologic study (number of motor units and rate of decay of motor units). Arch Neurol 1974; 30: 242–8

51. Brown WF, Jaatoul N. An electrophysiological estimation of the number of motor units and rate of decay of motor units in amyotrophic lateral sclerosis. Trans Am Neurol Assoc 1973; 98: 183–6

52. Carleton SA, Brown WF. Changes in motor unit populations in motor neuron disease. J Neurol Neurosurg Psychiatry 1979; 42: 42–51

53. Dantes M, McComas A. The extent and time course of motoneuron involvement in amyotrophic lateral sclerosis. Muscle Nerve 1991; 14: 416–21

54. Aggarwal A, Nicholson G. Detection of preclinical motor neuron loss in SOD1 mutation carriers using motor unit number estimation. J Neurol Neurosurg Psychiatry 2002; 73: 199–201

55. Brown WF. Functional compensation of human motor units in health and disease. J Neurol Sci 1973; 20: 199–209

56. Lambert E. Diagnostic value of electrical stimulation of motor nerves. Electroencephalogr Clin Neurophysiol Suppl 1962; 22: 9–16

57. Lambert E, Mulder D. Electromyographic studies in amyotrophic lateral sclerosis. Proc Staff Meet Mayo Clini 1957; 32: 441–6

58. Aggarwal A, Nicholson G. Normal complement of motor units in asymptomatic familial (SOD1 mutation) amyotrophic lateral sclerosis carriers. J Neurol Neurosurg Psychiatry 2001; 71: 478–81

59. Feeney SJ, McKelvie PA, Austin L, et al. Presymptomatic motor neuron loss and reactive astrocytosis in the SOD1 mouse model of amyotrophic lateral sclerosis. Muscle Nerve 2001; 24: 1510–19

60. Shefner JM, Brown RH Jr, Cole D, et al. Effect of neurophilin ligands on motor units in mice with SOD1 ALS mutations. Neurology 2001; 57: 1857–61

61. Doherty TJ, Brown WF. A method for the longitudinal study of human thenar motor units. Muscle Nerve 1994; 17: 1029–36

62. Gooch CL, Harati Y. Longitudinal tracking of the same single motor unit in amyotrophic lateral sclerosis. Muscle Nerve 1997; 20: 511–13

63. Chan KM, Stashuk DW, Brown WF. A longitudinal study of the pathophysiological changes in single human thenar motor units in amyotrophic lateral sclerosis. Muscle Nerve 1998; 21: 1714–23

64. Milner-Brown HS, Stein RB. The relation between the surface electromyogram and muscular force. J Physiol 1975; 246: 549–69

65. Venkatesh S, Shefner JM, Logigian EL. Does muscle reinnervation produce electromechanical dissociation in amyotrophic lateral sclerosis? Muscle Nerve 1995; 18: 1335–7

66. Felice KJ. A longitudinal study comparing thenar motor unit number estimates to other quantitative tests in patients with amyotrophic lateral sclerosis. Muscle Nerve 1997; 20: 179–85

67. Felice KJ. A longitudinal study comparing thenar motor unit number estimates to other quantitative tests in patients with amyotrophic lateral sclerosis. Muscle Nerve 1997; 20: 179–85

68. Bromberg MB, Forshew DA, Nau KL, et al. Motor unit number estimation, isometric strength, and electromyographic measures in amyotrophic lateral sclerosis. Muscle Nerve 1993; 16: 1213–19

69. Yuen EC, Olney RK. Longitudinal study of fiber density and motor unit number estimate in patients with amyotrophic lateral sclerosis. Neurology 1997; 49: 573–8

70. Felice KJ. Thenar motor unit number estimates using the multiple point stimulation technique: reproducibility studies in ALS patients and normal subjects. Muscle Nerve 1995; 18: 1412–16

71. Bromberg MB. Motor unit estimation: Reproducibility of the spike-triggered averaging technique in normal and ALS subjects. Muscle Nerve 1993; 16: 466–71

72. Bromberg MB, Fries TJ, Forshew DA, Tandan R. Electrophysiologic endpoint measures in a multicenter ALS drug trial. J Neurol Sci 2001; 184: 51–5

73. Bromberg MB, Abrams JL. Sources of error in the spike-triggered averaging method of motor unit number estimation (MUNE). Muscle Nerve 1995; 18: 1139–46

74. Smith BE, Stevens JC, Litchy WJ, et al. Longitudinal electrodiagnostic studies in amyotrophic lateral sclerosis patients treated with recombinant human ciliary neurotrophic factor. Neurology 1995; 45 (Suppl 4): A48(abstr)

75. Armon C, Brandstater ME. Motor unit number estimate-based rates of progression of ALS predict patient survival. Muscle Nerve 1999; 22: 1571–5

76. Armon C, Graves MC, Moses D, et al. Linear estimates of disease progression predict survival in patients with amyotrophic lateral sclerosis. Muscle Nerve 2000; 23: 874–82

77. Olney RK, Yuen EC, Engstrom JW. The rate of change in motor unit number estimates predicts survival in patients with amyotrophic lateral sclerosis. Neurology 1999; 52 (Suppl 2): A3

5

The corticomotoneuronal system in amyotrophic lateral sclerosis

Markus Weber

INTRODUCTION

There is now ample evidence that amyotrophic lateral sclerosis (ALS) represents a multisystem disorder and involves cortical areas outside the primary motor cortex[1,2]. However, the leading clinical features and majority of pathological abnormalities can be ascribed to the motor system (lower motor neurons (LMNs) in the brainstem and spinal cord, corticospinal tract and cortical (upper) motor neurons (UMNs) in the motor cortex). This preferential vulnerability of motor neurons as well as the relationship between upper and lower motor degeneration in ALS are incompletely understood, but human cortical and spinal motor neurons are amongst the largest and longest nerve cells in the nervous system. Their large size makes them particularly vulnerable to a variety of insults such as biochemical, oxidative and excitotoxic insults[3]. Pathologically the large corticospinal tract fibers and the large spinal motor neurons are predominantly affected[4]. The predominance of cases in which myelin pallor of the corticospinal tract is not demonstrable above the level of the medulla has led to the conclusion that in ALS UMN changes most commonly arise from an axonopathy with peripheral dying back[5]. Additionally, the degree of damage of pyramidal neurons in the motor cortex seems to be variable and sometimes undetectable[6]. Some autopsy studies have demonstrated loss or shrinkage of the large pyramidal motor neurons including Betz cells[7] but others revealed no Betz cell pathology[8,9] or an unchanged number of motor neurons in the ALS motor cortex[10]. However, neither this nor the 'dying back' features on autopsy prevent the cortical motor neuron and its surrounding cells from being affected, but rather raise the possibility that not neuronal death but metabolic dysfunction[10] or ultrastructural synaptic changes[11] of pyramidal cells are important pathogenetic mechanisms that may precede degeneration. On the other hand, corticospinal tract degeneration has been demonstrated in the progressive muscular atrophy variant of ALS[12], which implies that lack of clinical UMN signs does not rule out corticospinal tract damage. Although pathologic studies are a fundamental research tool, it is also clear that it is most difficult to reach meaningful conclusions regarding the temporal sequence of corticospinal dysfunction on the basis of autopsy studies. They are even more problematic if one wants to study a possible relationship of UMN and LMN degeneration[4].

While the discovery that 20% of familial ALS cases harbor a mutation in the antioxidant enzyme Cu/Zn superoxide dismutase (*SOD1*)[13–15] and the subsequent creation of a transgenic mouse model of ALS[16] as well as the use of organotypic models[17] and cell cultures[18] has led to a new area of research into the pathogenetic and pathophysiologic mechanisms of LMN degeneration in ALS[19], no comparable models are available to study disease of human corticomotoneurons.

This implies that only up-to-date neurophysiologic techniques and/or imaging methods are available to study corticospinal dysfunction and degeneration in ALS, which of course need to be applied in concert with other investigational methods, e.g. autopsy studies.

ANATOMY AND PHYSIOLOGY OF THE CORTICOMOTONEURONAL SYSTEM

Motor function in humans is subserved by several distinct anatomical regions which are interconnected. They include the primary motor cortex, also known as Brodman area 4, the premotor areas and supplementary motor cortex, basal ganglia, thalamus, cerebellum, brainstem and the reticular formation. The primary motor cortex is different from other regions of the cerebral cortex in that it is thicker but has a low cell density[20]. The spinal motoneurons (SMN) of the cord are the 'final common pathway' of the motor system to which the higher centers and pyramidal cells make direct or, more commonly, indirect connections. Compared to lower mammals there have been two key developments in the organization of the primate cortical control system. The first is the increasingly dominant role played by the motor cortex and corticospinal tract at the expense of other descending pathways such as the rubrospinal tract[21–23]. The second major development is the appearance of direct corticomotoneuronal connections (C-M) which make a monosynaptic linkage between the motor cortex and the spinal motoneurons[24], except those that innervate the external ocular muscles and Onuf's nucleus, whose cell bodies innervate the bladder wall. These two groups of spinal motor neurons are relatively spared in ALS. A recent stereologic study of Betz cells and neighboring pyramidal cells in humans has shown that the number of large Betz cells accounts for about 10% of the total number of pyramidal cells in layer V[25]. The distribution of cellular volumes of pyramidal cells exhibits a bimodal pattern, delineating two subpopulations[25]. The adult human corticospinal tract (medullary pyramids) contains roughly 1 million fibers; only 6% are unmyelinated. By contrast, in the macaque 38% of the pyramidal fibers are unmyelinated[26]. Although the corticospinal tract is derived from a large number of cortical regions (motor, premotor, supplementary motor, cingulated areas in the frontal lobe and postcentral gyrus of the parietal lobe[27], the C-M system originates exclusively from large pyramidal cells in the deepest part of layer V in the primary motor cortex. Glutamate is the primary excitatory neurotransmitter of the C-M system. All C-M connections are excitatory; inhibition is exerted through disynaptic pathways via spinal interneurons[28–30]. (See reference 30 for a comprehensive review of corticospinal function in man.) Each C-M synapses with many SMNs and each SMN receives input from many different C-M cells[31,32]. This arrangement of convergence and divergence is most abundant for the distal muscles, especially those responsible for hand and facial innervated musculature. It is what affords humans their amazing degree of independent finger movements which are an essential part of skilled hand function[33]. C-M control is largely responsible for delicate control of force, precision grip, angulation, rate of change of movement and muscle tension[34].

The pyramidal neurons have extensive spiny dendritic trees which collect an enormous number (up to 60 000) of different synaptic, excitatory and inhibitory inputs[35]. The pattern of excitatory amino acid receptors in the motor cortex differs from that of other regions. Whereas in non-motor cortical areas kainic acid binding is highest in laminae V and VI, it is lowest in the deep laminae V and VI of the motor cortex[36].

Several distinct types of inhibitory GABAergic interneurons have been identified by their immunohistochemical reactivity to the calcium binding proteins calbindin (CB), parvalbumin (PV) and calretinin (CR) [37–39]. These interneurons modulate the response of pyramidal neurons to excitatory inputs. They are also thought to provide intracellular calcium buffering, preventing hyperpolarization of cells, possibly protecting them from excitotoxic damage[40,41]. In the cat motor cortex it could be demonstrated that inhibitory circuits are – like excitatory receptors – laminar specific. Pyramidal neurons of superficial layers are controlled by a powerful local inhibitory circuit that operates through γ-aminobutyric acid (GABA)$_A$ (fast inhibitory postsynaptic potentials (fIPSP)) and GABA$_B$ (slow inhibitory postsynaptic potentials (sIPSP)) receptors, whereas sIPSPs mediated by GABA$_B$ receptors are weak or absent in layer V pyramidal cells, ensuring that these neurons can be brought to threshold rapidly during repeated synaptic excitatory input[42]. Two phases of intracortical inhibition have recently been revealed by a transcranial magnetic stimulation threshold paradigm in humans[43].

IN VIVO INVESTIGATIONAL METHODS OF THE MOTOR CORTEX

The utility of investigational methods in ALS would be manifold: first to elucidate the pathophysiology of UMN involvement in ALS; and second to serve as a sensitive marker for UMN involvement to obtain an early diagnosis and to monitor disease progression. Various imaging studies, using magnetic resonance imaging (MRI), positron emission tomography (PET), single photon emission computed tomography (SPECT), proton magnetic resonance spectroscopy (HMRS), functional MRI (fMRI) and more recently diffusion tensor imaging (DTI)[44,45] have given interesting information regarding UMN involvement in ALS. Although all techniques have a potential to detect cortical and corticospinal tract abnormalities, most if not all of them reveal changes that are not specific to ALS, and the range of values in control subjects and patients widely overlap[46,47]. Furthermore, most techniques focus on damage in terms of loss rather

than dysfunction. However, recent PET studies have provided evidence of cerebral microglial activation[2] and an fMRI study has shown reorganization of the motor cortex[48] which are important investigations into the pathophysiologic processes of UMNs. In this respect neurophysiologic testing is a powerful tool to study dysfunction and adds to the information obtained by imaging. In recent years a variety of neurophysiologic methods using transcranial magnetic stimulation (TMS) have been designed to investigate the integrity of the motor cortex and its descending pathways[49,50]. Most methods focus on the influence of UMN either on the discharge characteristics of single motor units or on the compound response of a target muscle or muscle group, thus depending on intact but potentially impaired functioning of C-Ms. While most of the routine measures and the triple stimulation technique have focused on detecting (subclinical) upper motor involvement and quantifying UMN loss, especially the functional studies such as double stimulation paradigms and peristimulus time histograms (PSTHs) have resulted in a clearer understanding of the pathophysiologic mechanisms underlying cortical dysfunction in ALS. They include changes in cortical excitability and selective involvement of certain cortical cell populations, which will be discussed later in this chapter.

CORTICAL EXCITABILITY AND TRANSCRANIAL MAGNETIC STIMULATION

It needs to be kept in mind that the responses in a target muscle depend on the global excitability of the motor pathway including large pyramidal cells, cortical excitatory and inhibitory interneurons and spinal motor neurons, most of which are affected to some degree in ALS. This implies that some of the discussed TMS techniques are not completely independent of LMN involvement. Studies using TMS with surface recording from the target muscle have shown a range of abnormalities. Some of these abnormalities can be interpreted as implying that the motor cortex in ALS is hyperexcitable. The increased excitation probably reflects a combination of hyperexcitability of the C-Ms and reduced inhibition due to dysfunction of cortical inhibitory interneurons[51]. One measure of excitability is the cortical threshold which is defined as the stimulus required to elicit reproducible responses of 50–100 µV in about 50% of 10–20 consecutive trials[52]. It is usually reliably reproducible and correlates inversely with the density and number of excitable C-Ms[53]. It is also likely that the threshold reflects the membrane excitability of pyramidal neurons, which is under the control of voltage gated ion channels. Several studies have demonstrated that the threshold is low in the beginning of the disease[54–58], implying that the motor cortex is hyperexcitable early on but increases as the disease progresses[54,59–63]. This is most evident in sequential studies[60,64–66]. The stimulus output curve that describes the relationship between TMS intensity and motor-evoked potential (MEP) amplitudes, thus reflecting the extent to which the spinal motoneuron pool is activated, is increased in early phases of the disease along with a tendency towards lowering of the threshold[57]. This suggests enhanced excitability of the C-M pathway. However, some investigators have found a normal threshold[60,67,68] or a lack of correlation with disease duration in cross sectional studies[69]. This lack of consistency in cross-sectional studies is not surprising, given the high interpatient variability of the threshold, which probably depends on many factors such as type of onset (limb versus bulbar)[70], or time point of study. The standard deviation of the threshold in an ALS population may be three times higher than that of a control group[69]. Furthermore, the time point of the study after symptom onset is highly variable within the studied populations and also amongst the studies, which makes it difficult if not impossible to compare the respective results. It is also clear that symptom onset is not equivalent to disease duration. For instance, pure UMN signs such as brisk

reflexes may not cause any clinical deficits. Similarly, cramps may well be the first symptom, preceding onset of weakness by years, but are not recognized as an early symptom.

Evidence that cortical inhibitory circuitry which is mediated through GABAergic interneurons is also impaired can be demonstrated through evoking the cortical silent period (CSP) (Figure 5.1). A single transcranial magnetic stimulus applied during a sustained voluntary contraction of a target muscle is followed by a long period of electromayogram (EMG) silence (up to 300 ms)[50]. This inhibitory period is highly stimulus-intensity dependent[71]. Spinal inhibitory mechanisms are considered to contribute only to the first 50–60 ms of the TMS-induced CSP, and most of the CSP results from cortical inhibitory mechanisms[50].

Compared to normal subjects the CSP is shortened in ALS[55,59,61,62,71–73]. Only a few studies did not confirm these findings[57,66,68]. The

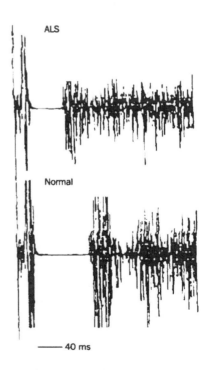

Figure 5.1 Silent period in a normal subject and an amyotrophic lateral sclerosis (ALS) patient

observation that the duration of the CSP is shorter than normal early on in the disease and shows progressive lengthening throughout the illness[60] underscores the view that change of cortical excitability is a dynamic process. This also explains contradictory findings as to whether the dependency of the CSP on stimulus intensity is preserved[71] or abolished[55,57,66].

Cortical excitability can also be studied with paired (double) transcranial magnetic stimulation (Figure 5.2). Normally, a subthreshold conditioning stimulus applied shortly before a test stimulus induces intracortical inhibition (ICI) if an interstimulus interval of 1–5 ms is used (early ICI), and intracortical facilitation (ICF) if an interstimulus interval of 7–20 ms is used (early ICF)[74]. Very short intervals (1.2–1.5 ms) also induce facilitation at the level of the motor cortex[75–77].

By contrast, two stimuli greater than the resting motor threshold given at an interstimulus interval of 50–200 ms induce a long latency (late ICI) which is probably also of cortical origin. ICI and ICF reflect the function of inhibitory and excitatory interneuronal circuits specifically at the cortical level[74,78]. The vast majority of double stimulation studies have shown that ICI is impaired in ALS[55–57,63,67,79–81] This does not seem to correlate with duration of illness, motor scores[67,68,79,80], or clinical features of UMN involvement[68]. However, it is most difficult to make meaningful conclusions in cross-sectional studies, as argued above. The effect of age on early ICI[82] and the variability of early ICI between different investigators (early ICI variance 17.3%) and sessions[83] also need be taken into account. In sequential studies it becomes clear that over time early and late ICI become significantly reduced[66]. Even more important, early facilitation may be increased in early stages of the disease and is lost with disease progression[61]. This is well in keeping with threshold and CSP studies and with recordings from single motor unit studies (see below) and points to the pivotal role of disturbed glutamatergic and GABAergic circuits. Imaging studies have also revealed *in vivo* evidence of disturbed glutamate metabolism[84] and loss of inhibitory GABAergic function[63]. Riluzole, which reduces glutamate and enhances GABAergic function, can reverse impaired intracortical inhibition[85]. However, it has no short-term influence on early ICI[67,80], but may influence early ICI after continuous intake of 3 months[81].

In summary, threshold studies as well as silent period and double stimulation studies reveal that cortical excitability is a dynamic process with a continuity of abnormalities in the early and late stages of the disease. This is well in accordance with the hypothesis of an excitotoxic mechanism[86,87] with excessive release of glutamate and/or impaired clearance due to excitatory amino acid transporter dysfunction[88]. In addition, coincidental loss of GABAergic interneurons as shown in anatomical studies[1,89] and an alteration in the expression of $GABA_A$ receptor unit subtypes in the motor cortex[90] may contribute to disturbed cortical excitability. However, it is not entirely clear whether increased excitability or impaired cortical inhibition is an early mechanism or a

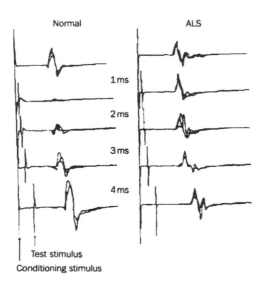

Normal   ALS

1 ms

2 ms

3 ms

4 ms

Test stimulus
Conditioning stimulus

Figure 5.2 Double stimulation paradigm showing intracortical inhibition in a control subject but not in an amyotrophic lateral sclerosis (ALS) patient. The subthreshold conditioning stimulus inhibits the response to the test stimulus at an interstimulus interval of 1–3 ms only in the control subject (left) but not in the ALS patient (modified from reference 79)

secondary event[57]. The physiologic studies favor a concept in which there is an early episode of glutamate-induced increased excitability and loss of inhibition as the disease progresses (see below).

DETECTING SUBCLINICAL UPPER MOTOR NEURON INVOLVEMENT AND QUANTIFYING OF UPPER MOTOR NEURON LOSS WITH TRANSCRANIAL MAGNETIC STIMULATION

The degree of UMN involvement and clinical signs in ALS patients is highly variable[6]. In patients who harbor the A4V *SOD* mutation, for instance, UMN signs are almost always absent[91], whereas other patients start off with pure UMN signs and develop LMN signs only after several years[92]. It would therefore be useful to have an objective measure of UMN involvement, first to obtain an early diagnosis in those patients lacking clinical UMN signs and second to monitor disease progression. Early studies have focused on measuring central motor conduction time[54,93]. It soon became clear that this parameter may be abnormal but is most often normal[60,70,93–96]. This is not surprising when it is considered that ALS is a neuronal axonal disorder and should not cause slowing of central conduction. If central motor conduction time (CMCT) is abnormal, it is only slightly prolonged, except for some patients, who harbor *SOD* mutations[97,98]. However, an interesting relationship between central conduction and strength of the cortical volley exists, which has given insight into pathophysiologic changes and will be discussed in the context of single motor unit studies.

It has been suggested that the ratio of the MEP amplitude or area to that of the evoked compound muscle action potential after electrical peripheral nerve stimulation could be used as a measure of functioning corticospinal tract fibers[99,100]. However, amplitude measurements depend on many factors, such as the amount of facilitation, moment-to-moment fluctuations of cortical excitability and the synchrony with which impulses arrive at the spinal motoneurons[101]. It is also known that spinal motoneurons may fire repeatedly in reponse to a magnetically induced descending volley in the corticospinal tract[102–104] and hence the MEP already desynchronized by temporal dispersion in the corticospinal tract may be rendered even more complex by multiple contributions from the same motor unit[60]. The only technique that overcomes the problem of MEPs desynchronized by temporal dispersion is the triple stimulation technique (TST) [101]. It appears that the TST is more sensitive than the routine measures to detect UMN involvement in ALS[105,106]. However, in the author's opinion no study has convincingly shown that if the revised El Escorial criteria[107] are consequently applied (e.g. a preserved reflex in a weak, wasted limb is an UMN sign) TMS studies are more sensitive than the clinical examination. Whether this also applies for the TST technique is presently unclear. Neither of the two TST studies has applied the revised El Escorial criteria published in 2000[107]. It is evident that the technique overcomes fundamental shortcomings of other amplitude measurements but longitudinal studies must show that parameters decline and it must be validated by another *in vivo* technique or by autopsy. Some of the imaging methods such as DTI and HMRS have the potential to detect cortical and spinal tract damage[47] and should be used in concert with TMS to detect and quantify UMN damage. However, the real value of TMS investigations is assessment of dysfunction in terms of *in vivo* pathophysiologic changes which cannot be analyzed by clinical examination or any other investigational method.

SINGLE MOTOR UNIT STUDIES AND CORTICOMOTONEURONAL DYSFUNCTION

A more sophisticated physiologic approach to investigating the C-M system in considerable detail is that of PSTHs[108–111]. PSTHs analyze modulations in the firing of a single voluntarily recruited motor unit in response to an imposed transcranial stimulus[102,109,111–117]. The primary peak in the PSTH reflects the initial rising phase of the composite excitatory postsynaptic potential (EPSP) generated in a single anterior horn cell[102,109,114,118,119]. This implies that *in vivo* information about physiologic properties can be obtained from the select group of C-Ms converging upon a single anterior horn cell which makes the PSTH method an ideal tool to study UMN pathophysiology in motor neuron disorders.

Method and theory underlying peristimulus time histograms

When a motor unit is voluntarily recruited it begins to fire steadily at about 10 Hz. According to the Henneman size principle, smaller motor neurons are recruited first[120]. For intrinsic hand muscles and forearm muscles this recruitment order is independent of whether the synaptic input is voluntary or evoked by a magnetic stimulus[121]. At threshold the composite EPSP of the anterior horn cell alters the membrane at a common trigger zone (the axon hillock) causing it to fire. If now an additional synaptic input, e.g. by transcranial magnetic stimulation, is introduced, the motor neuron may be brought to its firing level earlier than anticipated (Figure 5.3). These modulations in firing of a single motor unit in response to some imposed synaptic input can be studied using PSTHs.

In recording a PSTH a needle electrode is used to record the discharges from a single motor unit. If all discharges of 100–150 stimulus-triggered sweeps are collected into 1-ms bins and expressed as a peristimulus time histogram a sharp rise in the firing probability of this motor unit can be seen (Figure 5.4) which is referred to as the primary peak[102,109,114,119,122].

The primary peak

In healthy control subjects the primary peak is of short duration, is well synchronized and has an onset latency of approximately 20 ms followed by a phase of zero firing probability (suppression phase) (Figure 5.5a). The duration of this suppression phase depends on the stimulus intensity. Animal experiments using intracellular recordings can directly record the postsynaptic potentials in anterior horn cells while changes in firing frequency are simultaneously monitored[114]. They have shown that the increase in firing probability of the motor neuron is related to the rising edge of the EPSP. The onset latency and short duration of the primary peak in humans indicates activation of a fast-conducting, monosynaptic (C-M) projection originating from large pyramidal cells[110]. The primary peak consists of subpeaks reflecting the sequential arrival of subsequent descending

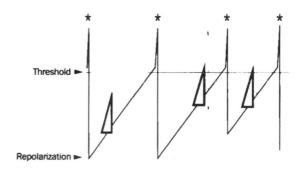

Figure 5.3 Model depicting the membrane excursions of the spinal motoneuron during voluntary, tonic contraction and how the neuron might respond to an intervening cortical or peripheral stimulus. Voluntary motor unit discharges (spike train) are indicated by asterisks (*). The shaded triangle indicates an excitatory postsynaptic potential (EPSP) of a given amplitude induced by a threshold cortical stimulus. The interrupted line indicates anticipated stimulation-induced firing of the motor unit. Three examples of an arrival of the EPSP at a given time on the interspike trajectory are illustrated. A stimulus-induced EPSP that arrives too soon after a preceding voluntary discharge is insufficient to bring the membrane potential to threshold (depicted in the first EPSP). With stimulus-induced EPSPs arriving progressively later, the membrane potential will first equal and then exceed the potential difference between the interspike trajectory and the threshold, and will bring the neuron to threshold (depicted in the second EPSP). When the interspike interval is shorter and the depth of post-spike repolarization is small (shown on the right side) the magnitude of an EPSP equals the potential difference earlier during a post-spike excursion

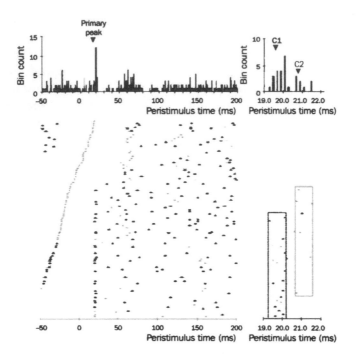

Figure 5.4   Primary peak in the peristimulus time histogram (PSTH) and raster displays of 100 sweeps with individual discharges underneath the PSTH in ascending order to show that stimulus-induced firing of the motor unit could only occur when the interval between the preceding voluntary discharge of the motor unit and the stimulus-induced firing was at least 30 ms (1-ms bins). The primary peak is also shown on the right, where discharges were collected into 0.2-ms bins between 19.0 ms and 22.0 ms. This shows that the primary peak is composed of two subcomponents labeled C1 and C2 (boxes in the raster display below)

volleys[102,109] They can be identified only by using 0.2-ms bin collections (Figure 5.4, right)[111,123]. Using threshold anodal scalp stimulation, the first subpeak is consistent with direct activation (D-wave) of pyramidal tract neurons whereas with threshold TMS a series of volleys named I_1, I_2 etc. to indicate their indirect trans-synaptic origin can be recorded[124,125]. The first subpeak occurs 1–2 ms later than the D-wave. Various measurements of the primary peak allow inferences regarding conduction speed in C-M fibers, extent of temporal dispersion/desynchronization of the descending volleys in the corticospinal tract, timing of excitatory or inhibitory effects on the motor neuron and the strength of the synaptic input (Table 5.1)[126].

The greatest advantage of the PSTH technique is that the above-mentioned physiologic properties of single anterior cells and their C-M input can be studied in humans by a non-invasive technique. However, only the anterior horn cells of the earliest recruited motor units can be studied which may not be representative of the whole muscle respecting its cortical representation[127]. While this may hold true in healthy subjects it is certainly not the case in anterior horn cell disorders, such as ALS, where the spinal motor neuron pool is diminished and low- and high-threshold motor units are amongst the first to be recruited. Furthermore, pairs of motor units from the same muscles in healthy subjects and in ALS patients behave in a similar manner, suggesting that the obtained PSTHs are representative of a larger group in the motor neuron pool[127]. This can be easily explained by the extensive system of divergence of C-M on to spinal motoneurons.

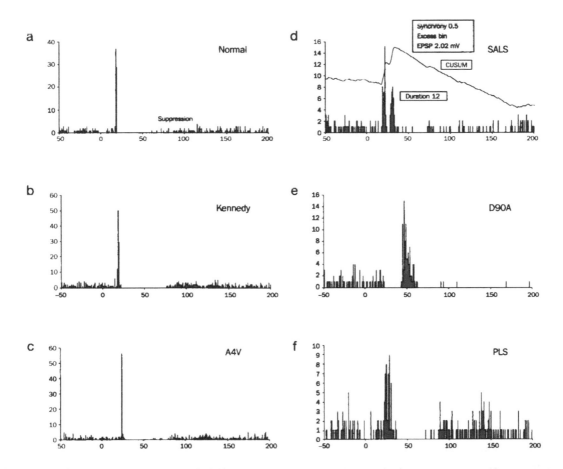

Figure 5.5   Peristimulus time histogram (PSTH) in a normal subject (a), patient with Kennedy's disease (b), amyotrophic lateral sclerosis (ALS) patients (A4V SOD mutation (c), sporadic ALS (SALS) (d), D90A *SOD* mutation (e) and a patient with primary lateral sclerosis (f). The primary peak is followed by a suppression phase during which the firing probability is zero (a). The cumulative sum analysis (CUSUM) helps to determine the onset of the primary peak. Its measurements are given in boxes (d, see also Table 5.1). In Kennedy's disease and A4V the primary peak is entirely normal. Double peak in SALS, profoundly delayed peak in D90A with a prepeak suppression phase, desynchronized peak of normal onset in primary lateral sclerosis (PLS). Note that the scales of the y-axes are different. Values of the parameters are given from a to f: onset latency (ms): 17, 17, 24,18, 45, 22; excess bins: 3, 3, 2, 11, 11, 7; duration (ms): 3, 3, 2, 15, 14, 9; amplitude (mV): 6.3, 5.9, 5.1, 6.8, 5.9, 4.8

PERISTIMULUS TIME HISTOGRAM STUDIES IN MOTOR NEURON DISORDERS

Evidence for a supraspinal origin of peristimulus time histogram abnormalities

The abnormalities in the primary peak are quite diverse in ALS[115,116,126–129]. The primary peak may be larger than normal, small or absent, large with an increased duration and temporal dispersion or its onset may be delayed (Figure 5.5). These abnormalities can be attributed to dysfunction of the C-Ms, because in the same anterior horn cell that produces an abnormal primary peak to cortical magnetic stimulation, the primary peak evoked by afferent Ia peripheral nerve stimulation is normal[112,129]. If anterior horn cell disease were responsible for the PSTH abnormality in ALS, the

Table 5.1	Definitions and inferences of primary peak measurements (from reference 126)	
Peak parameter	**Definition**	**Inference**
Excess bins (EB)	Bin exceeding the mean pre-stimulus background activity by more than 2 SD	
Onset latency (ms)	First EB after the stimulus	Conduction speed in corticomotoneuronal fibers; fiber diameter
Duration (ms)	Time interval between the first and the last EB terminated by a period of clear suppression (inhibition phase)	Correlates with the rising edge of the underlying EPSP; time required for temporal summation of descending volleys
Synchrony	Quotient of the number of EB within the PP divided by its duration	Index of dispersion/desynchronization of descending volleys arriving at the AHC
Amplitude (mV)	$\dfrac{\text{Bin count} \times \text{mean inter-spike interval}^{\#}}{10 \times \text{number of stimuli}}$	Estimate of the EPSP evoked at the AHC; strength of synaptic input to the AHC

EB, excess bin; EPSP, excitatory postsynaptic potential; PP, primary peak; AHC, anterior horn cell; #, the equation assumes a membrane potential excursion of 10 mV (–65 to –55 mV) at a firing rate of 10 Hz[114,119]

peripheral PSTH should be equally abnormal, since both Ia afferents and descending C-M fibers synapse on the same cell membrane. More direct evidence for a cortical mechanism of PSTH abnormalities was adduced by comparing a group of patients with ALS to a group with Kennedy's disease[117]. Kennedy's disease or spinobulbar muscular atrophy (SBMA) is an X-chromosomal recessive disorder which, in terms of the motor system, is restricted to the LMN[117,130–134]. In this study it could be demonstrated that the PSTHs in patients with Kennedy's disease despite profound electromyographic signs of LMN involvement were normal, which implies that the PSTH abnormalities in ALS are indeed supraspinal in origin (Figure 5.5b).

Changes over time

The most consistent abnormality of the primary peak is desynchronization and increased duration[115,127–129]. Another peculiar finding rarely seen in other UMN disorders such as stroke or multiple sclerosis is the occurrence of double peaks in ALS

(Figure 5.5d)[115,122]. The primary peak abnormalities follow a distinctive pattern and double peaks occur more probably as the disease progresses[65]. Initially the primary peak has a normal onset but it becomes desynchronized. Over time as C-M degeneration proceeds the onset is slightly delayed and desynchronization increases. Later, double peaks occur. Finally the primay peak loses the early component and the onset latency is profoundly delayed (Figure 5.6). Double peaks are most likely to reflect activation of a slowly conducting cortico-motoneuronal pathway[115,127] whose neurons are of smaller diameter than those of the fast-conducting corticospinal pathway originating from large pyramidal cells. Slowly conducting pathways have been demonstrated in the cat[135] and monkey[29] and in patients with idiopathic paraparesis using high-intensity electrical stimulation of the motor cortex and brainstem[136]. More recently an anatomical study provided evidence that the volume of pyramidal cells in the primary motor cortex follows a clear bi-modal pattern[25]. This is well in accordance with the finding that primary peak onset latencies reflecting conduction speed in cortical spinal fibers

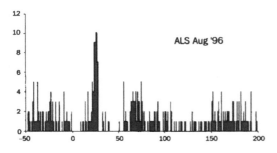

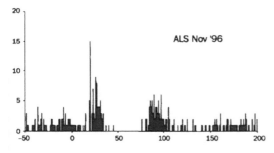

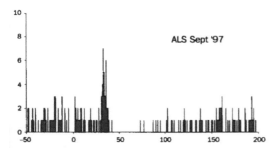

Figure 5.6 The peristimulus time histograms (PSTHs) were recorded from the same patient on three separate occasions. In August 1996 the primary peak has a normal onset latency at 22 ms but an increased number of excess bins[7] and duration (8 ms). With time the desynchronization increased (November 1996). A short-duration high component and a desynchronized component are discernible. In September 1997 the early components of the primary peak are entirely lost, causing a profound delay of the onset latency at 33 ms. Note that the scales for the y-axes (bin count) are different in each experiment. The major abnormality is the marked desynchronization of the primary peak in amyotrophic lateral sclerosis

are also bi-modal (Figure 5.7)[65,98]. This supports the conclusion that two different (slow- and fast-conducting) pathways exist in humans[115,127]. Alternatively, the origin of this slow-conducting pathway could be in the supplementary motor area,

since a MRI study[48] and a TMS study[64] have both shown that motor cortex activation shifts anteriorly in ALS patients compared to healthy control subjects. However, TMS is unlikely to excite pyramidal cells outside the motor cortex and the most likely explanation is that delayed peaks simply reflect the fact that smaller C-Ms of the primary motor cortex are relatively spared[7,98].

It is likely that the differential vulnerability of the slow- and fast-conducting pathways is related to the density and type of glutamate receptors[137,138]. Furthermore, neurofilament misfolding, a key feature of degenerating spinal motoneurons in ALS, is restricted to large, neurofilament-rich motor neurons[139–141]. Whether neurofilament misfolding is also a feature of large pyramidal cells is yet unknown, but needs to be examined.

As the number of descending volleys required for full depolarization of the anterior horn cell is determined by the strength of the individual descending volley, the appearance of desynchronized peaks of long duration is probably the result of weak descending volleys in degenerating corticospinal tract neurons requiring more temporal summation[142]. Thus the onset latency and duration of the primary peak is not exclusively a function of the length and conduction velocity of the motor pathway but reflects the time for temporal summation of arriving volleys at the anterior horn cell. This, however, can only explain modestly delayed onset latencies and conduction slowing[65]. Using a double-stimulation paradigm to study facilitatory I-wave interaction, it was confirmed that patients with normal CMCT had normal I wave summation, whilst patients with prolonged CMCTs had a significant reduction in facilitation[61]. This corresponds to the conduction failure in the corticospinal tract demonstrated by the triple stimulation technique[105]. By contrast, the profound conduction slowing seen in some patients with *SOD* mutations (e.g. D90A) and in late stages of the disease in sporadic ALS[65] is probably due to activation of a slowly conducting pathway[115,127].

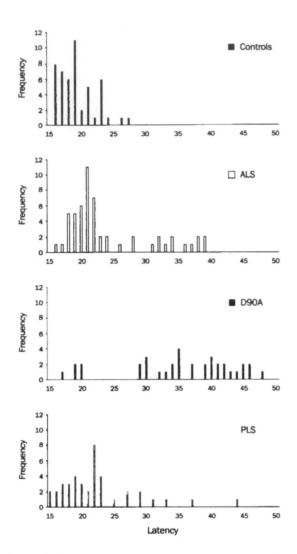

Figure 5.7 Histogram of the primary peak onset latencies. The vast majority of primary peaks in primary lateral sclerosis (PLS) and sporadic amyotrophic lateral sclerosis (ALS) have a normal or only slightly prolonged onset latency. In patients with the D90A mutation most of the primary peaks are profoundly delayed (≥29 ms). In both ALS populations the distribution appears to be bimodal

PERISTIMULUS TIME HISTOGRAMS IN PATIENTS WITH *SOD* MUTATIONS

ALS patients, homozygous for the D90A mutation, are unique in that the mean survival time is 13 years, roughly four times longer than in sporadic ALS cases[97,143]. Neurophysiologically the D90A

patients are characterized by very slow central motor conduction[97,127,144] which is unusual in ALS. The slowly progressive course and characteristic neurophysiologic findings in D90A homozygous cases make this particular mutation an ideal model to study upper motor neuron dysfunction in ALS[98]. The bimodal distribution of primary peak onset latencies together with a high threshold of delayed peaks to cortical stimulation provided further evidence that a slow-conducting C-M pathway is preserved in these ALS patients (Figure 5.7). Whether the fast-conducting corticospinal fibers in these patients are lost as originally thought[98] or just suppressed by abnormal intracortical or intraspinal inhibition[145] needs to be clarified by autopsy studies. A clear suppression phase preceding the primary peak (Figure 5.5e) which was never seen in sporadic ALS patients indicates that inhibitory mechanisms are preserved[98]. This concept has been recently confirmed by applying a paired stimulation paradigm in combination with C flumanezil PET which is a marker of cortical neuronal loss and might also reflect altered GABAergic inhibitory function. Intracortical inhibition and C flumanezil binding in sporadic ALS were significantly reduced compared to D90A patients[63]. These relatively preserved inhibitory mechanisms may provide additional resistance to the small-diameter motor neurons and are a good candidate for the postulated protecting factor in the D90A mutation[146,147].

In contrast to D90A patients, those patients harboring an A4V mutation progress very rapidly. Clinically, UMN signs are usually absent; however, pathologic evidence of mild cortical spinal tract damage may be present[91,148]. As to LMN involvement electromyographic signs of reinnervation, a typical finding in ALS, are also lacking[149].

In a comparative PSTH study (D90A, I113T, A4V) the primary peaks in A4V patients were characterized by normal onset and normal duration, indicating that the fast-conducting C-M pathway was activated[149]. Most importantly, the cortical threshold was significantly lowered and the size of the estimated EPSP amplitude, which is a reflection of the C-M synaptic strength, was larger than normal. This lends further support to the notion that excitation is increased early in the disease. The important implication is that even without clinical UMN signs or pathologic evidence of UMN corticospinal tract degeneration, dysfunction in terms of hyperexcitability may be overt. This has also been demonstrated in patients at early stages of the disease by a significantly lowered threshold associated with a steep MEP recruitment curve indicating increased corticospinal excitability[57]. Loss of the steep recruitment curve may reflect a change from cortical hyperexcitability to hypoexcitability. By the same token a low threshold is associated with an increased I1 volley in early stages which disappears with disease progression[61]. These findings also imply that the C-Ms may act negatively on the anterior horn cell supporting the idea that UMN dysfunction and LMN death are not independent processes[150–152]. The question also arises as to why A4V patients do not show signs of reinnervation[149]. The disease duration (mean 0.75 years) cannot account for that, since early signs of reinnervation occur within a few weeks after nerve damage[153]. It has been suggested that glutamate levels in the cerebrospinal fluid correlate with changes in cortical excitability[154]. Excitation can be ascribed at least in part to increased glutamate metabolism, for which abundant evidence exists in ALS[84,87,155]. The defective glutamate transporter responsible for glutamate excess is restricted to the motor cortex in ALS and more specifically to the primary motor cortex[156]. Increases in cortical glutamate concentrations have been demonstrated in transgenic ALS mice[157] and in humans with HMRS[84]. This is in keeping with excitotoxic neuronal damage in ALS. Human motor neurons preferentially express calcium-permeable α-amino-3-hydroxy-5-methyl-4-isoxazole propionic acid (AMPA) receptors[158]. Their activation can produce selective death of motor neurons in the spinal cord[159–161].

PERISTIMULUS TIME HISTOGRAMS IN PRIMARY LATERAL SCLEROSIS

In contrast to ALS, which requires the presence of UMN and LMN signs[107,162], primary lateral sclerosis (PLS) is a neurodegenerative disorder predominantly presenting with slowly progressive spinobulbar spasticity. The few reported autopsy studies are consistent with a primary C-M disease with secondary pyramidal tract degeneration[163–165]. Its nosologic status and relationship to other motor neuron syndromes, in particular ALS, is uncertain[166–169]. Descriptions of ALS developing many years after the onset of PLS have been well documented[92], indicating that PLS may form one end of the spectrum of motor neuron disease[170]. However, when degeneration of anterior horn cells develops in PLS it does so gradually[92,169,170]. MEP studies in PLS[54,168,170–174] reveal a similar spectrum of abnormalities as in ALS, but differ in that central motor conduction time in PLS is usually prolonged and the cortical threshold is typically high. This suggests that C-M function is impaired differently in PLS and ALS. Compared to ALS, primary peak in PLS was characterized by a significantly higher threshold and longer duration (Figure 5.5f)[175]. As discussed, the increased duration of the primary peak results from impaired, weak descending volleys (spatial summation)[176] and subsequent increased temporal summation, while the higher cortical threshold in PLS could be due to a much greater loss of low-threshold, large pyramidal cells than in ALS[7]. However, if the more extensive loss of large pyramidal cells, especially Betz cells, would exclusively account for the higher threshold in PLS, then one would expect a different distribution of primary peak onset latencies in ALS and PLS: a shift of onset latencies towards greater values and significantly more delayed primary peaks in PLS. However, the onset latency distribution is similar; additionally delayed primary peaks occur more often in ALS than in PLS, suggesting that fast- and slow-conducting connections in ALS are more easily activated than in PLS (Figure 5.7).

This indicates different excitability of pyramidal cells together with greater loss of C-M connections than in ALS. The latter is well in accordance with anatomical[165] and imaging studies[174,177], showing greater loss of precentral pyramidal neurons in PLS than in ALS. Most importantly, comparison with the PSTH data in D90A patients reveals that primary peak differences cannot be attributed to the longer disease duration of PLS but truly reflect different pathophysiologic properties of C-Ms (Figure 5.7). The conclusion would be that pathogenetic mechanisms leading to C-M degeneration are different in PLS and ALS.

SUMMARY

In summary, the greatest value of TMS studies lies not so much in detecting subclinical UMN damage, but in understanding dysfunction of the C-M system, which is unique to humans. Different TMS approaches have clearly shown that this system is affected early on and the large pyramidal cells as well as other inhibitory and excitatory interneurons may be involved. The changes are dynamic and depend on many factors which is the most likely explanation for conflicting results in various studies. An early phase of hyperexcitability which depends on alive yet dysfunctional C-Ms and interneurons is followed by a phase of hypoexcitability reflecting their degeneration. Large pyramidal cells are preferentially affected, which mirrors the situation at the anterior horn cell level and possibly points to the cell size as the common denominator of motor neuron degeneration. However, the intense somatotopical relationship of UMNs and LMNs in terms of divergence and convergence of C-M cells onto spinal motor neurons together with evidence of C-M hyperexcitability should raise the possibility that the C-M impacts negatively on the LMN, implying that the motor 'system' including the surrounding cells is affected and that UMNs and LMNs do not degenerate independently. Combining neurophysiology with other *in vivo*

techniques and autopsy will help to gain further insight into the C-M pathopysiology in ALS.

REFERENCES

1. Maekawa S, Al-Sarraj S, Kibble M, et al. Cortical selective vulnerability in motor neuron disease: A morphometric study. Brain 2004; 127: 1237–51
2. Turner MR, Cagnin A, Turkheimer FE, et al. Evidence of widespread cerebral microglial activation in amyotrophic lateral sclerosis: an [11C](R)-PK11195 positron emission tomography study. Neurobiol Dis 2004; 15: 601–9
3. Shaw PJ, Eggett CJ. Molecular factors underlying selective vulnerability of motor neurons to neurodegeneration in amyotrophic lateral sclerosis. J Neurol 2000; 247 (Suppl 1): I17–27
4. Terao S, Li M, Hashizume Y, et al. No transneuronal degeneration between human cortical motor neurons and spinal motor neurons. J Neurol 1999; 246: 61–2
5. Ince PG. Neuropathology. In: Brown RH, Meininger V, Swash M, eds. Amyotrophic Lateral Sclerosis. London: Martin Dunitz, 2000: 83–112
6. Adamek D, Tomik B, Pichor A, et al. The heterogeneity of neuropathological changes in amyotrophic lateral sclerosis. A review of own autopsy material. Folia Neuropathol 2002; 40: 119–24
7. Hudson AJ, Kiernan JA, Munoz DG, et al. Clinico-pathological features of primary lateral sclerosis are different from amyotrophic lateral sclerosis. Brain Res Bull 1993; 30: 359–64
8. Ince PG, Shaw PJ, Slade JY, et al. Familial amyotrophic lateral sclerosis with a mutation in exon 4 of the Cu/Zn superoxide dismutase gene: pathological and immunocytochemical changes. Acta Neuropathol (Berl) 1996; 92: 395–403
9. Troost D, Sillevis Smitt PA, de Jong JM, Swaab DF. Neurofilament and glial alterations in the cerebral cortex in amyotrophic lateral sclerosis. Acta Neuropathol (Berl) 1992; 84: 664–73
10. Gredal O, Pakkenberg H, Karlsborg M, Pakkenberg B. Unchanged total number of neurons in motor cortex and neocortex in amyotrophic lateral sclerosis: A stereological study. J Neurosci Methods 2000; 95: 171–6
11. Sasaki S, Iwata M. Ultrastructural change of synapses of Betz cells in patients with amyotrophic lateral sclerosis. Neurosci Lett 1999; 268: 29–32

12. Ince PG, Evans J, Knopp M, et al. Corticospinal tract degeneration in the progressive muscular atrophy variant of ALS. Neurology 2003; 60: 1252–8

13. Rosen DR, Siddique T, Patterson D, et al. Mutations in Cu/Zn superoxide dismutase gene are associated with familial amyotrophic lateral sclerosis [published erratum appears in Nature 1993; 364: 362] [see comments]. Nature 1993; 362: 59–62

14. Deng HX, Hentati A, Tainer JA, et al. Amyotrophic lateral sclerosis and structural defects in Cu,Zn superoxide dismutase. Science 1993; 261: 1047–51

15. Gurney ME, Liu R, Althaus JS, et al. Mutant CuZn superoxide dismutase in motor neuron disease. J Inherit Metab Dis 1998; 21: 587–97

16. Gurney ME, Pu H, Chiu AY, et al. Motor neuron degeneration in mice that express a human Cu,Zn superoxide dismutase mutation. Science 1994; 264: 1772–5

17. Corse AM, Bilak MM, Bilak SR, et al. Preclinical testing of neuroprotective neurotrophic factors in a model of chronic motor neuron degeneration. Neurobiol Dis 1999; 6: 335–46

18. Tikka TM, Vartiainen NE, Goldsteins G, et al. Minocycline prevents neurotoxicity induced by cerebrospinal fluid from patients with motor neurone disease. Brain 2002; 125: 722–31

19. Cleveland DW, Rothstein JD. From Charcot to Lou Gehrig: Deciphering selective motor neuron death in ALS. Nat Rev Neurosci 2001; 2: 806–19

20. Rockel AJ, Hiorns RW, Powell TP. The basic uniformity in structure of the neocortex. Brain 1980; 103: 221–44

21. Heffner RS, Masterton RB. The role of the corticospinal tract in the evolution of human digital dexterity. Brain Behav Evol 1983; 23: 165–83

22. Kuypers HGJM. Anatomy of descending pathways. In: Brookhart JM, Mountcastle VB, eds. Handbook of Physiology, Section 1, The Nervous System, Vol II, Motor Control, Part 1. Bethesda, MD: American Physiological Society 1981: 597–666

23. Evolution of the corticospinal tract in primates with special reference to the hand. In: Proceedings of the 3rd Interantional Congress of the Primatological Society, Zurich, Vol 2. Basel: Karger, 1971: 2–23

24. Lemon RN. The G. L. Brown Prize Lecture. Cortical control of the primate hand. Exp Physiol 1993; 78: 263–301

25. Rivara CB, Sherwood CC, Bouras C, Hof PR. Stereologic characterization and spatial distribution patterns of Betz cells in the human primary motor cortex. Anat Rec 2003; 270A: 137–51

26. DeMyer W. Number of axons and myelin sheaths in adult human medullary pyramids; study with silver impregnation and iron hematoxylin staining methods. Neurology 1959; 9: 42–7

27. Dum RP, Strick PL. The origin of corticospinal projections from the premotor areas in the frontal lobe. J Neurosci 1991; 11: 667–89

28. Jankowska E, Padel Y, Tanaka R. Disynaptic inhibition of spinal motoneurones from the motor cortex in the monkey. J Physiol 1976; 258: 467–87

29. Lemon RN, Werner WC, Benett KMB, Flament DA. The proportion of slow and fast pyramidal tract neurons producing post-spike facilitation of hand muscles in the conscious monkey. J Physiol (Lond) 1993; 459: 166 (abstr)

30. Porter R, Lemon RN. Corticospinal function and voluntary movement. Monographs of the Physiological Society No. 45. Oxford: Clarendon Press, 1993:122–209

31. Buys EJ, Lemon RN, Mantel GW, Muir RB. Selective facilitation of different hand muscles by single corticospinal neurones in the conscious monkey. J Physiol 1986; 381: 529–49

32. Fetz EE, Cheney PD. Postspike facilitation of forelimb muscle activity by primate corticomotoneuronal cells. J Neurophysiol 1980; 44: 751–72

33. Lemon RN. Neural control of dexterity: what has been achieved? Exp Brain Res 1999; 128: 6–12

34. Lemon RN, Johansson RS, Westling G. Corticospinal control during reach, grasp, and precision lift in man. J Neurosci 1995; 15: 6145–56

35. Cragg BG. The density of synapses and neurons in normal, mentally defective aging human brains. Brain 1975; 98: 81–90

36. Jansen KL, Faull RL, Dragunow M. Excitatory amino acid receptors in the human cerebral cortex: A quantitative autoradiographic study comparing the distributions of [3H]TCP, [3H]glycine, L-[3H]glutamate, [3H]AMPA and [3H]kainic acid binding sites. Neuroscience 1989; 32: 587–607

37. Celio MR. Calbindin D-28k and parvalbumin in the rat nervous system. Neuroscience 1990; 35: 375–475

38. Baimbridge KG, Celio MR, Rogers JH. Calcium-binding proteins in the nervous system. Trends Neurosci 1992; 15: 303–8

39. Conde F, Lund JS, Jacobowitz DM, et al. Local circuit neurons immunoreactive for calretinin, calbindin D-28k or parvalbumin in monkey prefrontal

cortex: distribution and morphology. J Comp Neurol 1994; 341: 95–116

40. Heizmann CW, Braun K. Changes in Ca(2+)-binding proteins in human neurodegenerative disorders. Trends Neurosci 1992; 15: 259–64

41. Ince P, Stout N, Shaw P, et al. Parvalbumin and calbindin D-28k in the human motor system and in motor neuron disease. Neuropathol Appl Neurobiol 1993; 19: 291–9

42. van Brederode JF, Spain WJ. Differences in inhibitory synaptic input between layer II-III and layer V neurons of the cat neocortex. J Neurophysiol 1995; 74: 1149–66

43. Fisher RJ, Nakamura Y, Bestmann S, et al. Two phases of intracortical inhibition revealed by transcranial magnetic threshold tracking. Exp Brain Res 2002; 143: 240–8

44. Kalra S, Arnold DL. Imaging: MRS, MRI, PET/SPECT: con. Amyotroph Lateral Scler Other Motor Neuron Disord 2002; 3 (Suppl 1): S73–4

45. Pioro EP. Imaging: MRS/MRI/PET/SPECT: pro. Amyotroph Lateral Scler Other Motor Neuron Disord 2002; 3 (Suppl 1): S71

46. Brooks BR, Bushara K, Khan A, et al. Functional magnetic resonance imaging (fMRI) clinical studies in ALS – paradigms, problems and promises. Amyotroph Lateral Scler Other Motor Neuron Disord 2000; 1 (Suppl 2): S23–32

47. Leigh PN, Simmons A, Williams S, et al. Imaging: MRS/MRI/PET/SPECT: Summary. Amyotroph Lateral Scler Other Motor Neuron Disord 2002; 3 (Suppl 1): S75–80

48. Konrad C, Henningsen H, Bremer J, et al. Pattern of cortical reorganization in amyotrophic lateral sclerosis: A functional magnetic resonance imaging study. Exp Brain Res 2002; 143: 51–6

49. Olney RK. Transcranial magnetic stimulation: pro. Amyotroph Lateral Scler Other Motor Neuron Disord 2002; 3 (Suppl 1): S111

50. Weber M, Eisen AA. Magnetic stimulation of the central and peripheral nervous systems. Muscle Nerve 2002; 25: 160–75

51. Eisen A, Weber M. Neurophysiological evaluation of cortical function in the early diagnosis of ALS. Amyotroph Lateral Scler Other Motor Neuron Disord 2000; 1 (Suppl 1): S47–51

52. Rothwell JC, Hallet M, Berardelli A, et al. Magnetic stimulation: Motor evoked potentials. In: Deuschl G, Eisen A, editors. Recommendations for the Practice of Clinical Neurophysiology: guidelines of the International Federation of Clinical Neurophysiol-ogy. International Federation of Clinical Neurophysiology, 1999: 99

53. Rossini PM. The anatomic and physiologic bases of motor-evoked potentials. Neurol Clin 1988; 6: 751–69

54. Caramia MD, Cicinelli P, Paradiso C, et al. Excitability changes of muscular responses to magnetic brain stimulation in patients with central motor disorders. Electroencephalogr Clin Neurophysiol 1991; 81: 243–50

55. Desiato MT, Caramia MD. Towards a neurophysiological marker of amyotrophic lateral sclerosis as revealed by changes in cortical excitability. Electroencephalogr Clin Neurophysiol 1997; 105: 1–7

56. Eisen A, Pant B, Stewart H. Cortical excitability in amyotrophic lateral sclerosis: A clue to pathogenesis. Can J Neurol Sci 1993; 20: 11–16

57. Zanette G, Tamburin S, Manganotti P, et al. Different mechanisms contribute to motor cortex hyperexcitability in amyotrophic lateral sclerosis. Clin Neurophysiol 2002; 113: 1688–97

58. Mills KR, Nithi KA. Corticomotor threshold is reduced in early sporadic amyotrophic lateral sclerosis [see comments]. Muscle Nerve 1997; 20: 1137–41

59. Desiato MT, Bernardi G, Hagi HA, et al. Transcranial magnetic stimulation of motor pathways directed to muscles supplied by cranial nerves in amyotrophic lateral sclerosis. Clin Neurophysiol 2002; 113: 132–140

60. Mills KR. The natural history of central motor abnormalities in amyotrophic lateral sclerosis. Brain 2003; 126: 2558–66

61. Quartarone A, Battaglia F, Majorana G, et al. Different patterns of I-waves summation in ALS patients according to the central conduction time. Clin Neurophysiol 2002; 113: 1301–7

62. Salerno A, Georgesco M. Interhemispheric facilitation and inhibition studied in man with double magnetic stimulation. Electroencephalogr Clin Neurophysiol 1996; 101: 395–403

63. Turner MR, Osei-Lah AD, Hammers A, et al. Abormal cortical excitability in sporadic but not homozygous D90A SOD1 ALS. J Neurol Neurosurg Psychiatry 2005; 76: 1279–85

64. de Carvalho M, Miranda PC, Luis ML, Ducla-Soares E. Cortical muscle representation in amyotrophic lateral sclerosis patients: Changes with disease evolution. Muscle Nerve 1999; 22: 1684–92

65. Weber M, Eisen A, Nakajima M. Corticomotoneuronal activity in ALS: Changes in the peristimulus

time histogram over time. Clin Neurophysiol 2000; 111: 169–77

66. Zanette G, Tamburin S, Manganotti P, et al. Changes in motor cortex inhibition over time in patients with amyotrophic lateral sclerosis. J Neurol 2002; 249: 1723–8

67. Schwenkreis P, Liepert J, Witscher K, et al. Riluzole suppresses motor cortex facilitation in correlation to its plasma level. A study using transcranial magnetic stimulation. Exp Brain Res 2000; 135: 293–9

68. Ziemann U, Winter M, Reimers CD, et al. Impaired motor cortex inhibition in patients with amyotrophic lateral sclerosis. Evidence from paired transcranial magnetic stimulation. Neurology 1997; 49: 1292–8

69. de Carvalho M, Evangelista T, Sales-Luis ML. The corticomotor threshold is not dependent on disease duration in amyotrophic lateral sclerosis (ALS). Amyotroph Lateral Scler Other Motor Neuron Disord 2002; 3: 39–42

70. Eisen A, Shytbel W, Murphy K, Hoirch M. Cortical magnetic stimulation in amyotrophic lateral sclerosis. Muscle Nerve 1990; 13: 146–51

71. Prout AJ, Eisen AA. The cortical silent period and amyotrophic lateral sclerosis. Muscle Nerve 1994; 17: 217–23

72. Siciliano G, Manca ML, Sagliocco L, et al. Cortical silent period in patients with amyotrophic lateral sclerosis. J Neurol Sci 1999; 169: 93–7

73. Uozumi T, Tsuji S, Murai Y. Motor potentials evoked by magnetic stimulation of the motor cortex in normal subjects and patients with motor disorders. Electroencephalogr Clin Neurophysiol 1991; 81: 251–6

74. Kujirai T, Caramia MD, Rothwell JC, et al. Corticocortical inhibition in human motor cortex. J Physiol 1993; 471: 501–19

75. Tokimura H, Ridding MC, Tokimura Y, et al. Short latency facilitation between pairs of threshold magnetic stimuli applied to human motor cortex. Electroencephalogr Clin Neurophysiol 1996; 101: 263–72

76. Ziemann U, Tergau F, Wischer S, et al. Pharmacological control of facilitatory I-wave interaction in the human motor cortex. A paired transcranial magnetic stimulation study. Electroencephalogr Clin Neurophysiol 1998; 109: 321–30

77. Ziemann U, Tergau F, Wassermann EM, et al. Demonstration of facilitatory I wave interaction in the human motor cortex by paired transcranial magnetic stimulation. J Physiol 1998; 511: 181–90

78. Ziemann U, Rothwell JC, Ridding MC. Interaction between intracortical inhibition and facilitation in human motor cortex. J Physiol 1996; 496: 873–81

79. Yokota T, Yoshino A, Inaba A, Saito Y. Double cortical stimulation in amyotrophic lateral sclerosis. J Neurol Neurosurg Psychiatry 1996; 61: 596–600

80. Sommer M, Tergau F, Wischer S, et al. Riluzole does not have an acute effect on motor thresholds and the intracortical excitability in amyotrophic lateral sclerosis. J Neurol 1999; 246 (Suppl 3): III22–26

81. Stefan K, Kunesch E, Benecke R, Classen J. Effects of riluzole on cortical excitability in patients with amyotrophic lateral sclerosis. Ann Neurol 2001; 49: 536–9

82. Peinemann A, Lehner C, Conrad B, Siebner HR. Age-related decrease in paired-pulse intracortical inhibition in the human primary motor cortex. Neurosci Lett 2001; 313: 33–6

83. Boroojerdi B, Kopylev L, Battaglia F, et al. Reproducibility of intracortical inhibition and facilitation using the paired-pulse paradigm. Muscle Nerve 2000; 23: 1594–7

84. Pioro EP, Majors AW, Mitsumoto H, et al. 1H-MRS evidence of neurodegeneration and excess glutamate + glutamine in ALS medulla. Neurology 1999; 53: 71–9

85. Desiato MT, Palmieri MG, Giacomini P, et al. The effect of riluzole in amyotrophic lateral sclerosis: a study with cortical stimulation. J Neurol Sci 1999; 169: 98–107

86. Leigh PN, Meldrum BS. Excitotoxicity in ALS. Neurology 1996; 47 (6 Suppl 4): S221–7

87. Shaw PJ. Calcium, glutamate, and amyotrophic lateral sclerosis: more evidence but no certainties [editorial; comment]. Ann Neurol 1999; 46: 803–5

88. Maragakis NJ, Dykes-Hoberg M, Rothstein JD. Altered expression of the glutamate transporter EAAT2b in neurological disease. Ann Neurol 2004; 55: 469–77

89. Nihei K, McKee AC, Kowall NW. Patterns of neuronal degeneration in the motor cortex of amyotrophic lateral sclerosis patients. Acta Neuropathol (Berl) 1993; 86: 55–64

90. Petri S, Krampfl K, Hashemi F, et al. Distribution of GABAA receptor mRNA in the motor cortex of ALS patients. J Neuropathol Exp Neurol 2003; 62: 1041–51

91. Cudkowicz ME, McKenna-Yasek D, Chen C, et al. Limited corticospinal tract involvement in amy-

otrophic lateral sclerosis subjects with the A4V mutation in the copper/zinc superoxide dismutase gene. Ann Neurol 1998; 43: 703–10

92. Bruyn RP, Koelman JH, Troost D, de Jong JM. Motor neuron disease (amyotrophic lateral sclerosis) arising from longstanding primary lateral sclerosis. J Neurol Neurosurg Psychiatry 1995; 58: 742–4

93. Schriefer TN, Hess CW, Mills KR, Murray NM. Central motor conduction studies in motor neurone disease using magnetic brain stimulation. Electroencephalogr Clin Neurophysiol 1989; 74: 431–7

94. Ingram DA, Swash M. Central motor conduction is abnormal in motor neuron disease. J Neurol Neurosurg Psychiatry 1987; 50: 159–66

95. Thompson PD, Day BL, Rothwell JC, et al. The interpretation of electromyographic responses to electrical stimulation of the motor cortex in diseases of the upper motor neurone. J Neurol Sci 1987; 80: 91–110

96. de Carvalho M, Scotto M, Lopes A, Swash M. Clinical and neurophysiological evaluation of progression in amyotrophic lateral sclerosis. Muscle Nerve 2003; 28: 630–3

97. Andersen PM, Forsgren L, Binzer M, et al. Autosomal recessive adult-onset amyotrophic lateral sclerosis associated with homozygosity for Asp90Ala CuZn-superoxide dismutase mutation. A clinical and genealogical study of 36 patients [published erratum appears in Brain 1998; 121: 187]. Brain 1996; 119: 1153–72

98. Weber M, Eisen A, Stewart HG, Andersen PM. Preserved slow conducting corticomotoneuronal projections in amyotrophic lateral sclerosis with autosomal recessive D90A CuZn-superoxide dismutase mutation. Brain 2000; 123: 1505–15

99. de Carvalho M, Turkman A, Swash M. Motor responses evoked by transcranial magnetic stimulation and peripheral nerve stimulation in the ulnar innervation in amyotrophic lateral sclerosis: The effect of upper and lower motor neuron lesion. J Neurol Sci 2003; 210: 83–90

100. Triggs WJ, Menkes D, Onorato J, et al. Transcranial magnetic stimulation identifies upper motor neuron involvement in motor neuron disease. Neurology 1999; 53: 605–11

101. Magistris MR, Rosler KM, Truffert A, et al. A clinical study of motor evoked potentials using a triple stimulation technique. Brain 1999; 122: 265–79

102. Day BL, Rothwell JC, Thompson PD, et al. Motor cortex stimulation in intact man. 2. Multiple descending volleys. Brain 1987; 110: 1191–209

103. Hess CW, Mills KR, Murray NM. Responses in small hand muscles from magnetic stimulation of the human brain. J Physiol 1987; 388: 397–419

104. Kiers L, Cros D, Chiappa KH, Fang J. Variability of motor potentials evoked by transcranial magnetic stimulation. Electroencephalogr Clin Neurophysiol 1993; 89: 415–23

105. Rosler KM, Truffert A, Hess CW, Magistris MR. Quantification of upper motor neuron loss in amyotrophic lateral sclerosis. Clin Neurophysiol 2000; 111: 2208–18

106. Komissarow L, Rollnik JD, Bogdanova D, et al. Triple stimulation technique (TST) in amyotrophic lateral sclerosis. Clin Neurophysiol 2004; 115: 356–60

107. Brooks BR, Miller RG, Swash M, Munsat TL. El Escorial revisited: Revised criteria for the diagnosis of amyotrophic lateral sclerosis. Amyotroph Lateral Scler Other Motor Neuron Disord 2000; 1: 293–9

108. Brouwer B, Ashby P. Corticospinal projections to upper and lower limb spinal motoneurons in man. Electroencephalogr Clin Neurophysiol 1990; 76: 509–19

109. Day BL, Dressler D, Maertens DN, et al. Electric and magnetic stimulation of human motor cortex: Surface EMG and single motor unit responses [published erratum appears in J Physiol (Lond) 1990; 430: 617]. J Physiol (Lond) 1989; 412: 449–73

110. de Noordhout AM, Rapisarda G, Bogacz D, et al. Corticomotoneuronal synaptic connections in normal man: An electrophysiological study. Brain 1999; 122: 1327–40

111. Mills KR. Corticomotoneuronal PSTH studies [editorial; comment]. Muscle Nerve 1999; 22: 297–8

112. Awiszus F, Feistner H. Comparison of single motor unit responses to transcranial magnetic and peroneal nerve stimulation in the tibialis anterior muscle of patients with amyotrophic lateral sclerosis. Electroencephalogr Clin Neurophysiol 1995; 97: 90–5

113. Eisen A, Entezari-Taher M, Stewart H. Cortical projections to spinal motoneurons: Changes with aging and amyotrophic lateral sclerosis. Neurology 1996; 46: 1396–404

114. Fetz EE, Gustafsson B. Relation between shapes of post-synaptic potentials and changes in firing probability of cat motoneurones. J Physiol (Lond) 1983; 341: 387–410

115. Kohara N, Kaji R, Kojima Y, et al. Abnormal excitability of the corticospinal pathway in patients

with amyotrophic lateral sclerosis: A single motor unit study using transcranial magnetic stimulation. Electroencephalogr Clin Neurophysiol 1996; 101: 32–41

116. Nakajima M, Eisen A, Stewart H. Diverse abnormalities of corticomotoneuronal projections in individual patients with amyotrophic lateral sclerosis. Electroencephalogr Clin Neurophysiol 1997; 105: 451–7

117. Weber M, Eisen A. Assessment of upper and lower motor neurons in Kennedy's disease: Implications for corticomotoneuronal PSTH studies [see comments]. Muscle Nerve 1999; 22: 299–306

118. Ashby P, Zilm D. Synaptic connections to individual tibialis anterior motoneurones in man. J Neurol Neurosurg Psychiatry 1978; 41: 684–9

119. Ashby P, Zilm D. Relationship between EPSP shape and cross-correlation profile explored by computer simulation for studies on human motoneurons. Exp Brain Res 1982; 47: 33–40

120. Henneman E, Somjen G, Carpenter DO. Functional significance of cell size in spinal motoneurons. J Neurophysiol 1965; 28: 560–80

121. Bawa P, Lemon RN. Recruitment of motor units in response to transcranial magnetic stimulation in man. J Physiol (Lond) 1993; 471: 445–64

122. Boniface SJ, Mills KR, Schubert M. Responses of single spinal motoneurons to magnetic brain stimulation in healthy subjects and patients with multiple sclerosis. Brain 1991; 114: 643–62

123. Kernell D, Chien-Ping W. Post-synaptic effects of cortical stimulation on forelimb motoneurones in the baboon. J Physiol (Lond) 1967; 191: 673–90

124. Burke D, Hicks R, Gandevia SC, et al. Direct comparison of corticospinal volleys in human subjects to transcranial magnetic and electrical stimulation. J Physiol 1993; 470: 383–93

125. Di Lazzaro V, Oliviero A, Pilato F, et al. Corticospinal volleys evoked by transcranial stimulation of the brain in conscious humans. Neurol Res 2003; 25: 143–50

126. Weber M, Eisen A. Peristimulus time histograms (PSTHs) – a marker for upper motor neuron involvement in ALS? Amyotroph Lateral Scler Other Motor Neuron Disord 2000; 1 (Suppl 2): S51–6

127. Mills KR. Motor neuron disease. Studies of the corticospinal excitation of single motor neurons by magnetic brain stimulation. Brain 1995; 118: 971–82

128. Awiszus F, Feistner H. Abnormal EPSPs evoked by magnetic brain stimulation in hand muscle

motoneurons of patients with amyotrophic lateral sclerosis. Electroencephalogr Clin Neurophysiol 1993; 89: 408–14

129. Nakajima M, Eisen A, McCarthy R, et al. Reduced corticomotoneuronal excitatory postsynaptic potentials (EPSPs) with normal Ia afferent EPSPs in amyotrophic lateral sclerosis. Neurology 1996; 47: 1555–61

130. Guidetti D, Motti L, Marcello N, et al. Kennedy disease in an Italian kindred. Eur Neurol 1986; 25: 188–96

131. Harding AE, Thomas PK, Baraitser M, et al. X-linked recessive bulbospinal neuronopathy: A report of ten cases. J Neurol Neurosurg Psychiatry 1982; 45: 1012–19

132. Kennedy WR, Alter M, Sung JH. Progressive proximal spinal and bulbar muscular atrophy of late onset. A sex-linked recessive trait. Neurology 1968; 18: 671–80

133. La Spada AR, Roling DB, Harding AE, et al. Meiotic stability and genotype–phenotype correlation of the trinucleotide repeat in X-linked spinal and bulbar muscular atrophy. Nat Genet 1992; 2: 301–4

134. Sperfeld AD, Karitzky J, Brummer D, et al. X-linked bulbospinal neuronopathy: Kennedy disease. Arch Neurol 2002; 59: 1921–6

135. Takahashi K. Slow and fast groups of pyramidal tract cells and their respective membrane properties. J Neurophysiol 1965; 28: 908–24

136. Ugawa Y, Kanazawa I. Motor-evoked potentials: Unusual findings. Clin Neurophysiol 1999; 110: 1641–5

137. Krampfl K, Schlesinger F, Wolfes H, et al. Functional diversity of recombinant human AMPA type glutamate receptors: Possible implications for selective vulnerability of motor neurons. J Neurol Sci 2001; 191: 19–23

138. Van Westerlaak MG, Joosten EA, Gribnau AA, et al. Differential cortico-motoneuron vulnerability after chronic mitochondrial inhibition in vitro and the role of glutamate receptors. Brain Res 2001; 922: 243–9

139. Beaulieu JM, Jacomy H, Julien JP. Formation of intermediate filament protein aggregates with disparate effects in two transgenic mouse models lacking the neurofilament light subunit. J Neurosci 2000; 20: 5321–8

140. Strong MJ, Strong WL, Jaffe H, et al. Phosphorylation state of the native high-molecular-weight neurofilament subunit protein from cervical spinal

cord in sporadic amyotrophic lateral sclerosis. J Neurochem 2001; 76: 1315–25

141. Wong NK, He BP, Strong MJ. Characterization of neuronal intermediate filament protein expression in cervical spinal motor neurons in sporadic amyotrophic lateral sclerosis (ALS). J Neuropathol Exp Neurol 2000; 59: 972–82

142. Eisen A, Nakajima M, Stewart H, Weber M. Excitability of the motor cortex in amyotrophic lateral sclerosis. Electroencephalogr Clin Neurophysiol Suppl 1999; 50: 175–82

143. Andersen PM, Nilsson P, Ala-Hurula V, et al. Amyotrophic lateral sclerosis associated with homozygosity for an Asp90Ala mutation in CuZn-superoxide dismutase. Nat Genet 1995; 10: 61–6

144. Andersen PM, Nilsson P, Keranen ML, et al. Phenotypic heterogeneity in motor neuron disease patients with CuZn-superoxide dismutase mutations in Scandinavia. Brain 1997; 120: 1723–37

145. Osei-Lah AD, Turner MR, Andersen PM, et al. A novel central motor conduction abnormality in D90A-homozygous patients with amyotrophic lateral sclerosis. Muscle Nerve 2004; 29: 790–4

146. Al Chalabi A, Andersen PM, Chioza B, et al. Recessive amyotrophic lateral sclerosis families with the D90A SOD1 mutation share a common founder: Evidence for a linked protective factor. Hum Mol Genet 1998; 7: 2045–50

147. Parton MJ, Broom W, Andersen PM, et al. D90A-SOD1 mediated amyotrophic lateral sclerosis: A single founder for all cases with evidence for a Cis-acting disease modifier in the recessive haplotype. Hum Mutat 2002; 20: 473

148. Ince PG, Tomkins J, Slade JY, et al. Amyotrophic lateral sclerosis associated with genetic abnormalities in the gene encoding Cu/Zn superoxide dismutase: Molecular pathology of five new cases, and comparison with previous reports and 73 sporadic cases of ALS. J Neuropathol Exp Neurol 1998; 57: 895–904

149. Stewart HG, Eisen A, Weber M, Andersen PM. Electrophysiological profiles in ALS patients with Cu,Zn-SOD mutations. Amyotrophic lateral sclerosis and other motor neuron disorders 2003; 4 (Suppl 1): 170

150. Eisen A, Weber M. The motor cortex and amyotrophic lateral sclerosis. Muscle Nerve 2001; 24: 564–73

151. Mochizuki Y, Mizutani T, Takasu T. Amyotrophic lateral sclerosis with marked neurological asymmetry: Clinicopathological study. Acta Neuropathol 1995; 90: 44–50

152. Probst A, Andersen PM, Weber M. A case of familial ALS with marked asymmetry. Amyotrophic lateral sclerosis and other motor neuron disorders, 2004; in press

153. Bendszus M, Wessig C, Solymosi L, et al. MRI of peripheral nerve degeneration and regeneration: Correlation with electrophysiology and histology. Exp Neurol 2004; 188: 171–7

154. Airapetian KV, Zavalishin IA, Nikitin SS, Barkhatova VP. [Physiopathological and chemopathological mechanisms of central motor disorders in amyotrophic lateral sclerosis]. Zh Nevrol Psikhiatr Im S S Korsakova 2000; 100: 33–6

155. Lin CL, Bristol LA, Jin L, et al. Aberrant RNA processing in a neurodegenerative disease: The cause for absent EAAT2, a glutamate transporter, in amyotrophic lateral sclerosis. Neuron 1998; 20: 589–602

156. Bristol LA, Rothstein JD. Glutamate transporter gene expression in amyotrophic lateral sclerosis motor cortex. Ann Neurol 1996; 39: 676–9

157. Andreassen OA, Jenkins BG, Dedeoglu A, et al. Increases in cortical glutamate concentrations in transgenic amyotrophic lateral sclerosis mice are attenuated by creatine supplementation. J Neurochem 2001; 77: 383–90

158. Williams TL, Day NC, Ince PG, et al. Calcium-permeable alpha-amino-3-hydroxy-5-methyl-4-isoxazole propionic acid receptors: A molecular determinant of selective vulnerability in amyotrophic lateral sclerosis. Ann Neurol 1997; 42: 200–7

159. Carriedo SG, Yin HZ, Weiss JH. Motor neurons are selectively vulnerable to AMPA/kainate receptor-mediated injury in vitro. J Neurosci 1996; 16: 4069–79

160. Roy J, Minotti S, Dong L, et al. Glutamate potentiates the toxicity of mutant Cu/Zn-superoxide dismutase in motor neurons by postsynaptic calcium-dependent mechanisms. J Neurosci 1998; 18: 9673–84

161. Terro F, Yardin C, Esclaire F, et al. Mild kainate toxicity produces selective motoneuron death with marked activation of CA(2+)-permeable AMPA/kainate receptors. Brain Res 1998; 809: 319–24

162. Brooks BR. El Escorial World Federation of Neurology criteria for the diagnosis of amyotrophic lateral sclerosis. Subcommittee on Motor Neuron Diseases/Amyotrophic Lateral Sclerosis of the World Federation of Neurology Research Group on Neuromuscular Diseases and the El Escorial 'Clinical limits of amyotrophic lateral sclerosis' workshop

contributors [see comments]. J Neurol Sci 1994; 124 (Suppl): 96–107

163. Beal MF, Richardson EP Jr. Primary lateral sclerosis: A case report. Arch Neurol 1981; 38: 630–3

164. Fisher CM. Pure spastic paralysis of corticospinal origin. Can J Neurol Sci 1977; 4: 251–8

165. Pringle CE, Hudson AJ, Munoz DG, et al. Primary lateral sclerosis. Clinical features, neuropathology and diagnostic criteria. Brain 1992; 115: 495–520

166. Forsyth PA, Dalmau J, Graus F, et al. Motor neuron syndromes in cancer patients [see comments]. Ann Neurol 1997; 41: 722–30

167. Rowland LP. Primary lateral sclerosis: Disease, syndrome, both or neither? [editorial; comment]. J Neurol Sci 1999; 170: 1–4

168. Swash M, Desai J, Misra VP. What is primary lateral sclerosis? [see comments]. J Neurol Sci 1999; 170: 5–10

169. Le Forestier N, Maisonobe T, Spelle L, et al. Primary lateral sclerosis: Further clarification. J Neurol Sci 2001; 185: 95–100

170. Le Forestier N, Maisonobe T, Piquard A et al. Does primary lateral sclerosis exist? A study of 20 patients and a review of the literature. Brain 2001; 124: 1989–99

171. Zhai P, Pagan F, Statland J, et al. Primary lateral sclerosis: A heterogeneous disorder composed of different subtypes? Neurology 2003; 60: 1258–65

172. Brown WF, Ebers GC, Hudson AJ, et al. Motor-evoked responses in primary lateral sclerosis. Muscle Nerve 1992; 15: 626–9

173. Salerno A, Carlander B, Camu W, Georgesco M. Motor evoked potentials (MEPs): Evaluation of the different types of responses in amyotrophic lateral sclerosis and primary lateral sclerosis. Electromyogr Clin Neurophysiol 1996; 36: 361–8

174. Kuipers-Upmeijer J, de Jager AE, Hew JM, et al. Primary lateral sclerosis: Clinical, neurophysiological, and magnetic resonance findings. J Neurol Neurosurg Psychiatry 2001; 71: 615–20

175. Weber M, Stewart H, Hirota N, Eisen A. Cortico-motoneuronal connections in primary lateral sclerosis (PLS). Amyotroph Lateral Scler Other Motor Neuron Disord 2002; 3: 190–8

176. Eisen A, Nakajima M, Weber M. Corticomotor-neuronal hyper-excitability in amyotrophic lateral sclerosis. J Neurol Sci 1998; 160 (Suppl 1): S64–8

177. Smith CD. Serial MRI findings in a case of primary lateral sclerosis. Neurology 2002; 58: 647–9

6

Conventional neurophysiology in amyotrophic lateral sclerosis

Mamede de Carvalho, Michael Swash

INTRODUCTION

Neurophysiological investigation in amyotrophic lateral sclerosis (ALS) has several roles. First, it is essential to confirm and test the clinical diagnosis by showing signs of widespread ongoing lower motor neuron (LMN) demise, in particular in non-clinically affected muscle, and by excluding other LMN conditions that resemble ALS. Second, it may be helpful in staging the disorder. Third, it can help in establishing the prognosis. Last, it is a useful tool for monitoring disease progression. Its role in diagnosis and follow-up has not been diminished by the appearance of new sophisticated imaging methods.

The importance of electromyography (EMG) in the diagnosis of this clinical disorder was recognized many years ago, in particular as a consequence of the work of Edward Lambert, who proposed a number of critical findings in EMG investigation to support the clinical diagnosis of ALS (Lambert's criteria)[1,2]. These are described below:

(1) Fibrillation and fasciculation potentials in muscles of the upper and lower extremities (three different muscles with different root and peripheral nerve innervation), or in extremities as well as in muscles innervated by cranial nerves;

(2) Reduction of the number and increase in the amplitude and duration of the motor unit potentials;

(3) Motor nerve conduction velocities which are normal when recorded from relatively unaffected muscles, and not less than 70% of average normal value, for age, when recorded from severely affected muscles;

(4) Normal sensory nerve conduction responses.

These criteria are still applicable. The relative preservation of the motor conduction velocities has been confirmed in several more recent papers[3,4]. However, the recent recognition of motor neuropathies mimicking ALS, some with conduction block[5–10], implies that these entities should be excluded in the EMG work-up of those with suspected ALS.

Another issue is the need for early diagnosis in the management of the disease, as well as for timely inclusion in clinical trials[11], or just to diminish the number of clinical investigations and the patient's anxiety. In the future, as more effective treatments become available, early diagnosis may become increasingly important[11]. Although the role of EMG in early diagnosis has not been systematically evaluated, it seems now to be the only method available to support that purpose, since LMN abnormalities are typically evident in EMG before they are clinically recognizable[12,13].

There is a length-dependent probability for the nerve–muscle anatomical unit to show signs of active denervation[14,15]. In other words, the distal muscles in any myotome tend to show more fibrillation and sharp-wave potentials (fibs-sw). Cranial innervated muscles do not often show fibs-sw[15,16], which might imply a later diagnosis for those patients presenting with bulbar features, if the strict Lambert criteria are used. On the other hand, weak and atrophic muscles show fibs-sw more consistently and in a greater number than strong muscles[2,16,17]. As a result, a large proportion of ALS patients fail to show classical findings in the initial EMG study, mainly because needle investigation may not show widespread active denervation early in the disease[18]. For these reasons, about one-third of ALS patients followed in one center did not meet the Lambert criteria[18] when investigated, although these criteria are thought to have a high specificity for ALS.

This question of the early diagnosis created the conditions for the establishment of the Escorial criteria[19]. These include both clinical and EMG features and define different degrees of certainty, which may be valuable when designing a new clinical trial. For definite ALS, the EMG criteria include reduced recruitment of large motor unit potentials (MUPs), with increased recruitment ratio and fibrillation potentials. For probable ALS, reduced numbers of large and unstable MUPs or reduced motor unit (MU) number and large macro-EMG MUP are required. To support possible LMN loss, less certain criteria were accepted, including one of the MUP features described above, fasciculation potentials (FPs), and decremental response on repetitive nerve stimulation. At least two muscles of different root and different cranial or peripheral nerve innervation in each region (bulbar, cervical, thoracic, lumbosacral) should show electrophysiologic evidence of either definite, probable or possible LMN degeneration for that region to be ranked as showing definite, probable or possible LMN degeneration. It was accepted that EMG signs could upgrade the clinical diagnosis. In addition, these criteria included the new concept of conduction block as inconsistent with the diagnosis of ALS.

The neurophysiologic part of the El Escorial criteria were criticized because they contain several flaws[20]. In particular, increased recruitment rate may not be found, owing to the upper motor neuron (UMN) involvement, the importance of FPs was undervalued and there were confusing definitions for establishing the criteria for definite or probable LMN degeneration.

It was felt that the classical El Escorial criteria should be revised to correct these drawbacks and to increase diagnostic sensitivity. The final report is known as the Revised El Escorial Criteria[21]. Electrophysiologic studies were considered essential to confirm LMN dysfunction in clinically affected regions, to detect evidence of LMN loss in clinically uninvolved regions and to exclude other pathophysiologic processes. The new criteria stated that EMG signs of LMN dysfunction required to support a diagnosis of ALS should be found in at least two of the four anatomical regions (bulbar/cranial motor neurons, cervical, thoracic, lumbosacral spinal cord). For the brainstem region it was considered sufficient to demonstrate EMG changes in one muscle. For the thoracic region it was sufficient to show EMG changes either in the paraspinal muscles at or below the T6 level or in the abdominal muscles. For the cervical and lumbosacral spinal cord regions, at least two muscles innervated by different roots and peripheral nerves must show EMG changes. To identify LMN dysfunction in a particular muscle, signs of active denervation (fibs-sw) and chronic denervation (large MUPs, reduced interference pattern with increased recruitment rate, unstable MUPs, or by using other quantitative methods) should be present. FPs were considered as supporting the diagnosis, particularly if they were complex and diffuse, but FPs were not regarded as specific to ALS itself. Nerve conduction studies were considered essential to exclude other conditions.

NEEDLE ELECTROMYOGRAPH INVESTIGATION

As many as 50–80% of the normal pool of MU may be lost before wasting and weakness become clinically apparent[22–24]. This reflects the capacity of MUs to expand their innervation field[25] by collateral sprouting which, at first, enables muscle strength to be preserved in the face of the continuing loss of anterior horn cells. Reinnervated muscle fibers tend to assume the same histologic characteristics as those of the reinnervating motor units. Denervated muscle fibers are reinnervated from the nearest nerve terminals, which causes clustering of muscles fibers innervated by the same MU, with the appearance of fiber-type grouping on histologic examination.

Needle EMG is essentially selective and does not evaluate all the MUs in a muscle. The concentric needle electrode has a small recording area (2.5 mm^2) which is less than the total area of a normal MU (which is 2–10 mm^2)[26]. The 'spiky' part of the MU is recorded from a very small area around the tip of the needle electrode (0.5 mm). However, needle EMG is a sensitive method to assess the characteristics of MU microanatomy. Reinnervation causes a change of individual MUP's electrical features, with a larger and more complex MUP. Moreover, type-grouping can be quantified by fiber density measurement using single-fiber EMG. Reinnervation results in MUPs of abnormal morphology, but the anatomical territory of the reinnervated MU, although larger[27], does not increase very much, as shown by scanning EMG studies[28,29], as result of anatomical constraints within the muscle[30]. The extent of the loss of LMNs can be assessed by observing the electrical activity on maximal muscle contraction and evaluating the interference pattern. Another important dimension is the ongoing reinnervation, causing unstable MUPs, as a result of slowed distal motor nerve conduction in newly, partially myelinated nerve fibers, immature end-plates and atrophic muscle fibers. Newly formed end-plates have a different composition of the acetylcholine receptor subunits, and a lower safety factor for neuromuscular transmission[31].

Active denervation

Insertional positive sharp-waves are probably the earliest sign of denervation, but it is difficult to support a diagnosis based on this insecure finding. Fibrillation and positive sharp-waves at rest, which are considered a cardinal sign of denervation[32], are non-specific findings that can be recorded in myopathies, as well as in neurogenic disorders. They represent action potentials generated by individual muscle fibers that have lost their nerve supply, either by axonal damage or by direct muscle fiber damage. Both fibrillation and positive sharp-waves appear to be generated from a biphasic intracellular action potential with a long hyperpolarization phase. The fibrillation potential simply propagates up to and beyond the recording electrode, while sharp-waves appear to be generated by spontaneous action potentials that encounter a needle-induced segment of crushed membrane[33].

In ALS these spontaneous potentials are more frequently observed in muscles that are moderately or severely weak, with clear signs of LMN loss[2,16,17]. The fibs-sw signs persist until the denervated muscle is either reinnervated by collateral nerve sprouts or completely transformed into a fibrous tissue, so they may be sparse in very wasted muscles. They tend to decrease in cold muscles[34], so temperature control is important not only for conduction studies but also for performing needle EMG.

The presence of abundant and diffuse fibs-sw is considered a poor prognostic sign[12]. Patients with bulbospinal neuronopathy (Kennedy's disease), Guamanian ALS and spinal muscular atrophy type III have less prominent fibs-sw[24,35], consistent with the slow progression profile of these conditions.

Fasciculation potentials

Fasciculations are typically observed in ALS and may be its presenting feature[36]. FPs are evident from the earliest clinical stages of the disease, even in muscles with normal strength, but generally become less evident in the end-stage, wasted muscles. They are not absolutely essential to the electrodiagnostic diagnosis, but FPs are so regularly observed that one rarely accepts the diagnosis if no FP is recorded[2]. It is important to recognize that FPs may arise in other neurogenic disorders, for example in root lesions associated with cervical spondylosis. Needle EMG may disclose FPs coming from deep layers of the muscle, although visual inspection detects only those arising in superficial layers.

Their site of origin and significance in relation to the pathogenesis of the disease has long been a controversial issue[17]. FPs are generated by MUs or parts of MUs, which fire irregularly. Probably, FPs are initiated along any neural portion of the MU, from the cell body to the terminal nerve fibers[17]. Norris recorded FPs from muscles innervated by adjacent but different myotomes that discharge almost synchronously, an observation that suggested a supraspinal origin for some FPs[37]. From a pathophysiologic stance fasciculations might be related to the excitotoxic hypothesis of the causation of ALS, at least early in disease progression[36]. There is good evidence that early in the course of the disease FPs may arise in the sick cell body of the motor neuron or at the proximal axon and that, later, their origin is probably distal, at the terminal nerve sprouts[17,38]. In ALS, FPs tend to be very complex and unstable, in particular when the muscle is weak, which may be helpful in the differential diagnosis[17,39]. The firing rate in ALS is about 0.3/s, and much lower in Kennedy's disease[40]. Possibly, in ALS, combined FPs may occur, facilitated by the UMN lesion[40]. Another unique marker of the FPs in ALS is the observation that two consecutive FPs may have different MU origins[41], an unusual occurrence in other neurogenic disorders, in which FPs tend to be due to repetitive firing of the same MU.

Transcranial magnetic stimulation studies have suggested that cortically driven FPs are probably not uncommon[42,43]. It is likely that this is a more frequent finding at an early phase of the disease progression, when fasciculations are more frequent, but we have also noted evoked FPs in weak muscles. The observation of evoked FPs when using threshold or even subthreshold stimulus intensity reinforces the hypothesis that these FPs originate in hyperexcitable motor cells, particularly as suprathreshold stimuli tend to evoke larger motor responses that may mask the FPs[43].

A number of healthy subjects have fasciculations, especially in calf and hand muscles, but these are rarely as prominent as those observed in ALS[44]. These FPs tend to have a simple morphology and a higher firing rate than the FPs associated with neurologic disorders[17,45]. FPs are also common is multiple motor neuropathy with conduction block (MMNCB), radiculopathies, cramp-fasciculation syndrome and electrolyte depletion, and in thyroid or parathyroid disorders.

Patients with denervation localized in one region and diffuse FPs should be strongly suspected of having ALS. A clinical–electrophysiological revaluation should be repeated 3–6 months later. With this strategy, it should be possible to shorten the time to diagnosis[16]. Ultrasound may add further information by detecting FPs from deep and superficial layers of the muscles[46], and surface electrodes are useful in providing more detailed information about their spatial and temporal distribution[47].

Other spontaneous activity

Cramps, a repetitive 200–300-Hz MUP discharge, accompanied by involuntary muscle contraction, are a very frequent early symptom in ALS, in general frequently induced by voluntary contraction. In our experience, sometimes they can be so disturbing that full contraction for EMG investigation of the interference pattern may be impossible in many muscles. They are not a specific finding, but when they occur in thoracic muscles it seems advisable to suspect ALS. Myokymic discharges may be associated with demyelination, but are rare in ALS, although they have been observed in Kennedy's disease.

Complex repetitive discharges, an abrupt train of simple or complex spikes of 5–150 Hz, are one example of non-specific spontaneous activity that occurs in situations of chronic denervation–reinnervation, or in myopathies. Its origin seems to be ephatic transmission through an excitatory loop between adjacent muscle fibers[48]. It may be observed in ALS, in particular in patients with slower progression. It is often found in the tongue[15].

Discharges resembling myotonic discharges occur extremely rarely in ALS. Such discharges, characteristic of membrane disturbance, may also be observed in patients with other long-lasting neurogenic disorders, such as radiculopathies.

Motor unit potential analysis

The morphology of MUPs should be studied with the muscle in slight contraction in terms of amplitude, duration, area and number of phases, as well as the firing pattern (recruitment ratio), relative number of the MUP relative to strength of contraction and stability. The cardinal signs of neurogenic change are the presence of larger, generally unstable, complex MUPs, with increased recruitment ratio. An increased number of satellite potentials is also often observed[49]. Increased MUP amplitude results from clustering of reinnervated muscle fibers. Increased MUP duration results from several different factors, including the number of innervated muscle fibers, end-plate dispersion, end-plate delay and slow conduction through terminal branches. Muscle fiber hypertrophy might increase both amplitude and duration. Possibly, changes in amplitude and area are more sensitive as an index of neurogenic change than increased duration. Giant MUPs (above 10 mV) are rarely observed in this progressive disorder, although they can sometimes be found in cases of slow progression, as in monomelic forms of ALS.

More commonly they are noticed in remote polio, spinal cord compression, congenital dysplasias of the spinal cord, syringomyelia, motor neuropathies, or in neurogenic thoracic outlet syndrome (Figure 6.1)[24]. In very progressive disorders, there is less time for surviving MUs to reach their full innervation potential before they die. In ALS, at an end-stage, small MUPs may be observed, possibly resulting from degeneration of distal nerve terminals through axonal dying-back pathology.

Ideally, all MUPs should be quantified in each muscle. However, since in ALS it is important to prove that the neurogenic process is diffuse, qualitative analysis may be acceptable, since a well-trained neurophysiologist may become proficient in evaluating the MUP changes[12]. The recruitment ratio is the ratio between the firing rate of the recruited MUP and the number of other MUPs that discharge at the same time; the normal value is between 3 and 5. This measurement is generally increased in ALS, and may be a sensitive measurement[12].

The stability (jiggle) may be better evaluated with a 500-Hz high-pass filter[50], giving important qualitative information. Unstable potentials

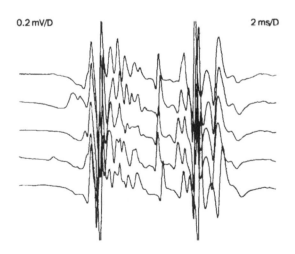

0.2 mV/D   2 ms/D

Figure 6.1 Very complex and relatively stable motor unit observed in a patient with cervical syringomyelia (high-pass filter of 500 Hz)

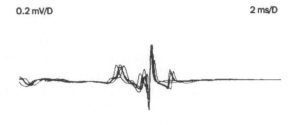

0.2 mV/D   2 ms/D

Figure 6.2   Complex and very unstable motor unit observed in an amyotrophic lateral sclerosis patient (high-pass filter of 500 Hz)

represent a process of ongoing reinnervation, secondary to recent denervation. MUP instability has many causes. In particular it is caused by the presence of immature axonal sprouts and motor endplates, and atrophic muscle fibers of slow propagation velocity (Figure 6.2)[29].

On full contraction, an incomplete interference pattern can be recorded, implying decompensation of the reinnervation process[51], which can be correlated with the loss of MUPs, with the remaining MUPs showing an increased firing rate. A typical neurogenic firing pattern is easily observed on full contraction. This latter technique is useful to differentiate MUP loss from poor central recruitment, e.g. poor co-operation or spasticity, in which only a few MUPs are recruited, firing at a slow rate.

Muscle investigation

Because the main purpose of the EMG is to show widespread loss of MUs, a number of sensitive muscles should be assessed in the routine EMG investigation. This issue is particularly critical in cranial-innervated muscles where fibs-sw are not so frequently observed[15]. Involvement of cranial muscles has a very important diagnostic significance in ALS, by excluding the diagnosis of spondylosis.

Orbicularis oris, masseter, trapezius, tongue (genioglossus) and sternomastoid muscles have been recommended for study in ALS, since these muscles are rostral to the cervical myotomes. However, it is very difficult to relax the tongue, in order to show fib-sw, and performing many insertions is much too aggressive in clinical practice. However, the tongue is probably a more sensitive muscle to study than the masseter, temporalis, frontalis and mentalis muscles, in showing fibs-sw[14,52]. The sternomastoid muscle seems more sensitive than the frontalis and masseter[53]. Qualitative EMG analysis showed that the sternomastoid muscle was abnormal in half of the bulbar-onset patients and two-thirds of spinal-onset patients, in which it is more sensitive than the tongue, although fibs-sw are not frequent in this muscle[54]. As the entire extramedullary pathway of the spinal accessory nerve is protected from cervical bony compression[55], neurogenic change in the sternocleidomastoid muscle is of major diagnostic importance. Although new quantitative methods can detect subtle neurogenic changes in cranial-innervated muscles, even in patients without bulbar signs[56], there is no unquestionable advantage over conventional MUP analysis.

In upper limbs, hand muscles are often involved early in ALS, and should be studied[57]. In particular the first dorsal interosseous is sensitive[13,15], very comfortably investigated in all patients, and more affected than the abductor digiti minimi, because in anterior horn cell disorders the thenar hand seems more severely affected than the hypothenar half[58–60]. Proximal muscles, such as the biceps, deltoid or the extensor digitorum communis are good options for obtaining information about more proximal myotomes. In lower limbs, the tibialis anterior regularly shows fibs-sw in ALS[13,15]; the more proximal vastus medialis or the gastrocnemius should be assessed in addition.

Study of thoracic paraspinal muscles[61] may be helpful in confirming ALS, but cervical and lumbar spinal muscles may be misleading, as degenerative changes in the elderly can cause abnormal MUPs in these muscles[62]. It should be noted that active denervation is more frequent in limb than in corresponding paraspinal muscles[14]. Abdominal muscles and internal intercostal muscles, activated during expiration, and diaphragm, activated during inspiration, are other useful muscles for testing. The superior part of the rectus abdominis has also been suggested as a useful muscle to study in the diagnosis of ALS (T8-12)[63].

ALS patients may present with acute ventilatory failure, caused by severe loss of MUs in the respiratory muscles[64]. Denervation of the respiratory muscles indicates impending respiratory failure[65]. Diaphragmatic involvement cannot be predicted from involvement of limb muscles in the same myotome. Thus, EMG of the diaphragm is essential, at least in the group of patients with probable respiratory involvement. We routinely perform diaphragmatic EMG in ALS patients. A concentric needle electrode is inserted through the eighth or ninth interspace at the anterior axillary line to reach the diaphragm (Figure 6.3).

In our experience[15] patients with lower-limb onset always show fibs-sw in lower limb muscles, and the same is almost always true for patients in whom the weakness commences in upper limbs, when fibs-sw are easily found in the first dorsal interosseous muscle. Regionally limited disease, in particular in the bulbar region, can raise problems regarding the confirmation of the diagnosis of ALS. The same is true for patients with limited lower limbs or C8-D1 LMN loss. However, the presence of widespread fibs-sw in lower limb or upper limbs, associated with diffuse fasciculation, supports the diagnosis of ALS[15]. It is important to understand that when one limb is affected, the next to be involved is often the homologous contralateral muscle, so this muscle deserves special attention during the needle study.

In patients with cervical and lumbar canal stenosis, ALS can be difficult to recognize. Nonetheless, the presence of diffuse fibs-sw and very unstable MUPs in the above conditions is rare, unless there is also severe pain with sensory loss. In these circumstances the clinical neurophysiologist should consider the clinical picture before reaching any conclusion. In addition, a second EMG investigation performed a few

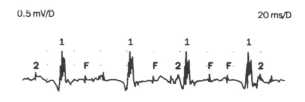

0.5 mV/D   20 ms/D

Figure 6.3 Interferential pattern of the diaphragm on full contraction of an amyotrophic lateral sclerosis patient with marked respiratory impairment, showing two motor units (1 and 2), one very complex (1), and fibrillation potentials (F)

months later will show progression, with more widespread involvement of additional myotomes, an essential feature of ALS. Neuroimaging is essential in ruling out clinically significant treatable spinal cord disease.

Spinal muscular atrophy is a condition generally causing a proximal, slow progressive weakness, starting at a young age; the most difficult differential diagnosis is with muscular dystrophy, not ALS. However, differential diagnosis between ALS and distal spinal muscular atrophy, a rare condition[66], can be more difficult. In these cases it can be rewarding to study less affected muscles, to see the very chronic giant MUPs.

In remote polio some wasted muscles may continue to show sparse fibs-sw, but in these patients almost all muscles show chronic changes, and giant MUPs are typically seen. Postpolio syndrome is a condition in which there is a late clinical progression, as a result of a further loss of MUs, probably caused by the normal aging process, in a limited functional pool of MUs. The differential diagnosis between postpolio and remote polio with no progression based on neurophysiologic grounds is virtually impossible, since fibs-sw and increased jitter are common in residual polio, not indicating progressive disease[67]. However, it is believed that the continuing motor unit loss with aging is more rapid in patients with previous polio than in healthy subjects[68].

Polymyositis and inclusion body myositis can clinically be mistaken for ALS but motor unit potential analysis will disclose myopathic potentials. It was previously thought that neurogenic potentials were found in inclusion body myositis, but this was not confirmed in newer studies using macro-EMG and quantitative motor unit analysis[69].

MOTOR CONDUCTION STUDIES

Motor conduction studies are essential in the diagnosis of ALS, in order to exclude axonal or demyelinating neuropathy, and motor neuropathies with conduction block[4-9].

Demyelinating neuropathies

Focal demyelination is the cause of weakness in patients with motor demyelinating neuropathies. Furthermore, focal demyelination may cause segmental slowing, increased threshold and ectopic discharges at the site of demyelination[70]. Paranodal segmental demyelination is the pathologic finding in focal demyelination. This causes dissipation of the action potential as a result of a decreased impedance of the pathologic region, when the nerve fiber is unable to achieve depolarization of the next node beyond the threshold, and conduction block occurs. Antibodies against the myelin, such as the anti-GM1 antibody, causing paranodal demyelination, or blocking the sodium channels, may be associated with focal demyelination.

Focal demyelination can be difficult to demonstrate, in particular because it may occur proximal to the most proximal stimulation site, or more distal than the distal stimulation point, and may therefore somewhat resemble axonal loss. Proximal focal demyelination can be suspected when a normal compound muscle action potential (CMAP) amplitude is recorded from a weak, non-atrophic muscle[70], in particular when the F-waves are very abnormal. In addition, proximal

conduction can be reliably measured in only a few nerves, and is more difficult when atrophy and small CMAPs introduce further technical difficulties. Root stimulation can be performed using high-voltage electrical stimulation, needle stimulation, or magnetic stimulation over the spine. However, the first two are poorly tolerated, and the stimulation obtained by the last method is not always maximal. Proximal stimulation of the lower limb nerves is not technically satisfactory. Pure motor neuropathies with no conduction block (CB), responsive to intravenous immunoglobulin (IVIg) might be associated with very proximal CB[71], although this is a very rare finding in our experience.

A different set of motor neuropathies with focal demyelination have been described, In multifocal motor neuropathy with CB[6-8], only the motor fibers are affected. The reason for this probably depends on the different ceramide composition of GM1 in motor and sensory nerve fibers[72]. In motor and sensory demyelinating neuropathy with CB[5] both the motor and sensory fibers are affected, although with motor predominance. Pure motor neuropathies have also been described in patients with monoclonal gammopathy[73-75], a rare condition.

A number of criteria have been proposed for the definition of abnormal CB. This is particularly relevant, since a 20% physiologic CB in motor fibers may often be observed from phase cancellation[70]. This is increased when there are small and dispersed motor responses. Ideally, CB should be identified by stimulation over short segments. A consensus definition of CB has been agreed[76]. Although such carefully defined criteria are necessary when CB is clinically relevant, it is almost always very marked. It is important to establish an early diagnosis of focal demyelination because very wasted muscles are less likely to benefit from treatment with IVIg[8].

Reports of several patients diagnosed with multifocal motor neuropathy with CB who have been found at autopsy to have loss of anterior horn cells and Bunina bodies in motor neurons has increased the difficulties of diagnosis and understanding in this field[77].

Motor conduction abnormalities in amyotrophic lateral sclerosis

An important technical point is the need to warm the limbs when studying nerve conduction in ALS patients, because the wasted limbs tend to be cold and a satisfactory temperature may be difficult to maintain.

Certain motor conduction abnormalities are well recognized in ALS. The distal motor latency may be increased – a feature that has been correlated with the degree of weakness, which has been correlated with slowly conducting, thin, distal, regenerated motor axons[4]. Mild to moderate slowing of conduction velocity may be found in wasted muscles in ALS, due to loss of myelinated motor nerve fibers, atrophy of axons, secondary changes in myelin or the predominance of thin regenerated axons in the nerves innervating wasted muscles[3,4,78]. Histological evidence of selective loss of large fibers has been noted[79], but in other studies no preferential involvement of fast conducting fibers was found[80], both the maximal and minimal motor conduction velocities are slowed[80], suggesting that faster and slower conducting motor fibers were similarly involved. This finding is consistent with the histologic finding of involvement of somatic extrafusal and intrafusal (gamma) motor fibers in the disease[81]. This slight reduction of the motor conduction velocities results from the random loss of fast conducting fibers, and not from preferential loss of this set of fibers[23]. In ALS, significant CB or temporal dispersion in not observed, even when the motor responses are of very small amplitude (Figure 6.4)[4].

CMAP amplitude may decrease as a consequence of a number of processes, such as axonal loss, neuromuscular junction disease, distal CB, or abnormal muscle fibers. In neurogenic conditions such as ALS, CMAP amplitude is the combined effect of denervation, muscle fiber atrophy and

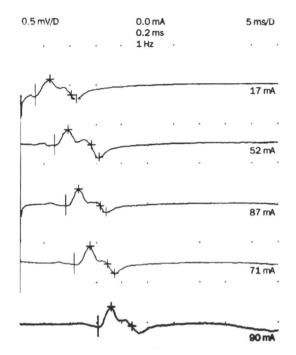

Figure 6.4 Motor conduction velocity of the ulnar nerve in an amyotrophic lateral sclerosis patient. The nerve was stimulated at the wrist, below and above the elbow, at the axilla and at Erb's point. In spite of a very small M-wave peak-to-peak amplitude (0.3 mV) no decrement of the amplitude was observed proximally, i.e. there was no conduction block

compensatory reinnervation. In ALS, there is a significant correlation between CMAP amplitude and the degree of muscle weakness and atrophy[4]. However, in very chronic conditions, such as old polio, the presence of a few giant remaining MUs may preserve normal mean CMAP amplitude in spite of moderate weakness.

SENSORY CONDUCTION STUDIES

Sensory potentials should be studied to confirm that the disease process does not involve sensory neurons and that the denervation process, therefore, is probably not localized at or distal to the dorsal root ganglia. There are a number of studies showing possible minor changes of the peripheral nerve sensory potentials in ALS[82]. Nevertheless, conventional electrophysiologic tests of sensory potential pathways are normal[4], and when these studies are abnormal, another diagnosis should be suspected. It should be remembered that sensory potentials decline in amplitude with age, and ALS usually affects older subjects. One exception is Kennedy's disease, in which abnormal sensory potentials are frequently observed[83].

More refined tests may discern some changes, as described using the near-nerve stimulation technique[82], measuring resistance to ischemia[84], or testing quantitatively the threshold to vibration[85]. Morphometry of the dorsal root ganglia showed some changes in sensory neurons[86] and loss of axons has been reported in the sural nerve[79], which may explain the abnormalities observed in some neurophysiologic investigations. The strength–duration time constant using a threshold tracking system has been used to analyze the function of sensory fibers in ALS; no abnormality was found[87].

The pioneering papers on somatosensory evoked potentials (SEPs) in ALS described a large number of abnormalities in these patients[88,89]. More recent papers using adequate methods to exclude spinal cord compression and peripheral delay describe fewer abnormalities[90,91]. However, a central delay might occur associated with dysfunction of the pyramidal control of the sensory system[92]. These abnormalities are probably more frequent in Guamanian ALS[35].

Table 6.1 summarizes the most important findings to confirm the diagnosis of ALS.

SPECIAL TESTS

F-waves

In UMN syndromes, F-waves are of increased amplitude, duration and, possibly, latency[93]. Although it is often stated that F-wave frequency is also increased, this assertion is poorly documented[93–95]. Using single-fiber recording it seems that in conditions with spasticity but no LMN

Table 6.1 Important findings to confirm the diagnosis of amyotrophic lateral sclerosis

	Essential	Important
(1) Cranial muscles (at least one)		
Fibs-sw		+
Fasciculations		+
Loss of MU	+	
Complex MU	+	
Instability	+	
(2a) Upper and (2b) lower limb muscles (at least two muscles innervated by different nerves and roots, in each limb)		
Fibs-sw	+	
Fasciculations		+
Loss of MU	+	
Complex MU	+	
Instability	+	
(3) Trunk muscles (at least one)		
Fibs-sw		+
Fasciculations		+
Loss of MU	+	
Complex MU	+	
Instability	+	
(4) Motor studies (at least one in each limb)		
No segmental demyelination	+	
CMAP amplitude		
> 50% of normal		
Normal DML		+
Normal F-waves		+
Normal CV		+
(5) Sensory studies (at least two in the most affected limb)		
Affected limb		
Normal SNAPs	+	

Fibs-sw, fibrillation and sharp-wave potential; MU, motor unit; CMAP, compound muscle action potential; DML, distal motor latency; CV, conduction velocity; SNAP sensory nerve action potential
Diagnosis (numbers refer to the categories above):
(A) 1 + (2a or 2b) + 4 + 5
(B) 3 + (2a or 2b) + 4 + 5
(C) 1 + 3 + 4 + 5
(D) 2a + 2b + 4 + 5

dysfunction there is an increased number of F-waves in responding neurons, but not an increase in the proportion of responding motor neurons[94].

In ALS the progressive loss of MUs is correlated with a decreased F-wave frequency[4]; this is more important in determining F-wave persistence than the clinical signs of UMN involvement, at least in upper limbs[95]. It is a common observation that, in severely weakened muscles in ALS, F-waves cannot be recorded. In ALS the number of responding motor units in a muscle recording is increased in spastic limbs as compared with limbs without UMN signs, although the F-wave frequency in individual MUs is not increased[95]. F-wave amplitude is frequently increased[96], which may be due to the presence of large remaining reinnervated MUs. F-waves show increased latency and dispersion, and there may be an increased frequency of repeater F-waves[4].

H-reflex

This is a monosynaptic response which assesses the integrity of both motor and sensory nerve fibers, and the nerve excitability at the spinal level. The most noticeable change in the presence of an UMN lesion is the presence of H-reflex responses in muscles other than the calf muscles. However, other changes may be observed, such as an increased H/M ratio, diminished inhibition of the H-reflex by simultaneous vibratory stimulation of the soleus muscle or its tendon, and lesser reduction of the amplitude of the H-reflex in a paired-stimulation paradigm[97].

In ALS patients, disinhibition of the LMN may be observed, as revealed by the last two tests above, in patients with or without clinical signs of an UMN lesion[97,98], suggesting a reduction of the pre- and post-synaptic inhibition, by Renshaw cells.

Repetitive nerve stimulation

Abnormal decrement of the motor response on RNS was documented in ALS many years ago[99], in particular in wasted muscles and in patients with rapidly progressive disorder. The decrement is usually less than 10%, and, as in myasthenia

gravis, it is enhanced after brief exercise, and is maximal after 3–5 stimuli. Probably, this abnormal decrement results from disturbed electrical conduction through immature nerve terminals and neuromuscular junctions[100]. Although of some interest, these decrement studies are not useful for diagnosis or follow-up in ALS.

Single-fiber electromyogram

With this technique the number of muscle fibers belonging to a single MU, within a radius of 300 μm from the tip of a single-fiber needle (fiber density), can be quantified. This number represents a correlate of fiber grouping observed in histologic samples[29]. This measurement is very sensitive in quantifying reinnervation[101].

Another possibility with this methodology is to determine the 'jitter', that is the variation in the interval between the firing onset of the action potentials of two repeatedly firing muscle fibers belonging to the same MU, which gives information about the stability of the neuromuscular transmission[29].

In staging studies[102] it has been demonstrated that, at an early phase of muscle involvement, when there is normal strength, no wasting and no fibs-sw in the concentric needle EMG study, and a full interference pattern on maximal contraction, the fiber density (FD) may be slightly increased, as is the jitter, fasciculation potentials (FPs) can be observed, and possibly MUPs of increased complexity may be documented. In more advanced phases, the FD and the jitter are clearly abnormal, at a phase where fibs-sw are found and full interference pattern is decreased. Finally, at an end-stage, the FD may decrease, representing a failure of the reinnervation process, which may not occur until there are less than 5% of the original neuronal pool surviving[23].

Macro-electromyogram

In this technique a modified needle electrode is used to record non-selectively from all muscles fibers of the same MU[103]. Enlargement of the macro-area is found in reinnervation, in general associated with an increased FD. This may be recorded at a very early stage of muscle involvement, although the FD may be abnormal before the macro-area has changed[28]. In end-stage wasted muscles, both FD and macro-EMG may show a lower than normal value.

In diseases with a slower progression than ALS, the FD and the macro-area can reach much higher values than observed in ALS, as seen in spinal muscular atrophy, hereditary sensory–motor neuropathy and polio survivors.

Studies of the respiratory muscles

Since the survival of the ALS patient is ultimately dependent on ventilatory function, neurophysiologic studies of the respiratory muscles are a potentially useful tool, whose utility has not been fully assessed. The most critical measurement would be the quantification of MU loss in the diaphragm, but this deep muscle is difficult to explore by needle EMG. As in any other muscle, its motor response to phrenic nerve stimulation is a crude approximation of its integrity.

Percutaneous electrical stimulation of the phrenic nerve in the neck is simple and non-invasive. The stimulation point should be at the posterior border of the sternomastoid muscle, either approximately 3 cm above the clavicle[104] or at the superior border of the cricoid or thyroid cartilage[105]. The most accepted position for surface recording is to place the active electrode 5 cm superior to the tip of the xiphoid process and the reference electrode on the costal margin, 16 cm from the active electrode[106]. The amplitudes of the motor responses vary with age, sex, height and chest circumference[107]. However, there is a poor correlation between phrenic nerve latency and age and height, and there is no significant gender-related latency difference[107]. Latencies show only a small interindividual variation and the side-to-side difference is also small[107]. The amplitude of phrenic nerve evoked action potentials, however,

has high interindividual variation. This is due to the variable depth of lung tissue separating the generator source from the diaphragm[106]. Nevertheless, there is only a small side-to-side variation in the CMAP amplitude[107]. The diaphragmatic motor response amplitude is highly correlated with transdiaphragmatic pressure[108]. Abnormally low motor responses suggest a weak diaphragm in ALS[107].

Surface EMG of the diaphragm is confounded by the high-frequency filtering effects of the skin and subcutaneous tissue and contamination by the electrical activity of adjacent muscles[107]. The thinness of the diaphragm (3–4 mm) and its movement during respiration creates some difficulty in using a needle EMG recording electrode. Nevertheless, it a useful technique, readily mastered, and can detect abnormal spontaneous activity in the diaphragm as well as abnormalities of MU potentials recorded during inspiration[105]. Reduced or discrete interference of MUs may occur on full inspiration, suggesting a significant degree of diaphragmatic motor neuronal loss[65,66,107]. The degree of diaphragm involvement is an indication of prognosis[107] and, possibly, the right time to suggest the need for non-invasive ventilation[66], in conjunction with functional pulmonary tests.

Collision techniques

In routine conduction studies only the fastest-conducting, large myelinated fibers are evaluated. The collision technique allows assessment of both the fast and the slow conducting motor fibers in a motor nerve[109,110]. This approach has shown that the minimum conduction velocity is also decreased in ALS[111], probably as a result of the presence of thin regenerating axons.

Electro-mechanical coupling

In reinnervation, of any cause, an increased twitch tension may be observed, as a consequence of the increased MUP area. However, in the later stages of ALS the twitch tension decreases in spite of an enlarged macro-EMG area, representing disturbed electromechanical coupling[112,113]. This could be caused by mitochondrial abnormalities, which have been described in muscles in ALS, causing abnormal muscle metabolism and associated abnormalities of calcium release and re-uptake in the sarcoplasmic reticulum. The dissociation between electrical signal and force output of motor units in ALS contributes to muscle weakness in the later stages of the disease, in addition to loss of motor units and corticospinal dysfunction. In selected cases, combined studies of MUP amplitude and motor unit force output could be helpful in monitoring the course of the disease and in studying the therapeutic effects of drugs[114].

Autonomic tests

In ALS autonomic nervous system involvement is rarely clinically evident, although it may be frequent but subclinical. In Guamanian ALS[115] and in ventilated end-stage patients[116] clinical autonomic manifestations are more frequently observed, and in this last group of patients autonomic dysfunction can contribute to sudden death. Laboratory tests can reveal mild autonomic dysfunction in ALS[117,118]. Cardiovascular sympathetic hyperactivity has been reported in ALS patients[119,120]. Sympathetic skin response studies have revealed abnormalities in ALS[121]. Other approaches to sweat gland function seem to support this observation[122,123]. These findings may be useful in the differential diagnosis from cervical spondylosis[124], and may perhaps lead to measures to prevent sudden death in ALS.

Threshold tracking

Strength-duration time constant studies using a threshold tracking system have confirmed abnormal function of motor fibers in ALS[87], which indicates that motor axons have irregular persistent sodium conduction. This is a complex technique with undetermined relevant diagnostic utility that

may be useful for studying excitatory manifestations in this condition.

Reflex studies

The involvement of inhibitory reflexes in ALS may be assessed by the study of several reflexes and the peripheral silent period. The masseter inhibitory reflex may reveal an increased area of the silent period, above all in patients with an exaggerated jaw jerk[125], by involvement of the corticobulbar facilitatory descending projections. These studies may be helpful to understand the precise neural pathway involvement. In addition, this technique might be useful to evaluate drug effects on the neural network, for example, in testing the changes induced by riluzole on the flexor reflexes[126].

Surface-electromyogram

The surface-EMG (sEMG) may well gain great popularity in the future, in particular when repeated studies are used to assess progression. In sEMG, the single muscle fiber action potential as the source, its firing pattern, as well as the physical aspects of volume conduction and recording configuration are considered. Using the unique patterns of spatial spread of MUPs recorded over the skin, MU classification and the determination of current density and polarity is performed non-invasively. With high-density surface electromyography, MUPs can be analyzed, permitting the detection of neurogenic MUPs, both by analysis of the raw signal itself and by analysis of extracted single MUPs[127]. Moreover, FPs may be analyzed regarding their complexity, origin and distribution in the muscle.

CONVENTIONAL PARAMETERS IN CLINICAL TRIALS

Ideally, surrogate markers used in clinical trials of any disorder should be sensitive, easily and quickly performed, well tolerated by the patient and highly reproducible, and they should correlate with conventional clinical findings. A number of neurophysiologic parameters could be applied to this goal.

Compound muscle action potential amplitude

LMN loss is probably the dominant cause of progressive weakness in ALS[128]. Quantitative evaluation of the LMN pool is therefore important. CMAP amplitude reflects the combined effect of denervation, muscle atrophy and compensatory reinnervation, and is an indirect measure of the number of innervated fibers[23]. The CMAP amplitude is maintained when collateral reinnervation effectively compensates for denervation and therefore does not distinguish the effect of loss of MU from collateral reinnervation. It has the advantage that it is not dependent on co-operation. CMAP amplitude measurement is non-invasive[129] and can be carried out in proximal and distal muscles. It is a simple, rapid and reliable measure, provided some care is taken in electrode positioning and temperature control[130]. Its underlying methodology is familiar and easily standardized in different laboratories[129].

In ALS, CMAP amplitude correlates well with muscle strength as determined by maximum voluntary isometric contraction[4,114], or as determined by electrical stimulation[128]. There is also a significant correlation between CMAP amplitude and the MU number estimation (MUNE)[114,131], as expected, since CMAP is a dependent variable for MUNE calculation. For these reasons, CMAP amplitude has been included as a variable in several ALS clinical trials[114]. However, CMAP amplitude measures do not enable detection of the effects of collateral reinnervation in masking MU loss, since successful reinnervation may maintain CMAP amplitude despite ongoing MU death[23,114]. This effect will be most marked when there is relatively extensive reinnervation, as in slowly progressive ALS. This will prevent the understanding of whether a given drug is working by enhancing collateral reinnervation or by slowing MU loss, or both. In addition, during reinnervation the synchronicity of MU and muscle fiber discharges is impaired, owing to anatomical reorganization of reinnervated MUs and, in particular, to the dysfunction of the immature neuromuscular junctions. Reinnervated MUPs often contain late components, causing temporal dispersion. Temporal dispersion, and phase cancellation, may cause a reduction in CMAP amplitude, independent of muscle fiber denervation, reducing the significance of any change in amplitude of the CMAP. Although the effect of temporal dispersion can be at least partially overcome if area measurement is used, the latter variable is no more sensitive than CMAP amplitude[132].

Neurophysiological index

De Carvalho and Swash have developed a multimetric index, the neurophysiologic index (NI) derived from the CMAP amplitude, F-wave frequency and distal motor latency of the ulnar nerve–abductor digiti minimi (ADM) system[4]. This is a sensitive parameter in evaluating progression in ALS patients[132].

The NI is sensitive to LMN loss and weakness in ALS, whether the disease is rapidly or slowly progressive[132]. A major advantage of the NI is that it is calculated from standard neurophysiologic measurements. It can therefore be used in any neurophysiologic laboratory, and requires no special equipment or expertise. It has been shown that it is more sensitive than CMAP amplitude[132] and with a rate of decay similar to MUNE[133]. It is reproducible in healthy controls[130] and in ALS patients (de Carvalho and Swash, unpublished data). It appears to be a useful measure in detecting progression.

Other techniques

In general, the F-wave frequency is reduced in weak muscles in ALS[4], but more studies are needed to apply them as a measurement of disease progression.

FD is not comfortable to the patient and, in addition, a period of training and experience is required by the examiner to achieve competence.

Macro-EMG is relatively complex and invasive. This technique was studied longitudinally for 6 months in one study, but was not sensitive in detecting change[131].

Successful longitudinal single motor unit tracking in patients with ALS, measuring change in functional innervation in a single motor unit, is possible. However, this is a technically challenging technique and is not recommended as a standard measure in sequential studies of ALS[134].

REFERENCES

1. Lambert EH, Mulder DW. Electromyographic studies in amyotrophic lateral sclerosis. Mayo Clin Proc 1957; 32: 441–6

2. Lambert EH. Electromyography in amyotrophic lateral sclerosis. In: Norris FH, Kurland LT, eds. Motor Neuron Diseases: Research in Amyotrophic Lateral Sclerosis and Related Disorders. New York: Grunne and Stratton, 1969: 135–53

3. Cornblath DR, Kuncl RW, Mellits ED, et al. Nerve conduction studies in amyotrophic lateral sclerosis. Muscle Nerve 1992; 15: 1111–15

4. De Carvalho M, Swash M. Nerve conduction studies in amyotrophic lateral sclerosis. Muscle Nerve 2000; 23: 344–52

5. Lewis RA, Sumner AJ, Brown MJ, Asbury AK. Multifocal demyelinating neuropathy with persistent conduction block. Neurology 1982; 32: 958–64

6. Parry GJ, Clarke S. Multifocal acquired demyelinating neuropathy masquerading as motor neuron disease. Muscle Nerve 1988; 11. 103–7

7. Pestronk A, Cornblath DR, Ilyas AA, et al. A treatable multifocal motor neuropathy with antibodies to GM1 ganglioside. Ann Neurol 1988; 24: 73–8

8. Bouche P, Moulonguet A, Younes-Chennoufi AB, et al. Multifocal motor neuropathy with conduction block: a study of 24 patients. J Neurol Neurosurg Psychiatry 1995; 59: 38–44

9. Evangelista T, de Carvalho M, Conceição I, et al. Motor neuropathies mimicking amyotrophic lateral sclerosis/motor neuron disease. J Neurol Sci 1996; 139 (Suppl): 95–8

10. Bentes C, de Carvalho M, Evangelista T, Sales-Luís ML. Multifocal motor neuropathy mimicking motor neuron disease: Nine cases. J Neurol Sci 1999; 169: 76–9

11. Swash M. Shortening the time to diagnosis in ALS: The role of electrodiagnostic studies. Amyotroph Lateral Scler 2000; 1 (Suppl 1): S67–72

12. Daube JR. Electrodiagnostic studies in amyotrophic lateral sclerosis and other motor neuron disorders. Muscle Nerve 2000; 23: 1488–502

13. Troger M, Dengler R. The role of electromyography (EMG) in the diagnosis of ALS. Amyotroph Lateral Scler 2000; 1 (Suppl 1): S33–40

14. Cappellari A, Brioschi A, Barbieri S, et al. A tentative interpretation of electromyographic regional differences in bulbar- and limb-onset ALS. Neurology 1999; 52: 644–6

15. de Carvalho M, Bentes C, Evangelista T, Sales-Luís M. Fibrillation and sharp-waves: Do we need them to diagnose ALS? Amyotroph Lateral Scler 1999; 1: 29–32

16. de Carvalho M. Pathophysiological significance of fasciculations in the early diagnosis of ALS. Amyotroph Lateral Scler 2000; 1 (Suppl 1): S43–6

17. de Carvalho M, Swash M. Fasciculation potentials: A study of amyotrophic lateral sclerosis and other neurogenic disorders. Muscle Nerve 1997; 21: 336–44

18. Behnia M, Kelly J. Role of electromyography in amyotrophic lateral sclerosis. Muscle Nerve 1991; 14: 1236–41

19. Brooks BR; and World Federation of Neurology Sub-Committee on Motor Neuron Diseases. El Escorial WFN criteria for the diagnosis of amyotrophic lateral sclerosis. J Neurol Sci 1994; 124: 965–1085

20. Wilbourn AJ. Clinical neurophysiology in the diagnosis of amyotrophic lateral sclerosis: The Lambert and the El Escorial criteria. J Neurol Sci 1998; 160 (Suppl 1): S25–9

21. Brooks BR, Miller RG, Swash M, Munsat TL. for the World Federation of Neurology Research Group on Motor Neuron Diseases. El Escorial revisited: revised criteria for the diagnosis of amyotrophic lateral sclerosis. Amyotroph Lateral Scler 2000; 1: 293–300

22. McComas AJ, Sica RE, Campbell MJ, Upton AR. Functional compensation in partially denervated

muscles. J Neurol Neurosurg Psychiatry 1971; 34: 453–60

23. Hansen S, Balantyne JP. A quantitative study of motor neurone disease. J Neurol Neurosurg Psychiatry 1978; 41:773–83

24. Daube JR. Electrophysiologic studies in the diagnosis and prognosis of MND. Neurol Clin 1985; 3: 473–93

25. Wohfart GL. Collateral regeneration from residual motor nerve fibers in ALS. Neurology 1957; 7: 124–34

26. Buchtal F, Guld C, Rosenfalk P. Multi-electrode study of the territory of a motor unit. Acta Physiol Scand 1957; 39: 83–103

27. Erminio F, Buchtal F, Rosenfalk P. Motor unit territory and muscle fiber concentraton in paresis due to peripheral nerve injury and anterior horn cell involvement. Neurology 1957; 9: 657–71

28. Stalberg E. Electrophysiological studies of reinnervation in amyotrophic lateral sclerosis. In: Rowland LP, ed. Human Motor Neuron Diseases. New York: Raven Press, 1982: 47–57

29. Stalberg E, Sanders BB. Neurophysiological studies in amyotrophic lateral sclerosis. In Smith RA, ed. Handbook of Amyotrophic Lateral Sclerosis. New York: Marcel Dekker, 1992: 209–36

30. Kugelberg E, Edstrom L, Abbruzzese M. Mapping of motor units in experimentally reinnervated rat muscle. Interpretation of histochemical and atrophic fiber patterns in neurogenic lesions. J Neurol Neurosurg Psychiatry 1970; 33: 319–29

31. Lindstrom JM. Acetylcholine receptors and myasthenia. Muscle Nerve 2000; 23: 453–77

32. Denny-Brown D, Pennybacker JB. Fibrillation and fasciculation in voluntary muscles. Brain 1938; 61: 311–32

33. Dumitru D. Electrophysiologic basis for single muscle fiber discharge morphology, Thesis, University of Nijmegen, 1999

34. Denys EH. The influence of temperature in clinical neurophysiology. Muscle Nerve 1991; 14: 795–811

35. Ahlskog JE, Litchy WJ, Peterson RC, et al. Guamanian neurodegenerative disease: electrophysiologic findings. J Neurol Sci 1999; 15: 28–35

36. de Carvalho M, Swash M. Cramps, muscle pain and fasciculations – not always benign? Neurology 2004; 63: 721–3

37. Norris FH. Synchronous fasciculations in motor neurone disease. Arch Neurol 1965; 13: 495–500

38. Roth G. The origin of fasciculations. Ann Neurol 1982; 12: 542–54

39. Janko M, Trontelj JV, Gersak K. Fasciculations in motor neuron disease: Discharge rate reflects extent and recency of collateral sprouting. J Neurol Neurosurg Psychiatry 1989; 52: 1375–81

40. Hirota N, Eisen A, Weber M. Complex fasciculations and their origin in amyotrophic lateral sclerosis and Kennedy's disease. Muscle Nerve 2000; 23: 1872–5

41. Shiga Y, Onodera H, Shimizu H, et al. Two consecutive fasciculation potentials having different motor unit origins are an electromyographically pathognomonic finding of ALS. Electromyogr Clin Neurophysiol 2000; 40: 237–41

42. Caramia MD, Cicinelli P, Paradiso C, et al. 'Excitability' changes of muscular responses to magnetic brain stimulation in patients with central motor disorders. Electroencephalogr Clin Neurophysiol 1991; 81: 243–50

43. de Carvalho M, Miranda PC, Lourdes Sales Luis M, Ducla-Soares E. Neurophysiological features of fasciculation potentials evoked by transcranial magnetic stimulation in amyotrophic lateral sclerosis. J Neurol 2000; 247: 189–94

44. Reed DM, Kurland LT. Muscle fasciculations in healthy population. Arch Neurol 1963; 9: 353–67

45. Trojaborg W, Buchthal F. Malignant and benign fasciculations, Acta Neurol Scand 1965; 41 (Suppl 13): 251–4

46. Walker FO, Donofrio PD, Harpold GJ, Ferrell WG. Sonographic imaging of muscle contraction and fasciculations: A correlation with electromyography. Muscle Nerve 1990; 13: 33–9

47. Howard RS, Murray NM. Surface EMG in the recording of fasciculations. Muscle Nerve 1992; 15: 1240–5

48. Trontelj JV, Stalberg E. Bizarre repetitive discharges recorded with single fibre EMG, J Neurol Neurosurg Psychiatry 1983; 46: 305–9

49. Partanen J, Nousiainen U. Motor unit potentials in a mildly affected muscle in amyotrophic lateral sclerosis, J Neurol Sci 1990; 95: 193–9

50. Stalberg E, Sonoo M. Assessment of variability in the shape of the motor unit action potential, the 'jiggle,' at consecutive discharges. Muscle Nerve 1994; 17: 1135–44

51. Emeryk-Szajewska B, Kopec J, Karwanska A. The reorganization of motor units in motor neuron disease. Muscle Nerve 1997; 20: 306–15

52. Preston DC, Shapiro BE, Raynor EM, Kothari MJ. The relative value of facial, glossal, and masticatory

muscles in the electrodiagnosis of amyotrophic lateral sclerosis. Muscle Nerve 1997; 20: 370–2

53. Finsterer J, Erdorf M, Mamoli B, Fuglsang-Frederiksen A. Needle electromyography of bulbar muscles in patients with amyotrophic lateral sclerosis: Evidence of subclinical involvement. Neurology 1998; 51: 1417–22

54. Li J, Petajan J, Smith G, Bromberg M. Electromyography of sternocleidomastoid muscle in ALS: A prospective study. Muscle Nerve 2002; 25: 725–8

55. Kang DX, Fan DS. The electrophysiological study of differential diagnosis between amyotrophic lateral sclerosis and cervical spondylotic myelopathy. Electromyogr Clin Neurophysiol 1995; 35: 231–8

56. Finsterer J, Fuglsang-Frederiksen A, Mamoli B. Needle EMG of the tongue: motor unit action potential versus peak ratio analysis in limb and bulbar onset amyotrophic lateral sclerosis. J Neurol Neurosurg Psychiatry 1997; 63:175–80

57. Swash M. Vulnerability of lower brachial myotomes in motor neurone disease: A clinical and single fiber EMG study. J Neurol Sci 1980; 47: 59–68

58. Wilbourn AJ, Seveeney PJ. Dissociated wasting of the medial and lateral hand muscles with motor neuron disease. Can J Neurol Sci 1994; 21 (Suppl 2): 59

59. Eisen A. Comments on the lower motor neuron hypothesis. Muscle Nerve 1993; 16: 870–2.

60. Kuwabara S, Mizobuchi K, Ogawara K, Hattori T. Dissociated small hand muscle involvement in amyotrophic lateral sclerosis detected by motor unit number estimates. Muscle Nerve 1999; 22: 870–3

61. Kuncl RW, Cornblath DR, Griffin JW. Assessment of thoracic paraspinal muscles in the diagnosis of ALS. Muscle Nerve 1988; 11: 484–92

62. Date ES, Mar EY, Bugola MR, Teraoka JK. The prevalence of lumbar paraspinal spontaneous activity in asymptomatic subjects. Muscle Nerve 1996; 19: 350–4

63. Eisen A. Clinical electrophysiology of the upper and lower motor neuron in amyotrophic lateral sclerosis, Semin Neurol 2001; 21: 141–54

64. de Carvalho M, Matias T, Coelho F, et al. Motor neuron disease presenting with respiratory failure. J Neurol Sci 1996; 139: 117–22

65. Stewart H, Eisen A, Road J, et al. Electromyography of respiratory muscles in amyotrophic lateral sclerosis. J Neurol Sci 2001; 191: 67–73

66. McLeod JG, Prineas JW. Distal type of chronic spinal muscular atrophy. Clinical, electrophysiological and pathological studies. Brain 1971; 94: 703–14

67. Ravits J, Hallett M, Baker M, et al. Clinical and electromyographic studies of postpoliomyelitis muscular atrophy, Muscle Nerve 1990; 13: 667–74

68. McComas AJ, Quartly C, Griggs RC. Early and late losses of motor units after poliomyelitis. Brain 1997; 120: 1415–21

69. Luciano CA, Dalakas MC. Inclusion body myositis: No evidence for a neurogenic component, Neurology 1997; 48: 29–33

70. Kimura J. Multifocal motor neuropathy and conduction block. In: Kimura J, Kaji R, eds. Physiology of ALS and related diseases. Amsterdam: Elsevier Science, 1997: 57–72

71. Pakiam AS, Parry GJ. Multifocal motor neuropathy without overt conduction block. Muscle Nerve 1998; 21: 243–5

72. Ogawa-Goto K, Funamoto N, Abe T, Nagashima K. Different ceramide compositions of gangliosides between human motor and sensory nerves. J Neurochem 1990; 55: 1486–93

73. Rowland LP, Defendini R, Sherman W, et al. Macroglobulinemia with peripheral neuropathy simulating motor neuron disease. Ann Neurol 1982; 11: 532–6

74. Parry GJ, Holtz SJ, Ben-Zeev D, Drori JB. Gammopathy with proximal motor axonopathy simulating motor neuron disease. Neurology 1986; 36: 273–6

75. Younger DS, Rowland LP, Latov N, et al. Lymphoma, motor neuron diseases, and amyotrophic lateral sclerosis. Ann Neurol 1991; 29: 78–86

76. Olney RK, Lewis RA, Putnam TD, Campellone JV. Consensus criteria for the diagnosis of multifocal motor neuropathy. Muscle Nerve 2003; 27: 117–21

77. Veugelers B, Theys P, Lammens M, et al. Pathological findings in a patient with amyotrophic lateral sclerosis and multifocal motor neuropathy with conduction block. J Neurol Sci 1996; 136: 64–70

78. Borg J. Conduction velocity and refractory period of single motor nerve fibers in motor neuron disease. J Neurol Neurosurg Psychiatry 1984; 47: 349–53

79. Bradley WG, Good P, Rasool CG, Adelman LS. Morphometric and biochemical studies of peripheral nerves in amyotrophic lateral sclerosis. Arch Neurol 1983; 41: 267–77

80. Ijima M, Arasaki K, Iwamoto H, Nakanishi T. Maximal and minimal motor nerve conduction velocities in patients with motor neuron diseases: Corre-

lation with age of onset and duration of illness. Muscle Nerve 1991; 14: 1110–15

81. Swash M, Fox KP. Pathology of the muscle spindle – effect of denervation. J Neurol Sci 1974; 22: 785–9

82. Shefner JM, Tyler RH, Krarup C,. Abnormalities in the sensory action potential in patients with amyotrophic lateral sclerosis. Muscle Nerve 1991; 14: 1242–6

83. Ferrante MA, Wilbourn AJ. The characteristic electrodiagnostic features of Kennedy's disease. Muscle Nerve 1997; 20: 323–9

84. Shahani B, Davies-Jones GA, Russell WR. Motor neurone disease. Further evidence for an abnormality of nerve metabolism. J Neurol Neurosurg Psychiatry 1972; 34: 185–91

85. Mulder DW, Bushek W, Spring E, et al. Motor neuron disease (ALS): Evaluation of detection thresholds of cutaneous sensation. Neurology 1983; 33: 1625–7

86. Kawamura Y, Dyck PJ, Shimura M, et al. Morphometric comparison of the vulnerability of motor and sensory neurons in amyotrophic lateral sclerosis. J Neuropathol Exp Neurol 1981; 40: 667–75

87. Mogyoros I, Kiernan MC, Burke D, Bostock H. Strength-duration properties of sensory and motor axons in amyotrophic lateral sclerosis. Brain 1998; 121: 851–9

88. Cosi V, Poloni M, Mazzini L, Callieco R. Somatosensory evoked potentials in amyotrophic lateral sclerosis. J Neurol Neurosurg Psychiatry 1884; 47: 857–61

89. Dasheiff RM, Drake ME, Brendle A, Erwin CW. Abnormal somatosensory evoked potentials in amyotrophic lateral sclerosis, Electroenceph Clin Neurophysiol 1985; 60: 306–15

90. Cascino GD, Ring SR, King PJL, et al. Evoked potentials in motor neuron disease. Neurology 1988; 38: 231–8

91. de Carvalho M, Conceição I, Alves M, Sales-Luís ML. Somatosensory evoked potentials in the differential diagnosis between spinal cord compression and amyotrophic lateral sclerosis, Acta Neurol Scand 1995; 92: 72–6

92. Georgesco M, Salerno A, Camu W. Somatosensory evoked potentials elicited by stimulation of lower-limb nerves in amyotrophic lateral sclerosis. Electroencephalogr Clin Neurophysiol 1997; 104: 333–42

93. Milanov IG. F-wave for assessment of segmental motoneurone excitability. Electromyogr Clin Neurophysiol 1992; 32: 11–15

94. Schiller HH, Stalberg E. F responses studied with single fiber EMG in normal subjects and spastic patients. J Neurol Neurosurg Psychiatry 1978; 41: 45–53

95. de Carvalho M, Swash M. The F-waves and the corticospinal lesion in amyotrophic lateral sclerosis. Amyotroph Lateral Scler 2002; 3: 131–6

96. Argyropoulos CJ, Panayiotopoulos CP, Scarpalezos S. F- and M-wave conduction velocity in amyotrophic lateral sclerosis. Muscle Nerve 1978; 1: 479–85

97. Drory VE, Kovach I, Groozman GB. Electrophysiologic evaluation of the upper motor neuron involvement in amyotrophic lateral sclerosis. Amyotroph Lateral Scler 2001; 2: 147–52

98. Raynor EM, Shefner JM. Recurrent inhibition is decreased in patients with amyotrophic lateral sclerosis. Neurology 1994; 44: 2148–53

99. Mulder DW, Lambert EH, Eaton LM. Myasthenic syndrome in patients with amyotrophic lateral sclerosis. Neurology 1959; 9: 627–31

100. Bernstein LP, Antel JP. Motor neuron disease decremental responses to repetitive nerve stimulation. Neurology 1981; 31: 202–4

101. Stalberg E, Schwartz MS, Trontelj JV. Single fiber electromyography in various processes affecting the anterior horn cell. J Neurol Sci 1975; 24: 403–15

102. Swash M, Schwartz MS. A longitudinal study of changes in motor units in motor neuron disease. J Neurol Sci 1982; 56: 185–97

103. Stalberg E. Macro EMG a new recording technique. J Neurol Neurosurg Psychiatry 1980; 43: 469–74

104. Swenson MR, Rubenstein RS. Phrenic nerve conduction studies. Muscle Nerve 1992; 15: 597–603

105. Newson-Davis J. Phrenic nerve conduction in man. J Neurol Neurosurg Psychiatry 1967; 30: 420–6

106. Bolton CF. AAEM Minimonograph # 40: Clinical neurophysiology of the respiratory system. Muscle Nerve 1993; 16: 809–18

107. De Carvalho M. Electrodiagnostic assessment of respiratory dysfunction in motor neuron disease. In: Daube J, Eisen A, eds. Handbook of Clinical Neurophyisiology in Motor Neuron Diseases. Amsterdam: Elsevier, 2004

108. Luo YM, Lyall RA, Harris ML, et al. Quantification of the esophageal diaphragm electromyogram with magnetic phrenic nerve stimulation. Am J Resp Crit Care Med 1999; 160: 1629–34

109. Ingram DA, Davis GR, Swash M. The double collision technique: A new method for measurement of the motor nerve refractory period distribution in man. Electroenceph Clin Neurophysiol 1987; 66: 225–34

110. Ingram DA, Davis GR, Swash M. Motor nerve conduction velocity distributions in man: Results of a new computer-based collision. Electroenceph Clin Neurophysiol 1987; 66: 235–43

111. Nakanishi T, Tamaki M, Arasaki K. Maximal and minimal motor nerve conduction velocities in amyotrophic lateral sclerosis. Neurology 1989; 39: 580–3

112. Dengler R, Konstanzer A, Küther G, et al. Amyotrophic lateral sclerosis: Macro-EMG and twitch forces of single motor units. Muscle Nerve 1990; 13: 545–50

113. Schmied A, Pouget J, Vedel JP. Electromechanical coupling and synchronous firing of single wrist extensor motor units in sporadic amyotrophic lateral sclerosis. Clin Neurophysiol 1999; 110: 960–74

114. de Carvalho M, Chio A, Dengler R, et al. Neurophysiologic measures in amyotrophic lateral sclerosis: Markers of progression in clinical trials. Amyotroph Lateral Scler Other Motor Neuron Disord 2005; 6: 17–28

115. Low PA, Ahlskog JE, Petersen RC, et al. Autonomic failure in Guamanian neurodegenerative disease. Neurology 1997; 49: 1031–4

116. Sato K, Namba R, Hayabara T, et al. Autonomic nervous disorder in motor neuron disease: A study of advanced stage patients. Intern Med 1995; 34: 972–5

117. Murata Y, Harada T, Ishizaki F, et al. An abnormal relationship between blood pressure and pulse rate in amyotrophic lateral sclerosis. Acta Neurol Scand 1997; 96: 118–22

118. Pisano F, Miscio G, Mazzuero G, et al. Decreased heart rate variability in amyotrophic lateral sclerosis. Muscle Nerve 1995; 18: 1225–31

119. Chida K, Sakamaki S, Takasu T. Alteration in autonomic function and cardiovascular regulation in amyotrophic lateral sclerosis. J Neurol 1989; 236: 127–30

120. Linden D, Diehl RR, Berlit P. Reduced baroreflex sensitivity and cardiorespiratory transfer in amyotrophic lateral sclerosis. Electroenceph Clin Neurophysiol 1998; 109: 387–90

121. Dettmers C, Fatepour D, Faust H, Jerusalem F. Sympathetic skin response abnormalities in amyotrophic lateral sclerosis. Muscle Nerve 1993; 16: 930–4

122. Kihara M, Takahashi A, Sugenoya J, et al. Sudomotor dysfunction in amyotrophic lateral sclerosis, Funct Neurol 1994; 9: 193–7

123. Santos-Bento M, de Carvalho M, Evangelista T, Sales Luis ML. Sympathetic sudomotor function and amyotrophic lateral sclerosis. Amyotroph Lateral Scler 2001; 2: 105–8

124. Shindo K, Watanabe H, Tanaka H, et al. A comparison of sympathetic outflow to muscles between cervical spondylotic amyotrophy and ALS. Amyotroph Lateral Scler 2002; 3: 233–8

125. Shimizu T, Komori T, Kato S, et al. Masseter inhibitory reflex in amyotrophic lateral sclerosis. Amyotroph Lateral Scler 2001; 2: 189–95

126. Riepe MW, Klappenbach G, Ludolph AC. Increase of flexor reflex latency in patients with amyotrophic lateral sclerosis treated with riluzole. J Neurol Neurosurg Psychiatry 1997; 62: 427

127. Drost G, Stegeman DF, Schillings ML, et al. Motor unit characteristics in healthy subjects and those with postpoliomyelitis syndrome: A high-density surface EMG study. Muscle Nerve 2004; 30: 269–76

128. Kelly JJ, Thibodeau L, Andres PL, Finison LJ. Use of electrophysiologic tests to measure disease progression in ALS therapeutic trials. Muscle Nerve 1990; 13: 471–9

129. de Carvalho M. Compound muscle action potential, Amyotroph Lateral Scler 2002; 3 (Suppl 1): S103–4

130. de Carvalho M, Lopes A, Scotto M, Swash M. Reproducibility of neurophysiological and myometric measurement in the ulnar nerve–abductor digiti minimi system. Muscle Nerve 2001; 24: 1391–5

131. Bromberg M, Fries T, Forshew D, Tandan R. Electrophysiological endpoint measures in a multicenter ALS drug trial. J Neurol Sci 2001; 184: 51–4

132. de Carvalho M, Scotto M, Lopes A, Swash M. Clinical and neurophysiological evaluation of progression in amyotrophic lateral sclerosis, Muscle Nerve 2003; 28: 630–3

133. de Carvalho M, Scotto M, Lopes A, Swash M. Quantitating progression in ALS. Neurology 2005; 64: 1784–5

134. Gooch CL, Harati Y. Longitudinal tracking of the same single motor unit in amyotrophic lateral sclerosis. Muscle Nerve 1997; 20: 511–13

7

The neuropsychology of amyotrophic lateral sclerosis

Jennifer Murphy, Cathy Lomen-Hoerth

WHY PERFORM NEUROPSYCHOLOGIC AND NEUROBEHAVIORAL TESTING IN AMYOTROPHIC LATERAL SCLEROSIS?

Traditionally amyotrophic lateral sclerosis (ALS) has been considered to spare cognition and behavior. A growing body of research now challenges this assumption, with evidence that a strong link exists between ALS and frontotemporal lobar dementia (FTLD). FTLD produces changes in behavior, executive function and language, while sparing memory. Patients with FTLD are at risk for developing ALS, and, conversely, a sizable percentage of patients with ALS exhibit co-morbid FTLD. In familial cases family members may manifest FTLD, ALS, or both.

A neuropsychologic and neurobehavioral evaluation provides clear confirmation of the presence of frontotemporal dementia or other dementia processes. The evaluation also can identify the more subtle cognitive and behavioral abnormalities that may be present. Because cognitive abnormalities in ALS are not exclusively due to a neurologic problem, a neuropsychologic assessment will help distinguish between a true brain-based change, clinical depression, pseudobulbar affect, or clinical sequelae of ALS that can impact cognitive function (e.g. lack of oxygenation at night, fatigue). Assessing patients' cognitive and behavioral function over the course of their disease progression allows for interventions for reversible causes of cognitive impairment or behavior problems, improved management of their disease, and identification of caregiver problems that may need addressing.

A LITERATURE REVIEW OF COGNITIVE ABNORMALITIES IN AMYOTROPHIC LATERAL SCLEROSIS

An association between dementia and ALS was first noted in the late 1800s (Raymond 1889; Marie 1892) and the literature has subsequently been reviewed by many investigators[1-4]. Mitsuyama and Takamiya[5] were the first to describe 'dementia with motor neuron disease' as a presenile dementia that later progressed to ALS. In 1994 the Lund group first used the term 'frontotemporal lobar dementia' with ALS, identifying three subtypes: frontal lobe degeneration type, Pick type and motor neuron disease (MND) type[6]. Since over the past few decades it has been well established that ALS does in fact involve a dementia syndrome, the debate has now turned to the nature and prevalence of cognitive and behavioral abnormalities in ALS.

THE NATURE OF COGNITIVE OR BEHAVIORAL CHANGES IN AMYOTROPHIC LATERAL SCLEROSIS

It has been well established that the cognitive and behavioral abnormalities seen in ALS are primarily a frontotemporal phenomenon with significant executive function impairment and behavioral alterations[7]. Attempts to define this syndrome have varied widely, with some investigations studying unselected patients, and others excluding or focusing on ALS patients with gross dementia features. Relatively few investigators employ clear criteria for diagnosing FTLD, such as the Neary criteria[8]; Table 7.1. As a result of these heterogeneous definitions, precise comparisons of neuropsychological and anatomic features are difficult. Even when explicit criteria are used, large proportions of patients have been classified as 'uncertain'[9], and neuropsychologic performance is not uniform across patients, with some patients performing normally and others not[10–13].

What is clear, however, is that dozens of studies have documented the presence of executive functioning deficits among ALS patients, with a sizable percentage of ALS patients being affected[10–12,14–17]. Frequently, these data reveal that non-demented patients possess the same executive function deficits seen in ALS patients with associated FTLD, but simply to a milder degree[18,19], suggesting a continuum of involvement. Broad cerebral circuits are required to process these executive function tasks, yet they rely heavily upon the frontal lobe. ALS patients have performed abnormally on a variety of executive function measures, including verbal and design fluency tasks[13,16,20], tests of verbal reasoning[13], visual attention[13], initiation of random movements on a joy-stick task[21] and problem solving on the Wisconsin Card Sorting Test[21,22]. Poor learning and recall have also been identified in

---

Table 7.1   Criteria for diagnosing frontotemporal lobar dementia

Core diagnostic features of frontotemporal dementia

A. Insidious onset and gradual progression
B. Early decline (within 2 years after onset) in social interpersonal conduct
C. Early impairment (within 2 years after onset) in regulation of personal conduct
D. Early (within 2 years after onset) emotional blunting
E. Early (within 2 years after onset) loss of insight

Core diagnostic features of primary non-fluent progressive aphasia

A. Insidious onset and gradual progression
B. Non-fluent spontaneous speech with one of the following: agrammatism, phonemic paraphasias, anomia

Core diagnostic features of semantic dementia

A. Insidious onset and gradual progression
B. Language disorder characterized by
   (1) Progressive, fluent, empty spontaneous speech
   (2) Loss of word meaning, manifest by impaired naming and comprehension
   (3) Semantic paraphasias and/or
C. Perceptual disorder characterized by
   (1) Prosopagnosia: impaired recognition of identity of familiar faces and/or
   (2) Associative agnosia: impaired recognition of object identity
D. Preserved perceptual matching and drawing reproduction
E. Preserved single word repetition
F. Preserved ability to read aloud and write to dictation orthographically regular words

non-demented ALS patients[12,21–23] but these particular deficits may have more to do with poor organization and retrieval than memory deficits per se. The most common deficit documented in ALS patients is a deficit in verbal fluency, and this pattern is seen in both demented and non-demented patients[3]. Neurobehaviorally, ALS patients also vary with regards to their frontotemporal lobar impairment. A significant proportion meet primary and supporting Neary criteria for FTLD[7,8,10], others have mild or moderate levels of behavioral or executive dysfunction, while still others appear normal[24]. Few studies have systematically measured the neurobehavioral impairments typically seen in FTLD dementia, but our laboratory has identified irritability, disinhibition, depression, apathy and agitation (in that order) as the most common complaints that caregivers see in ALS patients (manuscript in preparation). Even in a sample of ALS patients clearly diagnosed as non-demented ($n = 10$), neurobehavioral problems were rated by caregivers as progressively problematic, with 60% of the sample having increased behavioral problems over 1 year (Table 7.2). Mean scores reflected that by 1 year the group had mild-to-moderate eating disturbance, moderate-to-severe problems with sleep, moderate levels of depression and mild levels of anxiety (manuscript in preparation).

Functional imaging studies provide support for the neural mechanisms for these cognitive and behavioral abnormalities, documenting cerebral abnormalities that extend well beyond the primary, secondary and sensorimotor cortices. Structural imaging, positron emission tomography (PET) and single photon emission computed tomography (SPECT) data reveal a pattern of rather widespread cortical involvement in ALS, with a worsening of this pattern seen in cognitively or behaviorally abnormal ALS patients. Non-demented ALS patients have pronounced reductions in regional cerebral blood flow (rCBF) in frontal and anterior temporal cortices on PET[10], and non-demented patients with decreased verbal fluency scores have impaired

activation of the dorsolateral prefrontal cortex, premotor cortex, bilateral insular cortex and thalamus as compared with ALS patients who perform well on fluency measures[21]. When non-demented ALS patients are measured with functional magnetic resonance imaging (fMRI) when performing a verbal fluency task, impaired activation is seen in the middle and inferior frontal gyri and anterior cingulate gyrus, in addition to regions of the parietal and temporal lobes[25]. ALS patients with unknown cognitive status have reduced rCBF not only in primary and associated motor cortices but also anterior cingulate[12], and a subgroup of patients with verbal fluency deficits showed the same but heightened pattern of impairment, with additional hypometabolism in the right parahippocampal gyrus, anterior thalamic nucleus complex and anterior cingulate[26]. Mild-to-moderate cerebral atrophy has been documented in ALS patients with unknown cognitive status, with 50% of the sample having parietal atrophy, 38% insula atrophy,

Table 7.2 Progression of neuropsychiatric symptoms over 1 year		
Neurobehavioral symptom from the NPI	Baseline evaluation Mean score (SD) ($n = 8$)	Follow-up evaluation Mean score (SD) ($n = 8$)
Delusions	0.0 (0.0)	0.6 (1.9)
Hallucinations	0.0 (0.0)	0.0 (0.0)
Agitation	1.0 (1.7)	0.4 (0.7)
Depression	1.2 (1.1)	2.2 (2.2)
Anxiety	0.6 (1.9)	1.2 (2.7)
Elation	0.0 (0.0)	0.0 (0.0)
Apathy	0.2 (0.4)	0.7 (1.9)
Disinhibition	0.0 (0.0)	0.0 (0.0)
Irritability	0.9 (1.4)	1.2 (2.1)
Abnormal motor behavior	0.0 (0.0)	0.0 (0.0)
Sleep disturbance	0.7 (1.9)	3.0 (4.3)
Abnormal eating	0.2 (0.6)	1.9 (3.5)

32% frontal, 20% temporal and 12% occipital atrophy[27]. Investigations using SPECT reveal that patients without significant dementia signs have metabolic reduction in the frontal lobe[28], and those with neuropsychologic dysfunction have abnormal anterior cingulate metabolism[23] and frontal hypoperfusion[29]. ALS patients with diagnosed dementia have decreased uptake in the frontal lobe and some have additional abnormalities in temporal, parietal and right thalamic regions on PET[16,30,31].

Pathologic study of cognitively normal and abnormal ALS patients also supports the continuum hypothesis of the syndrome. All ALS patients display the characteristic ubiquitin-positive, tau-negative neural inclusions, and the density and extent of these inclusions are greater in ALS patients with dementia. Some ALS patients with dementia also possess superficial linear spongiosis of the first and second cortical layers, a pathologic feature common to several forms of FTD[32]. ALS patients with co-morbid FTLD pathology have also been identified as having heightened neuronal loss and gliosis in layers II and III of the frontal cortex and subcortical structures, inclusions in the hippocampal dentate granule cells, substantia nigra degeneration[33], amygdala involvement[34] and orbital, parahippocampal, ambiens and insular gyri involvement[12,35]. In particular, ubiquitin-positive inclusions have been identified in the motor neurons as well as in the frontal and temporal lobes in both familial and sporadic cases with co-morbid ALS and dementia[35-42]. In addition, white matter degeneration has also been identified, suggesting a loss of fibers from the temporal and parietal lobes[43].

PREVALENCE OF DEMENTIA AND MORE SUBTLE FRONTOTEMPORAL CHANGES IN AMYOTROPHIC LATERAL SCLEROSIS

Despite the reported links between FTLD and ALS, the prevalence of FTLD and associated cognitive changes in ALS has not yet been determined. Rates of cognitive and behavioral abnormalities among ALS patients have been artificially low in the past because Alzheimer's disease-based dementia criteria relied upon memory-heavy, orientation-based measures. FTLD had not been well characterized in the past and FTLD subtypes were frequently underdiagnosed because the earliest clinical symptoms are non-cognitive behavioral symptoms with relatively preserved orientation and memory function. Additionally, the rapid progression of the ALS disease out-paced the FTLD syndrome, frequently resulting in patient death before the frontotemporal neuron loss became severe. As a result, estimates of dementia rates among ALS patients have been documented at rates as low as 3% of sporadic cases and 15% of familial cases[44], while more recent studies using neuropsychologic measures have documented major cognitive deficits in rates as high as 28–48% and a mild dysexecutive syndrome occurring in 35% of ALS patients[11,29,45]. Our group examined an FTLD cohort and found that 15% met the criteria for definite ALS[46]. We then examined a large ALS cohort and found that approximately 50% of ALS patients had executive dysfunction with one-third of them meeting research criteria for FTLD[3].

SUBTYPING THE SPECTRUM OF FRONTOTEMPORAL CHANGE IN AMYOTROPHIC LATERAL SCLEROSIS

To characterize this continuum of frontotemporal abnormalities in ALS more clearly, we suggest that useful distinctions can be made between subgroups of abnormal ALS patients. A helpful nomenclature may be 'ALS with cognitive impairment (ALSci) for those ALS patients who perform 1.5 standard deviations below the mean on at least two executive function neuropyschological measures. A recent review offers the term 'behaviorally impaired' (ALSbi) to describe ALS patients who display frontal-lobe-based behavioral signs who do not meet full criteria for FTD[47]. Table 7.3 (partially adapted from reference 47) illustrates

Table 7.3   A proposed subtyping for frontotemporal changes seen in amyotrophic lateral sclerosis (ALS)

Terminology	Clinical characteristics
ALS	A pure motor system disorder as defined by the El Escorial criteria; no clinical evidence of frontotemporal dysfunction
ALSci (ALS with cognitive impairment)	Deficits (1.5 sd below the age-matched mean) on two or more neuropsychological tests of executive functioning, but insufficient to meet the Neary criteria for FTD
ALSbi (ALS with behavioral impairment)	Frontal lobe-type behavioral impairment in two or more areas, as measured by a standardized caregiver interview
ALS-FTD	ALS patient meeting Neary criteria for FTD

FTD, frontotemporal dementia

specific criteria to distinguish between ALSci, ALSbi and ALS-FTD. A separate group termed 'possible frontotemporal dementia (FTD)' identifies those behaviorally abnormal patients who have intermittent episodes of disinhibition or two conflicting informants, thus precluding a diagnosis of FTD. Using these definitions, we detected cognitive and behavioral abnormalities that varied in severity with 22% meeting Neary criteria for FTLD, 17% demonstrating more subtle behavioral disturbances (ALSbi) and 9% exhibiting subtle cognitive dysfunction (ALSci) (manuscript in preparation). Describing these patients as 'normal' also minimizes the significance of these subtle findings which can greatly impact clinical care.

DISTINGUISHING BETWEEN CLINICAL DEPRESSION AND COGNITIVE ABNORMALITIES IN AMYOTROPHIC LATERAL SCLEROSIS

Depression is a common problem for both ALS patients and their caregivers. A neuropsychologic evaluation for ALS patients therefore requires a clinical measure of depression to be able to distinguish adequately between clinical depression, executive function impairment and other neurobehavioral symptoms. Depression rates among ALS patients differ in the literature because of heterogeneous criteria and measurement tools. Rates range from 2% of patients having a major depressive disorder[48] to 11% with a 'clinical depression'[49], but with more patients (11–22%) displaying mild or subclinical levels of depression symptoms[50–52].

A substantial literature exists regarding how clinical depression affects attention span, memory, executive function, social behavior and inhibition. It is known that the mild-to-moderate levels of depression typically seen in ALS patients do not substantially or consistently mimic a dementia syndrome, although while actively depressed, patients can experience delayed response time, poor encoding of memory and limited attention span[53]. A series of investigations using large samples of patients have carefully controlled for the effects of depression, ruling out the explanation that depressive symptoms are causing the cognitive and behavioral abnormalities[11,20,29,54].

When depression symptoms are clinically identified, they can be clearly distinguished from the behavioral changes seen in a frank FTLD syndrome. FTLD behavioral changes are marked by disinhibition, poor personal conduct and poor insight into these changes, and these interpersonal problems are marked by an insidious onset and gradual progression (Table 7.1). Depressive symptoms, in contrast, are more likely to have a more distinct onset that is noticeable to the patient and family. Social withdrawal, poor hygiene and emotional blunting are common in both FTLD and depression, but a trained professional can rather easily distinguish between the unique natures of these two syndromes. Most depressed patients will readily articulate that they withdraw socially and are emotionally blunted because of sadness, lack of pleasurable feelings, excessive worry, poor energy, or hopelessness. Depressed patients can usually explain what losses or events contribute to their feelings, and there will be times when these feelings of sadness will remit and the patient's behavior will at least partially return to normal. An ALS patient with co-morbid FTLD, in contrast, will most often lack any insight into the fact that any changes have occurred at all, and they will probably deny the presence of sadness, loss of pleasurable feelings, or feelings of loss. FTLD behaviors will not remit over time but will worsen.

Repeated assessment of depression level in the clinic is essential also to ensure proper identification of this potentially treatable problem. Hopelessness must be carefully distinguished from depression, as it is a separate entity for the patient emotionally, may have a different treatment, and may involve higher levels of suffering for patients than depression[49]. It should be noted that some investigators have documented higher rates of depression and hopelessness in caregivers than in patients[48].

PSEUDOBULBAR AFFECT CAN MIMIC DEPRESSION

Pseudobulbar affect (PBA), also described as emotional lability or pathologic laughing and crying, is characterized by frequent episodes of laughing or crying, out of proportion or incongruous to the underlying emotion of happiness or sadness[55]. Studies have suggested that PBA occurs in up to 50% of patients with ALS[56]. While sharing some behavioral similarities with depression, PBA is distinct from depression and patients themselves often recognize the explosive occurrence of tearfulness or laughter as being inappropriate and not reflecting proportionate underlying feelings of despair or joy. In one previous study only 11 of 36 (31%) ALS patients with PBA had significant levels of depression[57]. The basic mechanisms underlying emotional control are unknown; however, lesions in a variety of areas of the brain, including the frontal and temporal lobes, have been associated with the occurrence of pathologic laughing and crying. By including a measure of PBA, clinicians can identify and treat the condition and avoid confusing this syndrome with depression or cognitive problems.

THE UTILITY OF A BRIEF COGNITIVE SCREEN IN THE CLINIC

Once ALS dementia had been identified as indistinguishable from classic FTLD, investigators began to recognize the utility of executive function-based neuropsychologic evaluations, comprehensive caregiver interviews using standardized neurobehavioral measures and Neary criteria for FTLD[9]. This comprehensive evaluation and diagnostic process involves a significant investment of time and money for clinics. However, many are now incorporating a brief screening process for patients in the clinic, and then referring patients identified as abnormal to a neuropsychologist for the complete diagnostic evaluation (described below).

The mini-mental status examination is the traditional measure used in neurology for screening dementia. Unfortunately, in patients with frontal lobe impairment, abnormalities are often not detected with this type of testing. Instead, verbal and written fluency tests have been identified as the most sensitive and reliable method to detect abnormalities in ALS patients. Fluency tests, together with a caregiver questionnaire that taps into frontotemporal behavioral changes, provide clinic staff with the tools to screen for patients at risk for abnormalities.

A variety of fluency tests have been used effectively in ALS populations, including the controlled oral word association test[58,59] and category fluency tests (e.g. naming animals)[58-60]. Typically, such verbal fluency tests require the patient spontaneously to generate words that begin with a certain letter for a 60-s period. Each test has individual merits and has standardized norms that can be applied to individual patients by sex, age and education[61]. One unique verbal fluency test is worthy of note because of its utility for the ALS population in particular. Abrahams' revised-Thurstone written fluency test provides controls for both dysarthria and limb progression by having patients write responses instead of vocalizing them, and by adjusting scores formulaically by adjusting for the speed with which they write[15].

When caregivers are explicitly questioned about day-to-day functioning, incidence rates of abnormalities increase substantially[9,45,62]. For initial screening purposes, several brief questionnaires exist that include explicit frontal lobe content. The Neuropsychiatric Inventory-Questionnaire version (NPI-Q)[63] possesses good reliability and validity and does not require a staff member to administer. The frontal behavior inventory (FBI) includes specific questions about frontal lobe abnormalities that are commonly seen in FTLD patients[64].

COMPONENTS OF A COMPLETE DIAGNOSTIC EXAMINATION

Patients suspected of cognitive or behavioral abnormality can be properly diagnosed by a clinical neuropsychologist using a battery of neuropsychologic tests, a measure of depression, a measure of PBA, and a caregiver-administered neurobehavioral interview. Investigators have successfully used a wide variety of neuropsychologic batteries to document the presence of dementia in ALS patients. An ALS dementia battery will necessarily include memory and visuospatial tests to evaluate the potential presence of Alzheimer's disease but of primary importance is the inclusion of a proportionally large number of executive functioning measures and the presence of a verbal fluency measure. Of note are those investigators who have had success employing creative ways to deal with upper limb impairment and dysarthria, for example using memory tests that do not require limb movement such as the Continuous Recognition Memory Test[65] or the Recognition Memory Test[66]. Our group has had success modifying tests such as the Wisconsin Card Sorting Test, which can be adapted so that patients can give verbal commands when limb movement is impaired, and a written adaptation of the California Verbal Learning Test[67].

Few ALS investigators have employed structured caregiver interviews to document the presence of a span of behavioral and psychiatric problems, yet it has been shown that behavioral quantification can be even more sensitive than cognitive testing when identifying FTLD[68]. Our clinic has had success using the NPI to identify patients' clinical needs and symptoms of FTLD dementia. The NPI is a measure of 12 neuropsychiatric behaviors: delusions, hallucinations, agitation, dysphasia, anxiety, apathy, irritability, euphoria, disinhibition, aberrant motor behavior, night-time behavior disturbances, and appetite and eating abnormalities[69] (see Table 7.2). The severity and frequency of each symptom is rated on the basis of scripted questions. The NPI is a sensitive measure of some of the behavioral disturbances in FTLD (e.g. disinhibition), and additional behavioral disturbances which are non-specific or exclusionary (e.g. sleep disturbance or hallucinations, respectively). Its ability to yield an objective number for each of the 12 areas makes it a useful measure for longitudinal comparison. The NPI is administered to a caregiver, usually the patient's spouse, without the patient being present. It is necessary to score this interview carefully on those behavioral changes that are related to dementia-caused phenomena and not physical manifestations of the motor neuron disease, because this measure was developed not for ALS patients but for detection of dementia. For example, sleep disturbance related to paralysis and restless legs, eating disturbance related to swallowing and choking, and normal-range agitation related to losing mobility would be scored a zero, because these problems are due to the ALS disease and not to a dementing syndrome.

HOW SHOULD THE EVALUATION RESULTS BE INTERPRETED?

The neuropsychologic and neurobehavioral results are best interpreted in the context of the Neary criteria, now widely accepted as the most useful diagnostic criteria for FTLD. Three subtypes of FTLD have been identified, and the core criteria for each of the subtypes are listed in Table 7.1.

WHAT ARE THE DIFFERENT SUBTYPES OF FRONTOTEMPORAL LOBAR DEMENTIA?

The basis of FTLD involves progressive degeneration of frontal or anterior temporal lobe neurons, but the clinical features differ among individuals. All have in common alterations in behavior, language or executive dysfunction and relative sparing of memory. The FTLD subtypes are currently divided into three categories (Figure 7.2):

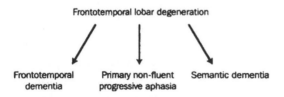

Figure 7.2   Subtypes of frontotemporal lobar degeneration

(1) Frontotemporal dementia (FTD), which is characterized by personality changes, behavioral problems, emotional blunting and loss of insight;

(2) Progressive non-fluent aphasia (PNFA), which presents with non-fluent speech and later may develop behavioral features;

(3) Semantic dementia (SD) involves fluent speech with semantic memory loss.

SUBTHRESHOLD DEMENTIA SYNDROMES IN AMYOTROPHIC LATERAL SCLEROSIS PATIENTS

As described above, the majority of ALS patients with cognitive and behavioral abnormalities do not meet the criteria for dementia. A sizable proportion of patients do possess executive function impairment and behavioral changes, however. As our understanding of these subclinical frontotemporal abnormalities evolves, investigators may find it useful to employ a standard set of criteria to diagnose executive dysfunction and behavioral abnormalities (Table 7.3).

THE PATIENT/CAREGIVER-LED APPROACH TO CLINICAL INTERVENTION

Patients and caregivers respond very differently when cognitive and behavioral changes are superimposed on an already overwhelming, everchanging terminal illness. Patients frequently have limited insight into the presence of changes and as a result it is either the family or a staff member who brings the issue to the clinician's attention. When caregivers approach clinic staff with concerns about a patient's behavior or thinking, staff can provide basic information about the range of changes commonly seen in ALS patients and they can suggest an evaluation. Examples of common caregiver complaints include irritability or aggression, emotional withdrawal, suspiciousness, poor hygiene, refusal to comply with treatment recommendations, or preventable falls and choking incidents. Regardless of whether the family chooses a full diagnostic evaluation and feedback/counseling session, they may experience considerable relief to receive basic education to understand that these changes are not uncommon. Educational materials developed for caregivers of FTLD[70] and head injury patients[71] have been helpful for caregivers of ALS-FTLD patients.

In our experience approximately a third of families choose not to address cognitive and behavioral changes directly, for a variety of reasons, and we encourage staff to respect each family's decision. Even in the presence of severe and disturbing cognitive and behavioral changes, families may feel that a sense of duty, respect, privacy, or cultural norms causes them to refuse evaluation or support from clinic staff. Other families deny the presence of changes that are noticed by staff, or they have a history of emotional instability or chaotic family relationships that renders them unable to address the issue.

In cases of executive dysfunction or mild-to-moderate behavioral change, caregivers may choose to refuse evaluation or intervention because they feel the changes are a minor issue as compared with the motor neuron changes they face. In such cases staff can be made aware that an evaluation has been refused but that the patient or family may at some time benefit from additional services (e.g. provision of written versions of clinical instructions, having the caregiver in the room for important discussions, or provision of additional caregiving resources).

WHAT TREATMENT CAN BE OFFERED?

Once a diagnosis has been made of either dementia or a subthreshold disorder of frontotemporal changes, the patient's individual needs can be addressed. A broad range of psychiatric and frontal lobe signs are seen in patients, and individual caregivers will experience distress in unique ways. Because virtually all requests for help come from the caregivers themselves, the first step in treatment is educating the caregiver. Caregivers will benefit from understanding that frontotemporal alterations are common among ALS patients and they have a biological basis rooted in cerebral changes that are associated with the motor neuron disease. Frequently caregivers are reassured to know that they are not to blame for patient's emotional withdrawal, decreased communication, emotional lability, irritability, poor motivation, suspiciousness, or aggression. 'Negative symptoms', those pertaining to a lack of behavior (e.g. not initiating loving contact), may not be able to be changed, and the caregiver can be encouraged to accept this change as a loss. 'Positive symptoms', or those changes that are new and troubling (hitting, rude language) may be effectively treated with a combination of psychotropic drugs and behavioral interventions.

Caregivers will also benefit from additional social work assistance to plan for support services for patients and cope with increased dependency as patients are less able to participate in making judgments about their care. Caregivers should be alerted to identify those patients who have exhibited the classic depression, anxiety and disinhibition symptoms of early FTD or the language impairment of SD or progressive non-fluent aphasia several years prior to their ALS onset. This group is more likely to have the more severe dementia that will complicate their care and are likely to require psychiatric medication and behavior management consultation to provide adequate care.

In terms of available psychotropic treatment, selective serotonin reuptake inhibitors (SSRIs) are found to be useful in FTLD patients because of serotonergic neuron depletion in the frontal lobe. Rigidity, agitation and compulsiveness are symptoms most commonly addressed successfully with SSRIs. Patients with more severe agitation and aggression may benefit from atypical antipsychotic medication. Physicians should consider stopping the use of anticholinergics, over-the-counter sedatives and antihistamines, as they may decrease blood flow to the frontal lobe.

FRONTOTEMPORAL DYSFUNCTION IN AMYOTROPHIC LATERAL SCLEROSIS: CLINICAL CORRELATES AND PROGNOSIS

Over a 2-year period our group has carefully tracked our 100-patient ALS cohort described above, collecting clinical information and survival data. Our data reveal that 28 of the original 100 patients now meet research criteria for FTLD based on neurobehavioral interviews and formal neuropsychologic testing. Nineteen patients are borderline in their behavior or language function and have not consented to detailed evaluation, and 53 patients are not suspected to have cognitive abnormalities based on word generation testing, behavioral observation or, in nearly half, formal evaluation[72]. Our data suggest, as do other investigations[15,22], that an important clinical correlate includes the presence of bulbar palsy. In our group, bulbar-onset patients were more than twice as likely to have received an FTLD diagnosis, and patients with obvious upper motor neuron signs were more than twice as likely to have an FTLD diagnosis than patients with soft upper motor signs. Additionally, family history of a neurodegenerative disease increased the risk of ALS-FTLD, suggesting that those patients with ALS-FTLD may be more likely to have genetic influences over the disease than ALS-only patients.

Our study suggests that the co-morbid diagnosis of FTLD may be associated with an adverse effect on survival. The median survival from symptom onset of ALS was 2 years 4 months for those with FTLD and 3 years 3 months for the 53 with normal executive and behavioral function. To test our clinical impression that poor compliance with treatment recommendations by ALS-FTLD patients may be a factor influencing shorter survival, we set criteria for compliance with non-invasive positive pressure ventilation (NPPV) and percutaneous endoscopic gastrostomy (PEG) recommendations and determined the frequency of compliance among the ALS and ALS-FTLD patients based on retrospective chart review. Compliance with recommendations for NPPV occurred in fewer patients with ALS-FTLD (five of 18, 28%) than in patients with ALS and normal behavioral function (14 of 23, 61%), ($z = 2.22$, one-tail $p < 0.02$). Similarly, compliance with recommendations for PEG occurred in fewer patients with ALS-FTLD (four of 16, 25%) than in patients with ALS and normal behavioral function (eight of 12, 67%), ($z = 2.01$, one-tail $p < 0.03$). However, bulbar onset and older age at onset are also associated with shorter survival and these two characteristics are more common in ALS-FTLD than in ALS alone, so larger cohorts of both groups are necessary to distinguish the effects of FTLD, bulbar onset, age and compliance on survival.

CONCLUSIONS

The concept that cognitive and behavioral dysfunction in ALS is rare can no longer be substantiated. Critical issues now include the prevalence of the dysfunction and the possible etiologic differences between those ALS patients who are cognitively and behaviorally normal and those with abnormalities. ALS may exist as a degenerative process of the motor system, in which degeneration of the frontotemporal lobar type can occur. When present, it may manifest as frontotemporal lobar degeneration (ALS-FTLD). In its more subtle manifestations, either a frontal dysexecutive syndrome or behavioral syndrome may occur, or both. It is intriguing, however, that frontal, temporal and parietal cortical atrophy, observed on neuroimaging, and disproportionate to that observed in age-matched controls, is seen across all ALS patients. These data suggest that the 'pure' phenotype of ALS in which the disease process is restricted to the motor neurons is in fact rare, and that the more common variant is a more complicated phenotype in which the neurodegeneration extends well outside the boundaries of the motor system.

Consensus on terminology is required in order to bring some order to what is becoming an increasingly complex picture. Approaching the same entity from a dementia perspective may ignore the complexity of ALS and vice versa, so groups of investigators from both specialties are needed to discuss the terminology and reach consensus. Do patients with ALSbi and ALSci progress to FTLD? Prospective studies are beginning to emerge[73] to answer these and other pressing questions.

REFERENCES

1. Neary D, Snowden JS, Mann DM. Cognitive change in motor neurone disease/amyotrophic lateral sclerosis (MND/ALS). J Neurol Sci 2000; 180: 15–20

2. Hudson AJ. Amyotrophic lateral sclerosis and its association with dementia, parkinsonism and other neurological disorders: a review. Brain 1981; 104: 217–47

3. Lomen-Hoerth C, Murphy J, Langmore S, et al. Are amyotrophic lateral sclerosis patients cognitively normal? Neurology 2003; 60: 1094–7

4. Bak TH, Hodges JR. Cognition, language and behavior in motor neurone disease: Evidence of frontotemporal dysfunction. Dement Geriatr Cogn Disord 1999; 10 (Suppl 1): 29–32

5. Mitsuyama Y, Takamiya S. Presenile dementia with motor neuron disease in Japan. A new entity? Arch Neurol 1979; 36: 592–3

6. Brun A, Gustafson L, Passant U. [A new kind of degenerative dementia. Localization, rather than type is significant in frontal lobe dementia]. Lakartidningen 1994; 91: 4751–7

7. Neary D. Dementia of frontal lobe type. J Am Geriatr Soc 1990; 38: 71–2

8. Neary D, Snowden JS, Northen B, Goulding P. Dementia of frontal lobe type. J Neurol Neurosurg Psychiatry 1988; 51: 353–61

9. Barson FP, Kinsella GJ, Ong B, Mathers SE. A neuropsychological investigation of dementia in motor neurone disease (MND). J Neurol Sci 2000; 180: 107–13

10. Talbot PR, Goulding PJ, Lloyd JJ, et al. Inter-relation between 'classic' motor neuron disease and frontotemporal dementia: neuropsychological and single photon emission computed tomography study. J Neurol Neurosurg Psychiatry 1995; 58: 541–7

11. Massman PJ, Sims J, Cooke N, et al. Prevalence and correlates of neuropsychological deficits in amyotrophic lateral sclerosis. J Neurol Neurosurg Psychiatry 1996; 61: 450–5

12. Kew JJ, Leigh PN, Playford ED, et al. Cortical function in amyotrophic lateral sclerosis. A positron emission tomography study. Brain 1993; 116: 655–80

13. Gallassi R, Montagna P, Ciardulli C, et al. Cognitive impairment in motor neuron disease. Acta Neurol Scand 1985; 71: 480–4

14. Abe K. Cognitive function in amyotrophic lateral sclerosis. Amyotroph Lateral Scler Other Motor Neuron Disord 2000; 1: 343–7

15. Abrahams S, Goldstein LH, Al-Chalabi A, et al. Relation between cognitive dysfunction and pseudobulbar palsy in amyotrophic lateral sclerosis. J Neurol Neurosurg Psychiatry 1997; 62: 464–72

16. Ludolph AC, Langen KJ, Regard M, et al. Frontal lobe function in amyotrophic lateral sclerosis: A neuropsychologic and positron emission tomography study. Acta Neurol Scand 1992; 85: 81–9

17. Hartikainen P, Helkala EL, Soininen H, Riekkinen P Sr. Cognitive and memory deficits in untreated Parkinson's disease and amyotrophic lateral sclerosis patients: A comparative study. J Neural Transm Park Dis Dement Sect 1993; 6: 127–37

18. Kilani M, Micallef J, Soubrouillard C, et al. A longitudinal study of the evolution of cognitive function and affective state in patients with amyotrophic lateral sclerosis. Amyotroph Lateral Scler Other Motor Neuron Disord 2004; 5: 46–54

19. Hanagasi HA, Gurvit IH, Ermutlu N, et al. Cognitive impairment in amyotrophic lateral sclerosis: evidence from neuropsychological investigation and event-related potentials. Brain Res Cogn Brain Res 2002; 14: 234–44

20. Gallassi R, Montagna P, Morreale A, et al. Neuropsychological, electroencephalogram and brain computed tomography findings in motor neuron disease. Eur Neurol 1989; 29: 115–20

21. Abrahams S, Goldstein LH, Kew JJ, et al. Frontal lobe dysfunction in amyotrophic lateral sclerosis. Brain 1996; 119: 2105–20

22. David AS. Neuropsychological measures in patients with amyotrophic lateral sclerosis. Acta Neurol Scand 1987; 75: 284

23. Strong MJ, Grace GM, Orange JB, et al. A prospective study of cognitive impairment in ALS. Neurology 1999; 53: 1665–70

24. Cavalleri F, De Renzi E. Amyotrophic lateral sclerosis with dementia. Acta Neurol Scand 1994; 89: 391–4

25. Abrahams S, Goldstein LH, Simmons A, et al. Word retrieval in amyotrophic lateral sclerosis: a functional magnetic resonance imaging study. Brain 2004; 127: 1507–17

26. Kew JJ, Goldstein LH, Leigh PN, et al. The relationship between abnormalities of cognitive function and cerebral activation in amyotrophic lateral sclerosis. A neuropsychological and positron emission tomography study. Brain 1993; 116: 1399–423

27. Poloni M, Patrini C, Rocchelli B, Rindi G. Thiamin monophosphate in the CSF of patients with amyotrophic lateral sclerosis. Arch Neurol 1982; 39: 507–9

28. Abe K. [Autosomal dominant ALS]. Ryoikibetsu Shokogun Shirizu 1999: 320–2

29. Portet F, Cadilhac C, Touchon J, Camu W. Cognitive impairment in motor neuron disease with bulbar onset. Amyotroph Lateral Scler Other Motor Neuron Disord 2001; 2: 23–9

30. Abe K, Fujimura H, Toyooka K, et al. Cognitive function in amyotrophic lateral sclerosis. J Neurol Sci 1997; 148: 95–100

31. Abrahams S, Leigh PN, Kew JJ, et al. A positron emission tomography study of frontal lobe function (verbal fluency) in amyotrophic lateral sclerosis. J Neurol Sci 1995; 129 (Suppl): 44–6

32. Wilson CM, Grace GM, Munoz DG, et al. Cognitive impairment in sporadic ALS: A pathologic continuum underlying a multisystem disorder. Neurology 2001; 57: 651–7

33. Mitsuyama Y. Presenile dementia with motor neuron disease in Japan: clinico-pathological review of 26 cases. J Neurol Neurosurg Psychiatry 1984; 47: 953–9

34. Mann DM, South PW, Snowden JS, Neary D. Dementia of frontal lobe type: neuropathology and immunohistochemistry. J Neurol Neurosurg Psychiatry 1993; 56: 605–14

35. Kato S, Oda M, Hayashi H, et al. Participation of the limbic system and its associated areas in the dementia of amyotrophic lateral sclerosis. J Neurol Sci 1994; 126: 62–9

36. Jellinger KA. Pick's disease with amyotrophic lateral sclerosis. J Neurol Sci 1997; 152: 227–8, 230

37. Hilton DA, Love S, Ferguson I, Newman P. Motor neuron disease with neurofibrillary tangles in a non-Guamanian patient. Acta Neuropathol (Berl) 1995; 90: 101–6

38. Machida Y, Tsuchiya K, Anno M, et al. Sporadic amyotrophic lateral sclerosis with multiple system degeneration: A report of an autopsy case without respirator administration. Acta Neuropathol (Berl) 1999; 98: 512–15

39. Kusaka H, Imai T. Pathology of motor neurons in amyotrophic lateral sclerosis with dementia. Clin Neuropathol 1993; 12: 164–8

40. Matsumoto S, Goto S, Kusaka H, et al. Ubiquitin-positive inclusion in anterior horn cells in subgroups of motor neuron diseases: a comparative study of adult-onset amyotrophic lateral sclerosis, juvenile amyotrophic lateral sclerosis and Werdnig–Hoffmann disease. J Neurol Sci 1993; 115: 208–13

41. Niizato K, Tsuchiya K, Tominaga I, et al. Pick's disease with amyotrophic lateral sclerosis (ALS): Report of two autopsy cases and literature review. J Neurol Sci 1997; 148: 107–12

42. Nakano I. Frontotemporal dementia with motor neuron disease (amyotrophic lateral sclerosis with dementia). Neuropathology 2000; 20: 68–75

43. Kiernan JA, Hudson AJ. Frontal lobe atrophy in motor neuron diseases. Brain 1994; 117: 747–57

44. Hudson AJ. Amyotrophic lateral sclerosis/parkinsonism/dementia: clinico-pathological correlations relevant to Guamanian ALS/PD. Can J Neurol Sci 1991; 18 (Suppl 3): 387–9

45. Rakowicz WP, Hodges JR. Dementia and aphasia in motor neuron disease: An underrecognised association? J Neurol Neurosurg Psychiatry 1998; 65: 881–9

46. Lomen-Hoerth C, Anderson T, Miller B. The overlap of amyotrophic lateral sclerosis and frontotemporal dementia. Neurology 2002; 59: 1077–9

47. Lomen-Hoerth C, Strong M. Frontotemporal dysfunction in ALS. In: Mitsumoto H, Przedborshi S, Gordon P, eds. ALS, 2nd edn. London: Taylor & Francis Group, 2006

48. Rabkin JG, Wagner GJ, Del Bene M. Resilience and distress among amyotrophic lateral sclerosis patients and caregivers. Psychosom Med 2000; 62: 271–9

49. Ganzini L, Johnston WS, Hoffman WF. Correlates of suffering in amyotrophic lateral sclerosis. Neurology 1999; 52: 1434–40

50. Houpt JL, Gould BS, Norris FH, Jr. Psychological characteristics of patients with amyotrophic lateral sclerosis (ALS). Psychosom Med 1977; 39: 299–303

51. Chio A, Gauthier A, Montuschi A, et al. A cross sectional study on determinants of quality of life in ALS. J Neurol Neurosurg Psychiatry 2004; 75: 1597–601

52. Trail M, Nelson ND, Van JN, et al. A study comparing patients with amyotrophic lateral sclerosis and their caregivers on measures of quality of life, depression, and their attitudes toward treatment options. J Neurol Sci 2003; 209: 79–85

53. Gainotti G, Marra C. Some aspects of memory disorders clearly distinguish dementia of the Alzheimer's type from depressive pseudo-dementia. J Clin Exp Neuropsychol 1994; 16: 65–78

54. Evdokimidis I, Constantinidis TS, Gourtzelidis P, et al. Frontal lobe dysfunction in amyotrophic lateral sclerosis. J Neurol Sci 2002; 195: 25–33

55. Dark FL, McGrath JJ, Ron MA. Pathological laughing and crying. Aust NZ J Psychiatry 1996; 30: 472–9

56. Gallagher JP. Pathologic laughter and crying in ALS: a search for their origin. Acta Neurol Scand 1989; 80: 114–17

57. Moore SR, Gresham LS, Bromberg MB, et al. A self-report measure of affective lability. J Neurol Neurosurg Psychiatry 1997; 63: 89–93

58. Benton AL, Hamsher KD. Multilingual Aphasia Examination. Iowa City, IA: AJA Associates, 1989

59. Spreen O, Strauss E. A Compendium of Neuropsychological Tests. New York: Oxford University Press, 1991

60. Morris JC, Heyman A, Mohs RC, et al. The Consortium to Establish a Registry for Alzheimer's Disease (CERAD). Part I. Clinical and neuropsychological assessment of Alzheimer's disease. Neurology 1989; 39: 1159–65

61. Lezak MD. Neuropsychological Assessement. 3rd edn. New York: Oxford University Press, 1995

62. Snowdon DA, Kemper SJ, Mortimer JA, et al. Linguistic ability in early life and cognitive function and Alzheimer's disease in late life. Findings from the Nun Study. J Am Med Assoc 1996; 275: 528–32

63. Kaufer DI, Cummings JL, Ketchel P, et al. Validation of the NPI-Q, a brief clinical form of the Neuropsychiatric Inventory. J Neuropsychiatry Clin Neurosci 2000; 12: 233–9

64. Kertesz A, Davidson W, Fox H. Frontal behavioral inventory: Diagnostic criteria for frontal lobe dementia. Can J Neurol Sci 1997; 24: 29–36

65. Hannay HJ, Levin HS, Grossman RG. Impaired recognition memory after head injury. Cortex 1979; 15: 269–83

66. Warrington EK. Recognition Memory Test. Windsor, UK: NFER-Nelson, 1984

67. Dellis DC, Kramer JH, Kaplan E, Ober BA. California Verbal Learning Test. San Antonio, TX: Psychological Corporation, 1987

68. Kertesz A, Davidson W, McCabe P, Munoz D. Behavioral quantitation is more sensitive than cognitive testing in frontotemporal dementia. Alzheimer Dis Assoc Disord 2003; 17: 223–9

69. Cummings JL. The Neuropsychiatric Inventory: Assessing psychopathology in dementia patients. Neurology 1997; 48 (5 Suppl 6): S10–16

70. Alliance FC. Fact Sheet: Frontotemporal Dementia, May, 2000

71. Alliance FC. Fact Sheet: Coping with Behavior Problems after Head Injury, July, 1996

72. Olney RK, Murphy J, Forshew D, et al. The effects of executive and behavioral dysfunction on the course of ALS. Neurology 2005; 65: 1774–7

73. Abrahams S, Leigh PN, Goldstein LH. Cognitive change in ALS: a prospective study. Neurology 2005; 64: 1222–6

Section 3

Genetics of amyotrophic lateral sclerosis and related disorders

8

Familial motor neuron diseases other than amyotrophic lateral sclerosis

Alice Brockington, Pamela J Shaw

INTRODUCTION

In this chapter we will discuss non-amyotrophic lateral sclerosis (ALS) forms of motor neuron degeneration that have a genetic basis. The conditions covered include the spinal muscular atrophies (SMAs), the hereditary motor neuropathies (HMNs), Kennedy's disease and the hereditary spastic paraplegias (HSPs). It is clear from the emerging concepts of cellular mechanisms of disease in these disorders that there is significant overlap with current understanding of disease pathogenesis in ALS, as highlighted in Table 8.1. We will not cover the hereditary motor and sensory neuropathies (HMSN)/Charcot–Marie–Tooth syndrome (CMT) disorders in which degeneration of sensory axons is a prominent feature. In addition, we will not cover ALS2 caused by mutations in alsin, which has many features in common with HSP. Alsin-related motor neuron degeneration is covered in Chapter 9 on the genetics of ALS.

SPINAL MUSCULAR ATROPHY

The classification of spinal muscular atrophy

SMA was first described independently by Werdnig and Hoffman in 1891. The term SMA

Table 8.1 Overlapping disease mechanisms in different types of motor neuron degeneration: amyotrophic lateral sclerosis (ALS)/motor neuron disease, spinal muscular atrophy (SMA) and hereditary spastic paraplegia (HSP)

Common problem of neurons with long axons

Axonal length up to 1 m
Axonal cytoplasm may be 1000 times that of the cell body
High energy requirements
Since protein manufacture, packaging and sorting are essentially restricted to the cell body – an exquisite dependence on intricate and efficient axonal transport mechanisms

Mitochondrial dysfunction

Morphologically and functionally abnormal mitochondria are seen in subtypes of HSP and ALS
An interlinking theme could be the problem of ATP deficiency at the distal ends of long axons

Intracellular trafficking and axonal transport mechanisms

Motor proteins, e.g. KIF5A, KIF1Bβ, p150 subunit of dynactin cause subtypes of HSP, CMT and ALS/MND, respectively
Microtubule dynamics, e.g. spastin
Intracellular trafficking of vesicles/endosomes, e.g. alsin, atlastin, spartin, maspardin
Secondary neurotrophic factor deficiency

Other

Protein aggregation
Defects in RNA handling and transcriptional regulation

CMT, Charcot–Marie–Tooth syndrome

encompasses a group of genetically determined pure lower motor neuron disorders. Degeneration of the anterior horn cells leads to a slowly progressive, symmetrical muscle weakness and wasting, with sparing of sensation, and absence of pyramidal tract involvement. As the bulbar musculature may be affected, and motor neuron degeneration is therefore not confined to the spinal cord, an alternative term 'hereditary motor neuronopathy' (HMN) was proposed, and both terms are currently in use. There are difficulties with the definition and classification of SMA, which are gradually being resolved with advances in understanding of the underlying genetic defects. Although they are by definition genetically determined, adult patients present not infrequently with what appears to be sporadic SMA, and a genetic basis is therefore unproven. In clinical practice, the neurodegenerative process has a predilection for motor neurons, but in some families, pyramidal tract and sensory involvement are also seen. Thus, SMA shows some overlap with other neurodegenerative diseases, such as hereditary spastic paraplegia (HSP), familial ALS, and CMT.

The most common type of SMA is proximal SMA of childhood, which is inherited in an autosomal recessive manner. It is the second most frequent lethal childhood autosomal recessive disease after cystic fibrosis. Patients develop predominantly proximal limb weakness, with sparing of the facial muscles and the diaphragm. Proximal SMA is divided into subtypes, according to severity and age of onset[1,2]. Type I SMA (OMIM no. 253300), or Werdnig–Hoffman disease, presents with severe generalized muscle weakness and hypotonia at birth, or by the age of 6 months. Affected children never sit or walk, and usually die from respiratory insufficiency by the age of 2 years. Type II (OMIM no. 253550) is an intermediate form. Onset of muscle weakness is before the age of 18 months, and patients can sit, but are never able to walk unaided, and survival is usually limited to adolescence. Type III SMA (OMIM no. 253400), or Wohlfart–Kugelberg–Welander dis-

ease, presents after the age of 18 months. Patients gain the ability to stand and walk, but often become wheelchair-bound during youth or adulthood. Life expectancy is thought to be normal. Onset of recessive proximal SMA has been described in adulthood, and this is sometimes designated type IV SMA. An adult-onset proximal SMA (Finkel type SMA, OMIM no. 182980), which shows autosomal dominant inheritance, is genetically distinct from proximal recessive SMA[3].

The distal SMAs (or distal hereditary motor neuronopathies) are a more diverse group of disorders. They usually present as a peroneal muscular atrophy syndrome, distinguished from the more common CMT, which causes a similar pattern of weakness, by the absence of sensory involvement. They have been classified in the past as a 'spinal' form of CMT. The overall clinical picture is of progressive weakness of the toes and feet, which extends to involve the distal upper limb muscles. Foot deformity is a common feature, and often unusual or additional features are present, including predominance in the hands, vocal cord paralysis, diaphragm paralysis and pyramidal tract signs. Harding proposed seven subtypes of distal HMN[4], on the basis of genetic and clinical criteria. This classification was reviewed by the European CMT consortium in 1998[5], but is constantly changing with the identification of novel clinical and genetic entities, the finding that previously delineated phenotypes show genetic heterogeneity and that single gene disorders can vary widely in phenotype (reviewed by Irobi et al.[6] and summarized in Table 8.2).

Proximal recessive spinal muscular atrophy of childhood

Chromosome 5q

Linkage analysis revealed that the three subtypes of proximal recessive SMA map to chromosome 5q13[7–10]. This region of chromosome 5 is complex, and characterized by low copy repeats, which may account for instability of this region, and

Name	OMIM	Gene / Linkage	Clinical features	Other name
SMA with respiratory distress (SMARD1)	604320	Mutations in *IGHMBP2* on chromosome 11q	Accounts for < 1% of infantile SMA. Intrauterine growth retardation, prematurity, a weak cry and foot deformities are often the earliest symptoms, progressing to respiratory distress and progressive muscular weakness with predominantly distal lower limb involvement. Death usually occurs by the age of 6 months	Distal HMN V Diaphragmatic spinal muscular atrophy
Autosomal recessive distal SMA	607088	Linkage to 11q13	Slowly progressive distal weakness of upper and lower limbs with a very variable age of onset. Diaphragmatic involvement is seen in more severely affected patients	
Jerash HMN	605726	Linkage to 9p21.1-p12	Consanguineous families in the Jerash region of Jordan were described, in which weakness and atrophy of the lower limbs associated with pyramidal features develops in childhood, and progresses to the upper limbs	
Autosomal dominant				
Distal SMA with lower limb predominance	158590	Mutations in *HSPB8* on chromosome 12q24	The age range of presentation of these patients is wide, but tends to be in the second to fourth decades. Predominant distal lower limb involvement progresses to involve all the muscle groups in the legs, and to mildly affect the upper limbs	Distal HMN II
Distal SMA with upper limb predominance	600794	Mutations in *GARS* on chromosome 7p14 and *BSCL2* on chromosome 11q12-14	Onset of hand weakness and wasting in the second decade, with slow progression to involve the feet, but patients remain ambulant into their sixties. In some patients, impaired vibration sense, or mild pyramidal features are seen	Distal HMN V
Congenital non-progressive SMA affecting the lower limbs	600175	Linkage to 12q23-24	Presents with congenital contractures of the lower limbs or delayed motor milestones, and non-progressive distal limb weakness predominantly affecting the lower limbs	Congenital benign SMA with contractures
Scapulo-peroneal SMA	181405	Linkage to 12q24.1-12q24.2	Scapuloperoneal atrophy of neurogenic origin with variable age of onset and progression. Clinical features vary between and within these pedigrees, and there is evidence of genetic anticipation. More severely affected patients may show absence of certain muscle groups, laryngeal palsy and progression to severe disability by adolescence	New England-type neurogenic scapuloperoneal amyotrophy
SMA with vocal cord paralysis	158580	Linkage to 2q14	Onset is in adolescence, with distal limb weakness, a husky voice due to laryngeal involvement and impaired vital capacity. The disease is slowly progressive and relatively benign	Distal HMN V

SMARD1, SMA with respiratory distress type I; *IGHMBP2*, immunoglobulin mu-binding protein 2; HMN, hereditary motor neuronopathy; *HSPB8*, heat shock protein B8; *GARS*, glycyl tRNA synthetase; *BSCL2*, Berardinelli–Seip congenital lipodystrophy 2

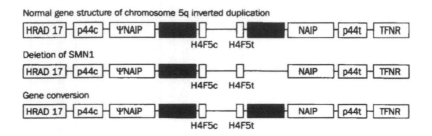

Figure 8.1   Representation of the spinal muscular atrophy critical region of chromosome 5q13, containing an inverted duplication of four genes: *H4F5*, *SMN*, *NAIP* and *BTF2p44*. This duplicate region is flanked by the genes *TFNR* and *HRAD17*

trigger frequent deletions or gene conversions[11]. Within the SMA critical region, there is a 500 kb inverted duplication[12], with four genes present in at least two copies, telomeric and centromeric: the survival motor neuron gene (*SMN*)[12], the neuronal apoptosis inhibitory protein gene (*NAIP*)[13], the gene encoding BTF2p44, a subunit of RNA polymerase II involved in transcription[14,15] and a putative RNA binding protein, H4F5[16] (Figure 8.1).

Homozygous deletion of the telomeric copies of all four genes have been described in patients with SMA[12–14,17]. The frequency of gene deletions is, however, much higher for *SMN1* than for *H4F5*, *NAIP* or *BTF2p44*, and it is now well established that mutations affecting *SMN1* cause 5q13-linked SMA. In a series of 525 patients with classical SMA, 96% were found to be linked to chromosome 5q13, all of which showed mutations in *SMN1*[18]. Furthermore, mice possess only one survival motor neuron gene (*Smn*), loss of which is embryonically lethal. However, *Smn*[–/–];*SMN2* mice that carry one or two copies of human *SMN2* develop a phenotype of motor neuron degeneration that resembles SMA type I[19,20].

The SMN gene

Duplication of *SMN* occurred more than 5 million years ago, before the separation of human and chimpanzee lineages[21]. Subsequent sequence divergence in *Homo sapiens* has led to five base pair differences between *SMN1*, and its centromeric homolog *SMN2*[12,22] (Figure 8.2). Three of the base pair differences are intronic; one, in exon 8, lies within the 3′ untranslated region, while that in exon 7 does not alter the amino acid sequence. The primary gene sequences of *SMN1* and *SMN2* therefore predict identical proteins. However, the translationally silent change in exon 7 decreases the activity of an exonic splicing enhancer, leading to skipping of exon 7 and a truncated protein in 80% of the transcript produced by *SMN2*. Homozygous absence of *SMN2*, found in about 5% of controls, has no clinical phenotype[12]. Of 5q13-linked SMA patients, 96% show homozygous absence of *SMN1* exon 7. This may occur through gene deletion, often a large deletion that includes the whole gene, or several genes within the SMA critical region. Alternatively, *SMN1* may be replaced by a copy of *SMN2* during DNA replication, a process known as gene conversion (see Figure 8.1)[23,24]. The remaining 4% of 5q13-linked SMA cases are compound heterozygotes with a deletion or gene conversion on one chromosome, and an intragenic 'subtle' mutation on the other.

Subtle mutations in spinal muscular atrophy

Thirty-one intragenic mutations have been described in SMA, which are summarized in Figure 8.3[18,25–29]. The majority of these produce a truncated protein, either through splice site

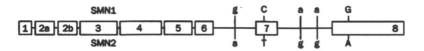

Figure 8.2   Single base pair differences that distinguish *SMN1* and *SMN2*

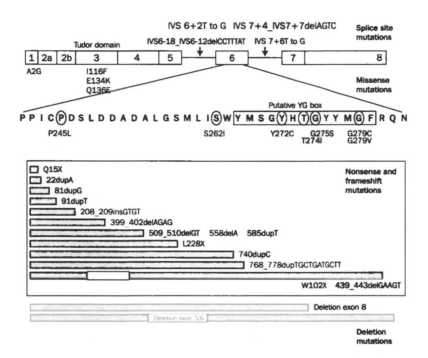

Figure 8.3   Schematic representation of the intragenic mutations in *SMN* that have been identified in spinal muscular atrophy patients. Nomenclature is based on the published sequence, and published nomenclature guidelines[25]. Nomenclature has varied in the literature in the past, and may differ from that used here. Eleven described missense mutations show clustering around the tudor domain in exon 3, and the tyrosine–glycine (YG)-rich region of exon 6. Nonsense, frameshift and deletion mutations are listed adjacent to a schematic representation of the resulting truncated protein product

mutations that disrupt exon 7, or through nonsense or frameshift mutations which introduce a stop codon. These mutations provide strong evidence that *SMN* is the SMA-determining gene, and that the region encoded by exons 6 and 7 is important, as it is disrupted in most types of mutation. However, they provide little information about the function of SMN. Missense mutations, on the other hand, show an interesting pattern of clustering that provides some insight into the functional domains of the SMN protein. A

tyrosine–glycine-rich sequence (the YG box) at the C-terminal of SMN encompasses five of the described missense mutations, and is a highly conserved sequence, identical in yeasts and nematodes. This region has homology to RNA-interacting proteins[30]. A further cluster of mutations is seen in the central region of SMN, which constitutes a so-called tudor domain. This is an evolutionarily conserved sequence of unknown function found in many eukaryotic proteins, and originally described for the *Drosophila* tudor protein[31].

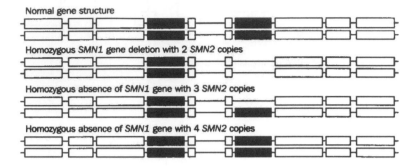

Figure 8.4   Homozygous *SMN1* deletions, with varying copy numbers of *SMN2* due to gene conversion events

Modifying factors in spinal muscular atrophy

SMN2

SMN2 produces only 20% of full-length protein. This is insufficient to rescue the phenotype in homozygous deletion of *SMN1*, but there is strong evidence that *SMN2* is a disease-modifying gene for SMA. A molecular basis for the wide variation in the SMA phenotype lies in the fact that homozygous absence of *SMN1* can be due to gene deletion or to conversion to *SMN2*. A patient may have anything from one to four copies of *SMN2*, leading to a progressive increase in the amount of full-length protein (Figure 8.4). Both the copy number of *SMN2*[32–34] and the protein levels of SMN[35] have been shown to correlate with severity of disease. However, the copy number of *SMN2* in types I, II and III SMA overlaps; therefore, this alone cannot expain the phenotypic variation of the disease, and other disease-modifying factors must exist.

NAIP and H4F5

The majority of type I SMA patients display large-scale 5q13 deletions, removing *SMN1* and adjacent microsatellite markers, whereas type III patients tend to have small deletions or gene conversions affecting only *SMN1*[36]. This suggests that an SMA-modifying locus distinct from *SMN1* lies in the 5q13 interval. *NAIP* is a good candidate as it functions as a negative regulator of apoptosis. *NAIP* deletion occurs in 45% of type I SMA patients, and 18% of type II and III patients[14], therefore loss of *NAIP* may lead to a more severe disease phenotype[13]. *H4F5* lies closer to *SMN1* than any other known gene. Homozygous deletions of this gene have been found in 90% of type I SMA cases, and it has also been proposed as a disease-modifying gene in SMA[16]. However, deletions of both *NAIP* and *H4F5* may simply reflect larger chromosomal deletions that involve both *SMN1* and *SMN2*, and their role in the pathogenesis of SMA is not confirmed.

THE SMN PROTEIN

SMN is a protein of 294 amino acids that is widely expressed. In SMA patients, the level of SMN is only moderately reduced in muscle and lymphoblasts, but reduced 100-fold in the spinal cord of type 1 patients[37]. It shows diffuse cytoplasmic expression, but within the nucleus is clustered in suborganelles called 'gems' (for 'gemini of coiled bodies'). These are similar in size and number to, and often associated with, Cajal or coiled bodies, which are known to have a role in mRNA metabolism[38]. The SMN protein oligomerizes, and associates with six proteins named Gemins,

Table 8.3	The Gemin family of proteins	
Protein	Comment	Reference
Gemin 2	Formerly SIP1	40
Gemin 3 (or DP103)	A DEAD-box helicase	41, 42
Gemin 4		43
Gemin 5 (or p175)	A WD repeat protein. (Tryptophan–aspartic acid, or WD, motifs are protein–protein interacting domains)	44
Gemin 6		45
Gemin 7		46

to form the SMN complex (Table 8.3). Self-association occurs through an oligomerization domain in exon 6, and appears to be essential for its activity[39].

The functions of survival motor neuron complex

The SMN complex interacts with several proteins, many of which are involved in RNA metabolism. These are ubiquitous cellular processes, which would suggest that the clinical features of SMA are caused by a particular vulnerability of motor neurons to defects in RNA handling. Alternatively, SMNs may have as yet unidentified functions that are specific to the motor neuron. The list of proteins reported to interact with SMNs also includes several which are not involved in RNA metabolism, including profilin, the FUSE binding protein, ZRP1 and p53. The functional significance of these interactions is currently unknown (reviewed by Gubitz et al.[40]).

Proteins and ribonucleoproteins involved in RNA processing

Nascent pre-mRNA transcripts are processed in the nucleus to produce mature mRNA by removal of introns. These splicing reactions are mediated by the spliceosome, which consists of five types of small nuclear RNA (snRNA), attached to specific proteins to form uridine-rich small nuclear ribonucleoproteins (U snRNPs): U1, U2, U4, U5 and U6. Assembly of snRNPs occurs in the cytoplasm, where snRNAs that are exported from the nucleus combine with the Smith antigen (Sm) core proteins (B/B′, D1, D2, D3, E, F and G). Formation of the Sm core is a prerequisite for several further processing steps of the U SnRNPs, including their import into the nucleus. Similarly, large numbers of small nucleolar RNAs (snoRNAs), within RNA–protein complexes called snoRNPs, direct cleavages and nucleotide modifications of pre-rRNA that are required for ribosome biogenesis. Pre-mRNA transcripts are also associated with heterogeneous nuclear RNP proteins (hnRNP proteins), which remain tightly bound to mRNA all the way to the ribosomes, and shuttle back and forth between the nucleus and the cytoplasm.

Cellular processes that involve alterations in RNA secondary structure, such as translation initiation and splicing, require the activity of the helicase superfamily of proteins. These are characterized by a common general function, an ATP-dependent nucleic acid unwinding, and many belong to the DEAD-box family, which possess a common tetrapeptide repeat Asp (D)–Glu (E)–Ala (A)–Asp (D).

Survival motor neuron complex and mRNA splicing

Within the cytoplasm, the SMN complex has a role in snRNP biogenesis. The Sm proteins interact with SMN itself via the tudor domain, and several of the Gemin proteins[41–48]. Experiments in vitro[49], in Xenopus oocytes[41,50] and mammalian somatic cells[51] have demonstrated an essential role for the SMN complex in the cytoplasmic assembly of spliceosomal snRNPs (recently reviewed by Yong et al.[52]). SMN has also been shown to have a function in pre-mRNA splicing in the nucleus, which appears to involve the regeneration of splicing components after rounds of splicing[51,53]. SMN mutations found in patients with SMA cause deficiencies in splicing regeneration activity[51] and interaction with Sm proteins[41,48,54], and Gemin 3[42]. However, in heterozygous *Smn* null mice, which display motor neuron degeneration resembling SMA, and have a 46% reduction in Smn protein levels in the spinal cord, splicing of candidate mRNAs in motor neurons appears to be unaffected[55]. Therefore, the function of pre-mRNA splicing may not explain motor neuron-specific pathology in SMA.

Survival motor neuron complex and transcriptional regulation

The SMN complex interacts with viral transcriptional activators[56], and with RNA polymerase II (pol II), which physically and functionally couples transcription, splicing and polyadenylation, an association mediated by RNA helicase A (RHA)[57]. Expression of a dominant-negative mutant of SMN causes accumulation of pol II and RHA in the nucleus, and inhibits transcription *in vivo*[57], suggesting a role for SMN in transcriptional regulation.

SMN and biogenesis of snoRNP

SMN binds directly to fibrillarin and GAR1, which are protein components of two classes of snoRNPs[58,59]. The SMN complex has a function in the biogenesis of snoRNPs, which are involved in post-transcriptional processing and modification of rRNA, similar to its role in snRNP biogenesis.

Motor neuron-specific functions of SMN

SMN has been shown to interact with two heteronuclear RNPs, hnRNP-R and hnRNP-Q, which are implicated in mRNA editing, transport and splicing. HnRNP-R is predominantly located in the axons of motor neurons, where it co-localizes with SMN, a finding which could provide a key to identifying a motor neuron-specific function of SMN[60]. In zebrafish, SMN-specific antisense morpholinos have been used to knock-down SMN protein levels in the developing embryo, which caused pathfinding defects specific to the motor axon[61]. Similarly, primary motor neurons isolated from a transgenic SMA mouse model exhibited reduced axon growth in culture[62], while overexpression of SMN and hnRNP-R in cultured PC12 cells promoted neurite outgrowth and modulated the localization of β-actin in neurites. This raises the possibility that SMN is involved in transport of mRNA molecules in motor axons.

DIFFERENTIAL DIAGNOSIS OF SPINAL MUSCULAR ATROPHY

Other disorders may present in infancy with hypotonia and a pattern of weakness identical to Werdnig–Hoffman disease, which are distinguished by associated features. The etiological relationship of these disorders to classical SMA has been clarified by testing for *SMN* mutations[63].

SMA with pontocerebellar hypoplasia presents with neonatal hypotonia, nystagmoid eye movements, cortical blindness and mental retardation. It is not caused by mutations in *SMN*[64–66].

SMA and arthrogryposis Arthrogryposis (congenital joint contractures) is caused by decreased fetal movements *in utero* that can occur in a number of conditions, including neuropathies, myopathies and oligohydramnios. Some infants with 5q13-linked SMA have arthrogryposis, the presence of which was previously regarded as an exclusion criterion for SMA[67].

SMA with arthrogryphosis and bone fractures is characterized by a pattern of weakness indistinguishable from SMA type 1, and congenital long-bone fractures[68,69]. It is genetically distinct from

SMN-related SMA, and may be autosomal recessive or X-linked recessive.

X-linked SMA/arthrogryphosis X-linked SMA/ arthrogryposis is linked to the short arm of chromosome X. Affected individuals have congenital joint contractures, facial dysmorphia, chest deformities, hypotonia and areflexia, and electromyogram (EMG) studies and muscle biopsy consistent with loss of anterior horn cells[70].

Lethal congenital contracture syndrome 1 (LCCS1) This is a syndrome of multiple congenital contractures with neuropathological changes resembling those of SMA, restricted to Finland[71]. The disorder is fatal in the third trimester, and has associated features of intrauterine growth retardation, fetal hydrops and facial abnormalities. Linkage has been established with chromosome 9p34[72].

Lethal congenital contracture syndrome 2 (LCCS2) A similar syndrome, affecting Israeli Bedouins, is distinguished by additional craniofacial/ocular findings, lack of hydrops, multiple pterygia, fractures and bladder distension. Linkage to both 5q13 and 9p34 were excluded[73].

AUTOSOMAL DOMINANT PROXIMAL SPINAL MUSCULAR ATROPHY

A missense mutation (P56S) in the vesicle-associated membrane protein (VAPB) gene on chromosome 20q13.3 has been identified in seven kindreds, with three different phenotypes of autosomal dominant motor neuron disease[74]. Some patients had an atypical slowly progressive ALS with tremor (ALS8), some had typical rapidly progressive familial ALS, while others presented with adult-onset proximal SMA (Finkel type). VAPB is a ubiquitously expressed protein that functions in endoplasmic reticulum (ER)–Golgi transport and secretion, and a mutation would be hypothesized to compromise intracellular membrane transport and secretion. The existence of disease-modifying genes is postulated to explain the different phenotypes caused by a single mutation.

DISTAL SPINAL MUSCULAR ATROPHY/HEREDITARY MOTOR NEURONOPATHIES

Spinal muscular atrophy with respiratory distress

In a series of 200 patients with infantile-onset SMA, Rudnik-Schoneborn *et al.*[75] found that approximately 1% had diaphragmatic weakness and did not have deletions of the *SMN* gene on chromosome 5q. This type of infantile SMA is characterized by severe respiratory distress and predominantly distal limb weakness[76]. SMA with respiratory distress (SMARD) was linked to chromosome 11q in two families (designated SMARD1)[77], but the disorder is genetically heterogeneous, as one family was not linked to this locus. SMARD1 is caused by mutations in the gene encoding immunoglobulin mu-binding protein 2 (IGHMBP2), which has RNA helicase activity, and is involved in pre-mRNA processing[78]. Mutations in the mouse homolog of this gene, *ighmbp2* are responsible for spinal muscular atrophy in the 'neuromuscular degeneration' (nmd) mouse, whose phenotype closely resembles SMARD1[79]. In infants presenting with respiratory distress and *IGHMBP2* mutations, the phenotypic characteristics are quite variable, including evidence of sensory and autonomic nerve involvement in some infants, and absence of anterior horn cell pathology in one[80,81]. The differing pathological involvement reported in peripheral nerves and spinal cords has a parallel in severe congenital SMA, in which lack of sensory and motor nerve excitability, axonal degeneration on sural nerve biopsy and relative preservation of anterior horn cells are seen[82]. These changes may therefore reflect an early-onset neuromuscular disorder of varying etiology.

Autosomal recessive distal spinal muscular atrophy

This disorder of slowly progressive distal limb weakness has a very variable age of onset. In the most severely affected patients, there is evidence of diaphragmatic involvement, with elevation of the hemidiaphragms on chest X-ray, and reduced vital capacity[83,84]. In a large consanguineous Lebanese family, the disorder has been mapped to chromosome 11q[84]. However, despite linkage to the same region, and clinical similarities to SMARD1, no mutations were found in these patients in *IGHMBP2*. Further linkage analysis in European families with autosomal recessive distal SMA narrowed the disease locus to a region on chromosome 11q13.3, which excludes the *IGHMBP2* gene[85]. A novel autosomal recessive distal SMA, described in families in the Jerash region of Jordan, is genetically distinct and linked to chromosome 9p21.1–p12. The gene involved is currently unknown.

Distal spinal muscular atrophy with upper limb predominance

Families with distal SMA with upper limb predominance (dHMN-V) often have members in whom there is evidence of mild sensory disturbance or pyramidal features such as brisk deep tendon reflexes or prolonged central motor conduction times[86–88]. dHMN-V was linked to chromosome 7p in a large Bulgarian family[88], to a region overlapping that identified in linkage studies of families with CMT type 2D, a progressive sensorimotor axonal neuropathy[89,90]. Sambuughin *et al.* identified a Mongolian family in which CMT2D and distal spinal muscular atrophy with upper limb predominance segregated in the same kindred. All affected members had weakness and wasting of the intrinsic muscles of the hands. Those with no sensory deficit and peroneal muscle weakness had a diagnosis of distal SMA, while in others CMT2D was diagnosed on the basis of a glove and stocking sensory loss. Both disorders in this family were linked to the same region of chromosome 7p[91]. Mutations were subsequently identified in the gene encoding glycyl tRNA synthetase (*GARS*) in CMT2D families, in families with dHMN-V and in the family with both disorders identified by Sambuughin's group[92]. Identification of the underlying genetic disorder has therefore confirmed that Charcot–Marie–Tooth type 2D (CMT2D) and distal spinal muscular atrophy with upper limb predominance are a single disorder. GARS is a member of the family of aminoacyl tRNA synthetases involved in diverse cellular processes, including charging tRNAs with their appropriate amino acids. As this defect would be expected to affect every protein bearing glycine, it is unknown why this disorder is specific to neurons. It may be that cells bearing long axons are more prone to ensuing pathology because of a reduction in protein product reaching axon termini, or that there is a specific need for glycine-rich proteins in affected neurons.

Linkage to chromosome 7p has been excluded in a large Austrian family with dHMN-V[93]. In this family and nine others, heterozygous mutations, N88S and S90L, were identified in the Berardinelli–Seip congenital lipodystrophy gene (*BSCL2*)[94]. The gene encodes seipin, an integral membrane protein of the endoplasmic reticulum, and null mutations cause Berardinelli–Seip congenital lipodystrophy. N88S and S90L mutations affect glycosylation of seipin, resulting in intracellular aggregate formation which is thought to underlie neurodegeneration. The same mutations were also identified in patients with Silver syndrome[95,96], a familial spastic paraplegia with amyotrophy of the hands, considered to be a variant of HSP. Again, the same genetic etiology causes two diseases with quite different phenotypes. The phenotype associated with *BSCL2* mutations has also recently widened: two families with N88S and S90L mutations have been described that, in addition to upper limb wasting, contain some individuals with lower limb-predominant distal amyotrophy in the absence of pyramidal tract signs, and some with a combination of spasticity and severe amyotrophy in the lower limbs[97].

Distal spinal muscular atrophy with lower limb predominance

Distal SMA with lower limb predominance (dHMN-II) is usually autosomal dominant, but sporadic cases are frequently described, which may reflect late-onset recessive disease, non-genetic etiology or new mutations[98–100]. A large Belgian pedigree was linked to chromosome 12q24[101], although genetic heterogeneity was again apparent, with one family not linked to chromosome 12q24 or to 7p14[102]. Heterozygous mutations were subsequently identified in four families, in the gene encoding the small heat shock 22-kDa protein 8 (HSPB8/HSP22)[103]. Missense mutations have recently also been identified in the interacting partner of HSP22, heat shock 27-kDa protein 1 (HSPB1/HSP27), both in patients with dHMN-II and in CMT2F families[104]. Most of the HSP22 and HSP27 mutations disrupt a conserved α-crystallin domain in these proteins. Functional studies have shown that HSP22 mutants show greater binding to HSP27, promoting the formation of intracellular aggregates[103]. HSP27 is involved in the organization of the neurofilament network, important for the maintenance of the axonal cytoskeleton and for transport, and mutant HSP27 alters neurofilament assembly[104].

Distal spinal muscular atrophy with vocal cord paralysis

Distal SMA with vocal cord paralysis (dHMN-VII), characterized by distal limb weakness and a husky voice due to laryngeal involvement, has been described in two large Welsh families thought to have a common ancestor[105,106]. It is linked in both families to chromosome 2q14[107]. Three conditions have been described with considerable phenotypic overlap with dHMN-VII: one family with distal SMA and vocal cord paral-

ysis also had sensorineural hearing loss[108], while HMSN type IIC[109] is characterized by progressive vocal cord paralysis, distal limb weakness and sensory loss. It is not known whether these disorders have the same genetic etiology. A third disorder, presenting with breathing difficulty due to vocal cord paralysis, progressive facial weakness and weakness and atrophy of the hands, has been found to be caused by a missense mutation in the gene encoding dynactin (DCTN1) on chromosome 2p13. This mutation is predicted to distort the folding of the dynactin microtubule binding domain, and lead to dysfunction of dynactin-mediated transport in peripheral nerves[110].

Congenital non-progressive spinal muscular atrophy affecting the lower limbs

This relatively benign disorder, described in three pedigrees in The Netherlands and Canada[111–113], has been shown by linkage analysis to map to chromosome 12q23-24[114]. Again, the disorder is genetically heterogeneous, as one family does not link to chromosome 12q23-24[114].

Scapuloperoneal spinal muscular atrophy

Distal muscle wasting in a scapuloperoneal distribution may be myopathic or neurogenic in origin. Several large pedigrees with EMG evidence of denervation have been described[115–117]. In the New England kindred, linkage has been established with chromosome 12q24.1-12q24.31[118]. This is a neighbor of the region of chromosome 12 to which a myopathic scapuloperoneal syndrome is linked[119], and many of the families described with scapuloperoneal SMA contain individuals with both myopathic and neurogenic changes on muscle biopsy. Congenital non-progressive SMA affecting the lower limbs maps to the same region as scapuloperoneal SMA. It is not yet known whether these disorders are allelic. Distal SMA with lower limb predominance also

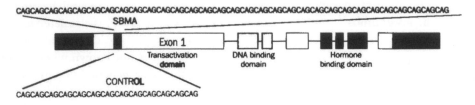

CAGCAGCAGCAGCAGCAGCAGCAGCAGCAGCAGCAGCAGCAGCAGCAGCAGCAGCAGCAGCAGCAGCAGCAGCAGCAGCAGCAGCAGCAGCAGCAGCAGCAGCAGCAGCAG

SBMA

Exon 1

Transactivation domain

DNA binding domain

Hormone binding domain

CONTROL

CAGCAGCAGCAGCAGCAGCAGCAGCAGCAGCAGCAGCAG

Figure 8.5   Structure of the androgen receptor gene, and location of the CAG repeat region

maps to chromosome 12q24, but these loci are separate.

KENNEDY'S DISEASE

Clinical features

Kennedy's disease, or spinobulbar muscular atrophy (SBMA) is an X-linked degenerative disorder of lower motor neurons, first described by Dr William Kennedy in 1968[120]. Initial symptoms of the disease are fasciculations and muscle cramps, followed by progressive weakness and atrophy of limb and bulbar musculature, predominantly affecting the proximal muscles. Upper motor neurons are not clinically affected, and tendon reflexes are therefore reduced or absent. Weakness of the lower facial and tongue muscles causes dysarthria and, in some patients, severe jaw weakness causes the mouth to hang open. Pharyngeal involvement causing dysphagia, and respiratory muscle weakness causing breathlessness, are less common. Perioral fasciculations, with 'quivering' of the chin, are characteristic of the disease.

Patients frequently have mild androgen insensitivity, causing gynecomastia, testicular atrophy, oligospermia and erectile dysfunction. The disease is only slowly progressive, and patients tend to become wheelchair dependent over two to three decades, although some may remain ambulatory until late in life, with a normal life expectancy. The extraocular muscles are spared in SBMA. Sensory symptoms are rare and mild; however, there is evidence that neurodegeneration is not exclusive

to motor neurons. Mild sensory loss to vibration is frequently present in the lower limbs, and sensory nerve conduction studies show decreased or absent sensory nerve potentials. Pathologic examination of the brain and spinal cord of patients with SBMA has confirmed that dorsal root ganglion cells are depleted.

Molecular pathophysiology

Clinical features of androgen insensitivity suggested a defect in androgen-receptor function. The SBMA gene defect was linked to chromosome Xq12-21 in 1986[121], and when the human androgen receptor gene was cloned and mapped to the same region, it became the candidate gene for SBMA[122]. The disease-causing mutation in SBMA was reported in 1991 by La Spada et al., who identified expansion of a trinucleotide CAG repeat in the androgen receptor (AR) gene from a normal length of 17 to 26 repeats, to a disease-associated length of 40 to 52 repeats[123]. The repeat encodes a long tract of glutamine residues, beginning at amino acid 58 (Figure 8.5). Disease severity and age of onset correlate with the size of the repeat expansion, although only a proportion of the clinical variability of the disease can be accounted for by repeat length, suggesting that as yet unidentified genetic factors also modify the disease[124–126]. Patients with minimally expanded polyglutamine tracts in the androgen receptor gene have been reported to have unusual clinical manifestations, including essential tremor[127], hypertrophic cardiomyopathy[128] and very late onset of muscular weakness[129].

Trinucleotide repeat disorders

Triplet repeat expansions have been found to cause 15 neurologic disorders, nine of which are neurodegenerative diseases that result from expansion of CAG repeats coding for polyglutamine (poly(Q)) tracts[130]. These include Huntington's chorea, dentatorubral-pallidoluysian atrophy and six subtypes of spinocerebellar ataxia. Shared features between these disorders suggest that there is a common mechanism underlying neuronal dysfunction and degeneration. In all the disorders, neurodegeneration occurs when the poly(Q) tract reaches a critical length of about 40 repeats. The length of the expanded repeat is unstable, and can change from one generation to the next, leading to the phenomenon of anticipation, although this is not a prominent feature of SBMA. This group of disorders tend to have a similar age of onset and rate of progression of disease, which correlate with the length of the poly(Q) tract. All are progressive neurologic disorders that affect only a subset of neurons, despite ubiquitous expression of the mutated protein.

The androgen receptor

The androgen receptor is a nuclear receptor in the steroid receptor superfamily. The protein, encoded by eight exons, contains three functional domains (Figure 8.5): a carboxy-terminal hormone-binding domain, a DNA-binding domain and an amino-terminal transactivation domain, which contains the polyglutamine tract. The androgen receptor is phosphorylated and bound to heat shock proteins in the cytoplasm. On ligand binding, it is transported to the nucleus, where it binds to DNA, and acts as a transcription factor.

Mechanisms of neurodegeneration

Expansion of the polyglutamine tract results in reduced target gene transactivation which may account for the clinical signs of reduced androgen sensitivity[131,132]. However, complete loss of androgen receptor function, in individuals with testicular feminization syndrome, does not lead to motor neuron degeneration. Reduction in AR function does not therefore appear to be the principal mechanism leading to motor neuron degeneration in SBMA, and it is thought that neurodegeneration in the polyglutamine diseases occurs through a toxic gain of function of the altered protein.

There is evidence that the polyglutamine repeats themselves are neurotoxic. Transgenic mice that express a polyglutamine repeat in the gene encoding hypoxanthine phosphoribosyl transferase, a gene that does not contain a polyglutamine tract in wild-type mice, develop a neurodegenerative disease with a unique profile. Thus, the polyglutamine tract is implicated as the neurotoxic entity, whilst the protein in which it is expressed is likely to modify the specific pattern of neurodegeneration seen in each disorder[133].

The toxicity of the mutant androgen receptor has been demonstrated in cell culture models[134]. In experimental animals, knockout of AR expression does not reproduce the phenotype of SBMA, which is reproduced only with expression of the mutant gene. Initial attempts to produce the SBMA phenotype in mice were unsuccessful, probably owing to low levels of expression of the transgene[135,136]. A neurodegenerative phenotype was reproduced with a truncated mutant AR gene under control of neuronal promoters[137], and with a very long pure CAG repeat under control of the AR promoter[138], but neither of these models of disease showed a gender difference in phenotype. A transgenic mouse model has since been developed with a full-length AR with very long repeat expansions, which phenotypically reproduces SBMA, and is more pronounced in males than in females[139]. There is evidence that toxicity of the mutant receptor is ligand dependent, as it occurs only with the higher androgen levels present in males. Castration of the transgenic male mice reduces symptom severity, whilst treatment of transgenic females with exogenous testosterone worsens their phenotype[139]. Ligand-dependent neurodegeneration is also seen in *Drosophila* expressing polyglutamine-expanded human AR[140].

Heterozygous female carriers of SBMA have been reported to show mild clinical manifestations of the disease such as muscle cramps, mild facial weakness and fasciculations, and neurophysiologic studies have shown mild changes of chronic denervation[141–143]. Carriers may escape the full manifestations of the disease through X-inactivation, or lyonization, whereby one of the two X-chromosomes undergoes transcriptional silencing, required for dosage compensation of X-linked genes[144]. An alternative explanation is that women are protected from disease by lower levels of circulating androgens, which would explain the observation that two women homozygous for the mutant AR developed only mild manifestations of the disease[145].

Mechanisms of toxic gain of function

Protein aggregation

Protein aggregates are a prominent neuropathologic feature of the polyglutamine diseases, and of many other neurodegenerative disorders, including Alzheimer's disease (AD), Parkinson's disease (PD) and ALS. Misfolding of the poly(Q) expanded proteins in SBMA and other polyglutamine diseases is thought to lead to formation of aggregates, which are seen as nuclear inclusions (NIs). NIs containing the amino-terminal epitopes of the mutant AR are found within motor neurons and certain non-neuronal tissues in patients with SBMA[146,147], and in cell culture and animal models of the disease[148].

The role of protein aggregation in the pathogenesis of neurodegeneration is, however, controversial. Aggregate formation could be a primary event underlying toxicity, aggregates may simply be markers of neuronal dysfunction, with no role in the degenerative process, or the formation of aggregates could be a cellular defence mechanism to reduce the intracellular concentration of a toxic protein. Circumstantial evidence that poly glutamine aggregates are the primary neurotoxic entity is seen in the fact that there is a remarkable correlation between the repeat length threshold for aggregate formation *in vitro*, and the repeat length that leads to human disease[149,150]. Further clues to the role of protein aggregation in SBMA are found by examining the other protein constituents of NIs, which include ubiquitin, proteasomes, molecular chaperones and transcription factors.

The ubiquitin–proteasome system

Misfolded, unassembled or damaged proteins within cells are polyubiquitinated, and degraded by cellular proteasomes. Molecular chaperones, which include the stress-induced heat-shock proteins (Hsp), and constitutively expressed heat-shock cognate proteins (Hsc) are a set of conserved proteins that stabilize and chaperone newly synthesized proteins, and are involved in intracellular protein degradation. The presence of ubiquitin, proteasomes and molecular chaperones within NIs implicates protein misfolding in disease pathogenesis. There is evidence that polyglutamine proteins may directly impair the ubiquitin–proteasome system, possibly by exceeding the capacity of proteasomes or sequestering molecular chaperones, which would then be unavailable to degrade other substrates[151]. Ubiquitin-dependent proteolysis has a central role in regulating fundamental cellular events, such as cell division and apoptosis; therefore, this is a potential mechanism linking protein aggregation to cellular dysregulation and cell death.

Transcription factors

Nuclear localization of mutant androgen receptor appears to be a requirement for neurotoxicity[139,140]. It is thought that nuclear accumulation of mutant polyglutamines may cause toxicity through interaction with transcription factors, to disrupt gene transcription. Down-regulation of gene transcription appears to be an early event in polyglutamine disease pathogenesis[152,153]. In the case of SBMA, interest has focused on CREB binding protein (CBP), which is sequestered by mutant polyglutamine[154]. CBP is a transcriptional co-activator that possesses histone acetyltransferase activity. Hyperacetylation of histones marks transcriptionally active regions of chromatin. As CBP is present in a functionally limiting level in cells, its sequestration by mutant polyglutamine could have widespread effects on gene expression. In neurons, CBP is a key component of neurotrophic factor signaling pathways[155,156]. including that of vascular endothelial growth factor (VEGF). Dysregulation of VEGF transcription has been implicated in motor neuron degeneration in a mouse model of ALS. Transgenic mice that overexpress mutant human AR have reduced spinal cord $VEGF_{164}$ protein levels, even in presymptomatic stages, and polyglutamine-expanded AR has been shown to interfere with CBP-mediated transcription of VEGF. Reversal of the histone acetylation defect caused by CBP sequestration, using histone deacetylase (HD) inhibitors, has been shown to reduce polyglutamine-associated cell death in both *Drosophila* and mouse models of HD[157,158].

Axonal transport

In immortalized motor neurons transfected with mutant AR, protein aggregates have been shown to be associated with impairment of distribution of the motor protein kinesin, and consequently in the distribution of mitochondria. This suggests that protein aggregation disrupts kinesin-mediated fast axonal transport[159].

HEREDITARY SPASTIC PARAPARESIS

HSP, first described in the 1880s, is a group of hereditary neurodegenerative or neurodevelopmental diseases that affects approximately 1 in 10 000 individuals. The main feature of the clinical phenotype is progressive lower limb spasticity due to degeneration of the corticospinal tracts within the spinal cord. HSP is most commonly inherited as an autosomal dominant trait. Autosomal recessive and X-linked recessive forms of HSP

also exist, but are less common. HSP may be classified on the basis of clinical phenotype or age at onset, but more recently increased knowledge of the genetic basis of HSP has allowed classification based on genetic mutations or linkage sites.

Clinically the HSP phenotype may be 'pure' in which the spastic paraparesis occurs in isolation or 'complicated' where the spastic paraparesis is one component of a much more complex neurological and/or systemic disorder. Some of the HSPs are clearly neurodegenerative, whereas others may be neurodevelopmental. HSP shows extreme genetic heterogeneity. To date more than 26 genetic loci have been identified and, as genes have been identified at 11 of these loci (Table 8.4), more precise genotype–phenotype correlations are becoming possible. The recent discovery of multiple genes is rapidly shaping new concepts of the cellular mechanisms of disease in HSP. It is apparent that motor neurons provide an extreme example of the potential difficulties for a cell in trafficking, transport and energy metabolism and that the longest axons of the central nervous system (CNS) may be specifically vulnerable to several distinct biochemical perturbations.

Clinical features

Pure hereditary spastic paraparesis

In pure HSP progressive spastic paraparesis is the major feature, but other clinical features may be observed including bladder disturbance, mild distal muscle wasting, pes cavus, dorsal column dysfunction, loss of ankle jerks and mild terminal dysmetria. Cranial nerve examination and bulbar function are usually reported to be normal in HSP. The most common presenting symptom in pure HSP is gait disturbance, the patient often complaining of lower limb stiffness, balance difficulties or a tendency to fall. In young children, delayed motor milestones or a tendency to walk on the toes may be the first indications of a problem. The major features apparent on neurologic examination consist of lower limb spasticity,

Table 8.4   Genetic classification of hereditary spastic paraparesis

Genome database designation	Chromosome	Inheritance	Phenotype	Genetic defect
SPG1	Xq28	X-linked	Complicated	L1CAM
SPG2	Xq22	X-linked	Both	PLP
SPG3	14q11.2	AD	Pure	Atlastin
SPG4	2p22	AD	Both	Spastin
SPG5	8p12-q13	AR	Pure	
SPG6	15q11.1	AD	Pure	NIPA1
SPG7	16q24.3	AR	Both	Paraplegin
SPG8	8q24	AD	Pure	
SPG9	10q23.3-24.2	AD	Complicated	
SPG10	12q13	AD	Pure	KIF5A
SPG11	15q13-15	AR	Both	
SPG12	19q13	AD	Pure	
SPG13	2q24-q34	AD	Pure	HSP60
SPG14	3q27-q28	AR	Complicated	
SPG15 (Kjellin)	14q	AR	Complicated	
SPG16	Xq11.2	X-linked	Pure	
SPG17 (Silver)	11q12-q14	AD	Complicated	BSCL2-seipin
SPG18	Pending			
SPG19	9q33-q34	AD	Pure	
SPG20 (Troyer)	13q12.3	AR	Complicated	Spartin
SPG21	15q22.31	AR	Complicated	Maspardin
SPG23	1q24-q32	AR	Complicated	

AD, autosomal dominant; AR, autosomal recessive

hyperreflexia and extensor plantar responses which may be accompanied by a mild pyramidal distribution weakness. A characteristic feature of HSP is that the patient's disability usually arises from prominent spasticity and any accompanying muscle weakness is often very mild.

There is considerable variation in age at onset and severity of the spastic paraparesis even within affected members of the same family, suggesting that further factors, genetic or environmental, also influence the phenotype observed in individual cases. The recorded age at onset of pure HSP ranges from infancy to the eighth decade[160]. The severity of HSP varies between families and, to a lesser extent, within the same family. Several studies have indicated that HSP with an early age of onset (< 35 years) tends to be associated with relatively slow disease progression, the majority of individuals retaining the ability to walk even in elderly life. In contrast, late-onset HSP (> 35 years), tends to show more rapid disease progression, and many patients become non-ambulant in the seventh and eighth decades of life[160–162]. HSP does not, in general, reduce life expectancy. It is also reported that approximately 25–30% of patients have a subclinical phenotype, i.e. symptoms that are so mild that the disorder may not be apparent without a neurologic examination.

Table 8.5   Additional clinical features which may be present in complicated hereditary spastic paraparesis (HSP)

Clinical feature	Subtype of HSP	Other comments
Amyotrophy	Peroneal muscular atrophy	Amyotrophy associated with an axonal sensory and motor neuropathy (AD)
	Silver syndrome	Severe wasting of the small muscles of the hand with sparing of the lower limb musculature. Linked to SPG17 (AD)
	Troyer syndrome	Distal wasting in the limbs with delayed development, spastic quadraparesis, pseudobulbar palsy, choreoathetosis and short stature. Linked to SPG20 (AR)
	Charlevoix–Saguenay syndrome	Similar to Troyer syndrome with additional ataxia, described in Quebec (AR)
	Resembling juvenile FALS	Childhood onset (AR)
Cardiac defects	—	Associated with mental retardation
Cerebellar signs	—	Dysarthria with a mild upper limb ataxia
Deafness	Sensorineural	X-linked
Dementia	Subcortical or cortical pattern	Dementia can occur in isolation with HSP, when it tends to be of the subcortical type, or be part of a much more complex phenotype (AR and AD). Linkage to SPG4 locus in a number of families
Endocrine dysfunction	Kallmann's syndrome	Hypogonadotrophic hypogonadism and anosmia
Epilepsy	—	Various epileptic seizure types have been descibed, including: absence, simple/complex partial, atonic, grand mal and myotonic
Extrapyramidal signs	Choreoathetosis Dystonia and rigidity	
	Mast syndrome	Dementia, dysarthria and athetosis in Amish people with onset in 2nd decade (AR)
Hyperekplexia	—	Neonatal hypertonia and an exaggerated startle response (AD)
Icthyosis	Sjögren–Larsson syndrome	Also with mental retardation and occasionally a pigmentary macular degeneration (AR)
Retinal changes	Optic atrophy Retinal degeneration	Pigmentation seen in SPG15
	Kjellin syndrome	Dysarthria, upper limb ataxia, dementia, retinal degeneration ± amyotrophy (AR)
Sensory neuropathy	Asymptomatic	Sensory neuropathy detected only on clinical examination
	Childhood onset	With painless ulcers and deformities secondary to neuropathic bone resorption
	Adult onset	Trophic skin changes and foot ulcers
Others	SPG1	Mental retardation, aphasia, a shuffling gait and adducted thumbs. Caused by mutations in L1CAM gene (X-linked)
	SPG9	Bilateral cataracts, gastroesophageal reflux and amyotrophy

AD, autosomal dominant; AR, autosomal recessive; FALS, familial amyotrophic lateral sclerosis

Complicated hereditary spastic paraparesis

In complicated HSP the spastic paraparesis is one component of a much more complex clinical disorder. Multiple clinical features have been described as a component of complicated HSP pedigrees and these are outlined in Table 8.5.

Some of the complicated HSP phenotypes are extremely rare, having been described only in single pedigrees. At some HSP loci, heterogeneity is seen, affected individuals showing either a pure or a complicated clinical phenotype. Certain complicated phenotypes with characteristic clinical features are associated with particular HSP loci. For example, HSP associated with cognitive impairment is most commonly described in patients with spastin (SPG4) mutations[163–165]. In patients with the SPG9 subtype of HSP there is a very distinctive clinical phenotype with the development of cataracts, severe gastroesophageal reflux and an axonal neuropathy in addition to the spastic paraparesis[166]. Pigmentary macular degeneration is an additional feature observed in patients with HSP at the SPG15 locus[167]. Peripheral neuropathy has been described in several subtypes of HSP including SPG11 and SPG14[168,169]. In the Silver variant of HSP (SPG17), striking amyotrophy and weakness of the hands is a characteristic feature[170]. Patients with Troyer syndrome (SPG20), a complicated type of autosomal recessive HSP, may have dysarthria, distal amyotrophy, short stature and developmental delay as additional clinical features[171].

The occurrence of epilepsy, cognitive impairment, amyotrophy and peripheral neuropathy are commonly seen in complicated HSP and these features will be described briefly below.

Epilepsy has been described in several reports as a feature complicating HSP[165,171–175]. Epilepsy has also been described in patients with spastin (SPG4) mutations, a common subtype of autosomal dominant HSP usually regarded as 'pure'[165,176,177]. There does not appear to be an association with particular types of seizures and myoclonic jerks; simple partial, complex partial and generalized tonic clonic seizures have all been reported in HSP pedigrees. Similarly, there is no consensus as to when in the course of the HSP seizures begin and there are descriptions of seizures both predating and post-dating the onset

of the spastic paraparesis, with variability also observed in members of the same family.

Dementia and cognitive impairment have been reported in complicated HSP pedigrees[163,165,178–181] and have also been described as an isolated accompaniment to spastic paraparesis in both autosomal dominant and autosomal recessive families[164,182–184]. The cognitive abnormalities observed – for example impairments of attention, perceptual speed, visuomotor coordination and forgetfulness – are in keeping with a subcortical type of dementia, and features suggesting major cortical involvement, e.g. dysphasia, agnosia and dyscalculia, are usually absent. Multiple families with dementia complicating HSP have been linked to SPG4[163–165]. Several studies have indicated that affected individuals in SPG4 pedigrees may have subclinical cognitive impairment discernible by neuropsychometric testing[185,186]. Other studies, which have incorporated careful evaluation of cognitive function, have also demonstrated asymptomatic deficits in some patients with otherwise pure HSP[187,188].

Distal amyotrophy is one of the commonest additional features seen in patients with HSP and may be observed in both autosomal dominant and autosomal recessive pedigrees. The mechanism of the amyotrophy appears to be heterogeneous, with anterior horn cell loss, axonal neuropathy and central axonopathy contributing in different families. Several well characterized syndromes of HSP with amyotrophy have been described. The commonest type of complicated HSP with amyotrophy is also known as peroneal muscular atrophy with pyramidal features or hereditary motor and sensory neuropathy (HMSN) type V[99,189,190]. It is usually transmitted as an autosomal dominant trait and develops in the second decade of life or later. Affected individuals have amyotrophy associated with axonal motor and sensory neuropathy as well as features of spastic paraparesis, and the relative severity of these features may vary between individuals.

Silver syndrome consists of autosomal dominant HSP complicated by striking amyotrophy of the hands[95]. There is variation in age at onset (ranging from childhood to late adult) and severity. Some Silver syndrome pedigrees are linked to the SPG17 locus, but others are not linked to this site, demonstrating that genetic heterogeneity exists even within this subtype of complicated HSP[170].

Troyer syndrome, originally described as a childhood-onset disorder in an Old Order Amish population, consists of autosomal recessive HSP complicated with amyotrophy of the hands and feet associated with pseudobulbar palsy, choreoathetosis, short stature and mental retardation[191,192]. Since the original description, other authors have suggested a broadening of the Troyer phenotype, and have classified families with later onset, lack of movement disorder, atrophy or partial agenesis of the corpus callosum and non-Amish origin under the Troyer syndrome[193-195]. The Troyer syndrome is linked to SPG20 and the gene encodes a protein named spartin[171]. Charlevoix–Saguenay syndrome, described in families from Quebec, appears similar to Troyer syndrome, but with the additional clinical feature of ataxia[196].

A further rare phenotype of recessive HSP complicated by amyotrophy is described, resembling juvenile onset familial amyotrophic lateral sclerosis[192,197]. In these pedigrees a childhood onset spastic paraparesis is observed with prominent wasting of the distal musculature. Neurophysiologic examination shows electromyographic changes in keeping with lower motor neuron degeneration[197].

Sensory neuropathy of either childhood or adult onset is also a common additional feature in complicated HSP. The severity of the neuropathy is variable. Some severe phenotypes have been described, with chronic painless cutaneous ulcers and neuropathic bone resorption occurring in early childhood[198]. Individuals with a less severe neuropathy may develop trophic skin changes and ulcers on the feet in adult life superimposed on a more chronic spastic paraparesis[199,200]. Schady and

Smith reported a family with asymptomatic sensory involvement detected on clinical examination and neurophysiologic assessment[201]. Sural nerve biopsy showed features of an axonal neuropathy with depletion of large and medium-sized myelinated fibres.

Pathology of hereditary spastic paraparesis

Detailed neuropathological findings have been reported in relatively few cases of HSP, possibly because life expectancy is not significantly reduced and patients usually die at home or in nursing care, often of unrelated causes[202]. The extent to which clinical and genetic heterogeneity in HSP is reflected in pathologic heterogeneity, therefore, remains to be defined. Furthermore, because genetic characterization has only recently emerged, few of the cases in whom pathology is reported have been genetically defined.

Spinal cord pathology

The core neuropathologic features of HSP were first described by Strümpell and confirmed in a series of subsequent reports[203-205] (Figure 8.6). The spinal cord shows pallor of the lateral and, more variably, the anterior corticospinal tracts with loss of axons and myelin which most

Figure 8.6   Pathology of hereditary spastic paraparesis: spinal cord section showing pallor and loss of axons of the corticospinal tracts and fasciculus gracilis

markedly affects the longest descending axons in the lumbosacral region. There is also pallor of the dorsal columns, particularly the medially placed fasciculus gracilis. Involvement of the spinocerebellar tracts is described in approximately 50% of cases. Depletion of Betz cells from the motor cortex is reported in some cases[206], but lower motor neurons in the spinal cord have usually been reported as appearing normal. Degeneration has occasionally been described in neurons of the dorsal nucleus of Clarke. A characteristic finding is more severe involvement of the distal part of the corticospinal tracts and dorsal columns so that the most marked changes in these tracts are observed in the lumbar and cervical cord, respectively. This has led to the suggestion that degeneration occurs as a 'dying back' axonopathy, affecting the most distal part of these long axons first. The pathogenesis of this degeneration is beginning to be unraveled and the involvement of different genes, encoding proteins of varying function, in different genetic subtypes of HSP indicates that there may be multiple molecular pathways which underlie the end result of long-tract degeneration[207].

A recent report described the distribution of spastin in the normal human CNS, as well as the molecular pathology of three cases of HSP with defined mutations in spastin[208]. Spastin was shown to be a neuronal protein with widespread distribution in the CNS. Within motor neurons, spastin was predominantly expressed in the cytoplasm of the cell body, with some extension of staining into the proximal neurites and axons. Some neuronal groups showed a nuclear staining pattern. In the spastin HSP cases, the expected distal axonal degeneration of the corticospinal tracts and fasciculus gracilis, together with a microglial reaction to the tract degeneration, were the principal findings with conventional staining techniques. Interestingly, although not prominently affected clinically in SPG4, the spinal cord lower motor neurons showed evidence of cytopathology, with the presence of hyaline inclusion bodies, some of which stained for α-tubulin. In addition, the anterior horn cells showed

variable loss of expression of non-phosphorylated neurofilament protein, β-tubulin, spastin and mitochondria from their perikarya, suggesting altered partitioning of cytoskeletal components and organelles. In addition, all three cases showed evidence of tau pathology, with neurofibrillary tangles, neuropil threads and glial tau pathology. This tau pathology was most prominent in the brainstem, but was also observed in some lower motor neurons and in areas outside the motor system.

Cerebral pathology

In many neuropathologic reports of pure HSP, cerebral structures, with the exception of Betz cells, are said to be uninvolved. However, subclinical involvement of other parts of the CNS is increasingly recognized and in particular there is emerging recognition of cognitive impairment on neuropsychologic testing, particularly in cases of HSP associated with a spastin gene mutation, as described earlier. The neuropathologic substrate of such cognitive impairment currently remains poorly defined. Ferrer and colleagues reported a case of HSP associated with the later development of severe mental impairment[209]. In addition to the typical spinal cord changes of HSP, this individual had developed prefrontal atrophy and loss of frontal white matter associated with atrophy of deep grey nuclei. Histologic examination demonstrated a loss of neurons in atrophic cortex including loss of calbindin D28k-immunoreactive neurons and parvalbumin-immunoreactive dendrites. White and co-workers described the neuropathologic findings in a patient with spastin-related HSP who developed late-onset dementia[163]. Two other members of this family also had cognitive decline. The spinal cord pathology was typical of HSP. Examination of the hippocampus revealed gross neuronal depletion from the pyramidal sector, with frequent tau-immunoreactive neurofibrillary tangles but without plaques. Ballooned neurons in the limbic cortex and neocortex labeled with tau, but not ubiquitin, and tau-positive glial inclusions were identified. The substantia nigra revealed neuronal loss with α-synuclein-immunoreactive Lewy body formation. The cerebral findings in this case were not typical of known tauopathies, but determination of whether such neurodegenerative cerebral pathology is a regular feature common to cases of spastin-associated HSP with cognitive impairment requires autopsy examination of further cases.

Muscle pathology

In autosomal recessive forms of HSP associated with mutation in the paraplegin gene (SPG7), muscle biopsies have shown ragged red fibers[210]. Scattered muscle fibers show negative histochemical reaction for cytochrome oxidase, but preserved or elevated succinate dehydrogenase activity and peripheral accumulation of mitochondria. These changes, which are typical of oxidative phosphorylation defects in muscle, support a role for mitochondrial dysfunction in the pathogenesis of paraplegin mutation-associated HSP[210,211]. Examination of skeletal muscle in autosomal dominant HSP linked to chromosome 8q (SPG8) did not reveal significant pathology[212]. Skeletal muscle has not been widely surveyed in other types of HSP, although it has been reported that muscle biopsies from some HSP patients in whom spastin and paraplegin mutations had been excluded showed biochemical evidence of impairment in mitochondrial respiratory chain function[213].

Diagnosis

Molecular genetic testing will undoubtedly become increasingly utilized in the diagnosis of HSP. Although 11 causative genes have now been identified, testing for mutations in these genes is not necessarily routinely available to the clinicians involved in patient care. Therefore, at present HSP is often a diagnosis of exclusion. It is clearly extremely important to exclude diagnoses in which there is be a treatable cause for the spastic paraparesis including vitamin B_{12} deficiency, multiple sclerosis, structural spinal cord disorders or dopa-responsive dystonia. It is also important to exclude other motor system disorders such as familial ALS, in which the clinical course and prognosis are likely to differ significantly from those in the spectrum of HSP. Conditions to be considered in the differential diagnosis of HSP are highlighted in Table 8.6.

Neurologic investigations in hereditary spastic paraplegia

Magnetic resonance imaging (MRI) in HSP may show a degree of spinal cord atrophy, but no other abnormalities are usually apparent. There are multiple reports, particularly from Japan, of mild-to-moderate atrophy of the corpus callosum. Several of these families have shown linkage to the SPG11 locus[214]. There are occasional reports of atrophy of other intracranial structures and of cerebral hemisphere white matter lesions[215,216]. However, marked atrophy or white matter changes on MRI require careful exclusion of other disorders. Nerve conduction studies and EMG are

Table 8.6 Differential diagnosis of hereditary spastic paraparesis

Multiple sclerosis

Cerebral palsy

Spondylotic spinal disease

Amyotrophic lateral sclerosis/motor neuron disease

Other structural spinal cord disorders, e.g. tumors, arteriovenous malformation

Arnold–Chiari malformation

Adrenoleukodystrophy/adrenomyeloneuropathy

Leukodystrophies, e.g. Krabbe disease, metachromatic leukodystrophy

Dopa-responsive dystonia

Subacute combined degeneration of the cord/vitamin B_{12} deficiency

Abetalipoproteinemia

Spinocereballar ataxias

HTLV-1 infection (tropical spastic paraparesis)

Neurosyphilis

Neurolathyrism

Vitamin E deficiency

Arginase deficiency

normal in the majority of cases of pure HSP[160,162,217-219]. The cerebrospinal fluid (CSF) is usually normal in HSP, although increased CSF protein has occasionally been reported in families with a complicated phenotype, and an elevated level of homocarnosine has been reported in one family with HSP complicated by progressive mental impairment and retinal pigmentation[220]. Central motor conduction times have been reported by several authors to show either unrecordable, or delayed, responses to the lower limbs, with usually normal values obtained for the upper limbs[215,217,221,222]. Somatosensory evoked potentials from the lower limbs have been reported to be small or absent[161,222,223].

Genetic testing is increasingly being applied in patients with HSP. The most useful molecular genetic test is screening for mutations in the spastin (SGP4) gene, which will be detected in approximately 40% of pedigrees with autosomal dominant HSP. Such mutation screening is, however, costly and time consuming, as mutations have been identified scattered throughout the spastin gene and therefore all 17 exons need to be analyzed, at least in the index cases[177,224]. Mutations in atlastin (SPG3A) will be detected in approximately 10–15% of families with autosomal dominant HSP[225]. Mutation screening is worthwhile, particularly in patients with an early-onset phenotype, as most reported cases with atlastin-related HSP have an age of onset of symptoms within the first decade of life.

The geneticts and molecular mechanisms of disease in hereditary spastic paraparesis

HSP is a disease that shows marked genetic heterogeneity. To date more than 23 genetic loci associated with subtypes of HSP have been identified and 11 causative genes found (Table 8.4). The majority of cases of HSP have autosomal dominant inheritance, but autosomal recessive and X-linked inheritance is observed in some pedigrees. This genetic complexity may converge to cause

Table 8.7   Emerging concepts of molecular mechanisms of disease in hereditary spastic paraparesis (HSP)

Cell recognition and signaling – SPG1, L1 CAM

Abnormalities of myelination – SPG2, PLP1

Mitochondrial disorder – protease and/or chaperone function – SPG7, paraplegin; SPG13, HSP60

Axonal transport/molecular trafficking defect – SPG4, spastin; SPG20, spartin; SPG10, KIF5A; SPG3A, atlastin; ?SPG 21, maspardin

Unknown – SPG6, NIPA1; SPG17, BSCL2 seipin

disruption in several different cellular processes that may underlie HSP and related phenotypes (Table 8.7).

Autosomal dominant hereditary spastic paraparesis

To date, ten autosomal dominant HSP (ADHSP) loci have been identified and the causative gene determined at six of these loci. The genes at SPG3A, SPG4, SPG6, SPG10, SPG13 and SPG17 have been identified as atlastin, spastin, NIPA1, the kinesin heavy chain gene KIF5A, heat shock protein 60 (hsp60) and seipin, respectively[94,225-229]. The genes at the remaining loci SPG8, SPG9, SPG12 and SPG19 are as yet unknown[166,230-234].

Atlastin-regulated hereditary spastic paraparesis

HSP linked to SPG3A on chromsome14q11.2 accounts for approximately 10% of cases of ADHSP[225]. Patients with atlastin-related HSP have a pure phenotype[225,235-240]. One of the distinguishing features of this subtype of HSP appears to be a young age of onset of symptoms, and most affected individuals manifest the disease in the first decade of life. Sometimes affected individuals have initially been misdiagnosed as having cerebral palsy. There are, however, occasional reports of adult-onset disease in patients with atlastin mutations[236,237]. Another possible distinguishing feature is the presence of distal amyotrophy in the upper and lower limbs and chronic neurogenic changes on EMG, implying involvement of lower motor neurons in the pathologic process[236]. Recently one pedigree has been described, with an R415W heterozygous substitution in exon 12, where penetrance was incomplete[239].

The SPG3A gene consists of 14 exons which encode a protein of 588 amino acid residues, with a predicted molecular weight of 63.5 kDa. Atlastin has conserved motifs for GTPase binding and hydrolysis and is structurally homologous to guanylate binding protein 1, a member of the dynamin family of large GTPases[225]. Its predicted structure also indicates that it is likely to be an integral membrane protein, with two transmembrane domains[241] (Figure 8.7). Dynamins are a group of proteins known to be involved in vesicle trafficking, including the formation of clathrin-coated vesicles from the plasma membrane and receptor-mediated endocytosis, Golgi membrane dynamics, and the maintenance and distribution of mitochondria[242–245]. Proteins in the dynamin group are also known to associate with cytoskeletal components including both actin and the microtubule network[246]. These functions are clearly important for neurotransmission, the action of neurotrophic factors and axonal transport. The atlastin protein is localized most abundantly in the CNS, where it is enriched in pyramidal neurons, particularly in layer V of the cortex, including the motor cortex, and in the hippocampus[241]. At the subcellular level, it has recently been shown to co-localize with the Golgi apparatus[244]. Interestingly, an intact Golgi apparatus is known to be required for normal axonal growth.

Seven mutations in atlastin, as well as multiple polymorphisms, have been reported to date[225,235–240]. Most are missense mutations which have been located in exons 4, 7 and 8 and, of these, only one (650G>A) disrupts the GTPase motif directly[240]. It has been speculated that the other missense mutations may exert their pathogenic effect by introducing an altered secondary

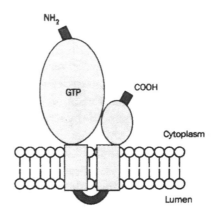

Figure 8.7   Predicted structure of atlastin protein

protein structure that disrupts GTPase activity by disturbing multimerization or protein–protein interactions[225]. One frameshift mutation has been described, predicted to encode a truncated protein that lacks the last 37 amino acid residues[235]. Five of the seven mutations described so far cluster in exons 7 and 8 and at present, therefore, this region of atlastin appears to be a hotspot for mutation.

It will be of interest in the future to explore the effects of atlastin mutations on the structure and function of the Golgi apparatus, axonal transport and growth, as well as parameters such as endocytosis and vesicle trafficking, as perturbations of these cellular functions could underlie the development of the distal axonopathy that develops in HSP.

Spastin-regulated hereditary spastic paraparesis

The gene responsible for SPG4, spastin, was identified in 1999[226]. Spastin is made up of 17 exons mapping to chromosome 2p21-p22, and encodes a protein with 616 amino acid residues and is ubiquitously expressed.

Clinical features

SPG4 is the most frequent form of autosomal dominant HSP, accounting for approximately 40% of cases. The age at onset for spastin-related

HSP is highly variable, demonstrating both inter- and intrafamilial variation. The mean age at onset of symptoms ranges from 25 to 41 years old in the published pedigrees. However, even within families, it is not uncommon to see age at onset of symptoms ranging over five or more decades.

Variation is seen also in the severity of the phenotype due to spastin mutations. Most affected individuals remain ambulant; however, the clinical extremes of the phenotype range from asymptomatic patients with detectable lower limb pyramidal signs found only when clinically examined, to a minority of severely affected patients who become chairbound or bedridden. It is estimated that up to 25% of individuals with spastin mutation are asymptomatic[177].

There is some evidence that disease progression and severity is worse in those with late-onset disease and that the frequency of features such as paresis, amyotrophy, dorsal column involvement and urinary disturbance increase with disease duration[177]. However, other authors have shown no correlation between severity of disease phenotype and age at onset[247]. Gender differences may influence the timing of onset of symptoms in spastin HSP[248]. In several reports there is a tendency for asymptomatic HSP individuals to be female[226,249].

The majority of HSP associated with spastin mutation is of a pure phenotype. However, there are now increasing reports of more complicated phenotypes caused by mutations in the spastin gene. Dementia complicating SPG4 has now been described in several families[163–165] and there are other less detailed reports of memory problems in some pedigrees[224,250]. McMonagle and colleagues demonstrated significantly lower CAMCOG scores and increased frequency of dementia in spastin HSP compared to non-spastin HSP and more recently reported the results of a longitudinal study which showed active progression of cognitive deterioration over a 3-year period in older patients with spastin-related HSP[186,251]. Their data suggest that there is evidence of cognitive impairment in all individuals with spastin muta-

tion when specifically sought. However, as with the rest of the phenotype, this is highly variable within and between families.

Epilepsy associated with spastin-related HSP has also been reported in several families. In one French family, affected family members have either spastic paraparesis alone or, in addition, epilepsy, a cortical-type dementia, or both[165]. The mutation in this family (Q193STOP) causes the translation of a mutant spastin protein truncated at approximately one-third of the normal protein length, missing the whole AAA cassette. In the second family, four out of 24 affected with spastic paraparesis have epilepsy[176]. In this family the mutation causes a frameshift at amino acid 427 and a premature truncation codon at 437, truncating the spastin protein within the AAA cassette. The reported seizure type varies, as does the timing of the onset of epilepsy in relation to onset of gait disturbance.

There are isolated reports of a variety of additional features complicating SPG4, including restless legs, myoclonus, atypical seizures, dysarthria, erectile dysfunction, severe constipation, ileus and fecal incontinence[247,250,252]. An interesting phenotype is described by Meijer et al. in an individual with a truncating mutation (Q434STOP) where, in addition to spastic paraparesis, the affected individuals showed ataxia, footdrop, dysarthria and nystagmus[250]. Mead et al. reported two siblings in a large autosomal dominant spastin pedigree complicated with epilepsy, who have a combination of HSP and multiple sclerosis[176]. The authors postulated that mutations in spastin might represent a susceptibility factor for multiple sclerosis.

Spastin-related HSP does not appear to have a distinctive clinical phenotype compared to other types of pure ADHSP. In addition, there is no clear correlation between the type of spastin mutation identified and the observed phenotype. The interfamilial variation in age at onset for spastin-related HSP does not correlate with the type or position of the mutation within the gene. Also, the presence of complicating factors such as epilepsy or dementia does not have an obvious correlation with genotype. No clear difference in disease phenotype between missense and truncating mutations has been demonstrated[177,224,253,254].

Molecular pathogenesis of spastin-related hereditary spastic paraparesis

Spastin shares homology with a large family of proteins known as the ATPases Associated with diverse cellular Activities (AAA), which are involved in a range of cellular processes including cell cycle regulation, gene expression, organelle biogenesis, vesicle-mediated protein transport and as molecular chaperones co-operating in the assembly, function and disassembly of protein complexes[255]. All the AAA proteins share a common functional domain known as the AAA cassette, which contains highly conserved motifs including Walker A, Walker B and the AAA minimal consensus domain. Outside the AAA cassette there is little homology between different AAA proteins. Spastin has been shown to possess a MIT (microtubule interacting and trafficking) domain[256] and also has nuclear localization sequences[257]. Spastin has particular homology with two other proteins, katanin and SKD1. Katanin is a microtubule-severing protein and is involved in the dynamic regulation of the microtubule cytoskeleton throughout the cell cycle, and SKD1 is an endosomal morphology and trafficking protein. There is evidence from cellular models generated in two laboratories that spastin may also be involved in regulating the microtubule cytoskeleton[258,259]. Microtubules are dynamic polymers of alpha and beta tubulin. They perform essential roles, forming the mitotic spindle in dividing cells, acting as 'railways' for transport of various cellular cargoes including membranous organelles such as mitochondria, and provide essential cytoskeletal support in all cells. When epitope-tagged wild-type spastin was overexpressed in both Cos-7 and HeLa cells it was seen to have a perinuclear/cytosolic punctate distribution. Overexpression of wild-type spastin was associated with a dramatic reduction in cell tubulin content and an increase in the amount of microtubule free ends was demonstrated. When mutant spastin was overexpressed, no decrease in cellular tubulin was seen. However, the spastin distribution changed to a filamentous pattern and co-localized with a subset of microtubules. It seems that missense mutations in spastin may lead to entrapment of the protein in a microtubule bound state[258,259]. Errico and colleagues went on to demonstrate that the N-terminal domain is necessary for targeting mutant spastin to microtubules[258]. They postulated that spastin is targeted by the N-terminus to microtubules and, once bound, undergoes ATP-dependent conformational change that disrupts the microtubules and frees the spastin molecule. If the AAA cassette is disrupted, the conformational change does not occur, and spastin remains bound to the microtubules. These data suggest that spastin, like katanin, may be acting as a microtubule-severing protein. A degree of controversy exists regarding the subcellular localization of spastin. Charvin and colleagues reported that spastin was located in the nuclei of neurons[260], whereas a more recent study of the human CNS detected spastin in the cytoplasm and/or the nucleus, depending on the neuronal subtype[208].

Of the mutations in the spastin gene published to date, approximately 11% are nonsense mutations, 26% frameshift with consequent premature termination codon, 28% missense and 35% splice site mutations. There is no particular 'hot spot' for mutation within the gene, with mutations throughout the length of the gene, making mutation screening a lengthy process. The majority are private mutations, with few occurring in more than one family. Most of the mutations are predicted to have a detrimental effect on the conserved AAA cassette, either by truncating the protein prior to or within the cassette sequence, by skipping of exons within the cassette or by causing amino acid changes within the cassette.

The broad mutational spectrum observed in spastin-related HSP initially suggested that axonal injury might be caused by a loss of function effect.

Further evidence to support haploinsufficiency, rather than a dominant negative or gain of function, as a disease mechanism comes from the fact that, as well as causing exon skipping, the splice site mutations lead to the formation of unstable mRNA. Haploinsufficiency implies that a 50% reduction in the expression of the spastin protein causes the disease. It seems that a critical threshold level of spastin may be necessary for axonal preservation. However, the demonstration of altered microtubule regulation in cells overexpressing missense spastin mutations suggests the possibility that a dominant negative pathogenic mechanism may be involved, at least in individuals with missense mutations[258,259]. Experiments using cellular models have shown that wild-type spastin associates with microtubules and that dissociation of spastin from microtubules during severing occurs in an ATPase-dependent manner. Spastin mutants with a missense mutation in the AAA cassette appear to bind constitutively to microtubules through the intact N-terminal microtubule binding domain and could easily prevent the normal action of wild-type spastin or otherwise block transport along the microtubule system. It is possible that more than one pathogenic mechanism may be involved, depending on the type of mutation. However, it seems likely that the pathogenesis of spastin-related HSP may be due to impairment of the fine regulation of the microtubule cytoskeleton in long axons. A recent study examined the gene expression profile of pathologically unaffected muscle tissue from patients with spastin mutations compared to normal and muscle-disease controls[261]. Dramatic and disease-specific alterations in the transcriptome were found with striking down-regulation of genes associated with microtubule protein and vesicle trafficking pathways in the presence of mutant spastin. Trotta and colleagues recently employed *Drosophila* transgenic methods for overexpression and RNA interference to investigate the role of spastin *in vivo*[262]. They found that the expression of spastin was enriched in axons and synaptic connections. Knockdown of spastin caused an aberrantly stabilized microtubule

cytoskeleton in neurons and defects in synaptic growth and neurotransmission. Spastin overexpression decreased stable microtubules and led to reduced synaptic strength. The misregulation of synaptic function caused by the reduction or overexpression of spastin could be rescued by pharmacologic modulation of microtubule stability by drugs, e.g. taxol and nocodazole. Errico and coworkers have recently extended their work examining the function of spastin in cellular models, and have demonstrated that spastin is enriched in cell regions containing dynamic microtubules[263]. In dividing cells, spastin is found in the spindle pole, the central spindle and the mid-body, whereas in immortalized motor neurons its expression is enriched in the distal axon and the branching points. They also demonstrated that spastin interacts with the centrosomal protein NA14 and cofractionated with γ-tubulin, a centrosomal marker.

Thus, current knowledge indicates that spastin is involved in regulating microtubule dynamics and rearrangement both in proliferating and in post-mitotic cells. It is thought likely that spastin influences microtubule dynamics in growth cones, thus regulating the stability of axons and axonal transport. Long axons such as those of the corticospinal tracts are likely to be most dependent on fine regulation of the microtubule transport system by the action of spastin.

The remaining autosomal dominant hereditary spastic paraparesis loci

Only a small number of families are so far described with mutations in SPG6, SGG10, SPG13 and SPG 17. This suggests that there may be another major locus for ADHSP still to be discovered.

Non-imprinted in Prader–Willi/ Angelman loci 1 (*NIPA1*)-related hereditary spastic paraparesis

SPG6 is located within a chromosomal region (15q11) which is deleted in Prader–Willi and

Angelman syndromes. In 2003, two families with ADHSP were described with the same T45R mutation in the *NIPA1* gene[227]. This mutation disrupts an interspecies conserved amino acid. The function of *NIPA1* is unknown, but it is highly expressed in neuronal tissues. Structural analysis of the encoded protein predicts that it possesses nine transmembrane domains, indicating that it may well be a membrane transporter or receptor[227]. The predicted protein does not contain AAA or GTPase domains and has no homology to other genes that cause HSP. The described T45R mutation is at the interface between the first transmembrane domain and the first putative outside loop. It has been speculated that the disease mechanism may involve altered signal transduction or small molecule transport. Many individuals with Prader–Willi or Angelman syndromes have deletions which include *NIPA1* and such individuals do not develop features of HSP. This suggests that the disease mechanism probably involves a dominant negative or gain of function rather than haploinsufficiency.

KIF5A-related hereditary spastic paraparesis

Within neurons, the microtubule cytoskeleton serves as the molecular transport system for intracellular cargo trafficking. Kinesins are a family of microtubule-associated proteins that serve as molecular motors that distribute intracellular cargoes including membranous organelles, e.g. mitochondria, synaptic vesicles, membrane proteins and prelysosomal organelles along microtubules in an anterograde direction. The kinesin heavy chain proteins KIF5A, KIF5B and KIF5C are part of a multisubunit complex (kinesin-1) that acts as a microtubule motor involved in anterograde fast axonal transport. KIF5A has an exclusively neuronal expression, enriched in motor neurons[264]. The heavy chain proteins represent the force-producing subunit of kinesin, possessing a motor domain that interacts with the microtubule track and hydrolyzes ATP. KIF5A is expressed in all

neurons and is distributed in the cell body, axons and dendrites.

A single family was described in 2002 with pure, autosomal dominant HSP associated with a missense mutation at an invariate asparagine residue (N256S) in the motor domain of the neuronal kinesin heavy chain protein KIF5A[228]. The mutation is predicted to cause loss of function or a dominant negative effect on the neuronal kinesin I motor. A similar mutation in yeast blocks microtubule-dependent stimulation of motor ATPase activity[265]. This defect would be predicted to cause abnormal fast axonal transport of cargoes vital for the distal axon. A homologous mutation in *Drosophila* larvae results in 'organelle jams' within axons of motor neurons[266]. Very recently a second ADHSP pedigree was described with a missense mutation (R280C) at an invariant arginine residue in exon 10, located in a region of the protein involved in microtubule binding activity[267]. Clinically affected members of this pedigree had pure HSP of childhood onset.

Heat-shock protein 60-related hereditary spastic paraparesis

The gene at the SPG13 locus has been identified as the mitochondrial chaperonin Hsp60 (heat shock protein). One family with a V72I substitution and AD pure HSP was described by Hansen and colleagues in 2002[229]. The use of a complementation assay showed that wild-type HSP60 and its co-chaperone HSP10, but not mutant (V72I) HSP60 could support the growth of *Escherichia coli* in which the homologous bacterial genes had been deleted[229]. HSP60 is thought to be a mitochondrial stress protein which is upregulated, for example, in the presence of an accumulation of unfolded proteins within the mitochondrial matrix[268].

Seipin-related hereditary spastic paraparesis/Silver syndrome

Silver syndrome is a disabling autosomal dominant form of HSP in which spastic paraparesis is complicated by amyotrophy of the hand muscles, especially the thenar muscles and sometimes the distal lower limb muscles[95]. In 2001, evidence of linkage was found to chromosome 11q12-q14 in some pedigrees with Silver syndrome, although genetic heterogeneity for this subtype of HSP was also apparent[170]. Neurophysiologic studies in these patients have suggested anterior horn cell or motor root involvement in addition to the corticospinal tract dysfunction[269]. Recently, heterozygous missense mutations in the Berardinelli–Seip congenital lipodystrophy type 2 (*BSCL2*) gene were found in two families, one with Silver syndrome and one with hereditary distal motor neuropathy[94]. The encoded protein has been termed seipin and the two mutations result in amino acid substitutions (N88S and S90L) in an *N*-glycosylation motif. These authors demonstrated that seipin was an integral membrane protein of the endoplasmic reticulum and that the disruption of glycosylation caused by the missense mutations resulted in protein aggregation. The clinical phenotype of this genetic disorder has recently been expanded to include patients with predominantly lower limb amyotrophy and those without signs of corticospinal tract pathology[97].

In 2001, it had been demonstrated that null mutations affecting seipin caused autosomal recessive Berardinelli–Seip congenital lipodystrophy type 2[270], which causes near absence of adipose tissue from early childhood and severe insulin resistance. It is at present not understood how mutant forms of seipin cause two such distinct clinical syndromes[271].

Other autosomal dominant hereditary spastic paraparesis

The genes associated with SPG8, SPG9, SGG12, and SPG19 await discovery. Spastic paraparesis at the SPG9 has been described in an Italian family in which the phenotype is complicated by bilateral cataracts, gastroesophageal reflux with vomiting and amyotrophy[166]. A further British family has been described with cataracts, learning difficulties and skeletal abnormalities[272,273]. In both families anticipation of age at onset is described, suggesting that SPG9 may represent a trinucleotide repeat disorder.

Autosomal recessive hereditary spastic paraparesis

Autosomal recessive HSP (ARHSP) is also clinically and genetically heterogeneous and is relatively rare compared to the dominantly inherited forms. ARHSP pedigrees have been linked to eight genetic loci, with both pure and complicated phenotypes described. The genes underlying three subtypes of ARHSP have been identified to date: SPG7 paraplegin[274], SPG20/Troyer syndrome spartin[171] and SPG21 maspardin[275]. The genes associated with SPG5, SPG11, SPG14, SPG15 and SPG23 await discovery.

Pure autosomal recessive hereditary spastic paraparesis

There are three loci for pure ARHSP – SPG5, SPG7 and SPG11 – although families with a complicated phenotype have also been described linking to the latter two loci. There is no apparent clinical difference between pure ARHSP and pure ADHSP.

Complicated autosomal recessive hereditary spastic paraparesis

Complicated ARHSP pedigrees have been linked to seven loci: SPG7, SPG11, SPG14, SPG15, SPG20, SPG21 and SPG23. At the SPG7 locus, HSP has been associated with a variety of features including optic atrophy, cortical and cerebellar atrophy, dysphagia, slowed speech, distal amyotrophy and sensorimotor neuropathy. Complicated HSP at the SPG11 has been associated with mixed motor sensory neuropathy, cerebellar dysfunction, mental retardation and abnormal brain imaging[168]. The latter consisted of atrophy or agenesis of the corpus callosum in two families, with additional periventricular white matter changes in one of these. In the one family linked to the SPG14 locus, the additional features co-segregating with the spastic paraparesis were a distal motor neuropathy and mild mental retardation[169]. Two families have been linked to the SPG15 locus. Pigmented macular degeneration, distal amyotrophy, mild cerebellar dysfunction and diffuse brain atrophy on MRI were the additional features described[167]. Troyer syndrome (SPG20) and Mast syndrome are also complicated, autosomal recessive forms of HSP, and are described below.

Paraplegin-related hereditary spastic paraparesis

Patients with SPG7-related HSP may have either a pure or a complicated phenotype. In the latter case the spastic paraparesis may be accompanied by a variety of other features including optic atrophy, cortical and cerebellar atrophy, dysphagia, dysarthria, distal amyotrophy or sensorimotor neuropathy[213,274].

The *SPG7* gene is 52 kb in size, comprising 17 exons, and the encoded protein, paraplegin, is a nuclear encoded mitochondrial metalloprotease. Paraplegin, like spastin (SPG4), is a member of the AAA protein family, and shares homology with spastin in the AAA cassette. However, outside of the 230 amino acid residue conserved AAA cassette, little homology is seen. Paraplegin is a nuclear encoded mitochondrial metalloprotease which is ubiquitously expressed, and initially its likely function was predicted by comparison with homologous proteins in yeast. Afg3p and Rca1p are AAA mitochondrial metalloproteases found in yeast and each share 55% amino acid homology with paraplegin. In yeast, Afg3p and Rca1p form a high molecular weight hetero-oligomeric complex in the inner mitochondrial membrane. These yeast proteins have both chaperone and proteolytic functions in the inner mitochondrial membrane and are involved in ATP synthase assembly, respiratory chain complex formation and the degradation of incompletely synthesized mitochondrial polypeptides[276–280]. Deletion or mutation of the conserved proteolytic site of either Afg3p or Rca1p leads to dysfunction of respiratory chain activity and an impaired ability to degrade incompletely synthesized mitochondrial polypeptides. From these studies of yeast homologs, it was predicted that paraplegin would function by forming multimeric complexes which have proteolytic and chaperone-like functions in the mitochondria, essential for the normal assembly and turnover of respiratory chain complexes. The amino terminus of paraplegin has a mitochondrial targeting sequence. Recent studies employing mouse knockout (Spg7–/–) and cellular models have further elucidated disease mechanisms caused by loss of function of paraplegin. The laboratory of Rugarli and colleagues have generated a paraplegin-deficient mouse[281]. The first detectable phenotype in the Spg7–/– mice is the appearance at 4 months of age of structurally abnormal enlarged mitochondria in synaptic terminals in the gray matter of the lumbar spinal cord. These mitochondrial abnormalities correlate in time with the onset of a significant functional motor deficit as assessed by rotarod performance, but precede signs of axonal degeneration by several months. Interestingly, although paraplegin is ubiquitously distributed, the morphologic abnormalities of mitochondria are restricted to the synaptic subset of these organelles. Clearly, mitochondrial dysfunction within axonal terminals could lead to problems with ATP generation, regulation of calcium homeostasis and oxyradical metabolism. The paraplegin knockout mice also develop accumulations of neurofilaments and organelles in swollen axons, indicating abnormalities in anterograde transport. Retrograde transport is delayed in symptomatic mice and this could clearly contribute to the axonal degeneration by affecting the transport of mitochondria, the trafficking of endosomes and the internalization of neurotrophic factors.

Atorino and co-workers have analyzed the function of paraplegin at the cellular level[282]. They demonstrated that paraplegin co-assembles with a homologous protein AFG3L2 into a high-molecular-weight complex within the inner mitochondrial membrane. Using fibroblasts from SPG7 patients they showed that this complex was defective in the presence of paraplegin mutations, with a resultant decrease in complex 1 activity of the mitochondrial respiratory chain and increased sensitivity of the cells to oxidative stress. Exogenous expression of wild-type paraplegin ameliorated both of these functional defects. The authors predicted that the complex 1 deficiency in HSP cells was likely to result from an inefficient folding process in the absence of a physiologic paraplegin-AFG3L2 complex and that the initial pathogenic mechanism was likely to arise from the combined effects of misfolded peptide accumulation and lack of chaperone activity on complex 1 assembly. Interestingly, there is evidence that different subsets of neurons have different complex 1 distributions, and this may account for selective vulnerability of restricted neuronal populations in paraplegin-related HSP.

Several families have so far been described with paraplegin mutations. All the mutations described in some way affect the conserved AAA domain, either by truncating the protein or by causing an in-frame deletion. One English pedigree has been described in which the proband was a compound heterozygote with both a 9 bp deletion (1450–1458del) and a missense change (1529C→T)[275]. The paraplegin missense change was inherited from a clinically normal mother, and the deletion was inherited from a father who was reported to be mildly affected with spastic paraparesis. The authors argued either that the father represented a manifesting heterozygote or that the deletion he carried was behaving in a dominant-negative manner.

Both pure and complicated HSP at the SPG7 locus have been associated with evidence of mitochondrial dysfunction on histochemical analysis of muscle[213,274]. As described above, mutation in a further nuclear-encoded mitochondrial protein, Hsp 60, has recently been identified as the cause for pure ADHSP at the SPG13 locus[229]. There is further evidence of mitochondrial dysfunction in HSP as respiratory chain complex I and IV

deficiencies have been reported in ADHSP and ARHSP, where both spastin and paraplegin mutations have been excluded as a cause[213,283]. Further studies of mitochondrial function in genetically defined subtypes of HSP should be pursued in the future.

Spartin-related hereditary spastic paraparesis – Troyer syndrome

Troyer syndrome, named after the family in which it was first identified, was originally described in 1967 in an Old Order Amish community[191], a genetically isolated population with an increased frequency of certain rare autosomal recessive disorders. It is an autosomal recessive, complicated form of HSP with the cardinal features of spastic paraparesis, pseudobulbar palsy, distal amyotrophy, mild developmental delay and subtle skeletal abnormalities including short stature. White matter abnormalities may be found in the cerebral hemispheres and thinning of the corpus callosum has been described on MRI[284]. In 2002, a frameshift mutation (1110delA) in SPG20 encoding spartin was found to be the genetic cause of this disorder[171]. The SPG20 gene comprises nine exons spanning a distance of 43.3 kb on chromosome 13q12.3. SPG20 encodes a protein of 666 amino acid residues (72.7 kDa) named spartin, which is ubiquitously expressed in adult tissues, with the highest expression in adipose tissue. Spartin shares homology with SNX15, VPS4 and Skd1, proteins known to be involved in endosomal morphology and dynamics and protein trafficking, suggesting that spastin may serve a similar role. Spartin also shares homology with the N-terminal region of spastin[256]. This region of spastin, known as the MIT (microtubule interacting and trafficking) domain is thought to be responsible for binding to microtubules. Thus, while detailed cell biologic studies to elucidate the intracellular functions of spartin are awaited, evidence presently available implicates spartin in endosomal trafficking and/or microtubule dynamics[285].

Maspardin-related hereditary spastic paraparesis – Mast syndrome

Mast syndrome is an autosomal recessive, complicated form of HSP accompanied by dementia, which is also found at relatively high frequency among the Old Order Amish community[181]. The phenotype may include developmental delay, pseudobulbar features, cerebellar and extrapyramidal signs, as well as MRI abnormalities consisting of thinning of the corpus callosum, cerebral atrophy and white matter demyelination. The neurologic abnormalities progress during adulthood. In 2003, 14 affected patients were found to be homozygous for a single basepair (601insA) insertion in the gene encoding the acid-cluster protein of 33 kDa (ACP33) which has been renamed maspardin[275]. This is a frameshift mutation that causes a truncated protein product which is likely to cause a loss of function effect. One previous study had reported the subcellular distribution of this protein in a CD4-positive T-cell line[286]. It appears that maspardin localizes to vesicles involved in the early endosome recycling pathway and to acidic organelles, suggesting that, at least in this type of cell, maspardin is partitioned between the cytosol and vesicles of the endosomal/trans-Golgi network. It is therefore predicted that maspardin may be involved in protein sorting and trafficking, and that defective trafficking might be important in disease pathogenesis. Further work is required to define precisely the role of maspardin within neurons.

X-linked hereditary spastic paraparesis

X-linked forms of HSP are relatively rare. There are three X-linked loci: SPG1, SPG2 and SPG16. The genes involved at the SPG1 and SPG2 loci have been known for some time and the molecular mechanisms of disease are relatively well understood. The gene at SPG16 is not yet known. One SPG16 family with a pure phenotype has been identified having a NOR insertion into Xq11.2[287]. One pedigree has been reported in whom linkage analysis excluded SPG1 and SPG2 and suggested a locus at Xq11.2-q23. The phenotype in this family was severe with mental retardation, upper limb involvement, visual impairment and bladder and bowel dysfunction in addition to spastic paraplegia[288]. A further complicated pedigree has had mutation in the SPG1 and SPG2 gene excluded[289]. It is at present uncertain whether these two families are both linked to SPG16 or whether there is a further X-linked locus to be confirmed.

L1 cell adhesion molecule-related hereditary spastic paraparesis

SPG1 is a rare developmental disorder of varying severity caused by mutations in the L1 cell adhesion molecule gene (*L1CAM*)[290]. In these patients there is usually a complex phenotype with mental retardation and congenital musculoskeletal abnormalities, most notably the absence of extensor hallucis longus, in addition to spastic paraparesis[291]. Mutations in *L1CAM* are also found in X-linked hydrocephalus, X-linked agenesis of the corpus callosum and the syndrome of MASA (mental retardation, aphasia, shuffling gait and adducted thumbs). The diseases are now considered to be part of a clinical syndrome with the acronym CRASH, for corpus callosum hypoplasia, retardation, adducted thumbs, spastic paraplegia and hydrocephalus[292].

L1CAM is a cell-surface, membrane-associated glycoprotein, a member of the immunoglobulin superfamily, which is expressed predominantly within neurons and Schwann cells[293]. It is a protein with complex extracellular and intracellular interactions and plays an important role in CNS development with involvement in neuronal adhesion, and axonal outgrowth and pathfinding[294]. L1CAM plays an essential role in corticospinal tract formation[295–298]. In knockout mice the normal anatomy of the corticospinal tracts is disrupted with failure of decussation of corticospinal axons across the midline at the level of the pyramids, a process normally stimulated by a chemorepellent molecule secreted by the ventral spinal cord known as Sema3A[299]. L1CAM is a component of the Sema3A receptor complex, and mice deficient in L1CAM fail to respond to Sema3A *in vitro*.

Proteolipid protein-related hereditary spastic paraparesis

SPG2 is caused by mutations in the proteolipid protein 1 (*PLP*) gene[300], which encodes PLP and its minor DM20 isoform, the major proteins of the myelin sheath. Both pure and complicated HSP phenotypes may be observed[301–305]. Complicated pedigrees have a cerebellar syndrome and mental retardation in addition to spastic paraparesis. Optic atrophy may also be found. Mutations in the *PLP* gene also cause Pelizaeus–Merzbacher disease (PMD), a severe dysmyelinating syndrome characterized by nystagmus, ataxia, spasticity, abnormal movements, optic atrophy and microcephaly, usually resulting in death during adolescence. The phenotype of disease caused by mutations in the *PLP* gene can be considered as a continuous spectrum with milder SPG2 at one end and the more severe PMD at the other. It is an intriguing question as to why mutations in a gene expressed in oligodendrocytes leads to axonal degeneration.

PLP is the major myelin protein of the CNS, accounting for approximately 50% of total myelin protein in the adult brain. DM20 is an alternatively spliced form of PLP, which lacks 35 amino acid residues. The function of the PLP and DM20 proteins has not been established with certainty, but they are likely to have an important function in stabilizing the structure of CNS myelin by forming the intraperiod line. It is possible that the two protein isoforms have different functions. The DM20 isoform appears earlier during development and is thought to play a role in glial cell development, while the PLP isoform is expressed later and may play a role in myelin assembly and

maintenance. Mutations in the PLP gene that do not affect the DM20 isoform are associated with the milder PMD phenotype or SPG2. Conversely, mutations which reduce the level of the DM20 isoform are associated with the more severe PMD phenotypes[306]. It has been suggested that PLP/DM20 may play an important role in glial/axon communication. *Plp* knockout mice develop normal myelin sheaths despite lack of PLP/DM20, but subsequently develop a severe axonopathy[307–309]. Recently, Edgar and colleagues have shown that absence of PLP/DM20 in oligodendrocytes resulted in early impairment of fast axonal transport and multifocal accumulations of membranous organelles, in a mouse model with a null mutation in *PLP*[310]. Axonal degenerative changes were found to be concentrated at the distal regions of long axons. This paper has importantly demonstrated a novel role for oligodendrocytes in the local regulation of function of underlying axons.

TREATMENT OF HEREDITARY SPASTIC PARAPARESIS

So far, increased knowledge of the molecular basis of HSP has had little impact on clinical practice. It is hoped that this situation will change as better animal models of disease are generated. At present symptomatic treatments can be used to alleviate spasticity, bladder dysfunction and the lower limb discomfort which can be troublesome features of HSP, but neuroprotective therapies to ameliorate the distal axonopathy are still awaited.

CONCLUSIONS

Common pathogenetic mechanisms in MN degeneration

The disease-causing genes identified in SMA, SBMA and HSP affect proteins that are often widely expressed, and involved in diverse cellular processes. These mutations nevertheless cause a highly selective degeneration of a subclass of neuronal cells. Their identification has revealed important insights into the causes of motor neuron vulnerability, and common pathogenetic mechanisms in motor neuron degeneration.

Defects in RNA handling and transcriptional regulation

Several mutations causing motor neuron degeneration occur in housekeeping genes involved in RNA handling and transcriptional regulation. SMN is necessary for the biogenesis of snRNPs, for pre-mRNA splicing, and is involved in transcriptional regulation. Mutant AR accumulates in the nucleus in SBMA, where it is thought to interact with transcription factors to disrupt gene transcription. GARS has diverse cellular functions, including tRNA processing, RNA splicing and trafficking, and rRNA synthesis, while IGHMBP2 has RNA helicase activity needed for pre-mRNA processing. Furthermore, missense mutations have been identified in the *senataxin* gene in families with an autosomal dominant juvenile-onset ALS (ALS4), and in two families with disease previously classified as distal SMA with pyramidal tract signs[311]. The senataxin protein contains a DNA/RNA helicase domain with significant homology to the IGHMBP2 protein. This provides strong evidence that motor neurons may be vulnerable to defects in gene transcription and RNA processing, and places SMA within a group of neurologic disorders, including fragile-X mental retardation and myotonic dystrophy, in which abnormalities of RNA handling appear to be central to the disease process.

Defects in axonal transport

Motor neurons contain ribosome-like structures in distal axons and growth cones. It is hypothesized that the axonal transport of mRNAs for some of the housekeeping genes may play an essential role in cell viability, and may explain the selective vulnerability of neurons with long axons to disruption of these functions. Abnormal axonal transport is implicated in other neurodegenerative disorders, including ALS and CMT, and has been demonstrated in both SMA and SBMA. The heat shock protein HSPB1/HSP27 is involved in organization of the neurofilament network, and the mutant protein disrupts neurofilament assembly. Mutations in dynactin I are predicted to disrupt dynactin-mediated transport. SMN interacts with HnRNP-R in axons, and may be involved in transport of mRNA molecules in motor axons, while protein aggregates of mutant AR disrupt kinesin-mediated fast axonal transport in SBMA. Several of the genetic defects underlying HSP are predicted to have a detrimental effect on intracellular transport and trafficking, axonal outgrowth or maintenance/regulation of the microtubule network (Table 8.7).

Protein aggregation

Protein aggregation is a common neuropathologic feature of many neurodegenerative disorders, including AD, PD and ALS, and may be a primary event underlying neurotoxicity in these disorders. Similarly, this pathologic process is implicated in SMA and SBMA. Aggregation of mutant protein is seen in motor neuron nuclei of patients with Kennedy's disease, due to misfolding of the mutant AR protein. Intracellular aggregate formation is promoted by N88S and S90L mutations of seipin, and by expression in cultured cells of mutant HSPB8/HSP22. Molecular pathological studies of spastin-related HSP have indictated that abnormal cytopathology includes protein aggregation[208].

Mitochondrial dysfunction

Particularly in relation to HSP, there is considerable interest in the potential role of mitochondrial dysfunction in the distal axon, in relation to disease pathogenesis. Two of the known HSP causative genes, paraplegin and HSP60, directly affect mitochondrial proteins, and defects in some of the other genes may impair the transport of mitochondria on the microtubule system to the distal axon. These two mechanisms may overlap in causing impaired ATP generation in the distal regions of long axons.

Relative vulnerability of motor neurons

In some families with SMA, lower motor neuron pathology is combined with evidence of sensory disturbance and pyramidal involvement. Indeed, in two cases, a single gene mutation can result in either SMA, or disorders in which the predominant pathology lies in sensory nerves, or in the upper motor neurons. dHMN-V may be caused by mutations in the *GARS* gene, or in *BSCL2*, while *GARS* mutations also underlie cases of CMT type 2D, and *BSCL2* mutations cause Silver syndrome. This suggests that different classes of neurons with long axons are vulnerable to similar pathogenetic mechanisms.

Selective vulnerability may arise from intrinsic properties of neurons with very long axons. The cell bodies of these neurons have to support axons of up to 1 m in length. These neurons are therefore highly metabolically active and are likely to be susceptible to any alteration of ATP generation. They are also exquisitely dependent on an intricate system of transport designed to ensure correct targeted delivery of cargoes over long distances. An interruption in the transport of vital cellular components to the distal axon could be responsible for the 'dying back' phenomenon observed in HSP. Mitochondria located in the distal regions of long axons may be particularly prone to malfunction because of the distance from the synthetic machinery predominantly located in the cell bodies. At present little is known about the factors determining the relative vulnerability of motor axons from upper versus lower motor neurons and why in some motor neuron degenerative disorders there is an upper motor neuron phenotype, in others a lower motor neuron phenotype, while some disorders cause degeneration of both upper and lower motor neuron axons.

HSP is an exemplary disease to study dysfunctional cellular programs initiating axonal degeneration. With the genes identified at 11 of the 23 known SPG loci, it is apparent that there is marked diversity in the function of genes associated with an HSP phenotype. Their functions include mitochondrial protein housekeeping, chaperoning, cytoskeleton regulation and intracellular transport, myelin formation and maintenance, neuron outgrowth and glial–axon communication.

The recent explosion in the identification of the genes underlying HSP heralds a new era in terms of diagnosing the condition. In a patient with ADHSP, screening of the spastin and atlastin genes will identify a mutation in approximately 50% of cases. Precise diagnosis enables appropriate counseling with regard to prognosis and implications for an individual's family. However, given the huge inter- and intrafamilial variation in age at onset of symptoms and severity seen in SPG4, the use of prenatal screening can be less clear-cut than with other inherited disorders. In the coming years there is hope that increased understanding of the neurodegenerative processes at work in HSP will lead to useful therapeutic interventions to slow disease progression.

The SMAs are a diverse group of single-gene disorders. Elucidation of the molecular pathogenesis of these diseases will lead to greater understanding of the factors influencing motor neuron survival, and this is likely to be applicable not only to SMA, but also to other diseases in which motor neurons are selectively vulnerable, including ALS and HSP.

REFERENCES

1. Zerres K, Rudnik-Schoneborn S. Natural history in proximal spinal muscular atrophy. Clinical analysis of 445 patients and suggestions for a modification of existing classifications. Arch Neurol 1995; 52: 518–23

2. Munsat TL, Davies KE. International SMA consortium meeting, 26–28 June 1992, Bonn, Germany. Neuromuscul Disord 1992; 2: 423–8

3. Kausch K, Muller CR, Grimm T, et al. No evidence for linkage of autosomal dominant proximal spinal

muscular atrophies to chromosome 5q markers. Hum Genet 1991; 86: 317–18

4. Harding AE. Inherited neuronal atrophy and degeneration predominantly of lower motor neurones. In: Poduslo JF, ed. Peripheral Neuropathy, Vol 2. Saunders, 1993: 1051–64

5. 2nd Workshop of the European CMT Consortium. 53rd ENMC International Workshop on Classification and Diagnostic Guidelines for Charcot–Marie–Tooth Type 2 (CMT2-HMSN II) and Distal Hereditary Motor Neuropathy (distal HMN-Spinal CMT) 26–28 September 1997, Naarden, The Netherlands. Neuromuscul Disord 1998; 8: 426–31

6. Irobi J, De Jonghe P, Timmerman V. Molecular genetics of distal hereditary motor neuropathies. Hum Mol Genet 2004; 13 (Suppl 2): R195–202

7. Brzustowicz LM, Lehner T, Castilla LH, et al. Genetic mapping of chronic childhood-onset spinal muscular atrophy to chromosome 5q11.2–13.3. Nature 1990; 344: 540–1

8. Gilliam TC, Brzustowicz LM, Castilla LH, et al. Genetic homogeneity between acute and chronic forms of spinal muscular atrophy. Nature 1990; 345: 823–5

9. Melki J, Sheth P, Abdelhak S, et al. Mapping of acute (type I) spinal muscular atrophy to chromosome 5q12–q14. The French Spinal Muscular Atrophy Investigators. Lancet 1990; 336: 271–3

10. Melki J, Abdelhak S, Sheth P, et al. Gene for chronic proximal spinal muscular atrophies maps to chromosome 5q. Nature 1990; 344: 767–8

11. Melki J, Lefebvre S, Burglen L, et al. De novo and inherited deletions of the 5q13 region in spinal muscular atrophies. Science 1994; 264: 1474–7

12. Lefebvre S, Burglen L, Reboullet S, et al. Identification and characterization of a spinal muscular atrophy-determining gene. Cell 1995; 80: 155–65

13. Roy N, Mahadevan MS, McLean M, et al. The gene for neuronal apoptosis inhibitory protein is partially deleted in individuals with spinal muscular atrophy. Cell 1995; 80: 167–78

14. Carter TA, Bonnemann CG, Wang CH, et al. A multicopy transcription-repair gene, BTF2p44, maps to the SMA region and demonstrates SMA associated deletions. Hum Mol Genet 1997; 6: 229–36

15. Burglen L, Seroz T, Miniou P, et al. The gene encoding p44, a subunit of the transcription factor TFIIH, is involved in large-scale deletions associated with Werdnig–Hoffmann disease. Am J Hum Genet 1997; 60: 72–9

16. Scharf JM, Endrizzi MG, Wetter A, et al. Identification of a candidate modifying gene for spinal muscular atrophy by comparative genomics. Nat Genet 1998; 20: 83–6

17. Thompson TG, DiDonato CJ, Simard LR, et al. A novel cDNA detects homozygous microdeletions in greater than 50% of type I spinal muscular atrophy patients. Nat Genet 1995; 9: 56–62

18. Wirth B. An update of the mutation spectrum of the survival motor neuron gene (SMN1) in autosomal recessive spinal muscular atrophy (SMA). Hum Mutat 2000; 15: 228–37

19. Monani UR, Sendtner M, Coovert DD, et al. The human centromeric survival motor neuron gene (SMN2) rescues embryonic lethality in Smn(-/-) mice and results in a mouse with spinal muscular atrophy. Hum Mol Genet 2000; 9: 333–9

20. Hsieh-Li HM, Chang JG, Jong YJ, et al. A mouse model for spinal muscular atrophy. Nat Genet 2000; 24: 66–70

21. Rochette CF, Gilbert N, Simard LR. SMN gene duplication and the emergence of the SMN2 gene occurred in distinct hominids: SMN2 is unique to Homo sapiens. Hum Genet 2001; 108: 255–66

22. Burglen L, Lefebvre S, Clermont O, et al. Structure and organization of the human survival motor neurone (SMN) gene. Genomics 1996; 32: 479–82

23. Campbell L, Potter A, Ignatius J, et al. Genomic variation and gene conversion in spinal muscular atrophy: implications for disease process and clinical phenotype. Am J Hum Genet 1997; 61: 40–50

24. Burghes AH. When is a deletion not a deletion? When it is converted. Am J Hum Genet 1997; 61: 9–15

25. Ogino S, Wilson RB. Genetic testing and risk assessment for spinal muscular atrophy (SMA). Hum Genet 2002; 111: 477–500

26. Martin Y, Valero A, del Castillo E, et al. Genetic study of SMA patients without homozygous SMN1 deletions: identification of compound heterozygotes and characterisation of novel intragenic SMN1 mutations. Hum Genet 2002; 110: 257–63

27. Skordis LA, Dunckley MG, Burglen L, et al. Characterisation of novel point mutations in the survival motor neuron gene SMN, in three patients with SMA. Hum Genet 2001; 108: 356–7

28. Tsai CH, Jong YJ, Hu CJ, et al. Molecular analysis of SMN, NAIP and P44 genes of SMA patients and their families. J Neurol Sci 2001; 190: 35–40

29. Sossi V, Giuli A, Vitali T, et al. Premature termination mutations in exon 3 of the SMN1 gene are asso-

ciated with exon skipping and a relatively mild SMA phenotype. Eur J Hum Genet 2001; 9: 113–20

30. Talbot K, Ponting CP, Theodosiou AM, et al. Missense mutation clustering in the survival motor neuron gene: A role for a conserved tyrosine and glycine rich region of the protein in RNA metabolism? Hum Mol Genet 1997; 6: 497–500

31. Talbot K, Miguel-Aliaga I, Mohaghegh P, et al. Characterization of a gene encoding survival motor neuron (SMN)-related protein, a constituent of the spliceosome complex. Hum Mol Genet 1998; 7: 2149–56

32. McAndrew PE, Parsons DW, Simard LR, et al. Identification of proximal spinal muscular atrophy carriers and patients by analysis of SMNT and SMNC gene copy number. Am J Hum Genet 1997; 60: 1411–22

33. Feldkotter M, Schwarzer V, Wirth R, et al. Quantitative analyses of SMN1 and SMN2 based on real-time lightCycler PCR: Fast and highly reliable carrier testing and prediction of severity of spinal muscular atrophy. Am J Hum Genet 2002; 70: 358–68

34. Wirth B, Herz M, Wetter A, et al. Quantitative analysis of survival motor neuron copies: identification of subtle SMN1 mutations in patients with spinal muscular atrophy, genotype–phenotype correlation, and implications for genetic counseling. Am J Hum Genet 1999; 64: 1340–56

35. Lefebvre S, Burlet P, Liu Q, et al. Correlation between severity and SMN protein level in spinal muscular atrophy. Nat Genet 1997; 16: 265–9

36. Rodrigues NR, Owen N, Talbot K, et al. Gene deletions in spinal muscular atrophy. J Med Genet 1996; 33: 93–6

37. Coovert DD, Le TT, McAndrew PE, et al. The survival motor neuron protein in spinal muscular atrophy. Hum Mol Genet 1997; 6: 1205–14

38. Liu Q, Dreyfuss G. A novel nuclear structure containing the survival of motor neurons protein. EMBO J 1996; 15: 3555–65

39. Lorson CL, Strasswimmer J, Yao JM, et al. SMN oligomerization defect correlates with spinal muscular atrophy severity. Nat Genet 1998; 19: 63–6

40. Gubitz AK, Feng W, Dreyfuss G. The SMN complex. Exp Cell Res 2004; 296: 51–6

41. Buhler D, Raker V, Luhrmann R, Fischer U. Essential role for the tudor domain of SMN in spliceosomal U snRNP assembly: Implications for spinal muscular atrophy. Hum Mol Genet 1999; 8: 2351–7

42. Charroux B, Pellizzoni L, Perkinson RA, et al. Gemin3: A novel DEAD box protein that interacts with SMN, the spinal muscular atrophy gene product, and is a component of gems. J Cell Biol 1999; 147: 1181–94

43. Charroux B, Pellizzoni L, Perkinson RA, et al. Gemin4. A novel component of the SMN complex that is found in both gems and nucleoli. J Cell Biol 2000; 148: 1177–86

44. Gubitz AK, Mourelatos Z, Abel L, et al. Gemin5, a novel WD repeat protein component of the SMN complex that binds Sm proteins. J Biol Chem 2002; 277: 5631–6

45. Pellizzoni L, Baccon J, Rappsilber J, et al. Purification of native survival of motor neurons complexes and identification of Gemin6 as a novel component. J Biol Chem 2002; 277: 7540–5

46. Baccon J, Pellizzoni L, Rappsilber J, et al. Identification and characterization of Gemin7, a novel component of the survival of motor neuron complex. J Biol Chem 2002; 277: 31957–62

47. Liu Q, Fischer U, Wang F, Dreyfuss G. The spinal muscular atrophy disease gene product, SMN, and its associated protein SIP1 are in a complex with spliceosomal snRNP proteins. Cell 1997; 90: 1013–21

48. Friesen WJ, Dreyfuss G. Specific sequences of the Sm and Sm-like (Lsm) proteins mediate their interaction with the spinal muscular atrophy disease gene product (SMN). J Biol Chem 2000; 275: 26370–5

49. Meister G, Buhler D, Pillai R, et al. A multiprotein complex mediates the ATP-dependent assembly of spliceosomal U snRNPs. Nat Cell Biol 2001; 3: 945–9

50. Fischer U, Liu Q, Dreyfuss G. The SMN-SIP1 complex has an essential role in spliceosomal snRNP biogenesis. Cell 1997; 90: 1023–9

51. Pellizzoni L, Kataoka N, Charroux B, Dreyfuss G. A novel function for SMN, the spinal muscular atrophy disease gene product, in pre-mRNA splicing. Cell 1998; 95: 615–24

52. Yong J, Wan L, Dreyfuss G. Why do cells need an assembly machine for RNA-protein complexes? Trends Cell Biol 2004; 14: 226–32

53. Meister G, Buhler D, Laggerbauer B, et al. Characterization of a nuclear 20S complex containing the survival of motor neurons (SMN) protein and a specific subset of spliceosomal Sm proteins. Hum Mol Genet 2000; 9: 1977–86

54. Pellizzoni L, Charroux B, Dreyfuss G. SMN mutants of spinal muscular atrophy patients are defective in binding to snRNP proteins. Proc Natl Acad Sci USA 1999; 96: 11167–72

55. Jablonka S, Schrank B, Kralewski M, et al. Reduced survival motor neuron (Smn) gene dose in mice leads to motor neuron degeneration: An animal model for spinal muscular atrophy type III. Hum Mol Genet 2000; 9: 341–6

56. Strasswimmer J, Lorson CL, Breiding DE, et al. Identification of survival motor neuron as a transcriptional activator-binding protein. Hum Mol Genet 1999; 8: 1219–26

57. Pellizzoni L, Charroux B, Rappsilber J, et al. A functional interaction between the survival motor neuron complex and RNA polymerase II. J Cell Biol 2001; 152: 75–85

58. Jones KW, Gorzynski K, Hales CM, et al. Direct interaction of the spinal muscular atrophy disease protein SMN with the small nucleolar RNA-associated protein fibrillarin. J Biol Chem 2001; 276: 38645–51

59. Pellizzoni L, Baccon J, Charroux B, Dreyfuss G. The survival of motor neurons (SMN) protein interacts with the snoRNP proteins fibrillarin and GAR1. Curr Biol 2001; 11: 1079–88

60. Rossoll W, Kroning AK, Ohndorf UM, et al. Specific interaction of Smn, the spinal muscular atrophy determining gene product, with hnRNP-R and gry-rbp/hnRNP-Q: A role for Smn in RNA processing in motor axons? Hum Mol Genet 2002; 11: 93–105

61. McWhorter ML, Monani UR, Burghes AH, Beattie CE. Knockdown of the survival motor neuron (Smn) protein in zebrafish causes defects in motor axon outgrowth and pathfinding. J Cell Biol 2003; 162: 919–31

62. Rossoll W, Jablonka S, Andreassi C, et al. Smn, the spinal muscular atrophy-determining gene product, modulates axon growth and localization of beta-actin mRNA in growth cones of motoneurons. J Cell Biol 2003; 163: 801–12

63. Zerres K, Wirth B, Rudnik-Schoneborn S. Spinal muscular atrophy – clinical and genetic correlations. Neuromuscul Disord 1997; 7: 202–7

64. Rudnik-Schoneborn S, Wirth B, Rohrig D, et al. Exclusion of the gene locus for spinal muscular atrophy on chromosome 5q in a family with infantile olivopontocerebellar atrophy (OPCA) and anterior horn cell degeneration. Neuromuscul Disord 1995; 5: 19–23

65. Rudnik-Schoneborn S, Sztriha L, Aithala GR, et al. Extended phenotype of pontocerebellar hypoplasia with infantile spinal muscular atrophy. Am J Med Genet 2003; 117A: 10–17

66. Chou SM, Gilbert EF, Chun RW, et al. Infantile olivopontocerebellar atrophy with spinal muscular atrophy (infantile OPCA + SMA). Clin Neuropathol 1990; 9: 21–32

67. Burglen L, Amiel J, Viollet L, et al. Survival motor neuron gene deletion in the arthrogryposis multiplex congenita–spinal muscular atrophy association. J Clin Invest 1996; 98: 1130–2

68. Kelly TE, Amoroso K, Ferre M, et al. Spinal muscular atrophy variant with congenital fractures. Am J Med Genet 1999; 87: 65–8

69. Borochowitz Z, Glick B, Blazer S. Infantile spinal muscular atrophy (SMA) and multiple congenital bone fractures in sibs: A lethal new syndrome. J Med Genet 1991; 28: 345–8

70. Kobayashi H, Baumbach L, Matise TC, et al. A gene for a severe lethal form of X-linked arthrogryposis (X-linked infantile spinal muscular atrophy) maps to human chromosome Xp11.3–q11.2. Hum Mol Genet 1995; 4: 1213–16

71. Herva R, Leisti J, Kirkinen P, Seppanen U. A lethal autosomal recessive syndrome of multiple congenital contractures. Am J Med Genet 1985; 20: 431–9

72. Makela-Bengs P, Jarvinen N, Vuopala K, et al. Assignment of the disease locus for lethal congenital contracture syndrome to a restricted region of chromosome 9q34, by genome scan using five affected individuals. Am J Hum Genet 1998; 63: 506–16

73. Landau D, Mishori-Dery A, Hershkovitz R, et al. A new autosomal recessive congenital contractural syndrome in an Israeli Bedouin kindred. Am J Med Genet 2003; 117A: 37–40

74. Nishimura AL, Mitne-Neto M, Silva HC, et al. A mutation in the vesicle-trafficking protein VAPB causes late-onset spinal muscular atrophy and amyotrophic lateral sclerosis. Am J Hum Genet 2004; 75: 822–31

75. Rudnik-Schoneborn S, Forkert R, Hahnen E, et al. Clinical spectrum and diagnostic criteria of infantile spinal muscular atrophy: Further delineation on the basis of SMN gene deletion findings. Neuropediatrics 1996; 27: 8–15

76. Bertini E, Gadisseux JL, Palmieri G, et al. Distal infantile spinal muscular atrophy associated with paralysis of the diaphragm: A variant of infantile spinal muscular atrophy. Am J Med Genet 1989; 33: 328–35

77. Grohmann K, Wienker TF, Saar K, et al. Diaphragmatic spinal muscular atrophy with respiratory distress is heterogeneous, and one form is linked to chromosome 11q13–q21. Am J Hum Genet 1999; 65: 1459–62

78. Grohmann K, Schuelke M, Diers A, et al. Mutations in the gene encoding immunoglobulin mu-binding protein 2 cause spinal muscular atrophy with respiratory distress type 1. Nat Genet 2001; 29: 75–7

79. Cox GA, Mahaffey CL, Frankel WN. Identification of the mouse neuromuscular degeneration gene and mapping of a second site suppressor allele. Neuron 1998; 21: 1327–37

80. Grohmann K, Varon R, Stolz P, et al. Infantile spinal muscular atrophy with respiratory distress type 1 (SMARD1). Ann Neurol 2003; 54: 719–24

81. Pitt M, Houlden H, Jacobs J, et al. Severe infantile neuropathy with diaphragmatic weakness and its relationship to SMARD1. Brain 2003; 126: 2682–92

82. Zerres K, Davies KE. 59th ENMC International Workshop: Spinal Muscular Atrophies: recent progress and revised diagnostic criteria, 17–19 April 1998, Soestduinen, The Netherlands. Neuromuscul Disord 1999; 9: 272–8

83. Pearn J, Hudgson P. Distal spinal muscular atrophy. A clinical and genetic study of 8 kindreds. J Neurol Sci 1979; 43: 183–91

84. Viollet L, Barois A, Rebeiz JG, et al. Mapping of autosomal recessive chronic distal spinal muscular atrophy to chromosome 11q13. Ann Neurol 2002; 51: 585–92

85. Viollet L, Zarhrate M, Maystadt I, et al. Refined genetic mapping of autosomal recessive chronic distal spinal muscular atrophy to chromosome 11q13.3 and evidence of linkage disequilibrium in European families. Eur J Hum Genet 2004; 12: 483–8

86. Lander CM, Eadie MJ, Tyrer JH. Hereditary motor peripheral neuropathy predominantly affecting the arms. J Neurol Sci 1976; 28: 389–94

87. O'Sullivan DJ, McLeod JG. Distal chronic spinal muscular atrophy involving the hands. J Neurol Neurosurg Psychiatry 1978; 41: 653–8

88. Christodoulou K, Kyriakides T, Hristova AH, et al. Mapping of a distal form of spinal muscular atrophy with upper limb predominance to chromosome 7p. Hum Mol Genet 1995; 4: 1629–32

89. Ellsworth RE, Ionasescu V, Searby C, et al. The CMT2D locus: Refined genetic position and construction of a bacterial clone-based physical map. Genome Res 1999; 9: 568–74

90. Ionasescu V, Searby C, Sheffield VC, et al. Autosomal dominant Charcot–Marie–Tooth axonal neuropathy mapped on chromosome 7p (CMT2D). Hum Mol Genet 1996; 5: 1373–5

91. Sambuughin N, Sivakumar K, Selenge B, et al. Autosomal dominant distal spinal muscular atrophy type V (dSMA-V) and Charcot–Marie–Tooth disease type 2D (CMT2D) segregate within a single large kindred and map to a refined region on chromosome 7p15. J Neurol Sci 1998; 161: 23–8

92. Antonellis A, Ellsworth RE, Sambuughin N, et al. Glycyl tRNA synthetase mutations in Charcot–Marie–Tooth disease type 2D and distal spinal muscular atrophy type V. Am J Hum Genet 2003; 72: 1293–9

93. Auer-Grumbach M, Loscher WN, Wagner K, et al. Phenotypic and genotypic heterogeneity in hereditary motor neuronopathy type V: A clinical, electrophysiological and genetic study. Brain 2000; 123: 1612–23

94. Windpassinger C, Auer-Grumbach M, Irobi J, et al. Heterozygous missense mutations in BSCL2 are associated with distal hereditary motor neuropathy and Silver syndrome. Nat Genet 2004; 36: 271–6

95. Silver JR. Familial spastic paraplegia with amyotrophy of the hands. J Neurol Neurosurg Psychiatry 1966; 29: 135

96. van Gent EM, Hoogland RA, Jennekens FG. Distal amyotrophy of predominantly the upper limbs with pyramidal features in a large kinship. J Neurol Neurosurg Psychiatry 1985; 48: 266–9

97. Irobi J, Van den Bergh P, Merlini L, et al. The phenotype of motor neuropathies associated with BSCL2 mutations is broader than Silver syndrome and distal HMN type V. Brain 2004; 127: 2124–30

98. Harding AE, Thomas PK. Hereditary distal spinal muscular atrophy. A report on 34 cases and a review of the literature. J Neurol Sci 1980; 45: 337–48

99. Dyck PJ, Lambert EH. Lower motor and primary sensory neuron diseases with peroneal muscular atrophy. II. Neurologic, genetic, and electrophysiologic findings in various neuronal degenerations. Arch Neurol 1968; 18: 619–25

100. McLeod JG, Prineas JW. Distal type of chronic spinal muscular atrophy. Clinical, electrophysiological and pathological studies. Brain 1971; 94: 703–14

101. Timmerman V, De Jonghe P, Simokovic S, et al. Distal hereditary motor neuropathy type II (distal HMN II): mapping of a locus to chromosome 12q24. Hum Mol Genet 1996; 5: 1065–9

102. De Angelis MV, Gatta V, Stuppia L, et al. Autosomal dominant distal spinal muscular atrophy: An Italian family not linked to 12q24 and 7p14. Neuromuscul Disord 2002; 12: 26–30

103. Irobi J, Van Impe K, Seeman P, et al. Hot-spot residue in small heat-shock protein 22 causes distal motor neuropathy. Nat Genet 2004; 36: 597–601

104. Evgrafov OV, Mersiyanova I, Irobi J, et al. Mutant small heat-shock protein 27 causes axonal Charcot–Marie–Tooth disease and distal hereditary motor neuropathy. Nat Genet 2004; 36: 602–6

105. Young ID, Harper PS. Hereditary distal spinal muscular atrophy with vocal cord paralysis. J Neurol Neurosurg Psychiatry 1980; 43: 413–18

106. Pridmore C, Baraitser M, Brett EM, Harding AE. Distal spinal muscular atrophy with vocal cord paralysis. J Med Genet 1992; 29: 197–9

107. McEntagart M, Norton N, Williams H, et al. Localization of the gene for distal hereditary motor neuronopathy VII (dHMN-VII) to chromosome 2q14. Am J Hum Genet 2001; 68: 1270–6

108. Boltshauser E, Lang W, Spillmann T, Hof E. Hereditary distal muscular atrophy with vocal cord paralysis and sensorineural hearing loss: A dominant form of spinal muscular atrophy? J Med Genet 1989; 26: 105–8

109. Donaghy M, Kennett R. Varying occurrence of vocal cord paralysis in a family with autosomal dominant hereditary motor and sensory neuropathy. J Neurol 1999; 246: 552–5

110. Puls I, Jonnakuty C, LaMonte BH, et al. Mutant dynactin in motor neuron disease. Nat Genet 2003; 33: 455–6

111. Frijns CJ, Van Deutekom J, Frants RR, Jennekens FG. Dominant congenital benign spinal muscular atrophy. Muscle Nerve 1994; 17: 192–7

112. Fleury P, Hageman G. A dominantly inherited lower motor neuron disorder presenting at birth with associated arthrogryposis. J Neurol Neurosurg Psychiatry 1985; 48: 1037–48

113. Adams C, Suchowersky O, Lowry RB. Congenital autosomal dominant distal spinal muscular atrophy. Neuromuscul Disord 1998; 8: 405–8

114. van der Vleuten AJ, van Ravenswaaij-Arts CM, Frijns CJ, et al. Localisation of the gene for a dominant congenital spinal muscular atrophy predominantly affecting the lower limbs to chromosome 12q23–q24. Eur J Hum Genet 1998; 6: 376–82

115. DeLong R, Siddique T. A large New England kindred with autosomal dominant neurogenic scapuloperoneal amyotrophy with unique features. Arch Neurol 1992; 49: 905–8

116. Kaeser HE. Scapuloperoneal muscular atrophy. Brain 1965; 88: 407–18

117. Emery ES, Fenichel GM, Eng G. A spinal muscular atrophy with scapuloperoneal distribution. Arch Neurol 1968; 18: 129–33

118. Isozumi K, DeLong R, Kaplan J, et al. Linkage of scapuloperoneal spinal muscular atrophy to chromosome 12q24.1–q24.31. Hum Mol Genet 1996; 5: 1377–82

119. Wilhelmsen KC, Blake DM, Lynch T, et al. Chromosome 12-linked autosomal dominant scapuloperoneal muscular dystrophy. Ann Neurol 1996; 39: 507–20

120. Kennedy WR, Alter M, Sung JH. Progressive proximal spinal and bulbar muscular atrophy of late onset. A sex-linked recessive trait. Neurology 1968; 18: 671–80

121. Fischbeck KH, Ionasescu V, Ritter AW, et al. Localization of the gene for X-linked spinal muscular atrophy. Neurology 1986; 36: 1595–8

122. Fischbeck KH, Souders D, La Spada A. A candidate gene for X-linked spinal muscular atrophy. Adv Neurol 1991; 56: 209–13

123. La Spada AR, Wilson EM, Lubahn DB, et al. Androgen receptor gene mutations in X-linked spinal and bulbar muscular atrophy. Nature 1991; 352: 77–9

124. La Spada AR, Roling DB, Harding AE, et al. Meiotic stability and genotype–phenotype correlation of the trinucleotide repeat in X-linked spinal and bulbar muscular atrophy. Nat Genet 1992; 2: 301–4

125. Doyu M, Sobue G, Mukai E, et al. Severity of X-linked recessive bulbospinal neuronopathy correlates with size of the tandem CAG repeat in androgen receptor gene. Ann Neurol 1992; 32: 707–10

126. Igarashi S, Tanno Y, Onodera O, et al. Strong correlation between the number of CAG repeats in androgen receptor genes and the clinical onset of features of spinal and bulbar muscular atrophy. Neurology 1992; 42: 2300–2

127. Kaneko K, Igarashi S, Miyatake T, Tsuji S. 'Essential tremor' and CAG repeats in the androgen receptor gene. Neurology 1993; 43: 1618–19

128. Kaneko K, Igarashi S, Miyatake T, Tsuji S. Hypertrophic cardiomyopathy and increased number of CAG repeats in the androgen receptor gene. Am Heart J 1993; 126: 248–9

129. Doyu M, Sobue G, Mitsuma T, et al. Very late onset X-linked recessive bulbospinal neuronopathy: Mild

clinical features and a mild increase in the size of tandem CAG repeat in androgen receptor gene. J Neurol Neurosurg Psychiatry 1993; 56: 832–3

130. Zoghbi HY, Orr HT. Glutamine repeats and neurodegeneration. Annu Rev Neurosci 2000; 23: 217–47

131. Lieberman AP, Harmison G, Strand AD, et al. Altered transcriptional regulation in cells expressing the expanded polyglutamine androgen receptor. Hum Mol Genet 2002; 11: 1967–76

132. Mhatre AN, Trifiro MA, Kaufman M, et al. Reduced transcriptional regulatory competence of the androgen receptor in X-linked spinal and bulbar muscular atrophy. Nat Genet 1993; 5: 184–8

133. Ordway JM, Tallaksen-Greene S, Gutekunst CA, et al. Ectopically expressed CAG repeats cause intranuclear inclusions and a progressive late onset neurological phenotype in the mouse. Cell 1997; 91: 753–63

134. Merry DE, Kobayashi Y, Bailey CK, et al. Cleavage, aggregation and toxicity of the expanded androgen receptor in spinal and bulbar muscular atrophy. Hum Mol Genet 1998; 7: 693–701

135. Bingham PM, Scott MO, Wang S, et al. Stability of an expanded trinucleotide repeat in the androgen receptor gene in transgenic mice. Nat Genet 1995; 9: 191–6

136. La Spada AR, Peterson KR, Meadows SA, et al. Androgen receptor YAC transgenic mice carrying CAG 45 alleles show trinucleotide repeat instability. Hum Mol Genet 1998; 7: 959–67

137. Abel A, Walcott J, Woods J, et al. Expression of expanded repeat androgen receptor produces neurologic disease in transgenic mice. Hum Mol Genet 2001; 10: 107–16

138. Adachi H, Kume A, Li M, et al. Transgenic mice with an expanded CAG repeat controlled by the human AR promoter show polyglutamine nuclear inclusions and neuronal dysfunction without neuronal cell death. Hum Mol Genet 2001; 10: 1039–48

139. Katsuno M, Adachi H, Kume A, et al. Testosterone reduction prevents phenotypic expression in a transgenic mouse model of spinal and bulbar muscular atrophy. Neuron 2002; 35: 843–54

140. Takeyama K, Ito S, Yamamoto A, et al. Androgen-dependent neurodegeneration by polyglutamine-expanded human androgen receptor in Drosophila. Neuron 2002; 35: 855–64

141. Sobue G, Doyu M, Kachi T, et al. Subclinical phenotypic expressions in heterozygous females of X-linked recessive bulbospinal neuronopathy. J Neurol Sci 1993; 117: 74–8

142. Meriggioli MN, Rowin J, Sanders DB. Distinguishing clinical and electrodiagnostic features of X-linked bulbospinal neuronopathy. Muscle Nerve 1999; 22: 1693–7

143. Mariotti C, Castellotti B, Pareyson D, et al. Phenotypic manifestations associated with CAG-repeat expansion in the androgen receptor gene in male patients and heterozygous females: A clinical and molecular study of 30 families. Neuromuscul Disord 2000; 10: 391–7

144. Ishihara H, Kanda F, Nishio H, et al. Clinical features and skewed X-chromosome inactivation in female carriers of X-linked recessive spinal and bulbar muscular atrophy. J Neurol 2001; 248: 856–60

145. Schmidt BJ, Greenberg CR, Allingham-Hawkins DJ, Spriggs EL. Expression of X-linked bulbospinal muscular atrophy (Kennedy disease) in two homozygous women. Neurology 2002; 59: 770–2

146. Li M, Miwa S, Kobayashi Y, et al. Nuclear inclusions of the androgen receptor protein in spinal and bulbar muscular atrophy. Ann Neurol 1998; 44: 249–54

147. Li M, Nakagomi Y, Kobayashi Y, et al. Nonneural nuclear inclusions of androgen receptor protein in spinal and bulbar muscular atrophy. Am J Pathol 1998; 153: 695–701

148. Wood JD, Beaujeux TP, Shaw PJ. Protein aggregation in motor neurone disorders. Neuropathol Appl Neurobiol 2003; 29: 529–45

149. Scherzinger E, Lurz R, Turmaine M, et al. Huntingtin-encoded polyglutamine expansions form amyloid-like protein aggregates in vitro and in vivo. Cell 1997; 90: 549–58

150. Scherzinger E, Sittler A, Schweiger K, et al. Self-assembly of polyglutamine-containing huntingtin fragments into amyloid-like fibrils: implications for Huntington's disease pathology. Proc Natl Acad Sci USA 1999; 96: 4604–9

151. Bence NF, Sampat RM, Kopito RR. Impairment of the ubiquitin–proteasome system by protein aggregation. Science 2001; 292: 1552–5

152. Lin X, Antalffy B, Kang D, et al. Polyglutamine expansion down-regulates specific neuronal genes before pathologic changes in SCA1. Nat Neurosci 2000; 3: 157–63

153. Luthi-Carter R, Strand A, Peters NL, et al. Decreased expression of striatal signaling genes in a

mouse model of Huntington's disease. Hum Mol Genet 2000; 9: 1259–71

154. McCampbell A, Taylor JP, Taye AA, et al. CREB-binding protein sequestration by expanded polyglutamine. Hum Mol Genet 2000; 9: 2197–202

155. Bonni A, Brunet A, West AE, et al. Cell survival promoted by the Ras-MAPK signaling pathway by transcription-dependent and -independent mechanisms. Science 1999; 286: 1358–62

156. Riccio A, Ahn S, Davenport CM, et al. Mediation by a CREB family transcription factor of NGF-dependent survival of sympathetic neurons. Science 1999; 286: 2358–61

157. Steffan JS, Bodai L, Pallos J, et al. Histone deacetylase inhibitors arrest polyglutamine-dependent neurodegeneration in Drosophila. Nature 2001; 413: 739–43

158. McCampbell A, Taye AA, Whitty L, et al. Histone deacetylase inhibitors reduce polyglutamine toxicity. Proc Natl Acad Sci USA 2001; 98: 15179–84

159. Piccioni F, Pinton P, Simeoni S, et al. Androgen receptor with elongated polyglutamine tract forms aggregates that alter axonal trafficking and mitochondrial distribution in motor neuronal processes. FASEB J 2002; 16: 1418–20

160. Harding AE. Hereditary 'pure' spastic paraplegia: A clinical and genetic study of 22 families. J Neurol Neurosurg Psychiatry 1981; 44: 871–83

161. Polo JM, Calleja J, Combarros O, Berciano J. Hereditary 'pure' spastic paraplegia: A study of nine families. J Neurol Neurosurg Psychiatry 1993; 56: 175–81

162. Schady W, Sheard A. A quantitative study of sensory function in hereditary spastic paraplegia. Brain 1990; 113: 709–20

163. White KD, Ince PG, Cookson M, et al. Clinical and pathological findings in hereditary spastic paraparesis with spastin mutation. Neurology 2000; 55: 89–94

164. Webb S, Coleman D, Byrne P, et al. Autosomal dominant hereditary spastic paraparesis with cognitive loss linked to chromosome 2p. Brain 1998; 121: 601–9

165. Heinzlef O, Paternotte C, Mahieux F, et al. Mapping of a complicated familial spastic paraplegia to a locus SPG4 on chromosome 2p. J Med Genet 1998; 35: 89–93

166. Seri M, Cusano R, Forabosco P, et al. Genetic mapping to 10q23.3-q24.2, in a large Italian pedigree, of a new syndrome showing bilateral cataracts, gas-troesophageal reflux, and spastic paraparesis with amyotrophy. Am J Hum Genet 1999; 64: 586–93

167. Hughes CA, Byrne PC, Webb S, et al. SPG15, a new locus for autosomal recessive complicated HSP on chromosome 14q. Neurology 2001; 56: 1230–3

168. Murillo F, Kobayashi H, Pegoraro E, et al. Genetic localization of a new locus for recessive familial spastic paraparesis to 15q13–15. Neurology 1999; 53: 50–6

169. Vazza G, Zortea M, Boaretto F, et al. A new locus for autosomal recessive spastic paraplegia associated with mental retardation and distal motor neuropathy, SPG14, maps to chromosome 3q27–q28. Am J Hum Genet 2000; 67: 504–9

170. Patel H, Hart PE, Warner TT, et al. The Silver syndrome variant of hereditary spastic paraparesis maps to chromosome 11q12–q14, with evidence for genetic heterogeneity within this subtype. Am J Hum Genet 2001; 69: 209–15

171. Patel H, Cross H, Proukakis C, et al. SPG20 is mutated in Troyer syndrome, an hereditary spastic paraplegia. Nat Genet 2002; 31: 347–8

172. Gigli GL, Diomedi M, Bernardi G, et al. Spastic paraplegia, epilepsy and mental retardation in several members of a family: a novel genetic disorder. Am J Med Genet 1993; 45: 711–16

173. Sommerfelt K, Kyllerman M, Sanner G. Hereditary spastic paraplegia with epileptic myoclonus. Acta Neurol Scand 1991; 84: 157–60

174. Webb S, Flanagan N, Callaghan N, Hutchinson M. A family with spastic paraparesis and epilepsy. Epilepsia 1997; 38: 495–9

175. Yih JS, Wang S-J, Su M-S, et al. Hereditary spastic paraplegia associated with epilepsy, mental retardation and hearing impairment. Paraplegia 1993; 31: 408–11

176. Mead SH, Proukakis C, Wood N, et al. A large family with hereditary spastic paraparesis due to a frame shift mutation of spastin (SPG4) gene: Association with multiple sclerosis in two affected siblings and epilepsy in other affected family members. J Neurol Neurosurg Psychiatry 2001; 71: 788–91

177. Fonknechten N, Mavel D, Byrne P, et al. Spectrum of SPG4 mutations in autosomal dominant spastic paraplegia. Hum Mol Genet 2000; 9: 637–44

178. Worster-Drought C, Greenfield JG, McMenemy W. A form of familial presenile dementia with spastic paralysis. Brain 1944; 67: 38–43

179. Manson J. Hereditary spastic paraplegia with ataxia and mental defect. Br Med J 1920; ii: 477

180. Sutherland JM. Familial spastic paraplegia. Its relation to mental and cardiac abnormalities. Lancet 1957; 2: 169–70

181. Cross HE, McKusick VA. The Mast syndrome: A recessively inherited form of pre-senile dementia with motor disturbances. Arch Neurol 1967; 16: 1–13

182. Arjundas G, Ramamurthi B, Chettur L. Familial spastic paraplegia (A review with four case reports). J Assoc Physicians India 1971; 19: 653–7

183. Pridmore S, Rao G, Abusah P. Hereditary spastic paraplegia with dementia. Aust NZ J Psychiatry 1995; 29: 678–82

184. Rothner AD, Yahr F, Yahr MD. Familial spastic paraparesis, optic atrophy and dementia: Clinical observations of affected kindred. NY State J Med 1976; 76: 756–8

185. Byrne PC, McMonagle P, Webb S, et al. Age-related cognitive decline in hereditary spastic paraparesis linked to chromosome 2p. Neurology 2000; 54: 1510–17

186. McMonagle P, Byrne PC, Fitzgerald B, et al. Phenotype of AD-HSP due to mutations in the SPAST gene. Comparison with AD-HSP without mutations. Neurology 2000; 55: 1794–800

187. Reid E, Grayson C, Rubinsztein DC, et al. Subclinical cognitive impairment in autosomal dominant 'pure' hereditary spastic paraplegia. J Med Genet 1999; 36: 797–8

188. Tedeschi G, Allocca S, Di Costanzo A, et al. Multisystem involvement of the central nervous system in Strumpell's disease. J Neurol Sci 1991; 103: 55–60

189. Harding AE, Thomas PK. Peroneal muscular atrophy with pyramidal features. J Neurol Neurosurg Psychiatry 1984; 47: 168–72

190. Mostacciuolo ML, Rampoldi L, Righetti E, et al. Hereditary spastic paraplegia associated with peripheral neuropathy: A distinct clinical and genetic entity. Neuromuscul Disord 2000; 10: 497–502

191. Cross HE, McKusick VA. The Troyer syndrome. A recessive form of spastic paraplegia with distal muscle wasting. Arch Neurol 1967; 16: 473–85

192. Harding AE. Hereditary spastic paraplegias. Semin Neurol 1993; 13: 333–6

193. Neuhauser G, Wiffler C, Opitz JM. Familial spastic paraplegia with distal muscle wasting in the Old Order Amish: Atypical Troyer syndrome or 'new' syndrome. Clin Genet 1976; 9: 315–23

194. Farag TI, El-Badramany MH, Al-Sharkawy S. Troyer syndrome: Report of the first 'non Amish'

195. Auer-Grumbach M, Fazekas F, Radner H, et al. Troyer syndrome: A combination of central brain abnormality and motor neuron disease? J Neurol 1999; 246: 556–61

196. Bouchard JP, Barbeau A, Bouchard R, Bouchard RW. Autosomal recessive spastic ataxia of Charlevoix–Saguenay. Can J Neurol Sci 1978; 5: 61

197. Bruyn RPM, Scheltens P. Autosomal recessive paraparesis with amyotrophy of the hands and feet. Acta Neurol Scand 1993; 87: 443–5

198. Cavanagh NPC, Eames RA, Galvin RJ, et al. Hereditary sensory neuropathy with spastic paraplegia. Brain 1979; 102: 79–94

199. Khalifeh RR, Zellweger H. Hereditary sensory neuropathy with spinal cord disease. Neurology 1963; 13: 406–11

200. Koenig RH, Spiro AJ. Hereditary spastic paraparesis with sensory neuropathy. Dev Med Child Neurol 1970; 12: 576–81

201. Schady W, Smith CML. Sensory neuropathy in hereditary spastic paraplegia. J Neurol Neurosurg Psychiatry 1994; 57: 693–8

202. Bruyn RPM, Scheltens P. Hereditary spastic paraparesis (Strümpell–Lorrain). In: de Jong JMBV, Vinken P, Bruyn RPM, Klawans H, eds. Handbook of Clinical Neurology. Amsterdam: Elsevier, 1991; 301–18

203. Strümpell A. Ueber eine bestimmte Form der primaren combinierten Systemerkrankung des Ruckenmarks. Arch Psychiatr Nervenkr 1886; 17: 217–38

204. Sack GH, Huether CA, Garg N. Familial spastic paraplegia – clinical and pathologic studies in a large kindred. Johns Hopkins Med J 1978; 143: 117–21

205. Schwartz G. Hereditary (familial) spastic paraplegia. Arch Neurol Psychiatry 1952; 68: 655–82

206. Schwartz G, Liu C. Hereditary (familial) spastic paraplegia: Further clinical and pathologic observations. Arch Neurol Psychiatry 1956; 75: 144–62

207. Reid E. Science in motion: Common molecular pathological themes emerge in the hereditary spastic paraplegias. J Med Genet 2003; 40: 81–6

208. Wharton SB, McDermott CJ, Grierson AJJ, et al. The cellular and molecular pathology of the motor system in hereditary spastic paraparesis due to mutation of the spastin gene. J Neuropathol Exp Neurol 2003; 62: 1166–77

209. Ferrer I, Olive M, Rivera R, et al. Hereditary spastic paraparesis with dementia, amyotrophy and

sibship and review. Am J Med Genet 1994; 53: 383–5

peripheral neuropathy. A neuropathological study. Neuropath Appl Neurobiol 1995; 21: 255–61

210. Casari G, De Fusco M, Ciarmatori S, et al. Spastic paraplegia and OXPHOS impairment caused by mutations in paraplegin, a nuclear-encoded mitochondrial metalloprotease. Cell 1998; 93: 973–83

211. McDermott CJ, Dayaratne RK, Tomkins J, et al. Paraplegin gene analysis in hereditary spastic paraparesis (HSP) pedigrees in north east England. Neurology 2001; 56: 467–71

212. Hedera P, DiMauro S, Bonilla E, et al. Phenotypic analysis of autosomal dominant hereditary spastic paraplegia linked to chromosome 8q. Neurology 1999; 53: 44–9

213. McDermott CJ, Taylor RW, Hayes C, et al. Investigation of mitochondrial function in hereditary spastic paraparesis. Neuroreport 2003; 14: 485–8

214. Casali C, Valente EM, Bertini E, et al. Clinical and genetic studies in hereditary spastic paraplegia with thin corpus callosum. Neurology 2004; 62: 262–8

215. Nielsen JE, Krabbe K, Jennum P, et al. Autosomal dominant pure spastic paraplegia: A clinical, paraclinical and genetic study. J Neurol Neurosurg Psychiatry 1998; 64: 61–6

216. Ormerod IEC, Harding AE, Miller DH, et al. Magnetic resonance imaging in degenerative ataxic disorders. J Neurol Neurosurg Psychiatry 1994; 57: 51–7

217. Schady W, Dick JPR, Sheard A, Crampton S. Central motor conduction studies in hereditary spastic paraplegia. J Neurol Neurosurg Psychiatry 1991; 54: 775–9

218. Mcleod JG, Morgan JA, Reye C. Electrophysiological studies in familial spastic paraplegia. J Neurol Neurosurg Psychiatry 1977; 40: 611–15

219. Thomas PK, Jefferys JGR, Smith IS, Loulakakis D. Spinal somatosensory evoked potentials in hereditary spastic paraplegia. J Neurol Neurosurg Psychiatry 1981; 44: 243–6

220. Sjaastad O, Berstad J, Gjesdahl P, Gjessing L. Homocarsinosis. 2. A familial metabolic disorder associated with spastic paraplegia, progressive mental deficiency, and retinal pigmentation. Acta Neurol Scand 1976; 53: 275–90

221. Claus D, Waddy HM, Harding AE, et al. Hereditary motor and sensory neuropathies and hereditary spastic paraplegia: A magnetic stimulation study. Ann Neurol 1990; 28: 43–9

222. Pelosi L, Lanzillo B, Perretti A, et al. Motor and somatosensory evoked potentials in hereditary spastic paraplegia. J Neurol Neurosurg Psychiatry 1991; 54: 1099–102

223. Aalfs CM, Koelman JHTM, Posthumus Meyjes FE, Ongerboer de Visser BW. Posterior tibial and sural nerve somatosensory evoked potentials: A study in spastic paraparesis and spinal cord lesions. Electroencephalogr Clin Neurophysiol 1993; 89: 437–41

224. Lindsey JC, Lusher ME, McDermott CJ, et al. Mutation analysis of the spastin gene (SPG4) in patients with hereditary spastic paraparesis. J Med Genet 2000; 37: 759–65

225. Zhao X, Alvarado D, Rainier S, et al. Mutations in a newly identified GTPase gene cause autosomal dominant hereditary spastic paraplegia. Nat Genet 2001; 29: 326–31

226. Hazan J, Fonknechten N, Mavel D, et al. Spastin, a novel AAA protein, is altered in the most frequent form of autosomal dominant spastic paraplegia. Nat Genet 1999; 23: 296–303

227. Rainier S, Chai J-H, Tokarz D, et al. NIPA1 gene mutations cause autosomal dominant hereditary spastic paraplegia (SPG6). Am J Hum Genet 2003; 73: 967–71

228. Reid E, Kloos M, Ashley-Koch A, et al. A kinesin heavy chain (KIF5A) mutation in hereditary spastic paraplegis (SPG10). Am J Hum Genet 2002; 71: 1189–94

229. Hansen JJ, Durr A, Cournu-Rebeix I, et al. Hereditary spastic paraplegia SPG13 is associated with a mutation in the gene encoding the mitochondrial chaperonin Hsp60. Am J Hum Genet 2002; 70: 1328–32

230. Fink JK, Wu C-tB, Jones SM, et al. Autosomal dominant familial spastic paraplegia: Tight linkage to chromosome 15q. Am J Hum Genet 1995; 56: 188–92

231. Hedera P, Rainer S, Alvarado D, et al. Novel locus for autosomal dominant hereditary spastic paraplegia, on chromosome 8q. Am J Hum Genet 1999; 64: 563–9

232. Reid E, Dearlove M, Rhodes M, Rubinsztein DC. A new locus for autosomal dominant 'pure' hereditary spastic paraplegia mapping to chromosome 12q13, and evidence for further genetic heterogeneity. Am J Hum Genet 1999; 65: 757–63

233. Reid E, Dearlove AM, Osborn O, et al. A locus for autosomal dominant 'pure' hereditary spastic paraplegia maps to chromosome 19q13. Am J Hum Genet 2000; 66: 728–32

234. Valente EM, Brancati F, Caputo V, et al. Novel locus for autosomal dominant pure hereditary spas-

tic paraplegia (SPG19) maps to chromosome 9q33–q34. Ann Neurol 2002; 51: 681–5

235. Tessa A, Casali C, Damiano M, et al. SPG3A: An additional family carrying a new atlastin mutation. Neurology 2002; 59: 2002–5

236. Dalpozzo F, Rossetto MG, Boaretto F, et al. Infancy onset hereditary spastic paraplegia associated with a novel atlastin mutation. Neurology 2003; 61: 580–1

237. Sauter SM, Engel W, Neumann LM, et al. Novel mutations in the atlastin gene (SPG3A) in families with autosomal dominant hereditary spastic paraplegia and evidence of late onset forms of HSP linked to the SPG3A locus. Hum Mutat 2004; 98: 1–7

238. Wilkinson PA, Hart PE, Patel H, et al. SPG3A mutation screening in English families with early onset autosomal dominant hereditary spastic paraplegia. J Neurol Sci 2003; 216: 43–5

239. D'Amico A, Tessa A, Sabino A, et al. Incomplete penetrance in an SPG3A-linked family with a new mutation in the atlastin gene. Neurology 2004; 62: 2138–9

240. Muglia M, Magariello A, Nicoletti G, et al. Further evidence that SPG3A gene mutations cause autosomal dominant hereditary spastic paraplegia. Ann Neurol 2002; 51: 794–5

241. Zhu PP, Patterson A, Lavoie B, et al. Cellular localisation, oligomerization, and membranous association of the hereditary spastic paraplegia (SPG3A) protein atlastin. J Biol Chem 2003; 278: 49063–71

242. Sever S, Muhlberg AB, Schmid SL. Impairment of dynamin's GAP domain stimulates receptor-mediated endocytosis. Nature 1999; 398: 481–6

243. Nicoziani P, Vilhardt F, Llorente A, et al. Role for dynamin in late endosome dynamics and trafficking of the cation-independent mannose 6-phosphate receptor. Mol Biol Cell 2000; 11: 481–95

244. Jones SM, Howell KE, Henley JR, et al. Role of dynamin in the formation of transport vesicles from the trans-Golgi network. Science 1998; 279: 573–7

245. Pitts KR, Yoon Y, Krueger EW, McNiven MA. The dynamin-like protein DLP1 is essential for normal distribution and morphology of the endoplasmic reticulum and mitochondria in mammalian cells. Mol Biol Cell 1999; 10: 4403–17

246. Ochoa GC, Slepnev VI, Neff L, et al. A functional link between dynamin and the actin cytoskeleton at podosomes. J Cell Biol 2000; 150: 377–89

247. Namekawa M, Takiyama Y, Sakoe K, et al. A large Japanese SPG4 family with a novel insertion mutation of the SPG4 gene: A clinical and genetic study. J Neurol Sci 2001; 185: 63–8

248. Morita M, Ho M, Hosler BA, et al. A novel mutation in the spastin gene in a family with spastic paraplegia. Neurosci Lett 2002; 325: 57–61

249. Scott WK, Gaskell PC, Lennon F, et al. Locus heterogeneity, anticipation and reduction of the chromosome 2p minimal candidate region in autosomal dominant familial spastic paraplegia. Neurogenetics 1997; 1: 95–102

250. Meijer IA, Hand CK, Cossette P, et al. Spectrum of SPG4 mutations in a large collection of North American families with hereditary spastic paraplegia. Arch Neurol 2002; 59: 281–6

251. McMonagle P, Byrne P, Hutchinson M. Further evidence of dementia in SPG4-linked autosomal dominant hereditary spastic paraplegia. Neurology 2004; 62: 407–10

252. Bantel A, McWilliams S, Auysh D, et al. Novel mutation of the spastin gene in familial spastic paraplegia. Clin Genet 2001; 59: 364–5

253. Higgins JJ, Loveless JM, Goswami S, et al. An atypical intronic deletion widens the spectrum of mutations in hereditary spastic paraplegia. Neurology 2001; 56: 1482–5

254. Hentati A, Deng H-X, Zhai H, et al. Novel mutations in spastin gene and absence of correlation with age at onset of symptoms. Neurology 2000; 55: 1388–90

255. Patel S, Latterich M. The AAA team: Related ATPases with diverse functions. Cell Biol 1998; 8: 65–71

256. Ciccarelli FD, Proukakis C, Patel H, et al. The identification of a conserved domain in both spartin and spastin, mutated in hereditary spastic paraplegia. Genomics 2003; 81: 437–41

257. Beetz C, Brodhun M, Moutzouris K, et al. Identification of nuclear localisation sequences in spastin (SPG4) using a novel tetra-GFP reporter system. Biochem Biophys Res Commun 2004; 318: 1079–84

258. Errico A, Ballabio A, Rugarli EI. Spastin, the protein mutated in autosomal dominant hereditary spastic paraplegia, is involved in microtubule dynamics. Hum Mol Genet 2002; 11: 153–63

259. McDermott CJ, Grierson AJ, Wood JD, et al. Hereditary spastic paraparesis: evidence of disrupted intracellular transport associated with spastin mutation. Ann Neurol 2003; 54: 748–59

260. Charvin D, Cifuentes-Diaz C, Fonknechten N, et al. Mutations of SPG4 are responsible for a loss of function of spastin, an abundant neuronal protein localized in the nucleus. Hum Mol Genet 2003; 12: 71–8

261. Molon A, Di Giovanni S, Chen YW, et al. Large-scale disruption of microtubule pathways in morphologically normal human spastin muscle. Neurology 2004; 62: 1097–104

262. Trotta N, Orso G, Rossetto MG, et al. The hereditary spastic paraplegia gene, spastin, regulates microtubule stability to modulate synaptic structure and function. Curr Biol 2004; 14: 1135–47

263. Errico A, Claudiani P, D'Addio M, Rugarli EI. Spastin interacts with the centrosomal protein NA14, and is enriched in the spindle pole, the midbody and the distal axon. Hum Mol Genet 2004; 13: 2121–32

264. Hirokawa N. Kinesin and dynein superfamily proteins and the mechanism of organelle transport. Science 1998; 279: 519–26

265. Hoyt MA, He L, Totis L, Saunders WS. Loss of function of Saccharomyces cerevisiae kinesin-related CIN8 and KIP1 is supressed by KAR3 motor domain mutations. Genetics 1993; 135: 35–44

266. Hurd DD, Saxton WM. Kinesin mutations cause motor neuron disease phenotypes by disrupting fast axonal transport in Drosophila. Genetics 1996; 144; 1075–85

267. Fichera M, Lo Giudice M, Flaco M, et al. Evidence of kinesin heavy chain (KIF5A) involvement in pure hereditary spastic paraplegia. Neurology 2004; 63: 1108–10

268. Zhao Q, Wang J, Levichkin IV, et al. A mitochondrial specific stress response in mammalian cells. EMBO J 2002; 21: 4411–19

269. Warner TT, Patel H, Proukakis C, et al. A clinical, genetic and cadidate gene study of Silver syndrome, a complicated form of hereditary spastic paraplegia. J Neurol 2004; 251: 1068–74

270. Magre J, Delepine M, Khallouf E, et al. Identification of the gene altered in Berardinelli–Seip congenital lipodystrophy on chromosome 11q13. Nat Genet 2001; 28: 365–70

271. Agarwal AK, Garg A. Seipin: A mysterious protein. Trends Mol Med 2004; 10: 440–4

272. Slavotinek AM, Pike M, Mills K, Hurst JA. Cataracts, motor system disorder, short stature, learning difficulties, and skeletal abnormalities: A new syndrome? Am J Med Genet 1996; 62: 42–7

273. Nigro CL, Cusano R, Scaranari M, et al. A refined physical and transcriptional map of the SPG9 locus on 10q23.3–q24.2. Eur J Hum Genet 2000; 8: 777–82

274. Casari G, De Fusco M, Ciarmatori S, et al. Spastic paraplegia and OXPHOS impairment caused by mutations in paraplegin, a nuclear-encoded mitochondrial metalloprotease. Cell 1998; 93: 973–83

275. Simpson MA, Cross H, Proukakis C, et al. Maspardin is mutated in Mast syndrome, a complicated form of hereditary spastic paraplegia associated with dementia. Am J Hum Genet 2003; 73: 1147–56

276. Tauer R, Mannhaupt G, Schnall R, et al. Yta10p, a member of a novel ATPase family in yeast, is essential for mitochondrial function. FEBS Lett 1994; 353: 197–200

277. Tzagoloff A, Yue J, Jang J, Paul M-F. A new member of a family of ATPases is essential for assembly of mitochondrial respiratory chain and ATP synthetase complexes in Saccharomyces cerevisiae. Mol Cell Biol 1994; 13: 5418–26

278. Paul M-F, Tzagoloff A. Mutations in RCA1 and AFG3 inhibit F1-ATPase assembly in Saccharomyces cerevisiae. FEBS Lett 1995; 373: 66–70

279. Langer T, Neupert W. Regulated protein degradation in mitochondria. Experimentia 1996; 52: 1069–76

280. Rep M, Grivell LA. The role of protein degradation in mitochondrial function and biogenesis. Curr Genet 1996; 30: 367–80

281. Ferreirinha F, Quattrini A, Pirozzi M, et al. Axonal degeneration in paraplegin-deficient mice is associated with abnormal mitochondria and impairment of axonal transport. J Clin Invest 2004; 113: 231–42

282. Atorino L, Sivestri L, Koppen M, et al. Loss of m-AAA protease in mitochondria causes complex 1 deficiency and increased sensitivity to oxidative stress in hereditary spastic paraplegia. J Cell Biol 2003; 163: 777–87

283. Piemonte F, Casali C, Carrozzo R, et al. Respiratory chain defects in hereditary spastic paraplegias. Neuromuscul Disord 2001; 11: 565–9

284. Proukakis C, Cross H, Patel H, et al. Troyer syndrome revisited. A clinical and radiological study of a complicated hereditary paraplegia. J Neurol 2004; 251: 1105–10

285. Crosby AH, Proukakis C. Is the transportation highway the right road for hereditary spastic paraplegia. Am J Hum Genet 2002; 71: 1009–16

286. Zeitlmann L, Sirim P, Kremmer E, Kolanus W. Cloning of ACP33 as a novel intracellular ligand of CD4. J Biol Chem 2001; 276: 9123–32

287. Tamagaki A, Shima M, Tomita R, et al. Segregation of a pure form of spastic paraplegia and NOR insertion into Xq11.2. Am J Med Genet 2000; 94: 5–8

288. Steinmuller R, Lantigua-Cruz A, Garcia-Garcia R, et al. Evidence of a third locus in X-linked recessive paraplegia. Hum Genet 1997; 100: 287–9

289. Claes S, Devriendt K, Van Goethem G, et al. Novel syndromic form of X-linked complicated spastic paraplegia. Am J Med Genet 2000; 94: 1–4

290. Jouet M, Rosenthal A, Armstrong G, et al. X-linked spastic paraplegia (SPG1), MASA syndrome and X-linked hydrocephalus result from mutations in the L1 gene. Nat Genet 1994; 7: 402–7

291. Kenwrick S, Ionasescu V, Ionasescu G, et al. Linkage studies of X-linked recessive spastic paraplegia using DNA probes. Hum Genet 1986; 73: 264–6

292. Fransen E, Lemmon V, Van Camp G, et al. CRASH syndrome: Clinical spectrum of corpus callosum hypoplasia, retardation, adducted thumbs, spastic paraparesis and hydrocephalus due to mutations in one single gene, L1. Eur J Hum Genet 1995; 3: 273–84

293. Joosten EA, Gribnau AA. Immunological localization of cell adhesion molecule L1 in developing rat pyramidal tract. Neurosci Lett 1998; 100: 94–8

294. Brummendorf T, Rathjen FG. Structure/function relationships of axon-associated adhesion receptors of the immunoglobulin superfamily. Curr Opin Neurobiol 1996; 6: 584–93

295. Dahme M, Bartsch U, Martini R, et al. Disruption of the mouse L1 gene leads to malformations of the nervous system. Nat Genet 1997; 17: 346–9

296. Cohen NR, Taylor JS, Scott LB, et al. Errors in corticospinal axon guidance in mice lacking the neural cell adhesion molecule L1. Curr Biol 1997; 8: 26–33

297. Fransen E, D'Hooge R, Van Camp G, et al. L1 knockout mice show dilated ventricles, vermis hypoplasia and impaired exploration patterns. Hum Mol Genet 1998; 7: 999–1099

298. Demyanenko GP, Tsai AY, Maness PF. Abnormalities in neuronal process extension, hippocampal development, and the ventricular system of L1 knockout mice. J Neurosci 1999; 19: 4907–20

299. Castellani V, Chedotal A, Schachner M, et al. Analysis of the L1-deficient mouse phenotype reveals cross-talk between Sema3A and L1 signaling pathways in axonal guidance. Neuron 2000; 27: 237–49

300. Saugier-Veber P, Munnich A, Bonneau D, et al. X-linked spastic paraplegia and Pelizaeus–Merzbacher disease are allelic disorders at the proteolipid protein locus. Nat Genet 1994; 6: 257–61

301. Johnson AW, McKusick VA. A sex-linked recessive form of spastic paraplegia. Am J Hum Genet 1962; 14: 83–94

302. Cambi F, Tang X-M, Cordray P, et al. Refined genetic mapping and proteolipid protein mutation analysis in X-linked pure hereditary spastic paraplegia. Neurology 1996; 46: 1112–17

303. Keppen LD, Leppert MF, O'Connel P, et al. Etiological heterogeneity in X-linked spastic paraplegia. Am J Hum Genet 1987; 41: 933–43

304. Bonneau D, Rozet J-M, Bulteau C, et al. X-linked spastic paraplegia (SPG2): Clinical heterogeneity at a single locus. J Med Genet 1993; 30: 381–4

305. Goldblatt J, Ballo R, Sachs B, Moosa A. X-linked spastic paraplegia: Evidence for homogeneity with a variable phenotype. Clin Genet 1989; 35: 116–20

306. Griffiths I, Klugmann M, Anderson T, et al. Current concepts of PLP and its role in the nervous system. Microsc Res Tech 1998; 41: 344–58

307. Boison D, Stoffel W. Disruption of the compacted myelin sheets of axons of the central nervous system in proteolipid protein-deficient mice. Proc Natl Acad Sci USA 1994; 91: 11709–13

308. Klugmann M, Schwab MH, Puhlhofer A, et al. Assembly of CNS myelin in the absence of proteolipid protein. Neuron 1997; 18: 59–70

309. Griffiths I, Klugmann M, Anderson T, et al. Axonal swellings and degeneration in mice lacking the major proteolipid of myelin. Science 1998; 280: 1610–13

310. Edgar JM, McLaughlin M, Yool D, et al. Oligodendroglial modulation of fast axonal transport in a mouse model of hereditary spastic paraplegia. J Cell Biol 2004; 166: 121–31

311. Chen YZ, Bennett CL, Huynh HM, et al. DNA/RNA helicase gene mutations in a form of juvenile amyotrophic lateral sclerosis (ALS4). Am J Hum Genet 2004; 74: 1128–35

9

Amyotrophic lateral sclerosis genetics with Mendelian inheritance

Peter M Andersen

INTRODUCTION

Familial amyotrophic lateral sclerosis (FALS) is today recognized as being a syndrome with considerable clinical and genetic heterogeneity, with ill-defined overlaps with other motor syndromes such as primary lateral sclerosis (PLS) and hereditary spastic paraparesis (HSP)/SPGs with only upper motor neuron (UMN) pathology, and progressive muscular atrophy (PMA), hereditary motor neuropathy (HMN) and Charcot–Marie–Tooth syndrome (CMT) with only lower motor neuron (LMN) or axonal pathology and occasional sensory or autonomic features (Figure 9.1). This chapter deals with the four genes known to cause Mendelian inherited amyotrophic lateral sclerosis (ALS). Non-Mendelian inherited ALS is described in Chapter 10, and the genetics of other familial motor neuron diseases in Chapter 8.

The first recorded case of familial amyotrophic lateral sclerosis

More than 20 years before J-M Charcot and A Joffroy coined the term amyotrophic lateral sclerosis in 1869 and 1873, F-A Aran published 11 cases of what he called 'progressive muscular atrophy'[1–3]. Case 7 was particularly interesting. A 43-year-old sea captain presented with cramps in the muscles of the upper extremities followed by the development of wasting and paresis of the arms. The disease became generalized, affecting also the lower limbs, and the patient died of bronchitis only 2 years after the onset of the first symptom. Aran reported that one of the patient's three sisters and two maternal uncles had died from a similar disease, but two sisters and three brothers showed no symptoms. The description by Aran was so detailed that later investigators have diagnosed case 7 as most likely to be FALS[4].

Charcot and Joffroy apparently ignored Aran's familial case, and though their own original description of ALS was based on only 20 cases, claimed that ALS was never hereditary (1873)[2]. This belief has unfortunately persisted in some textbooks of neurology.

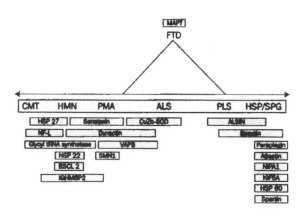

Figure 9.1 Genetic overlap in various motor syndromes

Table 9.1 Frequency of familial amyotrophic lateral sclerosis (FALS) in some epidemiologic studies

Study area	% FALS	n	Year	Reference
Germany	13.5	251	1959	5
Central Finland	11.6	36	1983	6
USA	9.5	1200	1995	7
Nova Scotia, Canada	5.8	52	1974	8
Wärmland, Sweden	5.6	89	1984	9
England	5.0	580	1988	10
USA	4.9	668	1978	11
Northern Sweden	4.7	128	1983	12
Sardinia, Italy	4.4	182	1983	13
Jutland, Denmark	2.7	186	1989	14
Hong Kong	1.2	84	1996	15
Finland	0.8	255	1977	16

The epidemiology of familial amyotrophic lateral sclerosis

Retrospective epidemiologic studies[5-16] (Table 9.1) have found 0.8–13.5% of ALS cases to have a family history of the disease. The ten-fold differences in frequency of FALS in these studies can partly be explained by different frequencies of disease genes in the populations studied. Remarkably, in only one of the listed studies is FALS defined[16]. In this book, FALS is defined as ALS existing in at least two blood-related individuals separated by not more than four generations. A number of factors can lead to under-representation of FALS cases (Table 9.2). Incomplete disease penetrance, and doctors' inattention and failure to record pertinent family history, are probably the most important. In a recent study of mutations in the CuZn superoxide dismutase gene (CuZn-SOD) among ALS patients in the Nordic countries, the referring neurologists were specifically asked whether the patient had a family history of ALS. Almost 17% of the 427 patients included in this study reportedly had a family history of ALS[17]. Another caveat of the epidemiologic studies listed in Table 9.1 are their retrospective nature

depending on old medical records or databases and absence of medical genealogic studies of the cause of deaths of the ALS patients' relatives. In an unpublished study of the medical genealogy of 153 randomly selected ALS patients in northern Sweden in the period 1983–1993, 17.4% were found to have a first-, second- or third-degree blood relative with ALS. In more than half the cases the relative's disease was unknown to the index patient. A traditionally performed epidemiologic study in the same geographic area had reported the frequency of FALS to be 4.7%[12].

The clinical differences between familial and sporadic amyotrophic lateral sclerosis

The poor recording of FALS has made it difficult to delineate any possible clinical differences between FALS and sporadic ALS (SALS). Frequently, SALS and FALS are claimed to be clinically indistinguishable in individual cases[10,18–21], but some group differences have been noted[10,21–24] (Table 9.3). In one study, FALS with extensive posterior column involvement was found in about 70% of autopsied FALS cases, although this has

Table 9.2 Factors that may lead to under-representation of familial amyotrophic lateral sclerosis (ALS) cases

Different diagnostic criteria used

Inadequate recording of pertinent family history in the patient's charts

The ALS disease expresses itself with different subtypes in different members of the family and is therefore not recognized as being one disease entity

Reluctance of the patient to report a hereditary disease

Loss of contact between different members of a family

Early death from other causes of an individual in the family who transmits the gene defect

The child develops ALS before the parent who transmitted the gene defect

Incomplete disease penetrance

Family members with ALS were misdiagnosed

Illegitimacy

Table 9.3 Characteristics of familial (FALS) compared to sporadic amyotrophic lateral sclerosis (SALS)

Earlier age of presentation[10,21,22]

Relative female preponderance (near unity)[10,21,22]

More frequent onset in the lower limbs[21,22]

Earlier and persistent absence of ankle reflexes[21]

Shorter survival time[10,21,22]

More frequent occurrence of sensory features at presentation[10]

Normally distributed age of onset in FALS compared with age-dependent incidence in SALS[23]

Finding of degeneration of the posterior columns, dorsal spinocerebellar tracts and nucleus dorsalis of Clarke in 70% of FALS[24]

---

rarely been detected clinically antemortem[24]. Based on genetic, pathoanatomic and clinical features, Horton *et al.* divided FALS into three major subtypes[24]:

I. Rapid, progressive loss of motor function with predominantly LMN features and a duration of less than 5 years. Neuropathologic changes are limited to the ventral horns and pyramidal tracts;

II. Clinically identical to (I), but at autopsy additional changes are found in the posterior columns, Clarke's column and spinocerebellar tracts;

III. Clinically distinguished by survival of more than 10 years but with the same pathologic features as found in (II).

There is general agreement that intrafamilial variation in site of onset (bulbar/upper limbs/truncus/lower limbs/diffuse) is common in FALS pedigrees and that, within the same family, cases with only LMN symptoms and signs (PMA), Charcot-classical type of ALS, progressive bulbar palsy

(PBP), flail arm syndrome (Vulpian–Bernhardt's form of ALS) and also PLS may be found[10,18–21].

Rare cases with frontotemporal dementia (in some cases preceeding the onset of motor symptoms) and ALS have been reported in pedigrees where other affected cases have been without obvious cognitive dysfunction. A few pedigrees in which all affected members develops both severe cognitive dysfunction as well as motor neuron dysfunction and loss have also been reported[25].

It is of importance to observe the variable age of onset of symptoms among members of the same family; an intrafamilial variation of 15–25 years is a common finding[10]. Also, the disease progression rate may differ markedly among different members of the same family[26], although in certain pedigrees the disease progression rate appears to be similar in all affected members[18].

It has been claimed that female patients may have longer survival than affected males[27], but this statement is based on small pedigrees with few affected members and has not been substantiated in larger samples[23,28]. A review of the world literature on FALS (84 families with 249 affected cases in 1989) found that, in contrast to the age-dependent incidence of SALS, the age of onset of FALS was normally distributed about a mean of

45.7 years (SD ± 11.3 years). Survival curves for FALS demonstrated a markedly skewed distribution with 74% surviving at 1 year, 48% at 2 years and 23% at 5 years. Age of onset, gender and site of onset were unrelated variables, and age of onset was the only predictor of survival[23].

Modes of inheritance of familial amyotrophic lateral sclerosis

ALS is not a rare disease and with a life-time risk of approximately 1:1000 in the Western world[29], the possibility exists that two family members might develop ALS from different causes, including enviromental influences. In this context the very rare occurrence of conjugal ALS should be mentioned to illustrate that the existence of ALS in more than one member of a family does not neccessarily imply a common genetic cause for a familial clustering of the disease.

Many FALS pedigrees contains only two sometimes remotely related affected blood relatives and it may be difficult to determine whether this reflects common genetic or environmental influences. The author has investigated a Finnish FALS pedigree where three siblings in one part of the pedigree had ALS caused by a CuZn-SOD mutation while two affected second-degree cousins-once removed tested negative for a CuZn-SOD mutation. In a Swedish FALS pedigree ALS was reported to exist in both the paternal and the maternal lines of the index patient. DNA analysis revealed the patient to carry a mutation in the CuZn-SOD gene which was also found in a young paternal cousin, the son of a diseased ALS patient. Surprisingly, the index patient was also found to have a maternally inherited CAG-trinucleotide expansion of the androgen receptor gene on the X-chromosome. Investigation and DNA analysis of the reported 'ALS cases' in the mother's family showed them to be four cases of spinobulbar muscular atrophy. Albeit probably rare, the possibility of different etiologic causes for ALS among affected members of a family should not be forgotten. This rare possibility complicates research into the cause of the disease; the evaluation of the effect of treatment among different members of the family raises ethical questions and makes genetic counseling difficult.

Three Mendelian patterns of inheritance have been recognized in adult-onset FALS. The most commonly reported is dominant inheritance with high if not complete penetrance (all carriers of the single gene defect will eventually develop ALS in an age-dependent manner specific for that gene defect in that particular family)[10,18,21,22,25–28]. Dominant inheritance with incomplete penetrance (some carriers of the single gene defect will – even though they live to advanced age – not develop ALS but may with 50% risk pass the gene defect on to their children), and recessive inheritance (the patient has inherited two identical gene defects, one from the mother and the other from the father who remain unaffected since they only have one defect gene each) have only rarely been reported[30].

No formal study of the frequency of the three different modes of inheritance exists but it is the author's experience from studying FALS pedigrees both in Europe and North America that families with dominant inheritance with incomplete penetrance (from biologic causes or for reasons listed in Table 9.2) are not infrequent and are often diagnosed as SALS cases. Many CuZn-SOD mutations have been found in apparent SALS cases or in FALS pedigrees with obvious reduced disease penetrance (see Tables 9.7 and 9.9 later). In fact, it may be that many SALS cases are FALS cases with very low disease penetrance. Supporting this notion, Williams et al. reported the mean age of onset in eight Australian families with low penetrance to be 60.8 years (i.e. comparable to what is reported for SALS in epidemiologic studies) contrasting with 47.8 years in a family with high penetrance[30].

It has proved to be difficult to find the genes predisposing to ALS. The age-dependent onset in adults, short disease duration, genetic heterogeneity, incomplete disease penetrance, misdiagnosis, etc. have hampered the availability of large pedigrees with multiple affected members in multiple generations, from whom DNA is available for genetic linkage analysis. The genetic studies in ALS have been restricted to the few available large pedigrees with Mendelian dominant or recessive inheritance with high penetrance and at present only four genes have been identified. Several additional gene loci are being studied (Figure 9.2).

GENES KNOWN TO CAUSE AMYOTROPHIC LATERAL SCLEROSIS

CuZn-SOD

In 1993 an international consortium reported the finding of 11 missense mutations in the gene encoding the enzyme CuZn-SOD (EC 1.15.1.1, superoxide: superoxide oxidoreductase, *SOD1*) in 13 of 18 FALS pedigrees[31]. The human CuZn-SOD gene spans about 11 kb of genomic DNA on the long arm of chromosome 21 with five small exons separated by four introns. The five exons code for 153 highly conserved amino acids which, together with a catalytic Cu ion and a stabilizing Zn ion form a subunit. Each subunit is also stabilized by an important disulfide bridge between amino acid residues C57 and C146. Two identical subunits combine through non-covalent binding to form the homodimeric CuZn-SOD enzyme. The only recognized function of CuZn-SOD is to catalyze the reduction of superoxide anion ($O_2^{\cdot-}$) to molecular oxygen (O_2) and hydrogen peroxide (H_2O_2), which in turn is further reduced to H_2O by glutathion peroxidases and catalase. CuZn-SOD is ubiquitously expressed in all cells in all organisms above bacteria, and constitutes about 0.5–1% of the soluble protein in the human brain and spinal cord. At the cellular level, it is found in the cytosol, nucleus and between the two mitochondrial membranes. In the mitochondrial matrix is the isoenzyme manganese-containing SOD (Mn-SOD, SOD2), and extracellularly in most body fluids the tetrameric CuZn-SOD (SOD3).

The discovery of mutations in CuZn-SOD in FALS sparked a worldwide search for mutations in the CuZn-SOD gene. Since 1993, a total of 125 mutations have been found, divided as follows: 114 mutations alter the amino acid sequence of CuZn-SOD and are assumed to cause disease (107 of them are listed in Table 9.4[32–92], an additional seven are in the process of being published). Also, six silent mutations and five intronic variants have been reported and are presumably non-causative. Two more intronic variants close to the border between intron 4 and exon 5 have been predicted either to introduce three novel amino acids FLQ between exon 4 and exon 5 (creating a CuZn-SOD monomer of 156 amino acids)[78] or introduce five novel amino acids FFTGP after exon 4, truncating the mutated polypeptide after amino acid number 123[79]. Of the 114 disease-associated mutations, 102 are missense mutations causing a change of one amino acid to another but keeping the polypeptide length of 153 amino acid residues. The 91 missense mutations are in 66 different codons throughout the five exons, including seven in exon 3, which codes for the catalytic site. The remaining 12 mutations are nonsense and deletion mutations that either introduce new nucleotides or remove nucleotides in the DNA sequence in exons 2, 4 or 5, or intron 4, as described. The result is a change of the length of the final polypeptide. The shortest of these mutant polypeptides is 121 and the longest 156 amino acid residues long[76,78]. Though most missense mutations are in exon 4 and the nonsense mostly in the beginning of exon 5, there is no obvious correlation between the mutated sites and conserved residues through evolution, enzymic stability or enzymic function[17,93]. Some mutants (H46R, D90A) are as stable as the native CuZn-SOD molecule, while others (L126X, G127X) are highly instable[17,94,95]. While most mutations have been found to cause a reduction in dismutation activity, the mutant protein of five mutations (L37R, L84F, A89V, D90A, G93A) have been found to possess essentially normal or only slightly reduced erythrocyte SOD activity[59,60,93,95]. These

Table 9.4   Summary of CuZn-SOD mutations associated with amyotrophic lateral sclerosis

Exon	No.	Codon	Amino acid change	Genotype	Sequence change	Country found	Principal reference
Disease-associated mutations							
I	1	4	Ala-Ser	A4S	GCC to TCC	Japan	32
1–23	2	4	Ala-Thr	A4T	GCC to ACC	Australia, Cyprus, Japan, USA	33
	3	4	Ala-Val	A4V	GCC to GTC	Canada, Italy, Sweden, USA	34
	4	6	Cys-Phe	C6F	TGC to TTT	Japan	35
	5	6	Cys-Gly	C6G	TGC to GGC	Japan	36
	6	7	Val-Glu	V7E	GTG to GAG	Japan	37
	7	8	Leu-Gln	L8Q	CTG to CAG	Austria	38
	8	8	Leu-Val	L8V	CTG to GTG	USA, UK	39
	9	10	Gly-Val	G10V	GGC to GGT	Korea	40
	10	12	Gly-Arg	G12R	GGC to CGC	Italy, Russia, USA	41
	11	14	Val-Gly	V14G	GTG to GGG	Sweden	17
	12	14	Val-Met	V14M	GTG to ATG	USA	42
	13	16	Gly-Ala	G16A	GGC to GCC	USA	43
	14	16	Gly-Ser	G16S	GGC to AGC	Japan	44
	15	19	Asn-Ser	N19S	AAT to AGT	Italy, France	45
	16	20	Phe-Cys	F20C	TTC to TGC	USA	39
	17	21	Glu-Lys	E21K	GAG to AAG	Scotland	46
	18	21	Glu-Gly	E21G	GAG to GGG	France, Spain	47
	19	22	Gln-Leu	Q22L	CAG to CTG	USA	39
II	20	37	Gly-Arg	G37R	GGA to AGA	Spain, Turkey, USA, Japan	31
24–55	21	38	Leu-Arg	L38R	CTG to CGG	France	47
	22	38	Leu-Val	L38V	CTG to GTG	Australia, Belgium, USA	31
	23	41	Gly-Asp	G41D	GGC to GAC	USA	31
	24	41	Gly-Ser	G41S	GGC to AGC	Italy, USA	31
	25	43	His-Arg	H43R	CAT to CGT	Australia, USA	31
	26	45	Phe-Cys	F45C	TTC to TGC	Italy	48
	27	46	His-Arg	H46R	CAT to CGT	France, Germany, Japan, Norway, USA	49
	28	47	Val-Phe	V47F	GTT to TTT	Italy	48
	29	48	His-Arg	H48R	CAT to CGT	USA	39
	30	48	His-Gln	H48Q	CAT to CAG	UK	50
	31	49	Glu-Lys	E49K	GAG to AAG	France	47
	32	54	Thr-Arg	T54R	ACA to AGA	USA	39
III	33	59	Ser-Ile	S59I	AGT to ATT	USA	39
56–79	34	65	Asn-Ser	N65S	AAT to AGT	Spain, USA, Zimbabwe (Caucasian)	51
	35	67	Leu-Arg	L67R	CTA to CGA	France	47
	36	72	Gly-Ser	G72S	GGT to AGT	England	52
	37	76	Asp-Val	D76V	GAT to GTT	Spain	53
	38	76	Asp-Tyr	D76Y	GAT to TAT	Canada, Denmark, New Zealand, UK	17
IV	39	80	His-Arg	H80R	CAT to CGT	Ireland	54
80–118	40	84	Leu-Phe	L84F	TTG to TTC	France, Italy, UK, USA	55
	41	84	Leu-Val	L84V	TTG to GTG	Japan, USA	56
	42	85	Gly-Arg	G85R	GGC to CGC	USA	31
	43	86	Asn-Ser	N86S	AAT to AGT	Japan, Scotland (Pakistan), Norway	57
	44	87	Val-Ala	V87A	GTG to GCG	USA	39
	45	87	Val-Met	V87M	GTG to ATG	USA	58
	46	88	Thr----	T88ΔTAD	del ACTGCTGAC	USA	39
	47	89	Ala-Thr	A89T	GCT to ACT	USA	39
	48	89	Ala-Val	A89V	GCT to GTT	Finland, Sweden, USA	59
	49	90	Asp-Ala	D90A	GAC to GCC	Australia, Belarus, Belgium, Canada, Estonia, Finland, France, Germany, Italy, Norway, Portugal, Russia, Spain, Sweden, Turkey, UK, USA	60
	50	90	Asp-Val	D90V	GAC to GTC	Japan	61
	51	93	Gly-Ala	G93A	GGT to GTC	Germany, USA	31
	52	93	Gly-Cys	G93C	GGT to TGT	USA	31
	53	93	Gly-Asp	G93D	GGT to GAT	Italy, USA	62
	54	93	Gly-Arg	G93R	GGT to CGT	UK	63
	55	93	Gly-Ser	G93S	GGT to AGT	Iceland, Japan, USA	64
	56	93	Gly-Val	G93V	GGT to GTT	UK, USA	65
	57	95	Ala-Thr	A95T	GCC to ACC	Italy	48
	58	95	Ala-Val	A95V	GCC to GTC	Ireland	66

Continued...

Table 9.4 Continued...

Exon	No.	Codon	Amino acid change	Genotype	Sequence change	Country found	Principal reference
	59	96	Asp-Asn	D96N	GAT to AAT	France	67
	60	97	Val-Leu	V97L	GTG to CTG	Italy	68
	61	97	Val-Met	V97M	GTG to ATG	USA	39
	62	100	Glu-Gly	E100G	GAA to GGA	New Zealand, UK, USA	31
	63	100	Glu-Lys	E100K	GAA to AAA	Afro-American, Germany	69
	64	101	Asp-Gly	D101G	GAT to GGT	Ireland	70
	65	101	Asp-His	D101H	GAT to CAT	Japan	71
	66	101	Asp-Asn	D101N	GAT to AAT	Pakistan/UK, Belarus	72
	67	104	Iso-Phe	I104F	ATC to TTC	Japan	73
	68	105	Ser---	S105ΔSL	delTCA CTC	Mexico, USA	39
	69	106	Leu-Val	L106V	CTC to GTC	Japan, USA	31
	70	108	Gly-Val	G108V	GGA to GTA	UK	74
	71	112	Ile-Met	I112M	ATC to ATG	Spain	51
	72	112	Ile-Thr	I112T	ATC to ACC	Spain, UK	62
	73	113	Ile-Thr	I113T	ATT to ACT	Australia, Canada, France, Italy, Japan, Norway, UK, USA	31
	74	115	Arg-Gly	R115G	CGC to GGC	Germany, USA	75
	75	118	Val-Lys...stop	V118KTGPX	delGinsAAAAC	UK	76
	76	118	Val-Leu	V118L	GTG to TTG	Japan	77
	77	118	Val-Leu	V118L	GTG to CTG	USA	39
	78	intron 4		V118VFLQ	T to G 10bp before exon 5	USA	78
	79	intron 4		V118VFFTGPX	A to G 11bp before exon 5	USA	79
V	80	124	Asp-Gly	D124G	GAT to GGT	USA	39
119–153	81	124	Asp-Val	D124V	GAT to GTT	Australia, USA	65
	82	125	Asp-His	D125H	GAC to CAC	UK	50
	83	126	Leu-......	L126GQRWKX	TTG to **G	Japan	80
	84	126	Leu-Ser	L126S	TTG to TCG	Japan	81
	85	126	Leu-stop	L126X	TTG to TAG	USA	79
	86	127	Gly-.....stop	G127GGQRWKX	insTGGG after bp1450	Denmark	82
	87	132	Glu-Aspstop	E132DX	insTT	UK	83
	88	133	Glu--	E133ΔE	delGAA	USA	65
	89	134	Ser-Asn	S134N	AGT to AAT	Japan	84
	90	139	Asn-Asp	N139D	AAC to GAC	France	85
	91	139	Asn-His	N139H	AAC to CAC	Spain	86
	92	139	Asn-Lys	N139K	AAC to AAA	USA	87
	93	140	Asp-Gly	A140G	GCT to GGT	USA	88
	94	141	Gly-Glu	G141E	GGA to GAA	Japan	89
	95	141	Gly-stop	G141X	GGA to TGA	USA	39
	96	144	Leu-Phe	L144F	TTG to TTC	Croatia, Germany, Italy, Serbia, Switzerland, USA	34
	97	144	Leu-Ser	L144S	TTG to TCG	USA	78
	98	145	Ala-Gly	A145G	GCT to GGT	Serbia	*
	99	145	Ala-Thr	A145T	GCT to ACT	USA	78
	100	146	Cys-Arg	C146R	TGT to CGT	Japan	69
	101	147	Gly-Asp	G147D	GGT to GAT	France	85
	102	147	Gly-Arg	G147R	GGT to CGT	USA	39
	103	148	Val-Gly	V148G	GTA to GGA	Germany, USA	34
	104	148	Val-Ile	V148I	GTA to ATA	Japan	90
	105	149	Ile-Thr	I149T	ATT to ACT	UK, USA	87
	106	151	Ile-Ser	I151S	ATC to AGC	USA	39
	107	151	Ile-Thr	I151T	ATC to ACC	Germany	91

Silent mutations

Exon	No.	Codon	Amino acid change	Genotype	Sequence change	Country found	Principal reference
	1	10	Gly	G10G	GGC to GGT	UK	76
	2	59	Ser	S59S	AGT to AGC	Italy, USA	65
	3.	116	Thr	T116T	ACA to ACG	New Zealand	92
	4	139	Asn	N139N	AAC to AAT	Sweden	17
	5	140	Ala	A140A	GCT to GCA	Israel, Sweden, USA	65
	6	153	Gln	Q153Q	CAA to CAG	Norway	17

* Keckarevic DP, personal communication

studies were performed in different cell systems using a variety of assays in different laboratories and the results are not directly comparable.

The finding of essentially normal SOD activity for some mutants combined with the discovery of a murine motor neuron disease in transgenic mice overexpressing human G93A SOD[96] and absence of motor degeneration in mice without CuZn-SOD[97] led to the conclusion that the mutant CuZn-SOD protein causes neurodegeneration by an acquired novel cytotoxic function. The proteotoxicity of mutant CuZn-SOD is further discussed in Chapter 11.

Regrettably, only few clinical data have been published for patients with CuZn-SOD mutations. An earlier 1996 review concluded that, with few exceptions, there were no clinical correlates between a specific mutation and phenotype[93]. Now more data are available and some of the mutants can be grouped according to survival time (Table 9.5), variability in site of onset (Table 9.6) and complete or incomplete disease penetrance (Table 9.7), with reservations for small numbers for some mutants. It is not clear why some mutants (A4V, G41S, G93A) are consistently associated with a very rapid disease *independently of site of onset*, while other mutants (G41D, H46R, A89V, homozygosity for D90A, E100K) are always associated with onset in the lower limbs and very slowly ascending paresis. It is the author's clinical experience that patients carrying any of the five latter mutations are remarkably similar in every aspect. In a third group of mutants, some individuals have very short survival while others in the same family survive for a decade or more. This is best illustrated by the G37R (survival range 2–36 years), I104F (3–38 years) and I113T (2–20 years)[98,99].

Without any obvious correlation with survival time, some mutants consistently have onset in the lower limbs (G37R, H46R, D76V, L84F, D90A homozygous, E100K) or upper limbs (L84V)[49,53,100]. Variable site of onset is the rule for many mutations (Table 9.6). For most mutants, there appears to be both intrafamilial and interfa-

milial variation in sites of onset with somewhat more frequent onset in the lower limbs than in ALS not associated with CuZn-SOD mutations. Bulbar onset has been claimed to be rare among patients with CuZn-SOD mutations[83,93] but has been reported in some patients (Table 9.6)[17,28].

The pedigrees used to find linkage to the CuZn-SOD gene were pedigrees with high penetrance. Unfortunately, only a few detailed pedigrees have been published and at present it is

Table 9.5 Disease survival time in amyotrophic lateral sclerosis associated with CuZn-SOD mutations (without artificial ventilation)

Fast (< 3 years)	Medium (3–10 years)	Slow (> 10 years)	Variable
A4T	G12R	G41D	E21G
A4V	G85R	H46R	G37R
C6F	G93V	D76V	L38V
C6G	E100G	A89V	D76Y
V7E	D101G	D90A hom	L84F
L8Q	D101N	G93C	L84V
G10V	G108V	G93D	N86S
G41S	N139H	G93S	D90A het
H43R	G141E	E100K	G93R
H48Q			I104F
D90V			I113T
G93A			L144F
D101H			L144S
D101Y			
L106V			
I112M			
I112T			
R115G			
L126X			
G127X			
A145T			
V148G			
V148I			

het, heterozygous; hom, homozygous

Table 9.6 Site of onset in amyotrophic lateral sclerosis associated with a CuZn-SOD mutation

Uniform	Variable	Bulbar onset
G10V	A4V	A4V
G12R	C6G	C6G
G37R	G41S	L8Q
H46R	N86S	D76Y
D76V	D90A het	D90A het
L84F	I112M	D101Y
L84V	I113T	I112M
D90A hom	L144F	V148I
E100K	V148I	I149T
E100G		I151T

het, heterozygous; hom, homozygous

Table 9.7 Disease penetrance in amyotrophic lateral sclerosis associated with a CuZn-SOD mutation

Complete (> 90% by age 70)	Incomplete
A4V	A4T
G37R	L8Q
L38V	N19S
G41S	E21G
H43R	N65S
H46R	D76Y
D76V	N86S
L84F	D90A het
L84V	G93S
N86K	A95T
D90A hom	I104F
E100G	S105L
D101H	I113T
G108V	L126S
G114A	N139H
L126GQRWKX	
G127GGQRWKX	
G141E	
L144F	
V148G	
V148I	

hom, homozygous; het, heterozygous

safe to state only that 17 mutations are associated with high if not complete penetrance (Table 9.7). Likewise, some mutations appear regularly to be inherited with reduced penetrance, sometimes obscuring the heredity of the disease and making genetic counseling difficult. This is particularly the case for the widespread I113T, which interestingly is also associated with a higher mean age of onset (58 years) than is most commonly reported for CuZn-SOD mutations (47 years)[28,101]. It is now well documented that I113T can pass asymptomatically from a patient down through to the grandchildren or even great-grandchildren before becoming manifest again[102,103]. The groupings listed in Tables 9.5 to 9.9 are based on available published data and may change as more patients are diagnosed and data published.

For many mutants no clinical data are available or the mutation has been found only in single patients, making characterization impossible at present.

The mean age at onset of the first symptom is 47 years for ALS patients with a CuZn-SOD mutation, 50.5 years for FALS and 56–58 years

for SALS both without the CuZn-SOD mutation[28,73,93,100,101]. The youngest onset of ALS in a patient with a CuZn-SOD mutation was 6 years (I104F)[98] and 18 years (G16S)[44], and the oldest 84 years (A4V; I113T)[28] and 94 years (D90A homozygous)[100]. The shortest survival time was 14 weeks (N86S homozygous)[104] and the longest 36 years (G37R)[28] and 38 years (I104F)[98]. There is surprisingly little variability in the mean age of onset for nearly all mutants, with the exception of L37R, V38L and G114A, with somewhat lower mean age of onset (perhaps biased by small numbers)[28] and I113T with somewhat higher age, as

Table 9.8 CuZn-SOD mutations associated with unusual features of amyotrophic lateral sclerosis

A4V
V14G
E21G
G41S
H46R
H48Q
L84F
D90A
G93S
E100G
I104F
V118L
I149T
I151T

Table 9.9 CuZn-SOD mutations reported in patients with apparently sporadic amyotrophic lateral sclerosis

A4V
L8V
G12R
V14G
G16S
N19S
E21K
H48Q
N65S
G72S
D76Y
H80R
L84F
N86S
N86D
A89V
D90A
G93S
A95T
V97L
D101N
S105ΔSL
L106P
I113T
V118L
V118KTGPX
E133ΔE
K136X
L144F

mentioned earlier. That the mutants have the same mean age of onset but very different disease progression rates, uniformity in site of onset or disease penetrance implies that onset of the disease and expression may be different processes.

While many patients with CuZn-SOD mutations reportedly are clinically identical to patients without CuZn-SOD mutations (patients with L84F, G108V, D125H and G127X can present with a phenotype completely in accordance with J-M Charcot's depictions of 1873)[17,39,74]; a predominantly LMN pattern is the rule for patients with a CuZn-SOD mutation[17,28,39,73,83,90,93]. No case with predominantly upper motor neuron (UMN) features has been reported. A feature that may be unique to ALS cases with CuZn-SOD mutations is very prolonged central motor conduction times upon transcranial magnetic stimulation of the motor cortex (MEP). Delayed central latency has been found in many cases with slowly progressing ALS heterozygous for D76Y or homozygous for D90A as well as in fast progressing cases heterozygous for G12R, G41S and N139H[41,86,100]. Some mutants may show features of involvement of other parts of the nervous system. Autonomic failure has been reported in cases

with G93S and V118L[64,77]. Sensory symptoms, paresthesias, lancinating pain in the back, localized neuralgic pain in the buttocks, hips or knees, ataxia, or bladder disturbance (in some cases progressing to incontinence) have been reported for some mutants (Table 9.8)[17,39,64,92,98,191]. In many instances (V14G, E21G, H46R, L84F, D90A, E100G) these atypical features have preceded the onset of motor symptoms and have caused difficulties and delay in arriving at the ALS diagnosis[89,92,100]. In H46R and in D90A homozygous patients, this preparetic disease phase may last for a few months to several years[49,100]. Autopsy studies have shown that in ALS patients with CuZn-SOD mutation the disease process is not confined to the motor systems and are types II or III according to the Horton classification[24,77].

The most common CuZn-SOD mutation globally is the D90A followed by the A4V (accounting for about half of all cases in the USA) and I113T[39,100]. Patients with the D90A SOD1 mutation have been found in almost every country where large numbers of patients have been screened for CuZn-SOD mutation (Table 9.4). The D90A is also the only one of the 114 mutations to show recessive inheritance and has as such been found in many apparently SALS cases (Table 9.9). Homozygosity for the D90A gives rise to an easily identifiable phenotype with an initially preparetic phase followed months to years later by slowly ascending creeping paresis and wasting, always beginning asymmetrically in the lower limbs[17,100]. After a mean of some 4 years from onset in the legs, paresis appears in the upper limbs and a year and a half later bulbar symptoms appear. With time bulbar symptoms have progressed to anarthria and aphagia, and some patients have shown slight pseudo-bulbar palsy. A few patients have also shown ataxia in the earlier stages of the diseases but it later disappears. At end-stage, the patient is completely tetraparalytic with generalized wasting, cachectic and in some cases with bladder incontinence. Dementia has not been seen in even very long surviving D90A cases, but was recently reported for a single case with L144F[105].

The background for the frequent finding of D90A homozygous ALS cases in Scandinavia is the occurrence of the D90A allele in heterozygous form in a substantial part of the population; 5% of the population in the large Torney Valley in northern Sweden are heterozygous carriers of D90A. In Finland alone it is estimated that there are > 99 000 heterozygous carriers of the D90A allele[100]. A few D90A homozygous ALS patients with the same characteristic phenotype have also

been found in Canada, southern France, Germany, southern Italy, Norway, Portugal, Russia and the USA[39,106]. A haplotype study has shown that all D90A homozygous cases have a common ancestor[107]. Surprisingly, a few D90A heterozygous ALS patients have been found in Belgium, Belarus, Great Britain, northern France, Spain, the USA as well as in the Scandinavian countries[39,60,76,106]. Most of these patients have presented a phenotype very different from the D90A homozygous cases with variable sites of onset, disease progression rates (survival time often less than 3 years) and disease penetrance, showing that the D90A allele can act in a dominant fashion like the D90V[61] and all other mutations. To explain the uniform phenotype and very slow progression found in all D90A homozygous cases it has been suggested that, in addition to the disease-causing two D90A SOD alleles, these patients also carry a protective or modifying gene which is co-inherited with the D90A CuZn-SOD alleles[17,106,107]. Studies are in progress to identify this modifying factor.

At present, only the D90A has been proven to show recessive inheritance, but homozygosity for three other mutations (L84F[47], N86S[104], L126S[108]) have been found in single individuals in heavily inbred families. In these families heterozygous individuals also develop ALS and the inheritance is therefore not recessive. Interestingly, the phenotype in two of these homozygous cases appears to be far more aggressive than in the heterozygous cases, suggesting a dose effect, as has also been found in transgenic mice with human SOD mutations[104,108].

Recently, two siblings with ALS were found to be carriers of both D90A and D96N CuZn-SOD alleles and the phenotype was rather similar to the D90A homozygous cases[67]. This is the only instance reported of compound heterozygosity in ALS, but the published pedigree is also consistent with dominant inheritance of D96N with incomplete penetrance, as has been shown for many other CuZn-SOD mutations (Table 9.7). To date, this is the only known family with D96N, and until the mutation has been found in more individuals it is not possible to state with certainty its mode of inheritance.

The prevalence of patients with CuZn-SOD mutations varies greatly from country to country and may partly explain the varying frequencies of FALS reported in different countries (Tables 9.1 and 9.4). No patient with a CuZn-SOD mutation has been found in Poland, and only nine mutations in a few patients in Germany, contrasting with four mutations in Scotland, six in Sweden and 22 in Japan. In Scotland, the I113T has been found in several FALS and apparently SALS cases (all shown to have the same common ancestor)[103], while in northern Scandinavia the D90A is very common, in particular in SALS cases[100]. Other mutations reported in apparent SALS are listed in Table 9.9. For only one of these, the H80R, has it been possible through paternity studies to show that it is a *de novo* mutation in one of the parents[54]. The others are likely to be FALS with low penetrance, though this has only been proven for N19S, D76Y, L84F, D90A and I113T. The high prevalence of the A4V in the Caucasian population in North America has, in a haplotype study, been shown to be unrelated to the three A4V families found in Italy and Sweden[17,68]. The widespread occurrence of A4V in both the USA and Canada implies that it must have been introduced with some of the first immigrants to North America. I113T is most commonly found in the UK and its former colonies, L144F is widespread in the Balkans and in northern Italy, while L84F is the most frequent mutation in central Italy. The most common mutation in Germany appears to be R115G, and in Japan H46R, though large epidmiological studies have not been performed[109]. Some mutations have been found in very different ethnic groups (H46R in Caucasians in eastern Norway, Germany and the USA, as well as in Japan; E100K in Afro-Americans as well as in Caucasians in eastern Germany) and are probably from separate mutational events in the past. While 22 mutations have been reported in the 128-million Japanese population, only recently were the first two mutations reported from Korea and China[40]. The global distribution of different mutations may change radically when mass screening is performed in all of Asia, including the Indian subcontinent, Africa and South America. The present knowledge is based mainly on screening a small proportion of the ALS patients in the industralized (Western) countries which accounts for less than 20% of the world population. The national differences in the reported prevalences of CuZn-SOD mutations is explained not only by the different ethnic backgrounds but also by whether only FALS cases were studied, the number of studied cases (in some countries as few as 30–40 cases have been studied) and the laboratory technique used to screen for mutation. Most laboratories have used single-stranded conformational polymorphism (SSCP) as the screening method, admitting that its sensitivity is only 85–90% depending on the polymerase chain reaction (PCR) conditions and primers used. Some laboratories have experienced difficulties detecting some mutations[17,70,80,109].

Screening for CuZn-SOD mutations has revealed that CuZn-SOD mutations are not found in diseases other than ALS[93], that the only CuZn-SOD polymorphism is the D90A[60] and that about a fifth to a sixth of all diagnosed FALS cases and a small percentage of apparently SALS cases carry a CuZn-SOD mutation (Table 9.10)[17,28,47,55,76,83,109,110]. The 114 mutations that cause a change in the CuZn-SOD polypeptide probably all cause disease, although for only a small part has statistical analysis shown linkage to ALS or been shown to cause a motor neuron disease when expressed in transgenic mice (G37R, G85R, G93A, G93D, D90A, G127X) or transgenic rats (H46R, G93A). The possibility that some mutants found in single patients (V14G, G16S, S134N) are coincidental findings cannot be excluded until further studies have been done.

In this context the finding of six silent mutations (mutations that cause a DNA nucleotide change but not a change in the resulting amino acid sequence, since some amino acids are coded

Table 9.10   Frequency of CuZn-SOD mutations

In apparently SALS	In FALS
7% (4/56) in Scotland[111]	23.5% (12/51) in Scandinavia[17]
6% (3/48) in Italy[68]	
4% (14/355) in Scandinavia[17]	23.4% (68/290) in the USA[28]
3% (5/155) in England[76]	21% (8/38)in the UK[55]
3% (5/175) in the UK[55]	20% (14/71) in the UK[83]
1% (1/87) in Spain[51]	18% (2/11) in Spain[51]
	14.3% (10/70) in France[47]
	12% (9/75) in Germany[110]

ALS, amyotrophic lateral sclerosis; SALS, sporadic ALS; FALS, familial ALS

for by more than one trinucleotide sequence) should be mentioned. Silent mutations are usually considered to be 'innocent bystanders' unrelated to the disease. One of the silent mutations, A140A, deserves special attention since it has now been found in affected cases in a Swedish FALS pedigree with reduced disease penetrance[17], in a Swedish SALS case, in an Israeli ALS case as well as in two US SALS cases[17,39,65], but never in any controls. A140A could be a coincidental finding, a marker for another disease gene, or – since the protein sequence is unaffected – the mutated mRNA sequence is cytotoxic.

Mutations in the CuZn-SOD gene were originally found in FALS pedigrees with typical ALS and dominant inheritance over several generations. The finding of ALS patients with CuZn-SOD mutations with atypical features, short, medium, long or variable survival times with different patterns of inheritance and in apparently SALS cases makes it plausible that similar variabilities may be the case for other FALS genes.

ALS2 and ALSIN

Recently a second gene was shown to cause a rare juvenile form of ALS called *ALS2* by some and

RFALS type 3 by others. In 1990 Tunisian researchers described three different forms of juvenile-onset ALS (mean 12 years, range 3–15 years) with slow progression and very long survival in 17 highly inbred families suggesting recessive inheritance[111].

Genetic linkage analysis of the single family with type 3 juvenile ALS linked the disease to chromosome 2q33 and recently a mutation in a new gene *ALS2* was shown to co-segregate with the disease[112]. *ALS2* is a very large gene of 34 exons coding for a new protein (by some termed Alsin[113]) of 184 kDa and 1657 amino acids in its long variant and – by alternate splicing after exon 4 – of 396 amino acids in a short variant. The short and long variants appear to be expressed in most tissues including neurons throughout the central nervous system (CNS), except in the liver, where the shorter transcript is predominantly expressed. The protein contains multiple domains that have homology to RanGEF and RhoGEF, suggesting that it is involved in membrane-proximity activities of small GTPases involved in vesicle transport and microtubule assembly.

In the Tunisian pedigree a homozygous deletion of nucleotide 261A in codon 46 in exon 3 was found[112]. The mutation causes a frameshift, the introduction of three novel amino acids and a premature stop codon in codon 50 dramatically truncating the polypeptide at only 49 amino acid residues[113].

Since then, eight more mutations have been reported in ALS2. In an inbred Kuwaiti family with juvenile-onset PLS a homozygous deletion of nucleotide 1548AG in codon 475 in exon 5 was found. This mutation causes a frameshift and the introduction of 70 novel amino acid residues followed by a stop codon[112]. In an inbred Saudi Arabian family with juvenile-onset PLS a homozygous deletion of two nucleotides in codon 623 in exon 9 causing a frameshift and truncation of 645 amino acid residues was reported[113]. The patients in Kuwait and Saudi Arabia have reportedly no LMN signs or symptoms (and therefore per definition do not fulfil ALS criteria), but present a very slowly evolving PLS-only phenotype. More recently, six more truncating Alsin mutations have been found in patients with infantile-onset slowly ascending hereditary spastic paraplegia. In most of these rare cases, spastic paraplegia started in the first 2 years of life and had progressed to the upper limbs by the end of the first decade. Eventually, the patients developed complete tetraplegia, anarthria, dysphagia and slow eye movements in the second decade of life. No sign of cognitive impairment has been reported in these patients. Clinical, neuroradiologic and neurophysiologic findings have been consistent with a relatively selective early involvement of the corticospinal and corticonuclear pathways and motor evoked potentials have demonstrated predominant involvement of the UMN system[114,115]. At present it is unclear whether these patients late in life may develop LMN features.

The nine Alsin gene mutations all cause premature truncation of the polypeptide and, since the patients are homozygous for the mutations, loss of protein function can be predicted. It is probable that full-length Alsin is required for the proper development and/or functioning of UMNs. The prevalence of *ALS2* in different subtypes of motor neuron disease is unknown at present but is probably rare. Mutations in *ALS2* have not been reported in patients with adult-onset typical ALS or PLS.

DNA/RNA α-helicase or senataxin

In a large Anglo-American family, Chance *et al.* found linkage to chromosome 9q34 of a high-penetrant autosomal dominant, childhood- or adolescent-onset (mean age 17 years) form of motor neuron disease with an essentially normal life span[116]. All patients show very slowly progressing symmetrical distal amyotrophy of all four limbs, sparing the bulbar and respiratory muscles. In addition, the patients may also show slight pyramidal signs including brisk deep tendon reflexes and pathologic Babinski responses. Postmortem examination showed severe loss of motor neurons in the brainstem and spinal cord.

The cause of this unusual syndrome was recently found to be a heterozygous L389S missense mutation in a novel gene called senataxin or *SETX*[117]. The senataxin protein is a large 302.8-kDa protein consisting of 2677 amino acid residues coded for by 24 exons. Its precise function is unknown at present. It contains an interesting DNA/RNA helicase domain with homology to IGHMBP2 – which is mutated in distal HMN type VI and juvenile spinal muscular atrophy with respiratory distress-1 (*SMARD1*) – and *RENT1*, two genes that encode proteins known to play roles in RNA housekeeping.

Genetic analysis of additional families with similar phenotypic features revealed a R2136H substitution in exon 19 in affected members of a Belgian family, and a T3I substitution in exon 3 in affected members of an Austrian family. Both families had earlier been diagnosed clinically as subtypes of CMT[117].

Reportedly, affected members with the SETX mutations eventually develop a severe motor handicap, whereas intellectual functions and longevity are unaffected. Adult patients with the R2136H mutation may show some sensory features as well. Interestingly, magnetic transcranial motor cortex stimulation (MEP) performed in five patients with the T3I mutation have revealed prolonged central motor conduction latencies to the upper and lower limbs, a neurophysiologic finding very similar to that reported in ALS patients with G12R, D76Y, L84F and D90A CuZn-SOD mutations[117]. This interesting syndrome has by some been designated ALS4 while others consider it a form of HMN with pyramidal signs. The clinical and genetic nosology of motor neuron disorders is complex and evolving. The ALS4 syndrome extends the phenotypic panoroma of the ALS syndrome (Figure 9.1).

VAPB

Recently Nishimura *et al.* mapped a large caucasian Brazilian FALS family of Portugese ancestry to a new ALS/MND locus on 20q13.3 (ALS8)[118]. ALS8 is inherited as an autosomal dominant disease with complete penetrance. In the first family reported, the age of onset varied from 25 to 45 years. Characteristic features are fasciculations, muscle cramps and tremor, and most patients have developed slowly progressing LMN paresis in the trunk and limbs. Wasting has been limited. Bulbar signs have been observed in some cases and pyramidal signs have been observed in only one case. According to the original report some cases appear not to have developed paresis even 10 years after the onset of other symptoms.

Illustrating the rapid advances in genetic research, the causative gene defect was recently identified as a heterozygous P56S missense mutation in a highly conservative domain of the ubiquitously expressed vesicle-associated membrane protein/synaptobrevin-associated membrane protein B/C (*VAPB*) gene in patients from this family[119]. Subsequently, the same mutation was identified in patients from six additional Brazilian kindreds but with different clinical courses, such as ALS8, adult-onset slowly progressive spinal muscular atrophy, progressive bulbar paresis as well as typical severe ALS with rapid progression and a survival time of less than 5 years[119]. A marked inter- and intrafamilial heterogeneity has been found in patients with the P56S *VAPB* mutation. The *VAPB* gene of six exons codes for a monomer of 243 amino acid residues; the functional protein is a 27.2-kDa homodimer but can also combine as a heterodimer with *VAPA*. This protein also can interact with VAMP1 and VAMP2. Members of the vesicle-associated proteins are intracellular membrane proteins that can associate with microtubules and have been found to have a function in transport of cytosolic vesicles, in particular in the endoplasmatic reticulum and the Golgi apparatus. These results suggest that clinically very variable cases of motor neuron disease may be caused by a dysfunction in intracellular membrane trafficking.

Other genetic loci being investigated

The finding that mutations in CuZn-SOD account for less than a quarter of all FALS cases

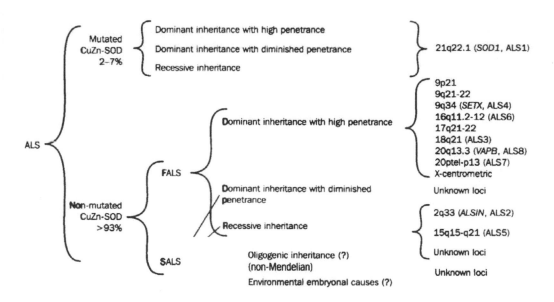

Figure 9.2 Loci linked to familial (FALS) and sporadic amyotrophic lateral sclerosis (SALS)

was a disappointment. A gene hunt to find other genes predisposing to ALS is being hampered by the lack of suitable pedigrees. A number of loci have been linked to FALS (Figure 9.2): 9q21-22 has been associated with ALS with frontal-lobe-type dementia in five pedigrees[120]; 16q11.2-12 linkage has been found in five Dutch, British and US pedigrees with dominantly inherited typical ALS, but the gene remains to be found[121-123]; 17q21-22 maps the gene encoding microtubule-associated protein tau (*MAPT*). Three affected members in a family with an exon 10 tau mutation showed ALS-like features with frontotemporal dementia, while other members developed frontotemporal dementia with parkinsonism. Age at onset was between 30 and 56 years and complete penetrance was found in three generations[124].

The 18q21 linkage has been found in a single large European FALS pedigree with dominant inheritance and complete penetrance. The phenotype is typical adult-onset ALS[125]. The 20p linkage has been found in a single North American FALS pedigree. The haplotype on chromosome 20 spans 6 cM (1 Mb), a region that encompasses 20–24 genes[122].

X-centromeric-linked dominant inheritance has been briefly reported in an American family with typical adult-onset ALS. Male patients were reported to have much earlier onset (> 20 years) than females in this family[126].

A 15q15-q21 linkage has been found in Tunisian pedigrees with juvenile ALS and a recessive inheritance pattern (juvenile ALS type 1)[127]. A third type of juvenile FALS in Tunisia has failed to show linkage to this locus or to 2q33, showing that there must be at least one more gene or genes involved in recessively inherited juvenile ALS.

REFERENCES

1. Charcot J-M, Joffroy A. Deux cas d'atrophie musculaire progressive avec lésions de la substance grise et des faisceaux antéro-latéraux de la moelle épinière. Arch Physiol Neurol Pathol 1869; 2: 744–60

2. Charcot J-M. Lecons sur les maladies du système nerveux. IInd series, collected by Bourneville 1873. In: Sigerson G, translator and ed. Charcot J-M. Lectures on the Diseases of the Nervous System, vol 2, series 2. London: New Sydenham Society, 1881: 163–204

3. Aran FA. Researches sur une maladie non encore décrite du système musculaire (atrophie musculaire progressive). Arch Gén Méd 1850; 24: 5–35, 172–214

4. Forbes H, Norris Jr. Adult spinal motor neuron disease. In: Vinken PJ, Bruyn GW, eds. Handbook of Clinical Neurology, vol 2. Amsterdam: North-Holland, 1975: 1–56

5. Haberlandt WF. Genetic aspects of amyotrphic lateral sclerosis and progressive bulbar paralysis. Acta Genet Med Gemellol 1959; 8: 369–73

6. Murros K, Fogelholm R. Amyotrophic lateral sclerosis in middle-Finland: an epidemiological study. Acta Neurol Scand 1983; 67: 41–7

7. Haverkamp LJ, Appel V, Appel SH. Natural history of amyotrophic lateral sclerosis in a database population. Brain 1995; 118: 707–19

8. Murray TJ, Pride S, Haley G. Motor neuron disease in Nova Scotia. Can Med Assoc J 1974; 110: 814–17

9. Gunnarsson L-G, Palm R. Motor neuron disease and heavy labour: An epidemiological survey of Värmland county, Sweden. Neuroepidemiology 1984; 3: 195–206

10. Li T-M, Alberman E, Swash M. Comparison of sporadic and familial disease amongst 580 cases of motor neuron disease. J Neurol Neurosurg Psychiatry 1988; 51: 778–84

11. Rosen AD. Amyotrophic lateral sclerosis. Clinical features and prognosis. Arch Neurol 1978; 35: 638–42

12. Forsgren L, Almay BGL, Holmgren G, Wall S. Epidemiology of motor neuron disease in northern Sweden. Acta Neurol Scand 1983; 68: 20–9

13. Giagheddu M, Puggioni G, Masala C, et al. Epidemiologic study of amyotrophic lateral sclerosis in Sardinia, Italy. Acta Neurol Scand 1983; 68: 394–404

14. Højer-Pedersen E, Christensen PB, Jensen NB. Incidence and prevalence of motor neuron disease in two Danish counties. Neuroepidemiology 1989; 8: 151–9

15. Fong KY, Yu YL, Chan YW, et al. Motor neuron disease in Hong Kong Chinese: Epidemiology and clinical picture. Neuroepidemiology 1996; 15: 239–45

16. Jokelainen M. Amyotrophic lateral sclerosis in Finland. II: Clinical characteristics. Acta Neurol Scand 1977; 56: 194–204

17. Andersen PM, Nilsson P, Keränen M-L, et al. Phenotypic heterogeneity in MND-patients with CuZn-superoxide dismutase mutations in Scandinavia. Brain 1997; 120: 1723–37

18. Kurland KT, Mulder DW. Epidemiological investigations of amyotrophic lateral sclerosis. Familial aggregations indicative of dominant inheritance. Part I and II. Neurology 1955; 5: 182–267

19. Emery AEH, Holloway S. Familial motor neuron diseases. In: Rowland LP, ed. Human Motor Neuron Diseases. New York: Raven Press, 1982: 139–45

20. Tandan R, Bradley WG. Amyotrophic lateral sclerosis. Part 1 and 2. Ann Neurol 1985; 18: 271–80, 419–31

21. Mulder DW, Kurland LT, Offord KP, Beard CM. Familial adult motor neuron disease: Amyotrophic lateral sclerosis. Neurology 1986; 36: 511–17

22. Veltema AN, Ross RAC, Bruyn GW. Autosomal dominant adult amyotrophic lasteral sclerosis: A six-generation Dutch family. J Neurol Sci 1990; 97: 93–115

23. Strong MJ, Hudson AJ, Alvord WG. Familial amyotrophic lateral sclerosis, 1850–1989: A statistical analysis of the world literature. Can J Neurol Sci 1991; 18: 45–58

24. Horton WA, Eldridge R, Brody JA. Familial motor neuron disease. Evidence for at least three different types. Neurology 1976; 26: 460–5

25. Gunnarsson L-G, Dahlbom K, Strandman E. Motor neuron disease and dementia reported among 13 members of a single family. Acta Neurol Scand 1991; 84: 429–33

26. Giménez-Roldán S, Esteban A. Prognosis in hereditary amyotrophic lateral sclerosis. Arch Neurol 1977; 34: 706–8

27. Espinosa RE, Okihiro MM, Mulder DW, Sayre GP. Hereditary amyotrophic lateral sclerosis. A clinical and pathologic report with comments on classification. Neurology 1962; 12: 1–7

28. Cudkowicz ME, McKenna-Vasek D, Sapp PE, et al. Epidemiology of mutations in superoxide dismutase in amyotrophic lateral sclerosis. Ann Neurol 1997; 2: 210–21

29. Bobowick AR, Brody JA. Epidemiology of motor-neuron diseases. N Engl J Med 1973; 288: 1047–55

30. Williams DB, Floate DA, Leicester J. Familial motor neuron disease: differing penetrance in large pedigrees. J Neurol Sci 1988; 86: 215–30

31. Rosen DR, Siddique T, Patterson D, et al. Mutations in CuZn superoxide dismutase gene are associated with familial amyotrophic lateral sclerosis. Nature 1993; 362: 59–62

32. Nakanishi T, Kishikawa M, Miyazaki A, et al. Simple and defined method to detect SOD-1 mutants from patients with familial amyotrophic lateral sclerosis by mass spectrometry. J Neurosci Methods 1998; 81: 41–4

33. Nakano R, Sato S, Inuzuka T, et al. A novel mutation in Cu/Zn superoxide dismutase gene in Japanese familial amyotrophic lateral sclerosis. Biochem Biophys Res Commun 1994; 200: 695–703

34. Deng H-X, Hentati A, Tainer JA, et al. Amyotrophic lateral sclerosis and structural defects in CuZn superoxide dismutase. Science 1993; 261: 1047–51

35. Morita M, Aoki M, Abe K, et al. A novel two-base mutation in the CuZn-superoxide dismutase gene associated with familial ALS in Japan. Neurosci Lett 1996; 205: 79–82

36. Kohno S, Takahashi Y, Miyajima H, et al. A novel mutation (Cys6Gly) in the Cu/Zn superoxide dismutase gene associated with rapidly progressing familial amyotrophic lateral sclerosis. Neurosci Lett 1999; 276: 135–7

37. Hirano M, Fujii J, Nagai Y, et al. A new variant CuZn superoxide dismutase (Val^7→Glu) deduced from lymphocyte mRNA sequences from Japanese patients with familial amyotrophic lateral sclerosis. Biochem Biophys Res Commun 1994; 204: 572–7

38. Bereznai B, Winkler A, Borasio GD, Gasser T. A novel SOD1 mutation in an Austrian family with amyotrophic lateral sclerosis. Neuromusc Disord 1997; 7: 113–16

39. Andersen PM, Sims KB, Xin WW, et al. Sixteen novel mutations in the gene encoding CuZn-superoxide dismutase in ALS. Amyotroph Lateral Scler Other Motor Neuron Disord 2003; 4: 62–73

40. Kim NH, Kim HJ, Kim M, Lee KW. A novel SOD1 gene mutation in a Korean family with amyotrophic lateral sclerosis. J Neurol Sci 2003; 206: 65–9

41. Penco S, Schjenone A, Bordo D, et al. A SOD1 gene mutation in a patient with slowly progressive familial ALS. Neurology 1999; 53: 404–6

42. Deng H-X, Tainer JA, Mitsumoto H, et al. Two novel SOD1 mutations in patients with familial

amyotrophic lateral sclerosis. Hum Mol Genet 1995; 4: 1113–16

43. Hung W-Y. American Society for Human Genetics Conference (abstract), Denver, CO, 1998

44. Kawamata J, Shimohama S, Takano S, et al. Novel G16S (GGC-AGC) mutation in the SOD-1 gene in a patient with apparently sporadic young-onset amyotrophic lateral sclerosis. Hum Mutat 1997; 9: 356–8

45. Mayeux V, Corcia P, Besson G, et al. N19S, a new SOD1 mutation in sporadic amyotrophic lateral sclerosis: No evidence for disease causation. Ann Neurol 2003; 53: 815–18

46. Jones CT, Swingler RJ, Brock DJH. Identification of a novel SOD1 mutation in an apparantly sporadic amyotrophic lateral sclerosis patient and the detection of Ile113Thr in three others. Hum Mol Genet 1994; 3: 649–50

47. Boukaftane Y, Khoris J, Moulard B, et al. Identification of six novel SOD1 gene mutations in familial amyotrophic lateral sclerosis. Can J Neurol Sci 1998; 25: 192–6

48. Gellera C, Castelotti B, Riggio MC, et al. Superoxide dismutase gene mutations in Italian patients with familial and sporadic amyotrophic lateral sclerosis: Identification of three novel missense mutations. Neuromusc Disord 2001; 11: 404–10

49. Aoki M, Ogasawara M, Matsubara Y, et al. Mild ALS in Japan associated with novel SOD mutation. Nat Genet 1993; 5: 323–4

50. Enayat ZE, Orrell RW, Claus A, et al. Two novel mutations in the gene for copper zinc superoxide dismutase in UK families with amyotrophic lateral sclerosis. Hum Mol Genet 1995; 4: 1239–40

51. Garcia-Redondo A, Bustos F, Juan Y, et al. Molecular analysis of the superoxide dismutase 1 gene in Spanish patients with sporadic or familial amyotrophic lateral sclerosis. Muscle Nerve 2002; 26: 274–8

52. Orrell RW, Marklund SL, de Belleroche JS. Familial ALS is associated with mutations in all exons of SOD1: A novel mutation in exon 3 (Gly72Ser). J Neurol Sci 1997; 153: 46–9

53. Segovia-Silvestre T, Andreu LA, Vives-Bauza C, et al. A novel exon 3 mutation (D76V) in the SOD1 gene associated with slowly progressive ALS. Amyotroph Lateral Scler Other Motor Neuron Disord 2002; 3: 69–74

54. Alexander MD, Traynor BJ, Miller N, et al. 'True' sporadic ALS associated with a novel SOD-1 mutation. Ann Neurol 2002; 52: 680–3

55. Shaw CE, Enayat ZE, Chioza BA, et al. Mutations in all five exons of SOD-1 may cause ALS. Ann Neurol 1998; 43: 390–4

56. Aoki M, Abe K, Houi K, et al. Variance of age at onset in a Japanese family with amyotrophic lateral sclerosis associated with a novel CuZn-superoxide dismutase mutation. Ann Neurol 1995; 37: 676–9

57. Maeda T, Kurahashi K, Matsunaga M, et al. On intra-familial clinical diversities of a familial amyotrophic lateral sclerosis with a point mutation of Cu/Zn superoxide dismutase (Asn86-Ser). No To Shinkei 1997; 49: 847–51

58. www.ALSOD.org

59. Jacobsson J, Jonsson, A, Andersen PM, et al. Superoxide dismutase in CSF from amyotrophic lateral sclerosis patients with and without CuZn-superoxide dismutase mutations. Brain 2001; 124: 1461–6

60. Andersen PM, Nilsson P, Ala-Hurula V, et al. Amyotrophic lateral sclerosis associated with homozygosity for an Asp90Ala mutation in CuZn-superoxide dismutase. Nat Genet 1995; 10: 61–6

61. Morita M, Abe K, Takahashi M, et al. A novel mutation Asp90Val in the SOD1 gene associated with Japanese familial ALS. Eur J Neurol 1998; 5: 389–92

62. Esteban J, Rosen DR, Bowling AC, et al. Identification of two mutations and a new polymorphism in the gene for CuZn- superoxide dismutase in patients with amyotrophic lateral sclerosis. Hum Mol Genet 1994; 3: 997–8

63. Elshafey A, Lanyon WG, Connor JM. Identification of a new missense mutation in exon 4 of the Cu/Zn superoxide dismutase (SOD-1) gene in a family with amyotrophic lateral sclerosis. Hum Mol Genet 1994; 2: 363–4

64. Kawata A, Kato S, Hayashi H, Hirai S. Prominent sensory and autonomic disturbances in familial amyotrophic lateral sclerosis with a Gly93Ser mutation in the SOD1 gene. J Neurol Sci 1997; 153: 82–5

65. Hosler BA, Nicholson GA, Sapp PC, et al. Three novel mutations and two variants in the gene for cu/zn superoxide dismutase in familial amyotrophic lateral sclerosis. Neuromuscul Disord 1996; 6: 361–6

66. Traynor BJ, Codd MB, Corr B, et al. Incidence and prevalence of ALS in Ireland, 1995–1997: A population-based study. Neurology 1999; 52: 504–9

67. Hand CK, Mayeux-Portas V, Khoris J, et al. Compound heterozygous D90A and D96N SOD1

mutations in a recessive amyotrophic lateral sclerosis family. Ann Neurol 2001; 49: 267–71

68. Gellera C, Testa D, Passariello P, et al. SOD1 gene mutations in amyotrophic lateral sclerosis Italian patients. P31 (abstr) 14th International Symposium on ALS/MND, Milan, Italy, 17–19 November 2003

69. Siddique T, Deng H-X. Genetics of amyotrophic lateral sclerosis. Hum Mol Genet 1996; 5: 1465–70

70. Yulug IG, Katsanis N, de Belleroche J, et al. An improved protocol for the analysis of SOD1 mutations, and a new mutation in exon 4. Hum Mol Genet 1995; 4: 1101–4

71. Sato T, Yamamoto Y, Nakanishi T, et al. Identification of two novel mutations in the Cu/Zn superoxide dismutase gene with familial ALS: Mass spectrometric and genomic analysis. J Neurol Sci 2004; 218: 79–83

72. Jones CT, Shaw PJ, Chari G, Brock DJH. Identification of a novel exon 4 SOD1 mutation in a sporadic amyotrophic lateral sclerosis patient. Mol Cell Probes 1994; 8: 329–30

73. Abe K, Aoki M, Ikeda M, et al. Clinical characteristics of familial amyotrophic lateral sclerosis with Cu/Zn superoxide dismutase gene mutations. J Neurol Sci 1996; 136: 108–16

74. Orrell RW, Jabgood JJ, Shepherd DI, et al. A novel mutation of SOD1 (Gly108Val) in familial amyotrophic lateral sclerosis. Eur J Neurol 1997; 4: 48–51

75. Kostrzewa M, Burck-Lehmann, Müller U. Autosomal dominant amyotrophic lateral sclerosis: A novel mutation in the CuZn superoxide dismutase-1 gene. Hum Mol Genet 1994; 3: 2261–2

76. Jackson M, Al-Chalabi A, Enayat ZE, et al. Copper/zinc superoxide dismutase 1 and sporadic amyotrophic lateral sclerosis: Analysis of 155 cases and identification of a novel insertion mutation. Ann Neurol 1997; 42: 803–7

77. Shimizu T, Kawata A, Kato S, et al. Autonomic failure in ALS with novel SOD1 gene mutation. Neurology 2000; 54: 1534–7

78. Sapp PC, Rosen DR, Hosler BA, et al. Identification of three novel mutations in the gene for CuZn superoxide dismutase in patients with familial amyotrophic lateral sclerosis. Neuromuscul Disord 1995; 5: 353–7

79. Zu JS, Deng H-X, Lo TP, et al. Exon 5 encoded domain is not required for the toxic function of mutant SOD1 but essential for the dismutase activity: Identification and characterization of two new SOD1 mutations associated with familial amy-

otrophic lateral sclerosis. Neurogenetics 1997; 1: 65–71

80. Pramatarova A, Goto J, Nanba E, et al. A two base-pair deletion in the SOD1 gene causes familial amyotrophic lateral sclerosis. Hum Mol Genet 1994; 3: 2061–2

81. Murakami T, Warita H, Hayashi T, et al. A novel SOD1 gene mutation in familial ALS with low penetrance in females. J Neurol Sci 2001; 189: 45–7

82. Hansen C, Gredal O, Werdelin L, et al. Novel 4-bp insertion in the CuZn-superoxide dismutase (SOD1) gene associated with familial amyotrophic lateral sclerosis. Hum Mutat 1998; (Suppl 1): S327–8

83. Orrell RW, Habgood JJ, Gardiner I, et al. Clinical and functional investigation of 10 missense mutations and a novel frameshift insertion mutation of the gene for copper–zinc superoxide dismutase in UK families with amyotrophic lateral sclerosis. Neurology 1997; 48: 746–51

84. Watanabe M, Aoki M, Abe K, et al. A novel missense mutation (S134N) of the Cu/Zn superoxide dismutase gene in a patient with familial motorneuron disease. Hum Mutat 1997; 9: 69–71

85. Jafari-Schluep HF, Khoris J, Mayeux-Portas V, et al. Groupe Francais d'Etude des Maladies du Motoneurone. [Superoxide dismutase 1 gene abnormalities in familial amyotrophic lateral sclerosis: Phenotype/genotype correlations. The French experience and review of the literature]. Rev Neurol (Paris) 2004; 160: 44–50

86. Nogales-Gadea G, Garcia-Arumi E, Andreu AL, et al. A novel exon 5 mutation (N139H) in the SOD1 gene in a Spanish family associated with incomplete penetrance. J Neurol Sci 2004; 219: 1–6

87. Pramatarova A, Figlewicz DA, Krizus A, et al. Identification of new mutations in the CuZn superoxide dismutase gene of patients with familial amyotrophic lateral sclerosis. Am J Hum Genet 1995; 56: 592–6

88. Naini A, Musumeci O, Hayes L, et al. Identification of a novel mutation in Cu/Zn superoxide dismutase gene associated with familial amyotrophic lateral sclerosis. J Neurol Sci 2002; 198: 17–19

89. Sato T, Nakanishi T, Yamamoto Y, et al. Rapid disease progression correlates with instability of mutant SOD1 in familial ALS. Neurology 2005; 65: 1954–7

90. Ikeda M, Abe K, Aoki M, et al. A novel point mutation in the CuZn superoxide dismutase gene in a patient with familial amyotrophic lateral sclerosis. Hum Mol Genet 1995; 4: 491–2

91. Kostrzewa M, Damian MS, Müller U. Superoxide dismutase 1: Identification of a novel mutation in a case of familial amyotrophic lateral sclerosis. Hum Genet 1996; 98: 48–50

92. Calder VL, Domigan NM, George PM, et al. Superoxide dismutase (Glu100Gly) in a family with inherited motor neuron disease: Detection of mutant superoxide dismutase activity and the presence of heterodimers. Neurosci Lett 1995; 189: 143–6

93. Radunovic A, Leigh PN. CuZn superoxide dismutase gene mutations in ALS. Correlation between genotype and clinical features. J Neurol Neurosurg Psychiatry 1996; 61: 565–72

94. Jonsson A, Ernhill K, Andersen PM, et al. Motor neuron disease in ALS patient and transgenic mice carrying Gly127insTGGG mutant human CuZn-superoxide dismutase. Brain 2003; 127: 73–88

95. Marklund SL, Andersen PM, Forsgren L, et al. Normal binding and reactivity of copper in mutant superoxide dismutase isolated from amyotrophic lateral sclerosis patients. J Neurochem 1997; 69: 675–81

96. Gurney ME, Pu H, Chiu AY, et al. Motor neuron degeneration in mice expressing a human CuZn superoxide dismutase mutation. Science 1994; 264: 1772–5

97. Reaume AG, Elliott JL, Hoffman EK, et al. Motor neurons in Cu/Zn superoxide dismutase-deficient mice develop normally but exhibit enhanced cell death after axonal injury. Nat Genet 1996; 13: 43–7

98. Ikeda M, Abe K, Aoki M, et al. Variable clinical symptoms in familial amyotrophic lateral sclerosis with a novel point mutation in the CuZn-superoxide dismutase gene. Neurology 1995; 45: 2038–42

99. Shaw CE, Enayat ZE, Powell JF, et al. Familial amyotrophic lateral sclerosis. Molecular pathology of a patient with a SOD1 mutation. Neurology 1997; 49: 1612–16

100. Andersen PM, Forsgren L, Binzer M, et al. Autosomal recessive adult-onset ALS associated with homozygosity for Asp90Ala CuZn-superoxide dismutase mutation. A clinical and genealogical study of 36 patients. Brain 1996; 119: 1153–72

101. Juneja T, Pericak-Vance MA, Laing NG, et al. Prognosis in familial amyotrophic lateral sclerosis: Progression and survival in patients with glu100gly and ala4val mutations in CuZn-superoxide dismutase. Neurology 1997; 48: 55–7

102. Suthers G, Laing N, Wilton S, et al. 'Sporadic' motoneuron disease due to familial SOD1 mutation with low penetrance. Lancet 1994; 344: 1773

103. Jones CT, Swingler RJ, Simpson SA, Brock DJH. Superoxide dismutase mutations in an unselected cohort of Scottish amyotrophic lateral sclerosis patients. J Med Genet 1995; 32: 290–2

104. Hayward C, Minns RA, Swingler RJ, Brock DJH. Homozygosity of Asn86Ser mutation in the CuZn-superoxide dismutase gene produces a severe clinical phenotype in a juvenile onset case of familial amyotrophic lateral sclerosis. J Med Genet 1998; 2: 174

105. Masé G, Ros S, Gemma A, et al. ALS with variable phenotypes in a six-generation family caused by leu144phe mutation in the SOD1 gene. J Neurol Sci 2001; 191: 11–18

106. Skvortsova VI, Limborska SA, Slominsky PA, et al. Sporadic ALS associated with the D90A CuZn-superoxide dismutase mutation in Russia. Eur J Neurol 2001; 8: 167–72

107. Al-Chalabi A, Andersen PM, Chioza B, et al. Recessive amyotrophic lateral sclerosis with the D90A SOD1 mutation shares a common founder: Evidence for a linked protective factor. Hum Mol Genet 1998; 13: 2045–50

108. Kato M, Aoki M, Ohta M, et al. Marked reduction of the Cu/Zn superoxide dismutase polypeptide in a case of familial ALS with the homozygous mutation. Neurosci Lett 2001; 312: 165–8

109. Niemann S, Joos H, Meyer T, et al. Familial ALS in Germany: Origin of the R115G SOD1 mutation by a founder effect. J Neurol Neurosurg Psychiatry 2004; 75: 1186–8

110. Jones CT, Swingler RJ, Simpson SA, Brock DJH. Superoxide dismutase mutations in an unselected cohort of Scottish amyotrophic lateral sclerosis patients. J Med Genet 1995; 32: 290–2

111. Hamida MB, Hentati F, Hamida CB. Hereditary motor system diseases (chronic juvenile amyotrophic lateral sclerosis). Brain 1990; 113: 347–63

112. Hadano S, Hand CK, Osuga H, et al. A gene encoding a putative GTPase regulator is mutated in familial amyotrophic lateral sclerosis. Nat Genet 2001; 29: 166–73

113. Yang Y, Hentati A, Deng H-X, et al. The gene encoding alsin, a protein with three guanine-nucleotide exchange factor domains, is mutated in a form of recessive ALS. Nat Genet 2001; 29: 160–5

114. Devon RS, Helm JR, Rouleau GA, et al. The first nonsense mutation in alsin results in a homogeneous phenotype of infantile-onset ascending spastic paralysis with bulbar involvement in two siblings. Clin Genet 2003; 64: 210–15

115. Lesca G, Eymard-Pierre E, Santorelli FM, et al. Infantile ascending hereditary spastic paralysis (IAHSP): Clinical features in 11 families. Neurology 2003; 60: 674–82

116. Chance PF, Rabin PA, Ryan SG, et al. Linkage of the gene for an autosomal dominant form of juvenile amyotrophic lateral sclerosis to chromosome 9q34. Am J Hum Genet 1998; 62: 633–40

117. Chen YZ, Bennett CL, Huynh HM, et al. DNA/RNA helicase gene mutations in a form of juvenile amyotrophic lateral sclerosis (ALS4). Am J Hum Genet 2004; 74: 1128–35

118. Nishimura AL, Mitne-Neto M, Silva HC, et al. A novel locus for late onset amyotrophic lateral sclerosis/motor neurone disease variant at 20q13. J Med Genet 2004; 41: 315–20

119. Nishimura AL, Mitne-Neto M, Silva HC, et al. A mutation in the vesicle-trafficking protein VAPB causes late-onset spinal muscular atrophy and amyotrophic lateral sclerosis. Am J Hum Genet 2004; 75: 822–31

120. Hosler BA, Siddique T, Sapp PC, et al. Linkage of familial amyotrophic lateral sclerosis with frontotemporal dementia to chromosome 9q21-q22. J Am Med Assoc 2000; 284: 1664–9

121. Ruddy DM, Parton MJ, Al-Chalabi A, et al. Two families with familial amyotrophic lateral sclerosis are linked to a novel locus on chromosome 16q. Am J Hum Genet 2003; 73: 390–6

122. Sapp PC, Hosler BA, McKenna-Yasek D, et al. Identification of two novel loci for dominantly inherited familial amyotrophic lateral sclerosis. Am J Hum Genet 2003; 73: 397–403

123. Abalkhail H, Mitchell J, Habgood J, et al. A new familial amyotrophic lateral sclerosis locus on chromosome 16q12.1-16q12.2. Am J Hum Genet 2003; 73: 383–9

124. Lynch T, Sano M, Marder KS, et al. Clinical characteristics of a family with chromosome 17-linked disinhibition–dementia–parkinsonism–amyotrophy complex. Neurology 1994; 44: 1878–84

125. Hand CK, Khoris J, Salachas F, et al. A novel locus for famillial amyotrophic lateral sclerosis, on chromosome 18q. Am J Hum Genet 2002; 70: 251–6

126. Hong S, Brooks SR, Hung WY, et al. X-linked dominant locus for late-onset familial amyotrophic lateral sclerosis. Soc Neurosci Abst 1998; 24: 478

127. Hentati A, Bejaoui K, Pericak-Vance MA, et al. Linkage of a commoner form of recessive ALS to chromosome 15q15-q22 markers. Neurogenetics 1998; 2: 55–60

10

Modifying genes in amyotrophic lateral sclerosis

Claire L Simpson, Ammar Al-Chalabi

INTRODUCTION

Ideas about disease causation have a long and varied history and are still in flux today. Until recently, most diseases were thought of as either genetic or sporadic. A good example of this kind of thinking is amyotrophic lateral sclerosis (ALS), in which work showing that 10% of individuals had a family history of ALS[1,2], was taken to mean that the remaining 90% had a non-genetic form of the disease. The discovery of *SOD1* gene mutations in 20% of those with a family history helped support this view of ALS, but between 2 and 7% of sporadic cases also carry *SOD1* mutations, and it is now becoming clear that the situation is not so simple.

Until recently, gene-hunting methods required large pedigrees showing a clear Mendelian pattern of inheritance. It is perhaps therefore not surprising that, of the robustly replicated genetic causes of ALS so far found, all are of familial disease conforming to a Mendelian pattern. For example, the earliest and best established of these, *SOD1* mutations, are of high penetrance and autosomal dominant. This is a self-fulfilling prophecy because gene hunting requires the selection of families with clear autosomal dominant inheritance, but this model cannot easily explain the finding of *SOD1* mutations in individuals with apparently sporadic ALS.

A more complete rationalization is that multiple genetic and environmental factors all contribute to a disease liability. Some factors will have a large effect, while others will be of small effect. If the cumulated effects increase the liability such that a certain threshold is exceeded, ALS follows. Familial clustering sometimes with and sometimes without Mendelian inheritance patterns would be a result. Another consequence would be the finding of affected individuals without a family history of ALS, but who carry genes that have a large effect. These are the same genes that are likely to cause classical Mendelian ALS because they greatly increase the liability to disease, bringing it close to the threshold required to develop ALS. All of these features are observed in ALS and in other diseases. This model of multiple genetic and environmental factors contributing to a disease liability is becoming recognized as the appropriate genetic model for most complex diseases. With this latest shift in our understanding of heredity, it is perhaps helpful to examine how we have arrived at this conclusion before exploring ALS as a complex disease.

THE HISTORY OF GENETIC IDEAS

Human interest in heredity can be traced at least to the ancient Babylonians and Assyrians, who practiced artificial pollination as far back as 2000 BC, showing an awareness that traits could be passed from parents to offspring. The Greek philosophers Hippocrates, Aristotle and Plato observed that some characteristics were frequently passed from parents to children[3] and believed semen was responsible for passing on traits[4]. In 1752, a mathematician called Maupertuis, with a strong interest in animal biology, observed that first-generation hybrids had traits from both parents[5,6]. He was also responsible for one of the first reports of an inherited genetic disorder, autosomal dominant postaxial polydactyly in a four-generation family[6,7]. It took until 1814 for the idea of recessive and dominant inheritance to appear, when Joseph Adams published *A Treatise on the Supposed Hereditary Properties of Diseases*[8]. He recognized the problems associated with consanguineous mating and the now familiar principles that some hereditary diseases can be expressed later in life or require some environmental factor in order to manifest.

Nearly a century later, Charles Darwin was serving as a naturalist aboard HMS Beagle (1831 to 1836). He laid out the theory of evolution in his book *On the Origin of Species by Means of Natural Selection, or the Preservation of Favoured Races in the Struggle for Life*[9] more commonly referred to as *The Origin of Species*. This theory described how the accumulation of small changes in continuous traits, such as height or beak length, might over many generations lead to new species. In other words, Darwin considered that continuous traits had a hereditary component.

At around the same time, Mendel published his *Experiments in Plant Hybridization*[10]. In it he proposed principles of heredity. His work on breeding pea plants and observing the passage of particular traits through the generations required hours of careful counting. Over the years 1856 to 1861 he raised over 10 000 pea plants which were highly inbred. He made various experimental crosses and counted the offspring, observing the transmission of seven traits: ripe seed shape, seed albumen color, seed-coat color, ripe pod shape, unripe pod color, position of flowers and length of stem. His work was remarkable for its attention to detail, and was an intellectual leap because of two things he noticed. First, if two parents with contrasting characters were crossed, the offspring was not a blend of the two parental types; it was like either one parent or the other. Second, certain crosses produced almost exact ratios of 3:1 of a 'dominant' character to a 'recessive' character. He was to deduce from this his laws of heredity. Sadly, his work was published in an obscure journal and forgotten until independently rediscovered three times by De Vries[11], Correns[12] and Tschermak[13]. An essential aspect of Mendel's theory was that it applied to discrete binary traits, such as wrinkled or round, pink or white, rather than to continuous traits.

QUANTITATIVE GENETICS

At this time, genetics was being born. The term 'genetics' was coined by William Bateson in 1905. He became the first Professor of Genetics in the world when he took the chair at Cambridge University. The problem that the early genetic pioneers faced was that evolution, a process dependent on heredity, applied to continuous traits, but Mendel's laws applied to discrete traits. There was therefore a paradox at the heart of genetics. How could inherited continuous traits be explained using Mendelian genetics? In 1918, RA Fisher finally squared this circle[14]. He proposed that continuous traits might be coded by three or more loci, with alleles at each locus acting not as dominant or recessive to each other, but simply having additive effects. For example, imagine that the Intelligence Quotient (IQ) is completely genetically determined by a single locus with two alleles, A and a. The A allele increases IQ by 5 units, while the a allele decreases it by 5 units. The mean IQ of a population is defined as 100, so someone with the Aa genotype will have an IQ of $100 + 5 - 5 = 100$. Someone with the aa genotype will have an IQ of $100 - 5 - 5 = 90$, and someone with the

AA genotype will be IQ 100 + 5 + 5 = 110. No other IQs will be possible because IQ is completely genetically determined in this thought experiment. How frequent will each IQ be? We will presume for simplicity that each allele is equally frequent. In this case, the possible genotypes in the offspring generation will be aa, aA, Aa and AA, each with frequency of 0.25. Two of these genotypes, aA and Aa, are in fact the same, so the different IQs will occur with relative frequencies of 1:2:1. If we now assume a second locus, with alleles B and b, also with these properties, then the possible IQs in the population become 80, 90, 100, 110 and 120, and the relative frequencies are 1:4:6:4:1. A third locus with alleles C and c makes IQs from 70 to 130 possible, with relative frequencies of 1:6:15:20:15:6:1. This is almost a normal distribution and if we add a little environmental variation, it is indistinguishable from a normal distribution. (It is in fact the binomial distribution, which taken to infinity is normal.) So, three or more loci and a little environmental variation can produce continuous traits that are normally distributed and yet determined by Mendelian genetics. In fact, even including dominance effects does not alter the fundamental result.

With these two models, a single locus of major effect, and multiple loci of smaller effect interacting with the environment, it is possible to explain the Mendelian inheritance of discrete traits, and the inheritance of continuous traits, respectively. What is still missing is an explanation of diseases or discrete traits that show a tendency to familial clustering, but which are non-Mendelian. Examples are diabetes, multiple sclerosis, Alzheimer's disease, Parkinson's disease and ALS. A modification of the multi-locus idea was proposed as an explanation by Falconer in 1965[15]. He suggested that diseases manifest when a threshold of liability is passed. The liability to disease is itself continuous and normally distributed, but towards the right of the distribution is a threshold, and individuals with disease liability beyond this threshold develop disease. The liability is therefore the continuous trait, and the amount of liability to disease that an individual has is determined by multiple genetic loci and environmental factors. The classic example of such a condition is cleft lip and palate. The rate at which the two palatal halves come together during development varies from person to person and is normally distributed. It does not matter how fast the plates come together, so long as they meet by a critical stage of development so that they can fuse into a single palate. Anything slower and there will be cleft lip and palate. Again, it does not matter how slow they are. If they are too slow, there will be a disease phenotype. So, the continuous underlying liability is transformed into a binary phenotype: affected or unaffected. There will be familial clustering because liability genes will be commoner among relatives, but it will not be obviously Mendelian because several loci and environmental factors contribute to phenotype. This model can be used to explain any disease in which there is an increased risk to relatives but in which most people in the pedigree are unaffected.

With these three models, it is possible to explain the genetics of all diseases. That is not to say that these are the only valid models, but they have proven a useful starting point from which to build up the statistical and laboratory methods required to find risk genes for non-Mendelian traits, modifying factors and continuous phenotypes. With this background, the evidence for putative genes modifying the risk of ALS, or its phenotype, can be assessed.

MODIFYING GENES

A phenotype is rarely the product of a single gene, even if it seems so at first. This is because the expression of one gene can alter the expression of another at transcription, at the level of molecular cell machinery, or based on the cell type, organ or system it is expressed in. Modifier genes may, for example, enhance or reduce a phenotype, produce novel phenotypes or mask the effect of a disease gene to produce an organism that resembles the wild type. In Mendelian diseases, this may be manifested as reduced penetrance, meaning that the disease has a reduced likelihood of occurring in individuals who carry the risk genotype. Age- or sex-dependent penetrance are common examples. Modifier genes mean that traits that are inherited in a dominant fashion on one genetic background can be recessive or co-dominant on another, even when the environment is the same. This is similar to the phenomenon of epistasis, in which an allele at one locus affects the phenotypic expression of a gene at another. Many other modifier effects are recognized, but all are examples of gene–gene or multiple gene–environment interactions.

Modifying genes and amyotrophic lateral sclerosis

We can therefore consider susceptibility to ALS as a spectrum of genetic and environmental risk, in which at one end, single genes of large effect cause Mendelian, dominant, familial ALS of high penetrance, and at the other, multiple genetic and environmental factors interact to cause isolated cases of apparently sporadic disease. Whereas genes of large effect can be found using traditional linkage studies, those causing sporadic disease or modifying phenotype are more easily found using association studies. Because of the high resolution and large numbers of people required to have sufficient power to perform an association study, until recently candidate gene approaches have been used rather than genome-wide scans. Table 10.1 summarizes the candidate genes which have been investigated in ALS as modifiers of risk or phenotype. Rather than list every single one of these in the text, we will discuss some of the most studied.

SOD1

In 1993, in one of the first linkage studies, mutations in SOD1 were identified as causing familial ALS, accounting for about 20% of familial cases[16,17]. Such mutations are also found in 2% or more of sporadic cases[18–20], lending weight to the

idea that liability to ALS is only partly derived from SOD1 mutations. The role of SOD1 in familial disease is covered in Chapter 9 but it also has much to tell us about modifier genes.

SOD1 mutations were first identified in autosomal dominant families. Well over 100 mutations in SOD1 are now known to exist, all behaving as dominant mutations. In 1995, the D90A mutation of SOD1 was reported in Scandinavia to cause recessive ALS[21]. Some families exist in which heterozygosity for D90A is associated with ALS, and a few heterozygous affected individuals with no family history of ALS have been described. There were two striking differences between the homozygous affected and heterozygous affected individuals in these reports. First, the homozygous individuals all came from the Torne Valley in northern Sweden and Finland, a remote region, while the heterozygous individuals came from other parts of the world, including southern Sweden, the UK, Belgium and France. Second, the phenotype of the homozygous individuals was predictable and relatively benign, consisting of a generally ascending spastic weakness, sometimes with extramotor involvement and long survival, while those with heterozygosity for D90A had a variable phenotype often with a classical aggressive course. Founder studies initially showed that the homozygous families from the Torne Valley had a single founder, around 40 to 50 generations previously, while the heterozygous families had a different founder. Higher-resolution studies have since shown that both groups shared the same founder about 500 generations previously, with the Torne Valley families becoming isolated at about 50 generations ago. The interpretation of these findings has been that D90A is a dominant mutation, as are all other SOD1 mutants, but a protective factor, tightly linked to SOD1 exists in the Torne Valley families, such that two copies of D90A are required for ALS to develop. No such linked protective factor has yet been identified.

An alternative interpretation, within the threshold liability model, is that all SOD1 mutations may act in an additive manner, to increase

Table 10.1 Candidate modifier gene studies in amyotrophic lateral sclerosis (ALS)

Gene	Description	Reason for investigation	Significance	References
ALAD	D-Aminolevulinic acid dehydratase	Susceptibility with lead exposure	No significant association found	22
ALS2	Alsin	Susceptibility	Causes early-onset familial ALS. No significant association found with sporadic disease	23–28
APEX	Apurinic endonuclease	Susceptibility	Possible	
APOE	Apolipoprotein E	Susceptibility, age at onset, survival, presentation	Not associated with increased susceptibility. May affect age of onset, presentation and survival	29–33
AR	Androgen receptor	Susceptibility	Causes Kennedy spinal and bulbar muscular atrophy but not associated with ALS	34
CCS	Copper chaperone for superoxide dismutase	Susceptibility	No significant association found	35
CNTF	Ciliary neurotrophic factor	Age at onset	Contradictory results in different studies, probably not significant	36–41
CYP2D6	Cytochrome p450, subfamily IID, polypeptide 6	Susceptibility	One study reports association, but was not able to be replicated	42, 43
DCTN1	Dynactin	Susceptibility	Significant association found in one small study, not yet replicated	44
DNCH1	Dynein heavy chain	Susceptibility	No significant association found	44–46
EAAT2	Excitatory amino acid transporter 2	Susceptibility	No significant association found	47–53
HexA	Hexosaminidase A	Susceptibility	Occasionally causes rare ALS-like syndrome	54
HFE	Hemochromatosis	Susceptibility	Contradictory results in different studies	55, 56
LIF	Leukemia inhibitory factor	Susceptibility	Single small study only	57, 58
LOX	Lysyl oxidase	Susceptibility	No significant association found	59
MAO-B	Monoamine oxidase B	Age at onset	Significant association found in one small study, not yet replicated	60
MAPT	Microtubule-associated protein tau	Susceptibility for ALS/parkinsonism–dementia complex	Probably not significant	61, 62
Mitochondrial DNA deletions		Susceptibility	Possible, only small studies carried out so far	63–69
NAIP	Neuronal apoptosis inhibitory protein	Age at onset	Single case in one study only. Probably not significant	70–73
ND2	Subunit 2 of mitochondrial NADH dehydrogenase (Complex I)	Susceptibility	Single study only. No significant association found	74

Continued...

Table 10.1   Continued...

Gene	Description	Reason for investigation	Significance	References
NEFH	Neurofilament, heavy chain	Susceptibility	Significant. ~1% ALS patients. not in controls. Multiple studies	75–79 56
PRPH	Peripherin	Susceptibility	Few mutations found, does not seem to be a common cause of ALS	80, 81
PSEN1	Presenilin-1	Susceptibility	Significant association found in one small study, not yet replicated	82
PVR	Poliovirus receptor	Susceptibility	Significant association with LMND found in one study, not yet replicated	83
SETX	Senataxin	Susceptibility	New familial gene, not yet tested in sporadics	84
SMN1/2	Survival of motor neuron 1/2	Susceptibility/survival	Contradictory results in different studies	73, 85, 86
Spastin and paraplegin	Hereditary spastic paraparesis	Susceptibility	No significant association found	87
SNCG	Persyn	Susceptibility	No significant association found	88
SOD1	Cu/Zn superoxide dismutase 1	Susceptibility	2–3% sporadic cases have mutations	16–20
SOD2	Manganese superoxide dismutase	Susceptibility	No significant association found	89
VAPB	Vesicle-associated membrane protein-associated protein B	Susceptibility	New familial gene, not yet tested in sporadics	90
VDR	Vitamin D receptor	Susceptibility with lead exposure	Not significant	22
VEGF	Vascular endothelial growth factor	Susceptibility	Single large study suggests susceptibility	91, 92

the risk of ALS. For most mutations, the effect is very large, such that only a small contribution from other factors is required to cause ALS, and the disease is therefore autosomal dominant with age-dependent penetrance. For D90A, the effect is smaller, perhaps a little over 50% of the liability threshold. For heterozygous individuals, a single copy would be insufficient to cause ALS unless other factors contributed sufficiently to cross the liability threshold. It would thus be polymorphic in the Torne Valley, as is seen. A second copy of D90A would be sufficient to cross the threshold as each contributes more than 50%,

so it would cause recessive ALS. Occasional affected heterozygotes with no family history should occur. In families living in regions with other strong contributing factors, it would appear to be a dominant trait. Evidence for this comes from the report of one of the French families with apparently dominant D90A-mediated ALS. They were subsequently found to have compound heterozygosity for a second *SOD1* mutation, N86S. *SOD1* mutations themselves may therefore be part of a general contribution to disease liability. What can explain the variability in age of onset or site of first symptoms?

It is likely that there are multiple components of ALS. *SOD1* mutation is a trigger for disease, but other factors influence the age at which it develops, where it first manifests and how rapidly it progresses. For example, the distribution in age of onset is quite wide, and similar for different *SOD1* mutations, whereas the rate of progression can be quite specific to a particular mutation. The A4V mutation, commonest in North America, is aggressive, with death often within 2 or 3 years of onset. D90A and I113T, on the other hand, are generally slowly progressive. Being female generally protects against ALS, with a 3:2 ratio of men to women affected. This is manifest as a decreased risk at all ages. In other words, part of the liability to disease is being male. Of all candidate genes studied as possible modifiers of age of onset or presentation, apolipoprotein E (*APOE*), known to influence age of onset in Alzheimer's disease and many other neurologic conditions, is perhaps the most illuminating, as it shows how study designs have been improving over the past few years, and that large numbers and stringent *p* values are required for replicable results.

APOE

APOE is required for catabolism of the components of triglyceride-rich lipoprotein. The remains of dietary lipids (chylomicron remnants) and very low-density lipoprotein (VLDL) are removed from the circulation by receptor-mediated endocytosis in the liver. Apolipoprotein E is a main apoprotein of the chylomicron, and binds to a specific receptor on liver cells and peripheral cells. There are three major alleles, E2, E3 and E4, although as many as 30 have now been identified[93]. Genetic variation in *APOE* has been implicated in many abnormalities of blood lipids and cardiovascular disease, but is also involved in neurologic diseases. The E4 allele has been associated with increased risk and earlier disease onset of late-onset familial and sporadic Alzheimer's disease[94], faster progression of disability and earlier disease onset in multiple sclerosis[95] and poorer recovery

after traumatic brain injury. The picture for *APOE* in ALS is less clear.

The first study examining *APOE* in ALS[29], showed no association between *APOE* and susceptibility, age at onset or prognosis. Although association between the E4 allele and bulbar onset was reported in two studies[30,31], a subsequent study found no such association[32]. Further studies also failed to show an effect of *APOE* on site of first symptoms[96,97]. A significant shortening of survival in patients carrying the E4 allele was reported in one study, which the authors felt was consistent with a role of apolipoproteins on neuronal survival and repair, rather than as a causal factor[33]. A family-based study design has been used to examine age of onset as a quantitative trait, showing that the age of onset for carriers of the E2 allele is about 3 years later than that for the other alleles[98].

Ciliary neurotrophic factor

Neurokines, also known as neuropoietins, are a small group of molecules which share structural similarities and employ common effector mechanisms in their target cells to cytokines. One of these is ciliary neurotrophic factor (CNTF), discovered because of its ability to promote the survival of parasympathetic neurons of the ciliary ganglion[99-101]. CNTF has a broad range of activities and can act upon several different neuronal populations[102].

Homozygous pmn/pmn mice display a progressive motor neuropathy and are a naturally occurring model of motor neuron degeneration. When treated with CNTF at symptom onset, these mice show prolonged survival, improved motor function and a reduction in the cellular changes associated with neural degeneration[103]. Knocking out the *CNTF* gene in mice produces progressive atrophy, loss of motor neurons, and decreased muscle strength[36]. These studies suggest that expression of *CNTF* is not essential for spinal motor neuron development but that it is necessary for postnatal maintenance of function.

About 2% of the human population are homozygous for mutations that inactivate *CNTF* and yet do not have overt problems[104,105]. Since null mutations in mice can lead to perinatal death or severe motor neuron loss[37], there have been many studies examining null mutations in humans as a possible risk factor for neurologic and psychiatric disorders. Such conditions include unipolar affective disorder, schizophrenia and Alzheimer's disease, none of which is associated with null mutations[106]. A possible role as a neuro-protective agent has been suggested in Hunting-ton's disease[107].

In ALS, most studies of null mutations in the CNTF gene have not demonstrated any associa-tion[38,39,104]. One which has suggested a role is a report of a patient with familial V148G SOD1-mediated ALS. He developed ALS at 25 years and survived only 11 months. The mutation in SOD1 was shared by his older unaffected sister and his mother, who developed ALS in her mid-fifties. The members of this family differed in their CNTF genotype. The son with young onset and rapid disease course was homozygous null for CNTF (–/–), his sister who remained unaffected at the time of the report was homozygous wild type (+/+) and his mother was heterozygous (+/–)[40]. This led to the suggestion that CNTF was modifying the age of onset of the SOD1 mutation. In order to explore this possibility, SOD1-G93A mice were crossed with CNTF (–/–) mice. The CNTF-deficient mice did indeed exhibit earlier disease onset than the mice with wild-type CNTF but the disease duration was similar in both cases. Eight CNTF (–/–) individuals with sporadic ALS were compared with 30 CNTF (+/+) individuals with sporadic ALS. Mean age of onset was about 8 years less in the CNTF null homozygotes than in those with wild-type alleles, although the confi-dence intervals overlapped. This was a well-designed series of experiments, but it is difficult to draw robust statistical conclusions, because of the rarity of CNTF null homozygotes in the ALS pop-ulation. A study of 400 ALS patients found no difference in age at onset, disease progression, duration or clinical presentation for those with

null mutations in CNTF[41], although again, not many homozygotes for CNTF null were available. On present evidence, it is difficult to conclude that CNTF is a major modifier of age of onset in ALS, but this cannot yet be excluded.

Vascular endothelial growth factor

Vascular endothelial growth factor (VEGF) regu-lates the growth of new blood vessels and induces vascular permeability. However, VEGF also has additional non-vascular functions. Neuronal axon pathfinding is mediated by semaphorins acting on neuropilin receptors. These receptors are also acted on by various members of the VEGF fam-ily[108,109], which implies a role for VEGF in neu-ronal growth and repair. Additionally, VEGF receptors have been discovered on neurons and astrocytes[110] and on the neural progenitor cells of the retina[111], which suggests that VEGF can act as a neurotrophic and neuroprotective factor in the central and peripheral nervous system.

Other proangiogenic growth factors such as basic fibroblast growth factor (bFGF) and platelet-derived growth factor (PDGF) have also been shown to be neurotrophic[112].

Transgenic mice with a deletion of the hypoxia-response element in the VEGF promoter (Vegfa$^{\delta/\delta}$) have reduced levels of VEGF in neural tissue, and induction of VEGF expression by hypoxia in the spinal cord and the brain is dimin-ished. At the age of 5 months, the transgenic ani-mals develop a progressive motor neuron degener-ation, reminiscent of ALS[91].

In a meta-analysis of almost 2000 individuals, in studies from Sweden, Belgium and the UK, subjects homozygous for two haplotypes in the VEGF promoter/leader sequence were found to have a 1.8 times increased risk of developing ALS[92]. These haplotypes are associated with a decrease in levels of circulating VEGF and reduc-tion in gene transcription. This is one of the largest association studies in ALS to date, and pro-vides good evidence for a true association of VEGF haplotype and susceptibility to ALS.

Neurofilaments and peripherin

The 10 nm diameter cytoplasmic intermediate filaments are divided into subclasses by their tissue distribution, biochemical properties and immunological specificity. All have three domains, consisting of a globular head, an α-helical rod with conserved domains for protein–protein interaction, and a globular tail. The tail domain tends to be the most variable. The type IV intermediate filament proteins include the three neurofilament proteins, classified as light (NEFL), medium (NEFM) and heavy (NEFH) chains. These proteins are the major intermediate filaments of most types of mature neuron and are particularly abundant in the axons of motor neurons. They are thought to play a critical role in supporting the long, thin processes. They assemble as heteropolymers, with NEFL forming the core and NEFM and NEFH decorating the outside. Phosphorylation of the tail causes extension and electrostatic repulsion, and is thought to regulate axonal caliber. The neurofilaments are largely distinguished on the basis of tail length, with NEFM and NEFH containing a repeated motif lysine-serine–proline (KSP), which is variably phosphorylated. NEFM contains 13 such repeats, whereas NEFH exists as two common variants, one with 44 and one with 45 repeats.

In ALS, neurofilaments form part of the aggregates which characterize the disease[113–116]. It remains unclear whether neurofilament accumulation is a cause, effect or bystander phenomenon of motor neuron degeneration in ALS[75,117–119]. The remarkable tail domain of NEFH has made it the subject of several studies in ALS. In the first, five people with ALS were found to have novel mutations in this domain of the NEFH gene[120]. A subsequent small study did not replicate this result, neither did a study of about 100 families[76,77]. An 84-bp insertion was found in a sporadic case[78]. A study of 530 cases and 447 controls from the UK and Scandinavia found four tail deletions in sporadic ALS and in a single family, although it was not possible to tell whether the deletion segregated

with disease[79]. In all studies in which it has been possible to determine genotype, disease-associated deletions have been paired with the longer wild-type NEFH allele, and the insertion was paired with the shorter. It is possible that the difference in tail lengths is one of the factors increasing susceptibility to ALS. Taking all cases from all these studies together, about 2000 people have been screened and NEFH deletions found in about 1% of isolated ALS cases.

Peripherin is a type III intermediate filament protein initially described as a cytoskeletal protein occurring in the mammalian peripheral nervous system[121]. A study of 149 sporadic and 40 familial cases of ALS, with 380 controls, identified seven mutations[80]. Two of these were not found in controls; there was one frameshift mutation, predicted to disrupt the protein, and another unlikely to have any functional effect. The frameshift mutation produced a truncated protein, which when transfected into SW13 cell cultures, was unable to self-assemble into neurofilament structures, disrupted NEFL assembly into the intermediate filament network and impeded assembly of NEFM into oligomeric structures.

Homozygosity for a Y141D mutation was found in a person with sporadic ALS[81]. Immunocytochemical analysis of the spinal cord revealed unusual large aggregates within spinal motor neurons containing peripherin and neurofilament proteins. In transfected mice, the mutant peripherin formed aggregates, suggesting that the mutation adversely affected peripherin assembly.

In the case of the intermediate filaments, there are pathologic and functional data to support association studies. It is likely that genetic variants of intermediate filaments can be a primary cause of ALS.

Dynein and dynactin

Intermediate filaments are not the only cytoskeletal structures in neurons. Microtubules and actin filaments interact with intermediate filaments to form a dense and dynamic scaffold for axonal support and transport. In microtubule-directed axonal transport, microtubule-activated ATPases known as dyneins are responsible for movement towards the (–) end of microtubules. Dyneins are large, multimeric proteins composed of two or three heavy chains complexed with indeterminate numbers of intermediate and light chains. Cytosolic dynein is involved in the movement of vesicles and chromosomes, and axonemal dynein is involved in the beating of cilia and flagella. Dynein requires a complex of microtubule-binding proteins that link the cargo to the microtubules. One of these complexes, dynactin, is a well-characterized heterocomplex of at least eight subunits, which enhances dynein-dependent motility. The dynamitin subunits of dynactin interact with the light chains of dynein.

Impaired retrograde axonal transport has been reported in *SOD1* mouse models of ALS[122]. Homozygous loss of the cytoplasmic dynein heavy chain 1 gene (*DNCHC1*) is lethal at an early stage of embryogenesis, but heterozygotes appear normal[123]. Two mouse phenotypes obtained by mutagenesis of this gene, 'Legs at odd angles' (*Loa*) and 'Cramping 1' (*Cra1*), exhibit an age-related progressive loss of muscle tone and motor ability. This does not affect lifespan, although homozygous mice are more severely affected, cannot feed or move, and die within 24 hours of birth[45]. The mice develop Lewy-like inclusion bodies, and significant loss of spinal anterior horn cells *in utero*. The mutations in *DNCHC1* in *Loa* and *Cra1* specifically cause a defect in fast retrograde transport that is observed only in alpha motor neurons. These observations are similar to the human pathology of ALS and other motor neuron degeneration phenotypes. Although no mutations have been found in human dynein associated with ALS[46], the numbers studied so far have been small.

Disruption of the dynactin complex in *Drosophila* results in an increase in the frequency and extent of synaptic retraction events at the neuromuscular junction[124], suggesting that dynactin is essential for stabilisztion of the synapse. Overexpressing dynamitin in postnatal motor neurons of transgenic mice disrupts the dynein–dynactin complex, resulting in an inhibition of retrograde axonal transport[125]. The mice develop a late-onset, slowly progressive neurodegenerative disease reminiscent of human ALS. In humans, a mutation has now been identified in the dynactin 1 gene (*DCTN1*) in a family with a slowly progressive, autosomal dominant form of motor neuron disease without sensory symptoms[126]. The mutation occurs in a highly conserved subunit of dynactin which binds directly to microtubules. In a study of 250 individuals with sporadic and familial ALS, and 150 controls, further heterozygous mutations were identified in dynactin in one person with sporadic ALS, and in two families[44]. It seems likely that, like intermediate filament mutations, genetic variants affecting axonal transport (particularly retrograde transport), increase susceptibility to ALS.

SMN

SMN and an associated protein, SMN-interacting protein-1 (SIP1) form a complex with several spliceosomal small nuclear ribonucleoproteins (snRNP)[127] and are implicated indirectly with general cellular RNA processing[128]. This complex has also been identified as important in the regulation of neuron-specific genes in neuronal development[129] and may be important in both neuronal and muscle function[130]. The region on chromosome 5q13 containing the *SMN* gene is duplicated, so that there are two copies of *SMN*, differing at two base pairs. The *SMN1* gene is the functional copy, although there is evidence that the *SMN2* gene product is able to compensate for loss of *SMN1* to some extent.

Mutations or deletions of *SMN1* are responsible for causing spinal muscular atrophy (SMA)[131]. Studies investigating *SMN* mutations in ALS have failed to find any association[70–72,85,132]. *SMN1* copy number has been examined with 27 of 167 cases, compared with seven of 167 controls, having one or three copies of the SMN1 gene[73]. It is not clear what mechanism could be responsible for a reduced or an increased number of *SMN1* genes having the same detrimental effect, and a replication of this finding is required before it can be accepted. More recently, studies have suggested a possible role for these genes as phenotype modifiers. *SOD1*-G86R mice crossbred on to different genetic backgrounds, have significantly delayed onset of disease on some backgrounds compared with others[133]. This effect is linked to a region on mouse chromosome 13 which is syntenic to human chromosome 5 and contains the mouse *SMN* gene.

SMN2 was examined in a study of 177 individuals with sporadic ALS and 66 with familial disease[86]. No deletions were found in ALS (although five of 14 individuals with a lower motor neuron syndrome had homozygous deletion). Another study of 110 cases and 100 controls found a significant association of homozygous *SMN2* deletion in cases (17 cases vs. four controls) and an effect on prognosis[86]. This could not be confirmed in a subsequent study, which found that 11 of 124 cases and 20 of 200 controls had homozygous *SMN2* deletion, with no effect on prognosis either[134].

It therefore seems unlikely on current evidence that *SMN* genes play an important role in human ALS, although it is possible that they will turn out to have a role in modifying disease.

CONCLUSION

The need for well-conducted, large-scale association studies in ALS is great. In sporadic ALS, only three genes have been examined to date in the detail required to draw reasonably firm conclusions, namely *SOD1*, *NEFH* and *VEGF*. All candidate gene studies are limited by their focus on small regions of the genome. As the techniques for large-scale association studies develop, and as protein and bioinformatics technologies improve, robust associations and gene pathways modifying phenotype will be found, bringing the prospects of diagnosis, therapeutic intervention and prevention nearer.

REFERENCES

1. Kurland LT, Mulder DW. Epidemiologic investigations of amyotrophic lateral sclerosis. 2. Familial aggregations indicative of dominant inheritance. I. Neurology 1955, 5: 182–96
2. Kurland LT, Mulder DW. Epidemiologic investigations of amyotrophic lateral sclerosis. 2. Familial aggregations indicative of dominant inheritance. Ii. Neurology 1955; 5: 249–68
3. Barthelmess A. Vererbungswissenschaft. Freiburg, Germany: Alber, 1952
4. Stubbe H. History of Genetics, from Prehistoric Times to the Rediscovery of Mendel's Laws. Cambridge, MA: MIT Press, 1972
5. Maupertuis PLM. Systeme de la nature: Essai sur la formation des corps organises. Erlangen, Germany, 1751
6. Maupertuis PLM. Lettres de m. De mauperituis. Dresden, Germany, 1752
7. Bowler PJ. The Mendelian Revolution: The Emergence of Hereditarian Concepts in Modern Science and Society. Baltimore, MD: Johns Hopkins University Press, 1989
8. Motulsky AG. Joseph Adams (1756–1818). Arch Intern Med 1959; 104: 490–6
9. Darwin C. On the Origin of Species by Means of Natural Selection, or the Preservation of Favoured Races in the Struggle for Life. London: John Murray, 1859
10. Mendel G. Experiments in plant hybridization. Verh Naturforsch Vereines Brunn 1865; 4: 3–47
11. De Vries H. Sur la loi de disjonction des hybrides. Compt Rend Acad Sci (Paris) 1990; 130: 845–7
12. Correns CG. Mendel's regel uber das verhalten der nachkommenschaft der rassen bastarde. Ber Dtsch Botan Ges 1900; 18: 158–68
13. Tschermak E. Uber kunstliche kreuzung bei pisum sativum. Ber Dtsch Botan Ges 1900; 18: 232–9
14. Fisher RA. The correlation between relatives on the supposition of mendelian inheritance. Trans R Soc Edinb 1918; 52: 399–433
15. Falconer DS. The inheritance of liability to certain diseases, estimated from the incidence among relatives. Ann Hum Genet 1965; 29: 51–76
16. Siddique T, Figlewicz DA, Pericak-Vance MA, et al. Linkage of a gene causing familial amyotrophic lateral sclerosis to chromosome 21 and evidence of genetic-locus heterogeneity. N Engl J Med 1991; 324: 1381–4

17. Rosen DR, Siddique T, Patterson D, et al. Mutations in Cu/Zn superoxide dismutase gene are associated with familial amyotrophic lateral sclerosis. Nature 1993; 362: 59–62

18. Jones CT, Swingler RJ, Brock DJ. Identification of a novel SOD1 mutation in an apparently sporadic amyotrophic lateral sclerosis patient and the detection of ile113thr in three others. Hum Mol Genet 1994; 3: 649–50

19. Andersen PM, Nilsson P, Keranen ML, et al. Phenotypic heterogeneity in motor neuron disease patients with CuZn-superoxide dismutase mutations in Scandinavia. Brain 1997; 120: 1723–37

20. Jackson M, Al-Chalabi A, Enayat ZE, et al. Copper/zinc superoxide dismutase 1 and sporadic amyotrophic lateral sclerosis: Analysis of 155 cases and identification of a novel insertion mutation. Ann Neurol 1997; 42: 803–7

21. Andersen PM, Nilsson P, Ala-Hurula V, et al. Amyotrophic lateral sclerosis associated with homozygosity for an asp90ala mutation in CuZn-superoxide dismutase. Nat Genet 1995; 10: 61–6

22. Kamel F, Umbach DM, Lehman TA, et al. Amyotrophic lateral sclerosis, lead, and genetic susceptibility: Polymorphisms in the delta-aminolevulinic acid dehydratase and vitamin D receptor genes. Environ Health Perspect 2003; 111: 1335–9

23. Hentati A, Bejaoui K, Pericak-Vance MA, et al. Linkage of recessive familial amyotrophic lateral sclerosis to chromosome 2q33-q35. Nat Genet 1994; 7: 425–8

24. Hosler BA, Sapp PC, Berger R, et al. Refined mapping and characterization of the recessive familial amyotrophic lateral sclerosis locus (ALS2) on chromosome 2q33. Neurogenetics 1998; 2: 34–42

25. Hadano S, Hand CK, Osuga H, et al. A gene encoding a putative GTPase regulator is mutated in familial amyotrophic lateral sclerosis 2. Nat Genet 2001; 29: 166–73

26. Yang Y, Hentati A, Deng HX, et al. The gene encoding alsin, a protein with three guanine-nucleotide exchange factor domains, is mutated in a form of recessive amyotrophic lateral sclerosis. Nat Genet 2001; 29: 160–5

27. Hand CK, Devon RS, Gros-Louis F, et al. Mutation screening of the ALS2 gene in sporadic and familial amyotrophic lateral sclerosis. Arch Neurol 2003; 60: 1768–71

28. Hayward C, Colville S, Swingler RJ, Brock DJ. Molecular genetic analysis of the apex nuclease gene in amyotrophic lateral sclerosis. Neurology 1999; 52: 1899–901

29. Mui S, Rebeck GW, McKenna-Yasek D, et al. Apolipoprotein E epsilon 4 allele is not associated with earlier age at onset in amyotrophic lateral sclerosis. Ann Neurol 1995; 38: 460–3

30. Al-Chalabi A, Enayat ZE, Bakker MC, et al. Association of apolipoprotein E epsilon 4 allele with bulbar-onset motor neuron disease. Lancet 1996; 347: 159–60

31. Moulard B, Sefiani A, Laamri A, et al. Apolipoprotein E genotyping in sporadic amyotrophic lateral sclerosis: Evidence for a major influence on the clinical presentation and prognosis. J Neurol Sci 1996; 139 (Suppl): 34–7

32. Siddique T, Pericak-Vance MA, Caliendo J, et al. Lack of association between apolipoprotein E genotype and sporadic amyotrophic lateral sclerosis. Neurogenetics 1998; 1: 213–16

33. Drory VE, Birnbaum M, Korczyn AD, Chapman J. Association of apoE epsilon4 allele with survival in amyotrophic lateral sclerosis. J Neurol Sci 2001; 190: 17–20

34. Garofalo O, Figlewicz DA, Leigh PN, et al. Androgen receptor gene polymorphisms in amyotrophic lateral sclerosis. Neuromuscul Disord 1993; 3: 195–9

35. Silahtaroglu AN, Brondum-Nielsen K, Gredal O, et al. Human CCS gene: Genomic organization and exclusion as a candidate for amyotrophic lateral sclerosis (ALS). BMC Genet 2002; 3: 5

36. Masu Y, Wolf E, Holtmann B, et al. Disruption of the cntf gene results in motor neuron degeneration. Nature 1993; 365: 27–32

37. DeChiara TM, Vejsada R, Poueymirou WT, et al. Mice lacking the cntf receptor, unlike mice lacking cntf, exhibit profound motor neuron deficits at birth. Cell 1995; 83: 313–22

38. Orrell RW, King AW, Lane RJ, Belleroche JS. Investigation of a null mutation of the cntf gene in familial amyotrophic lateral sclerosis. J Neurol Sci 1995; 132: 126–8

39. Takahashi R. [Deficiency of human ciliary neurotropic factor (CNTF) is not causally related to amyotrophic lateral sclerosis (ALS)]. Rinsho Shinkeigaku 1995; 35: 1543–5

40. Giess R, Holtmann B, Braga M, et al. Early onset of severe familial amyotrophic lateral sclerosis with a SOD-1 mutation: Potential impact of cntf as a candidate modifier gene. Am J Hum Genet 2002; 70: 1277–86

41. Al-Chalabi A, Scheffler MD, Smith BN, et al. Ciliary neurotrophic factor genotype does not influence clinical phenotype in amyotrophic lateral sclerosis. Ann Neurol 2003; 54: 130–4

42. Siddons MA, Pickering-Brown SM, Mann DM, et al. Debrisoquine hydroxylase gene polymorphism frequencies in patients with amyotrophic lateral sclerosis. Neurosci Lett 1996; 208: 65–8

43. Nicholl DJ, Bennett P, Hiller L, et al. A study of five candidate genes in Parkinson's disease and related neurodegenerative disorders. European study group on atypical parkinsonism. Neurology 1999; 53: 1415–21

44. Munch C, Sedlmeier R, Meyer T, et al. Point mutations of the p150 subunit of dynactin (dctn1) gene in ALS. Neurology 2004; 63: 724–6

45. Hafezparast M, Klocke R, Ruhrberg C, et al. Mutations in dynein link motor neuron degeneration to defects in retrograde transport. Science 2003; 300: 808–12

46. Ahmad-Annuar A, Shah P, Hafezparast M, et al. No association with common caucasian genotypes in exons 8, 13 and 14 of the human cytoplasmic dynein heavy chain gene (dnchc1) and familial motor neuron disorders. Amyotroph Lateral Scler Other Motor Neuron Disord 2003; 4: 150–7

47. Aoki M, Lin CL, Rothstein JD, et al. Mutations in the glutamate transporter eaat2 gene do not cause abnormal eaat2 transcripts in amyotrophic lateral sclerosis. Ann Neurol 1998; 43: 645–53

48. Lin CL, Bristol LA, Jin L, et al. Aberrant RNA processing in a neurodegenerative disease: The cause for absent eaat2, a glutamate transporter, in amyotrophic lateral sclerosis. Neuron 1998; 20: 589–602

49. Meyer T, Munch C, Volkel H, et al. The eaat2 (glt-1) gene in motor neuron disease: Absence of mutations in amyotrophic lateral sclerosis and a point mutation in patients with hereditary spastic paraplegia. J Neurol Neurosurg Psychiatry 1998; 65: 594–6

50. Jackson M, Steers G, Leigh PN, Morrison KE. Polymorphisms in the glutamate transporter gene eaat2 in European ALS patients. J Neurol 1999; 246: 1140–4

51. Meyer T, Fromm A, Munch C, et al. The RNA of the glutamate transporter eaat2 is variably spliced in amyotrophic lateral sclerosis and normal individuals. J Neurol Sci 1999; 170: 45–50

52. Honig LS, Chambliss DD, Bigio EH, et al. Glutamate transporter eaat2 splice variants occur not only in ALS, but also in AD and controls. Neurology 2000; 55: 1082–8

53. Flowers JM, Powell JF, Leigh PN, et al. Intron 7 retention and exon 9 skipping eaat2 mRNA variants are not associated with amyotrophic lateral sclerosis. Ann Neurol 2001; 49: 643–9

54. Drory VE, Birnbaum M, Peleg L, et al. Hexosaminidase a deficiency is an uncommon cause of a syndrome mimicking amyotrophic lateral sclerosis. Muscle Nerve 2003; 28: 109–12

55. Wang XS, Lee S, Simmons Z, et al. Increased incidence of the HFE mutation in amyotrophic lateral sclerosis and related cellular consequences. J Neurol Sci 2004; 227: 27–33

56. Yen AA, Simpson EP, Henkel JS, et al. Hfe mutations are not strongly associated with sporadic als. Neurology 2004; 62: 1611–12

57. Meyer MA, Potter NT. Sporadic ALS and chromosome 22: Evidence for a possible neurofilament gene defect. Muscle Nerve 1995; 18: 536–9

58. Giess R, Beck M, Goetz R, et al. Potential role of lif as a modifier gene in the pathogenesis of amyotrophic lateral sclerosis. Neurology 2000; 54: 1003–5

59. Chioza BA, Ujfalusy A, Csiszar K, et al. Mutations in the lysyl oxidase gene are not associated with amyotrophic lateral sclerosis. Amyotroph Lateral Scler Other Motor Neuron Disord 2001; 2: 93–7

60. Orru S, Mascia V, Casula M, et al. Association of monoamine oxidase B alleles with age at onset in amyotrophic lateral sclerosis. Neuromuscul Disord 1999; 9: 593–7

61. Poorkaj P, Tsuang D, Wijsman E, et al. Tau as a susceptibility gene for amyotropic lateral sclerosis-parkinsonism dementia complex of Guam. Arch Neurol 2001; 58: 1871–8

62. Kowalska A, Konagaya M, Sakai M, et al. Familial amyotrophic lateral sclerosis and parkinsonism-dementia complex – tauopathy without mutations in the tau gene? Folia Neuropathol 2003; 41: 59–64

63. Swerdlow RH, Parks JK, Cassarino DS, et al. Mitochondria in sporadic amyotrophic lateral sclerosis. Exp Neurol 1998; 153: 135–42

64. Dhaliwal GK, Grewal RP. Mitochondrial DNA deletion mutation levels are elevated in ALS brains. Neuroreport 2000; 11: 2507–9

65. Wiedemann FR, Manfredi G, Mawrin C, et al. Mitochondrial DNA and respiratory chain function in spinal cords of ALS patients. J Neurochem 2002; 80: 616–25

66. Gajewski CD, Lin MT, Cudkowicz ME, et al. Mitochondrial DNA from platelets of sporadic ALS

patients restores normal respiratory functions in rho(0) cells. Exp Neurol 2003; 179: 229–35

67. Mawrin C, Kirches E, Dietzmann K. Single-cell analysis of mtDNA in amyotrophic lateral sclerosis: Towards the characterization of individual neurons in neurodegenerative disorders. Pathol Res Pract 2003; 199: 415–18

68. Ro LS, Lai SL, Chen CM, Chen ST. Deleted 4977-bp mitochondrial DNA mutation is associated with sporadic amyotrophic lateral sclerosis: A hospital-based case–control study. Muscle Nerve 2003; 28: 737–43

69. Mawrin C, Kirches E, Krause G, et al. Single-cell analysis of mtDNA deletion levels in sporadic amyotrophic lateral sclerosis. Neuroreport 2004; 15: 939–43

70. Jackson M, Morrison KE, Al-Chalabi A, et al. Analysis of chromosome 5q13 genes in amyotrophic lateral sclerosis: Homozygous naip deletion in a sporadic case. Ann Neurol 1996; 39: 796–800

71. Orrell RW, Habgood JJ, de Belleroche JS, Lane RJ. The relationship of spinal muscular atrophy to motor neuron disease: Investigation of smn and naip gene deletions in sporadic and familial ALS. J Neurol Sci 1997; 145: 55–61

72. Parboosingh JS, Meininger V, McKenna-Yasek D, et al. Deletions causing spinal muscular atrophy do not predispose to amyotrophic lateral sclerosis. Arch Neurol 1999; 56: 710–12

73. Corcia P, Mayeux-Portas V, Khoris J, et al. Abnormal smn1 gene copy number is a susceptibility factor for amyotrophic lateral sclerosis. Ann Neurol 2002; 51: 243–6

74. Lin FH, Lin R, Wisniewski HM, et al. Detection of point mutations in codon 331 of mitochondrial NADH dehydrogenase subunit 2 in Alzheimer's brains. Biochem Biophys Res Commun 1992; 182: 238–46

75. Julien JP, Cote F, Collard JF. Mice overexpressing the human neurofilament heavy gene as a model of ALS. Neurobiol Aging 1995; 16: 487–90; discussion 490–2

76. Rooke K, Figlewicz DA, Han FY, Rouleau GA. Analysis of the ksp repeat of the neurofilament heavy subunit in familiar amyotrophic lateral sclerosis. Neurology 1996; 46: 789–90

77. Vechio JD, Bruijn LI, Xu Z, et al. Sequence variants in human neurofilament proteins: Absence of linkage to familial amyotrophic lateral sclerosis. Ann Neurol 1996; 40: 603–10

78. Tomkins J, Usher P, Slade JY, et al. Novel insertion in the KSP region of the neurofilament heavy gene in amyotrophic lateral sclerosis (ALS). Neuroreport 1998; 9: 3967–70

79. Al-Chalabi A, Andersen PM, Nilsson P, et al. Deletions of the heavy neurofilament subunit tail in amyotrophic lateral sclerosis. Hum Mol Genet 1999; 8: 157–64

80. Gros-Louis F, Lariviere R, Gowing G, et al. A frameshift deletion in peripherin gene associated with amyotrophic lateral sclerosis. J Biol Chem 2004; 279: 45951–6

81. Leung CL, He CZ, Kaufmann P, et al. A pathogenic peripherin gene mutation in a patient with amyotrophic lateral sclerosis. Brain Pathol 2004; 14: 290–6

82. Panas M, Karadima G, Kalfakis N, et al. Genotyping of presenilin-1 polymorphism in amyotrophic lateral sclerosis. J Neurol 2000; 247: 940–2

83. Saunderson R, Yu B, Trent RJ, Pamphlett R. A polymorphism in the poliovirus receptor gene differs in motor neuron disease. Neuroreport 2004; 15: 383–6

84. Chen YZ, Bennett CL, Huynh HM, et al. DNA/RNA helicase gene mutations in a form of juvenile amyotrophic lateral sclerosis (ALS4). Am J Hum Genet 2004; 74: 1128–35

85. Corcia P, Khoris J, Couratier P, et al. Smn1 gene study in three families in which ALS and spinal muscular atrophy co-exist. Neurology 2002; 59: 1464–6

86. Veldink JH, van den Berg LH, Cobben JM, et al. Homozygous deletion of the survival motor neuron 2 gene is a prognostic factor in sporadic ALS. Neurology 2001; 56: 749–52

87. McDermott CJ, Roberts D, Tomkins J, et al. Spastin and paraplegin gene analysis in selected cases of motor neurone disease (MND). Amyotroph Lateral Scler Other Motor Neuron Disord 2003; 4: 96–9

88. Flowers JM, Leigh PN, Davies AM, et al. Mutations in the gene encoding human persyn are not associated with amyotrophic lateral sclerosis or familial Parkinson's disease. Neurosci Lett 1999; 274: 21–4

89. Tomkins J, Banner SJ, McDermott CJ, Shaw PJ. Mutation screening of manganese superoxide dismutase in amyotrophic lateral sclerosis. Neuroreport 2001; 12: 2319–22

90. Nishimura AL, Mitne-Neto M, Silva HC, et al. A mutation in the vesicle-trafficking protein VAPB causes late-onset spinal muscular atrophy and amy-

otrophic lateral sclerosis. Am J Hum Genet 2004; 75: 822–31

91. Oosthuyse B, Moons L, Storkebaum E, et al. Deletion of the hypoxia-response element in the vascular endothelial growth factor promoter causes motor neuron degeneration. Nat Genet 2001; 28: 131–8

92. Lambrechts D, Storkebaum E, Morimoto M, et al. Vegf is a modifier of amyotrophic lateral sclerosis in mice and humans and protects motoneurons against ischemic death. Nat Genet 2003; 34: 383–94

93. de Knijff P, van den Maagdenberg AM, Frants RR, Havekes LM. Genetic heterogeneity of apolipoprotein E and its influence on plasma lipid and lipoprotein levels. Hum Mutat 1994; 4: 178–94

94. Corder EH, Saunders AM, Strittmatter WJ, et al. Gene dose of apolipoprotein E type 4 allele and the risk of Alzheimer's disease in late onset families. Science 1993; 261: 921–3

95. Chapman J, Vinokurov S, Achiron A, et al. ApoE genotype is a major predictor of long-term progression of disability in MS. Neurology 2001; 56: 312–16

96. Smith RG, Haverkamp LJ, Case S, et al. Apolipoprotein E epsilon 4 in bulbar-onset motor neuron disease. Lancet 1996; 348: 334–5

97. Bachus R, Bader S, Gessner R, Ludolph AC. Lack of association of apolipoprotein E epsilon 4 allele with bulbar-onset motor neuron disease. Ann Neurol 1997; 41: 417

98. Li YJ, Pericak-Vance MA, Haines JL, et al. Apolipoprotein E is associated with age at onset of amyotrophic lateral sclerosis. Neurogenetics 2004; 5: 209–13

99. Sendtner M, Kreutzberg GW, Thoenen H. Ciliary neurotrophic factor prevents the degeneration of motor neurons after axotomy. Nature 1990; 345: 440–1

100. Sendtner M, Arakawa Y, Stockli KA, et al. Effect of ciliary neurotrophic factor (cntf) on motoneuron survival. J Cell Sci Suppl 1991; 15: 103–9

101. Lo AC, Li L, Oppenheim RW, et al. Ciliary neurotrophic factor promotes the survival of spinal sensory neurons following axotomy but not during the period of programmed cell death. Exp Neurol 1995; 134: 49–55

102. Ip NY, Yancopoulos GD. The neurotrophins and cntf: Two families of collaborative neurotrophic factors. Annu Rev Neurosci 1996; 19: 491–515

103. Sendtner M, Schmalbruch H, Stockli KA, et al. Ciliary neurotrophic factor prevents degeneration of motor neurons in mouse mutant progressive motor neuronopathy. Nature 1992; 358: 502–4

104. Takahashi R, Yokoji H, Misawa H, et al. A null mutation in the human CNTF gene is not causally related to neurological diseases. Nat Genet 1994; 7: 79–84

105. Giess R, Goetz R, Schrank B, et al. Potential implications of a ciliary neurotrophic factor gene mutation in a German population of patients with motor neuron disease. Muscle Nerve 1998; 21: 236–8

106. Gelernter J, Van Dyck C, van Kammen DP, et al. Ciliary neurotrophic factor null allele frequencies in schizophrenia, affective disorders, and Alzheimer's disease. Am J Med Genet 1997; 74: 497–500

107. Emerich DF, Winn SR, Hantraye PM, et al. Protective effect of encapsulated cells producing neurotrophic factor cntf in a monkey model of Huntington's disease. Nature 1997; 386: 395–9

108. Fong GH, Rossant J, Gertsenstein M, Breitman ML. Role of the flt-1 receptor tyrosine kinase in regulating the assembly of vascular endothelium. Nature 1995; 376: 66–70

109. Soker S, Takashima S, Miao HQ, et al. Neuropilin-1 is expressed by endothelial and tumor cells as an isoform-specific receptor for vascular endothelial growth factor. Cell 1998; 92: 735–45

110. Lennmyr F, Ata KA, Funa K, et al. Expression of vascular endothelial growth factor (VEGF) and its receptors (flt-1 and flk-1) following permanent and transient occlusion of the middle cerebral artery in the rat. J Neuropathol Exp Neurol 1998; 57: 874–82

111. Yang K, Cepko CL. Flk-1, a receptor for vascular endothelial growth factor (VEGF), is expressed by retinal progenitor cells. J Neurosci 1996; 16: 6089–99

112. Sondell M, Lundborg G, Kanje M. Vascular endothelial growth factor has neurotrophic activity and stimulates axonal outgrowth, enhancing cell survival and Schwann cell proliferation in the peripheral nervous system. J Neurosci 1999; 19: 5731–40

113. Delisle MB, Carpenter S. Neurofibrillary axonal swellings and amyotrophic lateral sclerosis. J Neurol Sci 1984; 63: 241–50

114. Mizusawa H, Matsumoto S, Yen SH, et al. Focal accumulation of phosphorylated neurofilaments within anterior horn cell in familial amyotrophic lateral sclerosis. Acta Neuropathol (Berl) 1989; 79: 37–43

115. Matsumoto S, Kusaka H, Murakami N, et al. Basophilic inclusions in sporadic juvenile amyotrophic lateral sclerosis: An immunocytochemical and ultrastructural study. Acta Neuropathol (Berl) 1992; 83: 579–83

116. Troost D, Sillevis Smitt PA, de Jong JM, Swaab DF. Neurofilament and glial alterations in the cerebral cortex in amyotrophic lateral sclerosis. Acta Neuropathol (Berl) 1992; 84: 664–73

117. Collard JF, Cote F, Julien JP. Defective axonal transport in a transgenic mouse model of amyotrophic lateral sclerosis. Nature 1995; 375: 61–4

118. Julien JP. A role for neurofilaments in the pathogenesis of amyotrophic lateral sclerosis. Biochem Cell Biol 1995; 73: 593–7

119. Al-Chalabi A, Miller CC. Neurofilaments and neurological disease. Bioessays 2003; 25: 346–55

120. Figlewicz DA, Krizus A, Martinoli MG, et al. Variants of the heavy neurofilament subunit are associated with the development of amyotrophic lateral sclerosis. Hum Mol Genet 1994; 3: 1757–61

121. Portier MM, de Nechaud B, Gros F. Peripherin, a new member of the intermediate filament protein family. Dev Neurosci 1983; 6: 335–44

122. Murakami T, Nagano I, Hayashi T, et al. Impaired retrograde axonal transport of adenovirus-mediated E. coli lacz gene in the mice carrying mutant SOD1 gene. Neurosci Lett 2001; 308: 149–52

123. Harada A, Takei Y, Kanai Y, et al. Golgi vesiculation and lysosome dispersion in cells lacking cytoplasmic dynein. J Cell Biol 1998; 141: 51–9

124. Eaton BA, Fetter RD, Davis GW. Dynactin is necessary for synapse stabilization. Neuron 2002; 34: 729–41

125. LaMonte BH, Wallace KE, Holloway BA, et al. Disruption of dynein/dynactin inhibits axonal transport in motor neurons causing late-onset progressive degeneration. Neuron 2002; 34: 715–27

126. Puls I, Jonnakuty C, LaMonte BH, et al. Mutant dynactin in motor neuron disease. Nat Genet 2003; 33: 455–6

127. Liu Q, Fischer U, Wang F, Dreyfuss G. The spinal muscular atrophy disease gene product, smn, and its associated protein sip1 are in a complex with spliceosomal snrnp proteins. Cell 1997; 90: 1013–21

128. Lorson CL, Androphy EJ. The domain encoded by exon 2 of the survival motor neuron protein mediates nucleic acid binding. Hum Mol Genet 1998; 7: 1269–75

129. Campbell L, Hunter KM, Mohaghegh P, et al. Direct interaction of smn with dp103, a putative RNA helicase: A role for smn in transcription regulation? Hum Mol Genet 2000; 9: 1093–100

130. Fan L, Simard LR. Survival motor neuron (SMN) protein: Role in neurite outgrowth and neuromuscular maturation during neuronal differentiation and development. Hum Mol Genet 2002; 11: 1605–14

131. Lefebvre S, Burglen L, Reboullet S, et al. Identification and characterization of a spinal muscular atrophy-determining gene. Cell 1995; 80: 155–65

132. Moulard B, Salachas F, Chassande B, et al. Association between centromeric deletions of the smn gene and sporadic adult-onset lower motor neuron disease. Ann Neurol 1998; 43: 640–4

133. Kunst CB, Messer L, Gordon J, et al. Genetic mapping of a mouse modifier gene that can prevent ALS onset. Genomics 2000; 70: 181–9

134. Gamez J, Barcelo MJ, Munoz X, et al. Survival and respiratory decline are not related to homozygous smn2 deletions in ALS patients. Neurology 2002; 59: 1456–60

11

From genetic defects to molecular pathogenesis of memory and movement disorders

William H Stoothoff, Bradley T Hyman

INTRODUCTION

The primary focus of this chapter is to introduce the reader to neurodegenerative diseases linked to dementia or movement disorders in which a protein or proteins containing mutations have been identified as causative factors of the disease. Like amyotrophic lateral sclerosis (ALS), the disorders target specific regions of the central nervous system, neurotransmitter systems and subpopulations of neurons. The specific mechanisms for those vulnerabilities are still unknown, but together they illustrate a variety of molecular pathways, triggered perhaps by aggregation of specific proteins, that lead to neurodegenerative syndromes.

PARKINSON'S DISEASE

Parkinson's disease (PD) is a neurodegenerative disease that is marked primarily by the loss of dopaminergic neurons in the substantia nigra, and the occurrence of cytoplasmic inclusions termed Lewy bodies (LB) (Figure 11.1). The clinical features of PD are primarily movement disorders (i.e. bradykinesia, resting tremor and rigidity); however, cognitive decline accompanies PD symptoms in patients who have more widespread pathologic changes, a condition called diffuse Lewy body

a

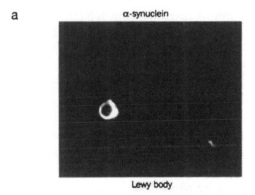

Lewy body

b

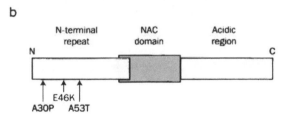

Figure 11.1 (a) Confocal microscope image showing a Lewy body from a Parkinsons's disease (PD)-affected patient's brain that was stained with anti-α-synuclein antibody. (b) Schematic diagram of α-synuclein illustrating the major identified protein domains. The three mutations that have been found in familial PD are identified with arrows in the N-terminus of the protein. See also Plate 7

disease. Recently, a number of different proteins have been shown to be present in LB including α-synuclein and ubiquitylated proteins (reviewed in reference 1).

Although the vast majority of PD cases are of unknown cause and are sporadic, a small number of PD cases are inherited. Several genes identified to date, including α-*synuclein*[2], *parkin*[3-5], ubiquitin C-terminal hydrolase L1 (*UCHL1*)[6], and *DJ-1*[7,8] either appear to be misfolded or are involved in the ubiquitin proteasome system (UPS), and implicate the UPS in the neurodegenerative process. Other genes, including *PINK1* and *LRRK2* (which are discussed below) are less clearly implicated in the UPS system.

Mutation or overexpression of α-synuclein leads to cytoplasmic inclusions of presumably misfolded α-synuclein recognized histologically as LB. These commonly contain both ubiquitin and α-synuclein[1]. Currently, three different mutations in the α-synuclein protein have been identified in families with PD. The A30P[9], A53T[10] and the recently described E46K[11] mutations each have a similar phenotype. Perhaps most interesting are several recently discovered kindreds in which an otherwise normal α-synuclein gene has been duplicated[12]. The end result of α-synuclein gene duplication is a pathology similar to that of mutated α-synuclein, and of sporadic PD. The mechanism by which this duplication leads to α-synuclein aggregates, pathologic changes and cell death is unclear.

In contrast, mutations in the *parkin* gene result in a recessive form of juvenile-onset PD; however, the affected neurons and brain regions do not contain LB as with other forms of PD. The parkin protein has been identified as an E3 ubiquitin ligase, which is directly involved in the UPS. Parkin has been implicated in metabolism of synuclein and a related protein, synphilin[13].

In one PD-affected kindred, an apparent autosomal dominant mutation in the *UCHL1* gene has been identified, but no other mutations have been found to date[6]. Surprisingly, a polymorphism in the *UCHL1* gene has been linked to a decrease in susceptibility for PD, at least in early life[14]. The apparent opposing effects of different amino acid substitutions in the same protein are not understood, and may provide insight into the role of UCHL1 in the pathogenesis of PD pathology. DJ-1 mutations lead to an adult-onset autosomal recessive form of PD[7,8]. DJ-1, however, does not have any clear motifs within its amino acid sequence, but DJ-1 has been suggested to act as a molecular chaperone for α-synuclein[15].

Two other genes implicated in heritable forms of PD are *PINK1*[16,17] and leucine-rich repeat kinase (*LRRK2*)[18]. The roles of these two proteins are not well understood in physiological or pathologic conditions; however, some data suggest possible roles for each. For instance, the PINK1 protein contains a mitochondrial-targeting sequence and a putative Ser/Thr protein kinase domain[19]. *LRRK2* was very recently identified as a gene containing mutations in a subset of autosomal dominant late-onset PD cases[18,20]. *LRRK2* encodes a kinase of unknown function.

Along with these genetic influences, certain environmental toxins can also cause specific loss of dopaminergic cells in the substantia nigra. The insecticides rotenone and paraquat, and the heroin-like 1-methyl-4-phenyl-1,2,3,6-tetrahydropyridine (MPTP) have all been used to recapitulate PD in mammalian animal models including mice and non-human primates[21]. These compounds have a common mechanism of action, in that they all inhibit mitochondrial complex I or III. Some of these treatments even induce intraneuronal inclusions that include α-synuclein, but are not structurally identical to LB[22]. These models have provided information into the possible mechanisms of cell death that may occur in PD.

The facts that mutations in proteins involved in the UPS and neurotoxins that affect the electron transport chain in mitochondria lead to cell death in similar brain regions and cause similar pathologic features suggest that there may be a link between the normal metabolism of proteins and the production of energy in affected cells. Further evidence of a link between protein metabolism and cellular dysfunction in PD has recently been demonstrated by the modulatory effect of the chaperone protein heat shock protein 70 (HSP 70)[23-26]. HSP70 is involved in aiding newly synthesized proteins and misfolded proteins in correct folding, and can pass some proteins off to HSP90 for further folding guidance[27]. Expression of HSP70 in *Drosophila melanogaster* attenuates the toxic effects of α-synuclein overexpression[26]. HSP70 overexpression was also shown to decrease the cellular aggregation of mutant α-synuclein and decrease cell death associated with α-synuclein toxicity in mammalian systems[25]. These results suggest that synuclein misfolding (and possibly subsequent aggregation) can directly damage and kill a cell, although whether aggregates *per se* are toxic remains controversial. Preventing protein misfolding and/or aggregation can prevent cell death induced by α-synuclein toxicity, and may provide therapeutic targets for treatment of the neurodegeneration that occurs in PD.

PROGRESSIVE SUPRANUCLEAR PALSY

Progressive supranuclear palsy (PSP) has both clinical and pathologic similarities to PD. PSP is a movement disorder characterized by axial dystonia, bradykinesia, falls, dysphagia and vertical gaze palsy[28]. Pathologically, PSP is characterized by a heterogeneous loss of neurons in specific subcortical areas. The areas most commonly affected are the subthalamic nucleus, globus pallidus interna and externa, pontine nuclei, periaqueductal gray matter, and the substantia nigra[29]. As a result of the different areas affected by the disease, the neurotransmitter systems affected by PSP include the dopaminergic, cholinergic, γ-aminobutyric acidergic (GABAergic), and norepinephrine systems[29].

On a cellular level, the hallmark of PSP is the presence of fibrillar lesions in neurons of the affected brain regions that are composed mainly of a hyperphosphorylated form of the microtubule-associated protein tau. This is the same molecule that leads to inclusions in frontotemporal dementia and in Alzheimer's disease (AD), but different neuronal populations are affected in PSP compared to these related disorders.

Tau is present in the brain in six major isoforms derived from alternative splicing of a single tau gene. The tau found in the neurofibrillary tangles (NFTs) from PSP brain are composed of tau that contains exon 10 (and hence a fourth microtubule-binding repeat domain) and that is phosphorylated throughout the molecule, which results in decreased tau–microtubule interaction[28,30]. Interestingly, there are also families that present with PSP that have no tau pathology, but instead ubiquitin-positive neuronal inclusions[31].

Because of the extensive tau pathology present in most PSP cases, it belongs to a larger family of neurodegenerative diseases that also have similar tau pathology, termed tauopathies. One genetic variant has been demonstrated to occur in a large number of sporadic PSP cases. In 1999 Baker *et al.*[32] demonstrated that there are two separate haplotypes (termed H1 and H2) that span the entire human *tau* gene. In a majority of the PSP cases genotyped in this and subsequent studies, the H1 haplotype was over-represented. To date, the causative polymorphism that occurs within the *tau* gene, or flanking the chromosomal region, has not been identified. However, the strong linkage data to the H1 haplotype strongly suggest that the tau gene, or a regulator of tau gene expression, is involved in the pathogenesis of PSP.

LOBAR DEGENERATIONS AND TAUOPATHIES

Other tauopathies include corticobasal degeneration (CBD), Pick's disease (PiD), and frontotemporal dementia (FTD). Most cases of CBD and PiD are sporadic and of unknown etiology, yet all involve tau lesions and neurodegeneration in affected brain areas. These variants of FTDs are late-onset dementias characterized by memory and language impairments, especially anomia, as well as the frequent occurrence of personality changes. The predominance of the atrophy is observed in the frontal and/or temporal lobes, and in many instances this atrophy is strikingly asymmetric.

Subcortical structures including the caudate can also be involved. The predominant pathologic feature is striking neuronal loss and gliosis, circumscribed frontal or temporal lobe atrophy, and inclusions that are immunopositive for tau and ubiquitin, such as Pick bodies. Rare familial forms occur, as well, with apparent autosomal dominant inheritance. For example, the autosomal dominantly inherited syndrome of frontotemporal dementia with parkinsonism linked to chromosome 17 (FTDP-17) has been shown to be caused by one of over 30 mutations identified in the tau gene (reviewed in reference 33).

As the name implies, FTDP-17 is characterized by the loss of neurons within the frontal and temporal lobes. Despite the fact that mutations all occur within the tau gene, there is a large degree of both cognitive and pathologic phenotype heterogeneity. For instance, different mutations can cause divergent behavioral phenotypes. The N279K mutation causes a PSP-like phenotype with concurrent dementia, while the V337M mutation often causes dementia coupled with psychotic disturbances[33]. The intronic +16 mutation, which alters exon 10 splicing, causes characteristic FTD and affective disorders, and has an age of onset between 40 and 60[34].

Further complicating the understanding of the effects of the tau mutations, several mutations have been shown to produce different clinical presentations, both among kindreds and even within the same families. For example, the P301S mutation causes epileptic seizures and FTDP in a German kindred[35], but a number of Japanese kindreds presented with parkinsonism[36]. Perhaps most strikingly, in a separate kindred, a father with the P301S mutation presented with FTD while his son, with the same mutation, presented with CBD[37]. The ΔN296 deletion mutation causes atypical PSP in homozygous individuals, while heterozygous individuals have incomplete penetrance and present with atypical PD[38].

The *tau* mutations associated with FTD in some instances cause changes in tau's amino acid sequence, but in many instances change its splicing patterns. The six different tau isoforms differ by the presence of zero, one, or two amino-terminal inserts (exons 2 and 3) and the presence of either three or four microtubule-binding repeats, with the second microtubule-binding repeat being encoded by exon 10 (reviewed in reference 39). The presence of the fourth microtubule-binding repeat increases tau's affinity for microtubules, while phosphorylation of tau generally decreases its affinity for microtubules. Tau normally localizes to axons and helps maintain the microtubule network, and its mistrafficking is postulated to be a cause of neuronal dysfunction.

The mutations in the tau gene that cause missense amino acid substitutions tend to cluster around the microtubule-binding domains of *tau*[33]. Interestingly, a few mutations encode either silent mutations or intronic mutations that affect the alternative splicing of the *tau* gene to increase the amount of 4-repeat tau expressed, while not affecting the amino acid make-up of tau. This implies that both the structure of tau, as well as the ratio between 3-and 4-repeat tau is critical in maintaining neuronal function[40].

Similar to the behavioral and cognitive phenotypes, the different *tau* mutations also correspond to distinct cellular and pathological phenotypes. The intronic mutations that alter the ratio of 3-repeat tau to 4-repeat tau lead to filamentous tau inclusions that contain mostly 4-repeat tau[33]. The three missense mutations that occur in exon 9 including K257T[41], L266V[42,43], and G272V[44,45] resemble Pick's disease. Further, the K257T mutation causes inclusions consisting mainly of 3-repeat tau while the L266V mutation causes inclusions with both 3- and 4-repeat tau present, with 4-repeat tau being present in neuronal lesions and 3-repeat isoforms being present in glial inclusions.

One common feature of all the FTDP-17 mutations is that they result in the deposition of tau into insoluble protein aggregates that contain tau in an abnormally phosphorylated state. Some mutations lead to the formation of NFT-like structures, while other mutations cause straight filaments or flame-shaped filaments. The mechanisms underlying the increased phosphorylation and aggregate formation are poorly understood, but it seems clear that altering the cellular distribution or balance of 3-repeat and 4-repeat tau is detrimental to neurons and is capable of compromising cell function and integrity.

ALZHEIMER'S DISEASE

AD is the most common neurodegenerative disease, with over 4 million Americans affected. AD is a progressive neurodegenerative disease that affects cognitive function and eventually leads to a near complete loss of higher order functioning. As the disease progresses, memory loss worsens (generally over years) until normal social and personal functioning are severely impaired. Along with progressive memory loss, AD patients often suffer from changes in personality in the later stages.

Neurons in limbic areas including the hippocampus, amygdala and entorhinal cortex, subcortical areas such as the nucleus basalis and the dorsal raphe, and cortical association cortices are most vulnerable. The motor system and primary sensory systems are relatively spared from pathology and neuron death.

AD is characterized by two major pathologic features: senile plaques (Figure 11.2) and NFTs (Figure 11.3). Senile plaques are extracellular lesions that occur in the neuropil in and around synapses. The major component of senile plaques is amyloid β (Aβ), which is a 40 or 42 amino acid residue proteolytic fragment of the amyloid precursor protein (APP). Aβ1-42, normally synthesized in smaller amounts than Aβ1-40, is more fibrillogenic and deposits to a greater extent in plaques. NFTs are intracellular lesions analogous to those seen in the tauopathies that are composed mainly of hyperphosphorylated tau; in AD, both

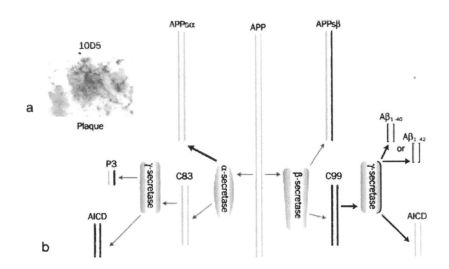

Figure 11.2   (a) Light microscope image of a plaque from an Alzheimer's disease (AD) brain section stained with 10D5 antibody, which recognizes the Aβ protein. Section was developed with HRP and DAB to visualize staining. (b) Diagram illustrating the different cleavage events that occur during amyloid precursor protein (APP) processing to yield the various end products. When APP is cleaved by α-secretase, the soluble APPsα is released into the extracellular space and the C83 fragment remains associated with the membrane. C83 is then cleaved by γ-secretase to yield the P3 and AICD fragment. Similarly, β-secretase cleaves APP to produce the soluble APPsβ and the membrane-associated C99 fragment. For reasons that are not understood, γ-secretase then cleaves the C99 fragment to produce either the Aβ1-40 or the more fibrillogenic Aβ1-42 peptide, along with the AICD fragment that is released into the intracellular space. See also Plate 8

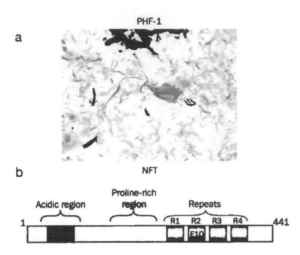

Figure 11.3 (a) Light microscope image of Alzheimer's disease (AD) affected brain section stained with PHF-1 antibody, which recognizes abnormally phosphorylated tau in neurofibrillary tangles (NFTs) in AD brain. Section was developed with DAB and HRP to visualize staining, and figure shows a plaque present in AD brain (b) Schematic diagram of tau protein showing the longest human isoform found in adult brain. The longest isoform is characterized by the presence of two amino-terminal inserts (exons 2 and 3) and a fourth microtubule-binding domain (exon 10), which are all alternatively spliced to give rise to the six isoforms of tau found in adult human brain. See also Plate 9

3-repeat and 4-repeat tau contribute to the NFT. NFTs are also ubiquitin immunoreactive.

The *APP* gene was identified in 1987 as the gene that encodes the full-length precursor of the amyloid peptide[46-49]. Since being cloned, it has been shown that *APP* mutants occur in a subset of familial AD (FAD) cases, which cause missense mutations in APP[50-54]. Specific mutations in the APP gene fall into three categories: those that increase the amount of total Aβ, those that increase Aβ1-42 production, or those that increase fibril formation. Each of these lead to an increase in Aβ plaque deposits.

The processing of the APP protein is a complex sequence of steps, dependent on numerous cleavage events mediated by secretases[55]. There are three separate secretases that can cleave APP and yield a variety of intracellular and extracellular products. The first step is cleavage in the extracellular N-terminal domain by either α- or β-secretase. If APP is cleaved first by α-secretase (a cell-surface metalloprotease), two proteolytic fragments are produced, termed APPsα (which is secreted) and C83 (which is membrane associated). γ-Secretase then cleaves the C83 fragment to yield the p3 fragment and the APP intracellular domain (AICD). Similarly, cleavage by β-secretase (memapsin 2; BACE) yields the extracellular secreted APPsβ and the membrane-associated C99 fragment. Cleavage of the C99 fragment by γ-secretase then yields either Aβ1-40 or the more fibrillogenic Aβ1-42, along with the intracellular AICD. Cleavage of C83 by γ-secretase leads to analogous products. The 20 mutations that occur in the APP protein all occur close to the cleavage sites for α-, β- and γ-secretases, or within the Aβmolecule[56].

Presenilin-1[57,58] and *presenilin-2*[59-62] were both identified as mutation-bearing genes in early-onset familial AD cases in 1995. *Presenilin-1* is located on chromosome 14q24.3. To date, there have been more than 100 mutations identified in different kindreds (reviewed in reference 63, see also www.alzforum.org). Fewer mutations in the *presenilin-2* gene have been identified. Identification of the homologous presenilin 1 (*PS1*) and presenilin 2 (*PS2*) genes as harboring multiple autosomal dominant AD mutations led to the discovery of the molecular identity of γ-secretase.

Data from cell culture studies demonstrated that presenilins were likely to be involved in processing of the APP protein, as cells from *PS1*-null animals showed markedly decreased Aβ production[64]. In normal brain, the amount of Aβ1-40 greatly exceeds the amount of Aβ1-42, although there is a small amount of Aβ1-42 produced even under physiologic conditions[65]. FAD-causing mutations in the *PS* genes cause an increase in the ratio of Aβ1-42 to Aβ1-40[66], indicating that changes in presenilin function affect γ-secretase activity. In accord with this, a direct interaction of PS1 and APP at the cell surface has been demonstrated[67].

These observations led to the suggestion that presenilin is the enzymatically active component of γ-secretase, via a novel mechanism: aspartate-mediated intramembranous cleavage of substrates[68, 69]. Presenilin is not sufficient for γ-secretase activity, and three other proteins have been identified that are necessary for proper γ-secretase activity. Nicastrin[70], APH-1[71, 72] and PEN-2[72, 73] appear to be critical components of the γ-secretase complex. Only presenilins have been identified as genetic causes of AD thus far, but this does not exclude nicastrin, APH-1, or PEN-2 from influencing pathological γ-secretase activity. Interestingly, Rozmahel et al.[74] found that alleles located at the nicastrin locus modify the PS knockout phenotype. This would indicate that nicastrin may influence the function and/or expression of PS or its substrates and may contribute to the pathogenic functioning of γ-secretase in disease states. APH-1, on the other hand, seems to be responsible for the proper formation and maturation of the presenilin and nicastrin complex, and may be involved in γ-secretase turnover[75]. In a similar manner, PEN-2 seems to be intimately linked to the levels of other γ-secretase proteins, as its expression level depends on and regulates the expression of both PS and nicastrin[73]. This led Steiner and colleagues[73] to speculate that the expression of the various members of the γ-secretase complex is coordinated with the expression levels of the other members of the complex. This again could mean that alterations in presenilin function/levels could be regulated by the other members of the secretase complex, and may prove to be additional risk factors associated with AD. In fact, recent data suggest that pharmacologic intervention can allosterically modulate the α-secretase complex to decrease the percentage of Aβ1-42[76].

In some ways the most important genetic risk for AD is APOE ε4[77-79]. In humans, three different isoforms (ApoE 2, 3 and 4) are encoded by separate alleles. One copy of the APOE ε4 allele is associated with a two- to three-fold increased risk of developing AD; two copies increase age-adjusted risk five- to ten-fold[77,78]. Epidemiologic data suggest that the APOE4 genotype might be present in as many as 50% of AD cases[80,81]. Of interest, inheritance of the relatively rare APOE2 allele is a protective genetic factor, decreasing the likelihood of AD almost two-fold and delaying its average age of onset[82,83].

ApoE proteins regulate the metabolism and distribution of lipids in cells. Glia are the primary source of central nervous system (CNS) ApoE[84-86]. ApoE receptors, including the low-density lipoprotein-related protein (LRP), are present on both neurons and glia[77, 87]. Therefore, ApoE may exert its influence directly on neurons, as well as having indirect effects by acting on the glial cells that surround neurons. Indeed, ApoE4 has been reported to bind Aβ peptides[79,88] and tau protein[89,90], in an isoform-specific manner, with ApoE4 binding most effectively. In humans, ApoE e4 is associated with increased amyloid deposition[77]. Data from transgenic mouse experiments support the view that ApoE has a role in Aβ clearance and in converting diffuse deposits of Aβ to the more permanent and more damaging tightly packed fibrils seen in a subset of plaques (thioflavine S plaques[91,92]).

Another possible contributor to increased Aβdeposition in AD is alterations in BACE protein, since the β-secretase enzymatic activity it performs appears to be the rate-limiting step in Aβ production. In several series of sporadic AD cases, BACE protein levels and activity are noted to be elevated in AD brain compared to controls[93,94]. Interestingly, brain BACE activity seems to increase with age, perhaps contributing to the age-related increased risk seen in AD[95]. Thus, BACE enzymatic activity is an attractive therapeutic target[96].

Despite the complexity involved in understanding how Aβ expression and metabolism are regulated, it is clear that increased deposition, especially of Aβ1-42, is detrimental to neurons. One mechanism by which Aβ may cause toxic injury to neurons is by sensitizing the cells to oxidative stress, and possibly by causing oxidative damage directly[97]. Plaques also are associated with local glial responses, disruption of the neuropil, distortion of axons and dendrites, and local neuronal loss[98].

The other major neuropathological hallmark of AD is NFTs (Figure 11.3). NFTs consist of a hyperphosphorylated form of tau that is redistributed from the axon to the somatodendritic compartment[99-102]. NFTs contain all six isoforms of tau, with no single isoform being over-represented[103]. Over 30 different phospho-epitopes have been identified in NFT tau from AD brain[39]. The mechanisms that underlie this hyperphosphorylation and cellular redistribution are currently not well understood. To date, no tau mutations have been identified in any AD cases.

Glycogen synthase kinase 3β (GSK3β) has been shown to be responsible for at least some of the phosphorylation events on tau. GSK3β is expressed in the brain, and within neurons[104]. GSK3β is known to phosphorylate numerous epitopes on tau, many of which are present in NFT tau[103]. Interestingly, GSK3β has also been localized to pretangle neurons and to microtubles[105]. In cultured cells treated with Aβ, GSK3β activity is increased, resulting in increased tau phosphorylation[106-108]. These results seem to indicate that tau phosphorylation and NFT formation result from toxic insults resulting from Aβ. However, a causal link between plaque formation and NFT formation and cell death has yet to be established *in vivo*.

Cdk5 is another putative tau kinase. Interestingly, Cdk5 is expressed in numerous tissue types, but one activator, p35, is largely expressed in the nervous system[109-112]. Cdk5 has also been localized to NFTs in AD brain[113,114]. Similar to GSK3β, Cdk5 is a Ser/Thr protein kinase that probably phosphorylates multiple sites on tau[115-118]. Indeed, Cdk5 activity is also increased in response to Aβ1-42 treatment of neurons[119,120]. Interestingly, in AD brain, p35 has been shown to be cleaved to a shorter p25 form that constitutively activates Cdk5 and mislocalizes the kinase[121]. Overexpression of p25 in a transgenic model led to tau phosphorylation and neuronal death[122]. This, together with the GSK3β data,

suggest that kinases that regulate tau phosphorylation may play important roles in mediating the neurodegenerative processes that occur in AD, although the roles they play in the cell death process are not clear.

The relationship between Aβ and tau is still not completely clear, but some experiments support Aβ overproduction as being upstream of tau abnormalities. Recently, Oddo *et al.*[123] utilized a triple transgenic AD mouse model to examine the effects of immunization against Aβ on both Aβ and tau pathology. This mouse model is based on a *PS-1* mutant knockin background, and contains mutant *APP* and tau transgenes incorporated into the genome. The mice display both Aβ and tau pathology, and neuronal death in many relevant brain areas. In *APP*-overexpressing mice, immunization with Aβ leads to decreased plaque load and even clearance of plaques[124-126]. Surprisingly, Aβ immunization also decreased the prevalence of early tau pathology, but did not affect late tau pathology. This implies that Aβ may initiate steps that lead to tau being aggregated and hyperphosphorylated. Genetic loci implicated in neurodegenerative diseases are shown in Table 11.1.

SUMMARY

PD, PSP, FTD and AD all have pathologic deposits, consistent with the accumulation of misfolded aggregated proteins. Mutations in genes that lead to these deposits, or in molecular pathways associated with those proteins, have been identified, causing autosomal dominant forms of these diseases. The more common 'sporadic' forms are identical in pattern, although frequently less aggressive clinically.

Today, there are animal models based upon overexpression of mutant disease-associated genes that mirror critical aspects of PD, FTD and AD. These models have been invaluable tools in addressing the cellular mechanisms involved in protein dysfunction, deposition and cell death. Animal models also provide an opportunity to test

Table 11.1   Genetic loci implicated in neurodegenerative diseases

Disease	Protein	Inheritance pattern	Chromosomal location	Putative function
Alzheimer's disease	APP	Autosomal dominant	21	Signaling molecule
	PS-1	Autosomal dominant	14	γ-Secretase
	PS-2	Autosomal dominant	1	γ-Secretase
	ApoE4	Increased risk	19	Cholesterol metabolism
Parkinson's disease	α-Synuclein	Autosomal dominant	4	Unknown
	Parkin	Autosomal dominant	6	E3 ubiquitin ligase
	UCHL-1	Autosomal dominant	4	Ubiquitin C-terminal hydrolase
	PINK1	Autosomal recessive	1	Mitochondrial kinase
	DJ-1	Autosomal recessive	1	Protein chaperone
	LRRK-2	Autosomal dominant	12	Kinase
PSP	Tau	Linkage to H1 haplotype	17	—
FTDP-17	Tau	Autosomal dominant	17	Microtubule binding

PSP, progressive supranuclear palsy; FTDP, frontotemporal dementia with parkinsonism linked to chromosome 17

new treatments, and examine their effects on the development or resolution of pathologic features of that disease.

Therapeutic intervention to halt or reverse the course of neurodegenerative disease is the ultimate goal of both basic and clinical research on neurodegeneration. Despite the fact that these neurodegenerative diseases involve different genes and cellular processes and pathways, there are likely commonalities among the degenerative processes that occur in the diseases. For example, the cell death pathways in PD, FTD and AD might be initiated at different points, or by different upstream events, but the final downstream events that lead to cell dysfunction and death may converge on common pathways. If this is the case, then a neuroprotective treatment paradigm that intervened in the final stages of the pathway might have beneficial effects on a number of different neurodegenerative conditions. For example, if aggregation of proteins proves to be a toxic insult, then therapies designed to prevent the aggregation of proteins could serve as a treatment in numerous conditions. Further elucidation of the underlying genetic predispositions, and protective factors, for these closely related neurodegenerative diseases promises to lead to new therapeutic approaches.

REFERENCES

1. Lim KL, Dawson VL, Dawson TM. The cast of molecular characters in Parkinson's disease: felons, conspirators, and suspects. Ann NY Acad Sci 2003; 991: 80–92

2. Munoz E, Oliva R, Obach V, et al. Identification of Spanish familial Parkinson's disease and screening for the Ala53Thr mutation of the alpha-synuclein gene in early onset patients. Neurosci Lett 1997; 235: 57–60

3. Hattori N, Matsumine H, Asakawa S, et al. Point mutations (Thr240Arg and Gln311Stop) [correction of Thr240Arg and Ala311Stop] in the Parkin gene. Biochem Biophys Res Commun 1998; 249: 754–8

4. Hattori N, Kitada T, Matsumine H, et al. Molecular genetic analysis of a novel Parkin gene in Japanese families with autosomal recessive juvenile parkinsonism: Evidence for variable homozygous deletions in the Parkin gene in affected individuals. Ann Neurol 1998; 44: 935–41

5. Lucking CB, Abbas N, Durr A, et al. Homozygous deletions in parkin gene in European and North

African families with autosomal recessive juvenile parkinsonism. The European Consortium on Genetic Susceptibility in Parkinson's Disease and the French Parkinson's Disease Genetics Study Group. Lancet 1998; 352: 1355–6

6. Leroy E, Boyer R, Auburger G, et al. The ubiquitin pathway in Parkinson's disease. Nature 1998; 395: 451–2

7. Bonifati V, Rizzu P, Squitieri F, et al. DJ-1 (PARK7), a novel gene for autosomal recessive, early onset parkinsonism. Neurol Sci 2003; 24: 159–60

8. Bonifati V, Rizzu P, van Baren MJ, et al. Mutations in the DJ-1 gene associated with autosomal recessive early-onset parkinsonism. Science 2003; 299: 256–9

9. Kruger R, Kuhn W, Muller T, et al. Ala30Pro mutation in the gene encoding alpha-synuclein in Parkinson's disease. Nat Genet 1998; 18: 106–8

10. Polymeropoulos MH, Lavedan C, Leroy E, et al. Mutation in the (alpha)-synuclein gene identified in families with Parkinson's disease. Science 1997; 276: 2045–2047

11. Zarranz JJ, Alegre J, Gomez-Esteban JC, et al. The new mutation, E46K, of alpha-synuclein causes Parkinson and Lewy body dementia. Ann Neurol 2004; 55: 164–73

12. Ibanez P, Bonnet AM, Debarges B, et al. Causal relation between alpha-synuclein gene duplication and familial Parkinson's disease. Lancet 2004; 364: 1169–71

13. Chung KK, Zhang Y, Lim KL, et al. Parkin ubiquitinates the alpha-synuclein-interacting protein, synphilin-1: implications for Lewy-body formation in Parkinson disease. Nat Med 2001; 7: 1144–50

14. von Bohlen und Halbach O, Schober A, Krieglstein K. Genes, proteins, and neurotoxins involved in Parkinson's disease. Prog Neurobiol 2004; 73: 151–77

15. Shendelman S, Jonason A, Martinat C, et al. DJ-1 is a redox-dependent molecular chaperone that inhibits alpha-synuclein aggregate formation. PLoS Biol 2004; 2: e362

16. Valente EM, Abou-Sleiman PM, Caputo V, et al. Hereditary early-onset Parkinson's disease caused by mutations in PINK1. Science 2004; 304: 1158–60

17. Healy DG, Abou-Sleiman PM, Gibson JM, et al. PINK1 (PARK6) associated Parkinson disease in Ireland. Neurology 2004; 63: 1486–8

18. Zimprich A, Biskup S, Leitner P, et al. Mutations in LRRK2 cause autosomal-dominant Parkinsonism with pleomorphic pathology. Neuron 2004; 44: 601–7.

19. Valente EM, Salvi S, Ialongo T, et al. PINK1 mutations are associated with sporadic early-onset parkinsonism. Ann Neurol 2004; 56: 336–41

20. Paisan-Ruiz C, Jain S, Evans EW, et al. Cloning of the gene containing mutations that cause PARK8-linked Parkinson's disease. Neuron 2004; 44: 595–600

21. Kahle PJ, Haass C, Kretzschmar HA, Neumann M. Structure/function of alpha-synuclein in health and disease: Rational development of animal models for Parkinson's and related diseases. J Neurochem 2002; 82: 449–57

22. Maries E, Dass B, Collier TJ, et al. The role of alpha-synuclein in Parkinson's disease: Insights from animal models. Nat Rev Neurosci 2003; 4: 727–38

23. Klucken J, Shin Y, Hyman BT, McLean PJ. A single amino acid substitution differentiates Hsp70-dependent effects on alpha-synuclein degradation and toxicity. Biochem Biophys Res Commun 2004; 325: 367–73

24. McLean PJ, Klucken J, Shin Y, Hyman BT. Geldanamycin induces Hsp70 and prevents alpha-synuclein aggregation and toxicity in vitro. Biochem Biophys Res Commun 2004; 321: 665–9

25. Klucken J, Shin Y, Masliah E, et al. Hsp70 reduces alpha-synuclein aggregation and toxicity. J Biol Chem 2004; 279: 25497–502

26. Auluck PK, Chan HY, Trojanowski JQ, et al. Chaperone suppression of alpha-synuclein toxicity in a Drosophila model for Parkinson's disease. Science 2002; 295: 865–8

27. Barral JM, Broadley SA, Schaffar G, Hartl FU. Roles of molecular chaperones in protein misfolding diseases. Semin Cell Dev Biol 2004; 15: 17–29

28. Kertesz A, Munoz D. Relationship between frontotemporal dementia and corticobasal degeneration/progressive supranuclear palsy. Dement Geriatr Cogn Disord 2004; 17: 282–6

29. Rajput A, Rajput AH. Progressive supranuclear palsy: Clinical features, pathophysiology and management. Drugs Aging 2001; 18: 913–25

30. Feany MB, Ksiezak-Reding H, Liu WK, et al. Epitope expression and hyperphosphorylation of tau protein in corticobasal degeneration: differentiation from progressive supranuclear palsy. Acta Neuropathol (Berl) 1995; 90: 37–43

31. Kertesz A, Kawarai T, Rogaeva E, et al. Familial frontotemporal dementia with ubiquitin-positive, tau-negative inclusions. Neurology 2000; 54: 818–27

32. Baker M, Litvan I, Houlden H, et al. Association of an extended haplotype in the tau gene with progressive supranuclear palsy. Hum Mol Genet 1999; 8: 711–15

33. Forman MS. Genotype–phenotype correlations in FTDP-17: Does form follow function? Exp Neurol 2004; 187: 229–34

34. Janssen JC, Warrington EK, Morris HR, et al. Clinical features of frontotemporal dementia due to the intronic tau 10(+16) mutation. Neurology 2002; 58: 1161–8

35. Sperfeld AD, Collatz MB, Baier H, et al. FTDP-17: An early-onset phenotype with parkinsonism and epileptic seizures caused by a novel mutation. Ann Neurol 1999; 46: 708–15

36. Yasuda M, Yokoyama K, Nakayasu T, et al. A Japanese patient with frontotemporal dementia and parkinsonism by a tau P301S mutation. Neurology 2000; 55: 1224–7

37. Bugiani O, Murrell JR, Giaccone G, et al. Frontotemporal dementia and corticobasal degeneration in a family with a P301S mutation in tau. J Neuropathol Exp Neurol 1999; 58: 667–77

38. Pastor P, Pastor E, Carnero C, et al. Familial atypical progressive supranuclear palsy associated with homozygosity for the delN296 mutation in the tau gene. Ann Neurol 2001; 49: 263–7

39. Johnson GV, Stoothoff WH. Tau phosphorylation in neuronal cell function and dysfunction. J Cell Sci 2004; 117: 5721–9

40. Zhukareva V, Trojanowski JQ, Lee VM. Assessment of pathological tau proteins in frontotemporal dementias: Qualitative and quantitative approaches. Am J Geriatr Psychiatry 2004; 12: 136–45

41. Pickering-Brown S, Baker M, Yen SH, et al. Pick's disease is associated with mutations in the tau gene. Ann Neurol 2000; 48: 859–67

42. Hogg M, Grujic ZM, Baker M, et al. The L266V tau mutation is associated with frontotemporal dementia and Pick-like 3R and 4R tauopathy. Acta Neuropathol (Berl) 2003;106(4):323–36

43. Kobayashi T, Ota S, Tanaka K, et al. A novel L266V mutation of the tau gene causes frontotemporal dementia with a unique tau pathology. Ann Neurol 2003; 53: 133–7

44. Hutton M, Lendon CL, Rizzu P, et al. Association of missense and 5'-splice-site mutations in tau with the inherited dementia FTDP-17. Nature 1998; 393: 702–5

45. Spillantini MG, Crowther RA, Kamphorst W, et al. Tau pathology in two Dutch families with mutations in the microtubule-binding region of tau. Am J Pathol 1998; 153: 1359–63

46. Robakis NK, Wisniewski HM, Jenkins EC, et al. Chromosome 21q21 sublocalisation of gene encoding beta-amyloid peptide in cerebral vessels and neuritic (senile) plaques of people with Alzheimer disease and Down syndrome. Lancet 1987; 1: 384–5

47. Tanzi RE, Gusella JF, Watkins PC, et al. Amyloid beta protein gene: cDNA, mRNA distribution, and genetic linkage near the Alzheimer locus. Science 1987; 235: 880–4

48. Goldgaber D, Lerman MI, McBride WO, et al. Isolation, characterization, and chromosomal localization of human brain cDNA clones coding for the precursor of the amyloid of brain in Alzheimer's disease, Down's syndrome and aging. J Neural Transm Suppl 1987; 24: 23–8

49. Kang J, Lemaire HG, Unterbeck A, et al. The precursor of Alzheimer's disease amyloid A4 protein resembles a cell-surface receptor. Nature 1987; 325: 733–6

50. Goate A, Chartier-Harlin MC, Mullan M, et al. Segregation of a missense mutation in the amyloid precursor protein gene with familial Alzheimer's disease. Nature 1991; 349: 704–6

51. Murrell J, Farlow M, Ghetti B, Benson MD. A mutation in the amyloid precursor protein associated with hereditary Alzheimer's disease. Science 1991; 254: 97–9

52. Yoshioka K, Miki T, Katsuya T, et al. The 717Val→Ile substitution in amyloid precursor protein is associated with familial Alzheimer's disease regardless of ethnic groups. Biochem Biophys Res Commun 1991; 178: 1141–6

53. Naruse S, Igarashi S, Kobayashi H, et al. Missense mutation Val→Ile in exon 17 of amyloid precursor protein gene in Japanese familial Alzheimer's disease. Lancet 1991; 337: 978–9

54. van Duijn CM, Hendriks L, Cruts M, et al. Amyloid precursor protein gene mutation in early-onset Alzheimer's disease. Lancet 1991; 337: 978

55. Hardy J, Selkoe DJ. The amyloid hypothesis of Alzheimer's disease: Progress and problems on the road to therapeutics. Science 2002; 297: 353–6

56. Kowalska A. Amyloid precursor protein gene mutations responsible for early-onset autosomal dominant Alzheimer's disease. Folia Neuropathol 2003; 41: 35–40

57. Cruts M, Backhovens H, Wang SY, et al. Molecular genetic analysis of familial early-onset Alzheimer's

disease linked to chromosome 14q24.3. Hum Mol Genet 1995; 4: 2363–71

58. Sherrington R, Rogaev EI, Liang Y, et al. Cloning of a gene bearing missense mutations in early-onset familial Alzheimer's disease. Nature 1995; 375: 754–60

59. Rogaev EI, Sherrington R, Rogaeva EA, et al. Familial Alzheimer's disease in kindreds with missense mutations in a gene on chromosome 1 related to the Alzheimer's disease type 3 gene. Nature 1995; 376: 775–8

60. Li J, Ma J, Potter H. Identification and expression analysis of a potential familial Alzheimer disease gene on chromosome 1 related to AD3. Proc Natl Acad Sci USA 1995; 92: 12180–4

61. The structure of the presenilin 1 (S182) gene and identification of six novel mutations in early onset AD families. Alzheimer's Disease Collaborative Group. Nat Genet 1995; 11: 219–22

62. Levy-Lahad E, Wasco W, Poorkaj P, et al. Candidate gene for the chromosome 1 familial Alzheimer's disease locus. Science 1995; 269: 973–7

63. Lleo A, Berezovska O, Growdon JH, Hyman BT. Clinical, pathological, and biochemical spectrum of Alzheimer disease associated with PS-1 mutations. Am J Geriatr Psychiatry 2004; 12: 146–56

64. De Strooper B, Saftig P, Craessaerts K, et al. Deficiency of presenilin-1 inhibits the normal cleavage of amyloid precursor protein. Nature 1998; 391: 387–90

65. Tamaoka A, Odaka A, Ishibashi Y, et al. APP717 missense mutation affects the ratio of amyloid beta protein species (A beta 1-42/43 and a beta 1-40) in familial Alzheimer's disease brain. J Biol Chem 1994; 269: 32721–4

66. Scheuner D, Eckman C, Jensen M, et al. Secreted amyloid beta-protein similar to that in the senile plaques of Alzheimer's disease is increased in vivo by the presenilin 1 and 2 and APP mutations linked to familial Alzheimer's disease. Nat Med 1996; 2: 864–70

67. Berezovska O, Ramdya P, Skoch J, et al. Amyloid precursor protein associates with a nicastrin-dependent docking site on the presenilin 1-gamma-secretase complex in cells demonstrated by fluorescence lifetime imaging. J Neurosci 2003; 23: 4560–6

68. Wolfe MS, Xia W, Moore CL, et al. Peptidomimetic probes and molecular modeling suggest that Alzheimer's gamma-secretase is an intramembrane-cleaving aspartyl protease. Biochemistry 1999; 38: 4720–7

69. Wolfe MS, Xia W, Ostaszewski BL, et al. Two transmembrane aspartates in presenilin-1 required for presenilin endoproteolysis and gamma-secretase activity. Nature 1999; 398: 513–17

70. Yu G, Nishimura M, Arawaka S, et al. Nicastrin modulates presenilin-mediated notch/glp-1 signal transduction and betaAPP processing. Nature 2000; 407: 48–54

71. Lee SF, Shah S, Li H, et al. Mammalian APH-1 interacts with presenilin and nicastrin and is required for intramembrane proteolysis of amyloid-beta precursor protein and Notch. J Biol Chem 2002; 277: 45013–19

72. Francis R, McGrath G, Zhang J, et al. aph-1 and pen-2 are required for Notch pathway signaling, gamma-secretase cleavage of betaAPP, and presenilin protein accumulation. Dev Cell 2002; 3: 85–97

73. Steiner H, Winkler E, Edbauer D, et al. PEN-2 is an integral component of the gamma-secretase complex required for coordinated expression of presenilin and nicastrin. J Biol Chem 2002; 277: 39062–5

74. Rozmahel R, Mount HT, Chen F, et al. Alleles at the Nicastrin locus modify presenilin 1-deficiency phenotype. Proc Natl Acad Sci USA 2002; 99: 14452–7

75. Gu Y, Chen F, Sanjo N, et al. APH-1 interacts with mature and immature forms of presenilins and nicastrin and may play a role in maturation of presenilin–nicastrin complexes. J Biol Chem 2003; 278: 7374–80

76. Lleo A, Berezovska O, Herl L, et al. Nonsteroidal anti-inflammatory drugs lower Abeta42 and change presenilin 1 conformation. Nat Med 2004; 10: 1065–6

77. Rebeck GW, Reiter JS, Strickland DK, Hyman BT. Apolipoprotein E in sporadic Alzheimer's disease: Allelic variation and receptor interactions. Neuron 1993; 11: 575–80

78. Strittmatter WJ, Saunders AM, Schmechel D, et al. Apolipoprotein E: High-avidity binding to beta-amyloid and increased frequency of type 4 allele in late-onset familial Alzheimer disease. Proc Natl Acad Sci USA 1993; 90: 1977–81

79. Strittmatter WJ, Weisgraber KH, Huang DY, et al. Binding of human apolipoprotein E to synthetic amyloid beta peptide: Isoform-specific effects and implications for late-onset Alzheimer disease. Proc Natl Acad Sci USA 1993; 90: 8098–102

80. Hyman BT, Gomez-Isla T, Briggs M, et al. Apolipoprotein E and cognitive change in an elderly population. Ann Neurol 1996; 40: 55–66

81. Raber J, Huang Y, Ashford JW. ApoE genotype accounts for the vast majority of AD risk and AD pathology. Neurobiol Aging 2004; 25: 641–50

82. Corder EH, Saunders AM, Risch NJ, et al. Protective effect of apolipoprotein E type 2 allele for late onset Alzheimer disease. Nat Genet 1994; 7: 180–4

83. West HL, Rebeck GW, Hyman BT. Frequency of the apolipoprotein E epsilon 2 allele is diminished in sporadic Alzheimer disease. Neurosci Lett 1994; 175: 46–8

84. Snipes GJ, McGuire CB, Norden JJ, Freeman JA. Nerve injury stimulates the secretion of apolipoprotein E by nonneuronal cells. Proc Natl Acad Sci USA 1986; 83: 1130–4

85. Oropeza RL, Wekerle H, Werb Z. Expression of apolipoprotein E by mouse brain astrocytes and its modulation by interferon-gamma. Brain Res 1987; 410: 45–51

86. Mouchel Y, Lefrancois T, Fages C, Tardy M. Apolipoprotein E gene expression in astrocytes: Developmental pattern and regulation. Neuroreport 1995; 7: 205–8

87. Bu G, Maksymovitch EA, Nerbonne JM, Schwartz AL. Expression and function of the low density lipoprotein receptor-related protein (LRP) in mammalian central neurons. J Biol Chem 1994; 269: 18521–8

88. Sanan DA, Weisgraber KH, Russell SJ, et al. Apolipoprotein E associates with beta amyloid peptide of Alzheimer's disease to form novel monofibrils. Isoform apoE4 associates more efficiently than apoE3. J Clin Invest 1994; 94: 860–9

89. Huang DY, Weisgraber KH, Goedert M, et al. ApoE3 binding to tau tandem repeat I is abolished by tau serine262 phosphorylation. Neurosci Lett 1995; 192: 209–12

90. Strittmatter WJ, Saunders AM, Goedert M, et al. Isoform-specific interactions of apolipoprotein E with microtubule-associated protein tau: Implications for Alzheimer disease. Proc Natl Acad Sci USA 1994; 91: 11183–6

91. Bales KR, Verina T, Cummins DJ, et al. Apolipoprotein E is essential for amyloid deposition in the APP(V717F) transgenic mouse model of Alzheimer's disease. Proc Natl Acad Sci USA 1999; 96: 15233–8

92. Holtzman DM, Bales KR, Tenkova T, et al. Apolipoprotein E isoform-dependent amyloid deposition and neuritic degeneration in a mouse model of Alzheimer's disease. Proc Natl Acad Sci USA 2000; 97: 2892–7

93. Fukumoto H, Cheung BS, Hyman BT, Irizarry MC. Beta-secretase protein and activity are increased in the neocortex in Alzheimer disease. Arch Neurol 2002; 59: 1381–9

94. Li R, Lindholm K, Yang LB, et al. Amyloid beta peptide load is correlated with increased beta-secretase activity in sporadic Alzheimer's disease patients. Proc Natl Acad Sci USA 2004; 101: 3632–7

95. Fukumoto H, Rosene DL, Moss MB, et al. Beta-secretase activity increases with aging in human, monkey, and mouse brain. Am J Pathol 2004; 164: 719–25

96. Turner RT 3rd, Loy JA, Nguyen C, et al. Specificity of memapsin 1 and its implications on the design of memapsin 2 (beta-secretase) inhibitor selectivity. Biochemistry 2002; 41: 8742–6

97. McLellan ME, Kajdasz ST, Hyman BT, Bacskai BJ. In vivo imaging of reactive oxygen species specifically associated with thioflavine S-positive amyloid plaques by multiphoton microscopy. J Neurosci 2003; 23: 2212–7

98. Urbanc B, Cruz L, Le R, et al. Neurotoxic effects of thioflavin S-positive amyloid deposits in transgenic mice and Alzheimer's disease. Proc Natl Acad Sci USA 2002; 99: 13990–5

99. Kowall NW, Kosik KS. Axonal disruption and aberrant localization of tau protein characterize the neuropil pathology of Alzheimer's disease. Ann Neurol 1987; 22: 639–43

100. Kosik KS, Finch EA. MAP2 and tau segregate into dendritic and axonal domains after the elaboration of morphologically distinct neurites: An immunocytochemical study of cultured rat cerebrum. J Neurosci 1987; 7: 3142–53

101. Grundke-Iqbal I, Iqbal K, Quinlan M, et al. Microtubule-associated protein tau. A component of Alzheimer paired helical filaments. J Biol Chem 1986; 261: 6084–9

102. Grundke-Iqbal I, Iqbal K, Tung YC, et al. Abnormal phosphorylation of the microtubule-associated protein tau (tau) in Alzheimer cytoskeletal pathology. Proc Natl Acad Sci USA 1986; 83: 4913–17

103. Johnson GV, Bailey CD. Tau, where are we now? J Alzheimers Dis 2002; 4: 375–98

104. Woodgett JR. Molecular cloning and expression of glycogen synthase kinase-3/factor A. EMBO J 1990; 9: 2431–8

105. Pei JJ, Braak E, Braak H, et al. Distribution of active glycogen synthase kinase 3beta (GSK-3beta) in brains staged for Alzheimer disease neurofibrillary changes. J Neuropathol Exp Neurol 1999; 58: 1010–19

106. Takashima A, Honda T, Yasutake K, et al. Activation of tau protein kinase I/glycogen synthase kinase-3beta by amyloid beta peptide (25–35) enhances phosphorylation of tau in hippocampal neurons. Neurosci Res 1998; 31: 317–23

107. Takashima A, Yamaguchi H, Noguchi K, et al. Amyloid beta peptide induces cytoplasmic accumulation of amyloid protein precursor via tau protein kinase I/glycogen synthase kinase-3 beta in rat hippocampal neurons. Neurosci Lett 1995; 198: 83–6

108. Takashima A, Noguchi K, Michel G, et al. Exposure of rat hippocampal neurons to amyloid beta peptide (25–35) induces the inactivation of phosphatidyl inositol-3 kinase and the activation of tau protein kinase I/glycogen synthase kinase-3 beta. Neurosci Lett 1996; 203: 33–6

109. Shetty KT, Kaech S, Link WT, et al. Molecular characterization of a neuronal-specific protein that stimulates the activity of Cdk5. J Neurochem 1995; 64: 1988–95

110. Tomizawa K, Matsui H, Matsushita M, et al. Localization and developmental changes in the neuron-specific cyclin-dependent kinase 5 activator (p35nck5a) in the rat brain. Neuroscience 1996; 74: 519–29

111. Ino H, Chiba T. Intracellular localization of cyclin-dependent kinase 5 (CDK5) in mouse neuron: CDK5 is located in both nucleus and cytoplasm. Brain Res 1996; 732: 179–85

112. Matsushita M, Tomizawa K, Lu YF, et al. Distinct cellular compartment of cyclin-dependent kinase 5 (Cdk5) and neuron-specific Cdk5 activator protein (p35nck5a) in the developing rat cerebellum. Brain Res 1996; 734: 319–22

113. Yamaguchi H, Ishiguro K, Uchida T, et al. Preferential labeling of Alzheimer neurofibrillary tangles with antisera for tau protein kinase (TPK) I/glycogen synthase kinase-3 beta and cyclin-dependent kinase 5, a component of TPK II. Acta Neuropathol (Berl) 1996; 92: 232–41

114. Augustinack JC, Sanders JL, Tsai LH, Hyman BT. Colocalization and fluorescence resonance energy transfer between cdk5 and AT8 suggests a close association in pre-neurofibrillary tangles and neurofibrillary tangles. J Neuropathol Exp Neurol 2002; 61: 557–64

115. Trinczek B, Biernat J, Baumann K, et al. Domains of tau protein, differential phosphorylation, and dynamic instability of microtubules. Mol Biol Cell 1995; 6: 1887–902

116. Lew J, Qi Z, Huang QQ, et al. Structure, function, and regulation of neuronal Cdc2-like protein kinase. Neurobiol Aging 1995; 16: 263–8; discussion 268–70

117. Hosoi T, Uchiyama M, Okumura E, et al. Evidence for cdk5 as a major activity phosphorylating tau protein in porcine brain extract. J Biochem (Tokyo) 1995; 117: 741–9

118. Scott CW, Vulliet PR, Caputo CB. Phosphorylation of tau by proline-directed protein kinase (p34cdc2/p58cyclin A) decreases tau-induced microtubule assembly and antibody SMI33 reactivity. Brain Res 1993; 611: 237–42

119. Liu T, Perry G, Chan HW, et al. Amyloid-beta-induced toxicity of primary neurons is dependent upon differentiation-associated increases in tau and cyclin-dependent kinase 5 expression. J Neurochem 2004; 88: 554–63.

120. Alvarez A, Toro R, Caceres A, Maccioni RB. Inhibition of tau phosphorylating protein kinase cdk5 prevents beta-amyloid-induced neuronal death. FEBS Lett 1999; 459: 421–6

121. Patrick GN, Zukerberg L, Nikolic M, et al. Conversion of p35 to p25 deregulates Cdk5 activity and promotes neurodegeneration. Nature 1999; 402: 615–22

122. Cruz JC, Tseng HC, Goldman JA, et al. Aberrant Cdk5 activation by p25 triggers pathological events leading to neurodegeneration and neurofibrillary tangles. Neuron 2003; 40: 471–83

123. Oddo S, Billings L, Kesslak JP, et al. Abeta immunotherapy leads to clearance of early, but not late, hyperphosphorylated tau aggregates via the proteasome. Neuron 2004; 43: 321–32

124. Schenk D, Barbour R, Dunn W, et al. Immunization with amyloid-beta attenuates Alzheimer-disease-like pathology in the PDAPP mouse. Nature 1999; 400: 173–7

125. Bacskai BJ, Kajdasz ST, Christie RH, et al. Imaging of amyloid-beta deposits in brains of living mice permits direct observation of clearance of plaques with immunotherapy. Nat Med 2001; 7: 369–72

126. Bacskai BJ, Kajdasz ST, McLellan ME, et al. Non-Fc-mediated mechanisms are involved in clearance of amyloid-beta in vivo by immunotherapy. J Neurosci 2002; 22: 7873–8

Section 4

Pathogenic mechanisms

12

Transgenic mouse and mutagenesis models

Ludo Van Den Bosch, Wim Robberecht

INTRODUCTION

Different model systems have helped to gain insights into the pathogenic mechanisms underlying motor neuron death, the hallmark of neurodegenerative diseases, such as amyotrophic lateral sclerosis (ALS), spinal muscular atrophy (SMA) and X-linked spinal and bulbar muscular atrophy (SBMA). Mouse models with spontaneous or induced mutations and transgenic mice (over) expressing (mutant) genes recapitulate different aspect of these human diseases. Although the exact mechanisms leading to selective motor neuron death in these mice are not yet elucidated, rodent models have been of great value to delineate pathogenic mechanisms that could be important. These mechanisms are very diverse and include oxidative stress, aggregate formation, deficiencies in axonal transport, excitotoxicity, inflammation, growth factor depletion and defective RNA processing. As selective motor neuron death is always the end result of these pathogenic mechanisms, it appears that these processes are more pronounced in motor neurons and/or that motor neurons are extremely vulnerable to these stresses. However, one always has to keep in mind that models remain models. As a consequence, it is important to envisage the limitations of these animal models. We will end this chapter with some important remarks about possible problems and pitfalls when working with these mouse models for neurodegenerative diseases.

OXIDATIVE STRESS AND FORMATION OF AGGREGATES

In 1993, mutations in the superoxide 1 gene (*SOD1*) were discovered that account for 10–20% of familial ALS cases[1]. Shortly after this discovery, a transgenic mouse overexpressing mutant (G93A) SOD1 was created by insertion of multiple copies of human genomic *SOD1* into the mouse genome[2]. These transgenic mice showed progressive hindlimb weakness leading to paralysis and death. The moment of disease onset and the lifespan of these mice were related to the level of overexpression of mutant SOD1, while overexpression of non-mutated SOD1 gave no overt phenotype. Transgenic mice that (over)expressed human SOD1 containing other mutations (G37R or G85R) or mutant (G86R) mouse SOD1 showed a similar phenotype to that of the mutant (G93A) SOD1 mouse line[3-5]. Selective expression of mutant SOD1 in motor neurons[6] or in glial cells[7] was not sufficient to induce pathology, indicating that interplay between different cell types is necessary for motor neuron death. This concept was further illustrated by the creation of chimeric mice with mixtures of normal cells and cells that

Table 12.1 Overview of therapeutic interventions that increased the lifespan of transgenic mutant SOD1 mice/rats by at least 10%

Treatment	Survival of control (days)	Survival of treated (days)	Difference in survival (treated − control) (days)	Difference in survival (%) (relative to lifespan controls)	References
Anti-excitotoxic					
2-MPPA	190	219	29	15	Ghadge et al., 2003[9]
RPR119990	158	178	20	13	Canton et al., 2001[10]
Riluzole	134	148	14	11	Gurney et al., 1996[11]
Ceftriaxone	122	135	13	11	Rothstein et al., 2005[12]
NBQX	130	143	13	10	Van Damme et al., 2003[13]
Anti-inflammatory					
Celecoxib	112	140	28	25	Drachman et al., 2002[14]
Rofecoxib	126	152	26	21	Klivenyi et al., 2004[15]
Celecoxib	126	150	24	19	Klivenyi et al., 2004[15]
Minocycline	130	151	21	16	Van Den Bosch et al., 2002[16]
Minocycline	126	139	13	10	Zhu et al., 2002[17]
Growth factors					
AAV-IGF	123	160	37	30	Kaspar et al., 2003[18]
VEGF-ICV	121	143	22	18	Storkebaum et al., 2005[19]
LV-VEGF	127	146	19	15	Azzouz et al., 2004[20]
AAV-GDNF	122	139	17	14	Wang et al., 2002[21]
Others					
Creatine	144	169	25	18	Klivenyi et al., 1999[22]
Arimoclomol	125	148	23	18	Kieran et al., 2004[23]
zVAD-fmk	126	153	27	22	Li et al., 2000[24]

express mutant SOD1. In these animals, non-neuronal cells that do not express mutant SOD1 delayed degeneration and significantly extended survival of mutant SOD1-expressing motor neurons[8].

Since its creation, the mutant SOD1 mouse models have been extensively studied. These transgenic mice proved that mutant SOD1 caused selective motor neuron death by a gain of function. Moreover, these mice were used both to study the pathogenic changes that occur during the disease process, as well as to test possible drugs (Table 12.1). Mutant SOD1 transgenic mice were also crossbred with other transgenic mice to learn about the pathogenic mechanisms involved. Using this strategy, it was shown that SOD1-mediated oxidative abnormalities were not the primary cause of mutant SOD1 toxicity. SOD1 is an enzyme that requires copper to catalyze the conversion of toxic superoxide radicals into hydrogen peroxide and oxygen. Copper plays a crucial role in the normal and/or aberrant enzymatic activity of the enzyme, and copper loading of SOD1 is performed by a specific copper chaperone (CCS). Crossbreeding of transgenic mutant (G93A) SOD1 mice with knockout mice lacking the CCS, did not influence the lifespan of mutant (G93A) SOD1 mice[25]. Another argument that oxidative stress is not the initiating factor was supported by the transgenic mouse overexpressing mutant SOD1 in which the four essential histidines that bind copper were mutated (SOD1-Quad). Two of these mutations are known human mutations causing ALS, and the SOD1-Quad mice developed age-dependent motor neuron loss despite the lack of copper binding by SOD1[26].

Alternatively, the 'gain of function' of mutant SOD1 could be the formation of intracellular SOD1 aggregates[27]. A perfect correlation between the formation of these aggregates and selective motor neuron death was found after intranuclear injection of constructs expressing mutant SOD1 into cultured motor neurons[28]. The formation of SOD1 aggregates and the selective motor neuron death could be influenced by expression of the heat shock protein, HSP70, indicating that increasing the chaperoning activity could be protective against mutant SOD1-induced motor neuron death[29]. Moreover, both motor neuron death and aggregate formation could be prevented by inhibiting Ca^{2+}-permeable AMPA receptors or by providing the cells with additional Ca^{2+}-binding proteins[30], indicating an important role for excitotoxicity (see below).

SOD1 aggregates were found in ALS patients with SOD1 mutations, as well as in the different mutant SOD1 mouse models. They were present both in neurons and in surrounding glial cells[27]. The formation of SOD1 aggregates was one of the first pathological signs, and the abundance increased as a function of the disease process[31]. Furthermore, detergent-insoluble forms of SOD1 could be detected in the brainstem and spinal cord of the different transgenic mouse models[26]. Despite these results, it is still an open question whether the formation of SOD1 aggregates is the cause of ALS. On the other hand, the formation of aggregates could be a harmless side-effect of the presence of mutant SOD1 or it could even be protective by sequestering aberrant SOD1.

SBMA, also known as Kennedy's disease, is caused by polyglutamine repeat expansions in the androgen receptor (AR) and is characterized by nuclear aggregates and a selective loss of motor neurons. Only males are affected, while female carriers are usually asymptomatic. To determine the basis of AR polyglutamine neurotoxicity, a number of transgenic mice were created of which some demonstrated a late-onset, progressive motor neuron loss, as well as sexual difference of phenotype (for a review, see reference 32). Studies with these transgenic mice showed that nuclear translocation of the polyglutamine-containing AR into the nucleus was essential to induce neurodegeneration. This process was dependent on testosterone and could be inhibited by overexpression of HSP70[33,34]. The nuclear polyglutamine-containing AR binds to cAMP-responsive element binding protein (CBP) and inhibits transcription mediated by this transcription factor. This could lead to a lower expression of vascular endothelial growth factor (VEGF), as expression of this growth factor is dependent on the CBP transcription factor[35]. A shortage of VEGF could be a universal mechanism leading to motor neuron death as is illustrated by the lowered VEGF expression that is implicated in the pathology of the $VEGF^{\delta/\delta}$ mouse and in ALS (see below).

Furthermore, loss of detergent solubility and formation of aggregates is a common phenomenon in a large number of neurodegenerative diseases. Mutant SOD1 and polyglutamine-containing AR share this property with the β-amyloid peptide in Alzheimer's disease (AD), tau in AD and in frontotemporal dementia with parkinsonism (FTDP), α-synuclein in Parkinson's disease and proteins harboring expansions of polyglutamine tracts as occurs in Huntington's disease.

DISTURBANCE OF AXONAL TRANSPORT

Intermediate filaments

Neurofilaments

Neurofilaments (NFs) are the most abundant intermediate filaments in neurons and consist of three subunits: NF-L, NF-M and NF-H. Accumulation of NFs and concomitant slowing of slow anterograde axonal transport were reported in the mutant (G93A) SOD1 mouse model[36]. Moreover, NF accumulations were found in both familial and sporadic ALS cases[37–39]. In ALS patients, mutations in the KSP phosphorylation domain of NF-H were found in a limited number of ALS patients[40]. Over the years, a large number of transgenic mice with modifications related to NFs were made, in order to determine the role of these intermediate filaments in the pathology of motor neurons (for reviews, see references 41 and 42).

Knockout mice for these different subunits alone, or double transgenic mice deficient in two NF subunits, did not show a clear phenotype, although in some of these mice a loss of motor axons was detected. Also, overexpression of the different NF subunits did not induce motor neuron death. In some of these transgenic mice NF accumulations in neuronal cell bodies were found, but this did not induce motor neuron death.

However, NF abnormalities can induce selective motor neuron death *in vivo* as indicated by a transgenic mouse expressing a mutant NF-L. Leucine at position 394 was mutated into a proline and this caused a dominant motor neuron disease in mice[43]. These transgenic mice showed massive, selective degeneration of motor neurons accompanied by accumulations of NFs, although no effect on the lifespan of these mice was reported. This mouse model became highly relevant after the discovery of NF-L mutations causing a dominantly inherited motor neuropathy, Charcot–Marie–Tooth disease[44,45].

Another example of a transgenic NF mouse with motor dysfunction overexpressed the 3′ untranslated region (UTR) of NF-L. These mice developed an age-dependent, slowly progressive deterioration of motor function, while no motor neuron loss could be detected. Insertion of a 36-bp c-*myc* in the destabilizing element of the 3′ UTR aggravated this phenotype[46]. Although the relevance and the exact mechanism leading to this phenotype is not yet clear, *in vitro* studies suggested that the 3′ UTR of NF-L induced co-aggregation of NF-L with mutant SOD1 protein[47].

The importance of NF content and organization in motor neuron disease is further indicated by crossbreeding experiments of different NF transgenic mice with mutant SOD1 mice. Eliminating NFs by deletion of NF-L extended the lifespan of mutant (G85R) SOD1 mutant mice by 12%, despite an early loss of 15% of motor neurons in these mice[48]. Elevating the synthesis of NF-L or NF-H slowed disease in mutant SOD1 mice and extended survival of the mutant (G93A) mice by 16% and 18%, respectively[49]. Crossbreeding of the mutant (G37R) mice with transgenice mice overexpressing NF-H with 43 KSP or 44 KSP repeats increased the lifespan by 65% or by 21%, respectively[50].

A disturbance of the NF network could also be the underlying mechanism responsible for the phenotype induced by mutations in HSP27 and/or HSP22. Mutations in both of these small heat shock proteins are associated with distal heridatary motor neuropathies and Charcot–Marie–Tooth disease[51,52]. In cultured cells, mutant HSP27 dramatically disturbed the integrity of the NF network[51]. A dramatic, age-dependent upregulation of HSP27 and αB-crystallin was observed in the mutant SOD1 mice[53] and these small heat shock proteins co-fractionated with insoluble SOD1[26]. Although the exact significance of these findings is not yet clear, these upregulated small heat shock proteins could play a role as molecular chaperones and/or as stabilizers of elements involved in axonal transport.

Peripherin

Another intermediate filament protein that could be involved in selective motor neuron death is peripherin. This is mostly expressed in the peripheral nervous system and is upregulated in both the peripheral and the central nervous system after injury and by inflammatory cytokines. Transgenic mice that overexpress wild-type peripherin developed motor dysfunctions very late in their life (after 2 years). This phenotype was accompanied by the loss of motor axons and by the appearance of peripherin inclusion bodies in the motor neurons. The onset of motor dysfunction and axonal loss was dramatically accelerated by the absence of NF-L, as revealed by crossbreeding of peripherin-overexpressing mice with NF-L knockout mice. These double transgenic mice also showed a dramatic loss of motor neurons[54]. The exact mechanism underlying this peripherin-mediated neurodegeneration is not yet clarified.

Upregulation or suppression of peripherin expression had no effect on disease onset, mortality and loss of motor neurons in mutant (G37R) SOD1 mice, indicating that peripherin is not a contributing factor to motor neuron disease in this mouse model[55]. However, this does not exclude a role for peripherin in ALS, as illustrated by the recent discovery in ALS patients of a frameshift deletion and a mutation in the peripherin gene[56,57].

Microtubules

Tubulin-specific chaperone E and tau

In mice, a motor syndrome was found in transgenic mouse models that contained mutations in proteins playing a role in microtubule structure and/or stability. Microtubules are long polar polymers, consisting of α- and β-tubulin that are part of the cytoskeleton and play an important role in axonal transport.

The tubulin-specific chaperone E gene (*Tbce*) has an effect on microtubule stability and/or on the polymerization dynamics of microtubules. In the pmn mouse, point mutations were identified in the *Tbce* gene on chromosome 13[58]. However, in humans a deletion in *Tbce* is responsible for hypoparathyroidism–retardation dysmorphism syndrome (HRD or Sanjad–Sakati syndrome, SSS) or autosomal recessive Kenny–Caffey syndrome (AR-KCS). Although neurologic symptoms are part of the HRD/SSS phenotype, this syndrome is clinically variable, involves multiple tissues and is quite different from the disease observed in the pmn mouse.

Other mouse models that show a motor phenotype, were generated by making changes in the microtubule-associated protein tau. This axonal phosphoprotein establishes short crossbridges between axonal microtubules and thereby supports intracellular trafficking, including axonal transport. In neurons affected by a tauopathy, tau is hyperphosphorylated and is located not only in axons but also in cell bodies and dendrites. Tau is the major component of the intracellular filamentous deposits found in a number of neurodegenerative diseases including AD, while mutations in tau are associated with frontotemporal dementia with parkinsonism (FTDP)[59]. Several tau transgenic mice showed a progressive motor phenotype with muscle atrophy and paresis. The motor axons had dilatations that contained accumulation of NFs, mitochondria and vesicles[60]. Overexpression of mutant tau also induced age-dependent accumulation of insoluble filamentous tau aggregates in neuronal perikarya of the spinal cord, a motor phenotype and a reduced lifespan[61].

These examples indicate that mouse models also have their limitations in that the phenotypes observed in mice do not always exactly replicate the disease process in humans (see Limitations of mouse models).

Dynein and dynamitin

Two mouse mutants, Legs at odd angles (Loa) and Cramping 1 (Cra1) arose in two independent mutagenesis experiments in the offspring of *N*-ethyl-*N*-nitrosourea (ENU)-treated mice. These mice manifest progressive motor neuron disorders and show remarkable similarities to specific features of human pathology, including Lewy body-like inclusions containing SOD1, NFs and ubiquitin. Two different point mutations in dynein were found in the Loa and Cra1 mice[62]. Dynein is a motor protein complex that is involved in retrograde transport and moves in the minus-end direction along microtubules.

Similarly, disruption in postnatal motor neurons of the dynactin complex, an activator of cytoplasmic dynein that makes it more processive[63], produced a late-onset, progressive motor neuron disease in mice. This disruption was obtained by overexpression of dynamitin, the p50 subunit of dynactin, leading to neurofilamentous swellings in motor axons and inhibition of retrograde axonal transport[64]. In humans, a dominant point mutation in dynactin was found as the cause of a lower motor neuron disorder that starts with vocal cord paralysis[65]. Impairment of retrograde axonal transport could also be involved in ALS as indicated by the observation that this process was disturbed in mutant SOD1 transgenic mice[66,67].

Unexpectedly, crossbreeding of the Loa mice with mutant (G93A) SOD1 mice significantly extended the lifespan of the mutant (G93A) SOD1 mice by 28%[66]. Defects in retrograde transport were no longer found in motor neurons cultured from these double transgenic mice[66]. These experiments indicate that axonal transport is restored by combining the dynein mutation with a *SOD1* mutation, although the exact explanation for these intriguing findings is not yet clear.

EXCITOTOXICITY

Glutamate-induced, AMPA receptor-mediated excitotoxicity contributes to the selective motor neuron degeneration in ALS. The most important argument is that riluzole, the only effective drug for the treatment of ALS patients, interferes with glutamate release[68]. Moreover, AMPA receptor antagonists prolonged survival of mutant (G93A) SOD1 mice[10,13]. Also interference with glutamate metabolism by inhibiting glutamate carboxypeptidase II significantly increased the lifespan in this mouse model[9].

Excitotoxicity could explain the selectivity of motor neuron death, as motor neurons have a low Ca^{2+} buffering capacity in combination with a large number of Ca^{2+}-permeable AMPA recep-

tors[69–72]. In addition, concomitant GABAergic stimulation and chloride influx could aggravate this AMPA receptor-mediated excitotoxic motor neuron death[73].

The low Ca^{2+}-buffering capacity of motor neurons is due to the low expression of Ca^{2+}-binding proteins[74]. Providing motor neurons with extra Ca^{2+}-binding proteins by overexpressing parvalbumin protected them against excitotoxicity *in vitro*[75]. Moreover, crossbreeding of parvalbumin overexpressing mice with mutant (G93A) SOD1 mice prolonged survival by 11%[76].

The Ca^{2+}-permeability of the AMPA receptor is determined by the GluR2 subunit in the receptor complex. Receptors containing at least one GluR2 subunit have a very low Ca^{2+} permeability compared to GluR2-lacking receptors[77]. The low permeability to Ca^{2+} is due to the presence of a positively charged arginine at position 586 (Q/R site) instead of the genetically encoded neutral glutamine. This arginine residue at the Q/R site is introduced by editing of the GluR2 pre-mRNA[78]. Under normal conditions, the editing efficiency at the Q/R site is virtually 100%, but incomplete editing has been reported to occur in motor neurons of ALS patients[79]. Moreover, mice overexpressing GluR2 with an asparagine (GluR2-N) at the Q/R site, were reported to develop a motor neuron syndrome late in life[80]. GluR2 knockout mice have been generated, but they were reported to have normal brain morphology and no overt motor neuron degeneration[81]. This suggests that a low GluR2 level is not sufficient to cause ALS, but it could be a modifier of motor neuron degeneration in ALS. In line with this is the observation that GluR2 deficiency significantly accelerated the motor neuron degeneration and shortened the lifespan of mutant (G93A) SOD1 mice by 15%[82]. Providing motor neurons with extra GluR2 subunits also did not induce a phenotype. Crossbreeding of these GluR2-overexpressing mice with the late-onset variant of the mutant (G93A) SOD1 mice resulted in a 14% increase of the lifespan of these double transgenic mice[83].

Another pathologic mechanism that could contribute to excitotoxicity is the selective loss in the spinal cord of the glial glutamate receptor GLT-1. GLT-1 is responsible for the clearance of glutamate and is dramatically decreased in ventral spinal cords from both end-stage mutant (G85R) SOD1 mice[3] and mutant (G93A) rats[84]. Crossbreeding GLT-1-overexpressing mice with mutant SOD1 mice delayed disease onset but did not prolong survival[85]. Treatment of the mutant SOD1 mice with ceftriaxone, an antibiotic that induced GLT-1 expression, significantly increased the lifespan of these mice by 11%[12].

INFLAMMATION

Although it is not yet clear whether inflammation plays a crucial role in motor neuron degeneration, evidence in humans indicates that microglial activation is a widespread phenomenon in ALS patients[86,87]. The involvement of microglial activation in motor neuron degeneration was found in a transgenic mouse with general overexpression of the cytokine interleukin-3 (IL-3). This induced a clear motor phenotype[88] due to progressive motor neuron loss, and these mice also showed muscular atrophy leading to hindlimb paralysis at 7 months of age. Restricted overexpression of IL-3 in astrocytes also induced a motor phenotype[89]. Although the exact mechanism leading to this motor neuron degeneration is not yet clarified, it was suggested that an autoimmune reaction with excessive stimulation of microglia was involved.

A role for inflammation in ALS was indicated by the marked microglial activation observed in the spinal cord of mutant (G93A) SOD1 mice[90,91] and the significant effect of anti-inflammatory drugs on the survival of different mutant SOD1 mice (Table 12.1). Both minocycline[16,17,92] as well as cyclo-oxygenase (COX)-2 inhibitors[14,93] significantly increased the lifespan of different mutant SOD1 mouse models. The therapeutic effect of minocycline is not due to its strong inhibition of the extracellular matrix proteinase MMP9[94], as

crossbreeding of mutant (G93A) SOD1 mice with transgenic mice deficient for MMP9 did not increase survival[90].

Another indication that inflammation could play an important role, at least in the mouse model for ALS, is that chronic application of lipopolysaccharide to mutant (G37R) mice stimulated inflammation, exacerbated disease progression and significantly shortened the lifespan of these mice[95].

GROWTH FACTOR DEFICIENCY

Culturing motor neurons is critically dependent on the presence of different growth factors. Motor neuron survival *in vivo* can also be selectively disturbed by the absence of neurotrophic factors, as illustrated by the phenotype of the transgenic mice in which the gene for ciliary neurotrophic factor (CNTF) was deleted. CNTF is a cytosolic protein, expressed at high levels in myelinating Schwann cells, promoting survival of motor neurons *in vitro*. These knockout mice had no pathologic phenotype during the postnatal weeks, but developed atrophy and loss of motor neurons with increasing age[96].

Another indication that selective motor neuron death can be induced by an insufficiency of growth factors was the phenotype of the VEGF[δ/δ] transgenic mouse. This mouse model was created by deleting the hypoxia-response element (HRE) in the promoter region of the gene encoding VEGF. This modification induced an adult-onset, slowly progressive motor neuron loss leading to muscle atrophy and a motor phenotype[97]. Crossbreeding of VEGF[δ/δ] mice with mutant (G93A) SOD1 transgenic mice resulted in earlier motor neuron loss and a reduction of the lifespan of these double transgenic mice by 14%[98], indicating that low VEGF levels accelerated motor neuron degeneration in the mutant (G93A) SOD1 mouse model. The effect of VEGF is at least partially due to its direct neuroprotective effect on motor neurons, as was shown both *in vitro*[97-99] and *in vivo* by crossbreeding mutant (G93A) SOD1 mice with mice overexpressing the VEGF receptor 2 (also termed Flk-1). Overexpression of this receptor not only delayed the onset of motor impairment by 21%, but also prolonged survival of the mutant (G93A) SOD1 mice by 8%[19]. In conclusion, our studies show that a low VEGF level can induce selective motor neuron death, probably due to the lack of neuroprotection, although indirect, vascular effects of VEGF cannot be completely excluded.

In contrast to CNTF and VEGF, knockout mice that lack other growth factors such as insulin-like growth factor I (IGF-I), brain-derived neurotrophic factor (BDNF) or glia-derived neurotrophic factor (GDNF), did not show age-related, selective motor neuron loss and/or motor dysfunctions[100–102]. This indicates that the selective loss of motor neurons is not a general consequence of neurotrophic factor shortage, although compensatory effects in these transgenic mice cannot be excluded.

RNA PROCESSING DEFECTS

A common denominator of a number of motor neuron diseases is that proteins playing a role in RNA metabolism are involved. As a consequence, it was suggested that lower motor neurons are selectively vulnerable to defects in RNA metabolism[103].

Spinal muscular atrophy (SMA) is caused by the deletion of or by mutations in the telomeric copy of *SMN1*. SMA patients develop weakness primarily in proximal muscle groups and inefficient respiration develops due to degeneration of motor neurons in the spinal cord. SMN is involved in various cellular processes, including cytoplasmic assembly of spliceosomal small nuclear ribonucleoproteins, pre-mRNA processing and activation of transcription. Knockout of the murine *SMN* gene, which is present in a single copy, caused early embryonic lethality, demonstrating the essential role of SMN[104]. Heterozy-

gous SMN+/- mice showed a significant decrease of motor neurons, but did not present an SMA phenotype[105]. Knockdown of SMN in zebrafish caused defects in axonal outgrowth as well as pathfinding defects[106]. Two other approaches were used to generate an SMA mouse model: creation of transgenic mice by introduction of the human *SMN2* on an SMN-/- background[107,108] and generation of conditional knockout mice in which exon 7 has been targeted by using the Cre-loxP system[109,110]. These mouse models replicated at least some aspects of SMA and could become very useful for investigating the pathogenesis of this disease.

A spontaneous autosomal recessive mutation in the mouse genome gives rise to the neuromuscular degeneration (nmd) mouse line. These mutant mice develop a progressive motor neuron disease, in which muscle atrophy is secondary to motor neuron loss. Homozygous nmd mice become progressively paralysed and rarely survive longer than 4 weeks after birth. A mutation that creates a cryptic splice donor site was found in intron 4 of the immunoglobulin μ-binding protein 2 (*Ighmbp2*) gene. The consequence of this mutation is that the majority of the Ighmbp2 transcripts are aberrantly spliced. This results in an Ighmbp2 protein truncated at the C-terminus. This mouse model became highly relevant after the discovery of *Ighmbp2* mutations in patients suffering from spinal muscular atrophy with respiratory distress (SMARD) type 1[111]. SMARD is an autosomal recessive motor neuron disease that affects infants. Patients present with respiratory distress due to diaphragmatic paralysis and progressive muscle weakness with predominantly distal lower limb muscle involvement.

A third example of abnormal RNA metabolism leading to selective motor neuron death is related to PQPB-1. This protein is a transcription and/or RNA processing factor that was discovered because of its interaction with ataxin-1, a polyglutamine disease gene product responsible for spinocerebellar ataxia. Overexpression of PQPB-1 in mice resulted in a late-onset and progressive motor neuron disease-like phenotype. Pathologic examination revealed motor neuron loss in the spinal cord[112].

The involvement of defects in RNA metabolism was further suggested by the discovery of missense mutations in the *senataxin* gene of patients suffering from ALS4. ALS4 is an early-onset, autosomal dominant form of ALS, characterized by slow disease progression, limb weakness, severe muscle wasting and pyramidal signs associated with degeneration of motor neurons in brain and spinal cord. Mutations in *senataxin* were also found in patients with ataxia–ocular apraxia 2. Although the exact function of *senataxin* remains unknown, homology with other genes indicates that mutations in *senataxin* may cause degeneration of motor neurons through dysfunction of the helicase activity or of other steps in RNA processing[113].

Last but not least, mutations in the gene encoding the glycyl-tRNA synthetase (*GARS*) cause dominant Charcot–Marie–Tooth disease 2D and distal SMA type V[114], while mutations in the tyrosyl-tRNA synthetase (YARS) gene are responsible for dominant intermediate Charcot–Marie–Tooth (type C) disease[115]. Both GARS and YARS are members of the family of aminoacyl-tRNA synthetases responsible for charging tRNAs with their cognate amino acids. How mutations in such ubiquitously expressed genes lead to such a highly specific phenotype (i.e. peripheral neuropathy/neuronopathy) is not yet clear.

LIMITATIONS OF MOUSE MODELS

It is clear from the above-mentioned experiments, that mouse models for motor neuron diseases and models generated in mutagenesis screens have largely contributed to our insights in the pathomechanisms of motor neuron degeneration. It is also clear that cellular models, however useful, have their limitations. Animal models, although almost always closer to the human disease, have their limitations too. These should not be

discarded. Some of them are inherent to the animal's anatomy, physiology, longevity, genetics, etc. The corticospinal tract in a mouse is not the corticospinal tract of a human; mice have a higher metabolism; the lifespan of a mouse is shorter than that of humans; mice have fewer genes than humans, etc. Others are secondary to the overexpression of the disease-causing gene: the mutant *SOD1* levels in a mutant (G93A)/SOD1-overexpressing mouse are higher than the level of mutant *SOD1* in a heterozygous patient. Yet other limitations to what mice experiments teach us are due to the completely different experimental design with which we approach mouse models, as compared to how we approach human patients.

Of the very long list of limitations of animal models for ALS, we here mention two: (1) the mouse as a model to study the interaction between biologic factors; and (2) the mouse as a model to study potential treatments.

Cell biologic and animal studies have demonstrated the multiple molecular pathways, both in the motor neuron and in surrounding cells, involved in the mechanism of motor neuron degeneration. To prove the *in vivo* relevance of these molecules in a specific disease model such as the mutant SOD1 mouse, researchers have relied on crossbreeding the mutant (G93A) SOD1 or (G37R) SOD1 mice with a different transgenic mouse, lacking or overexpressing the gene product of interest. Crossbreeding experiments have thus demonstrated the role of parvalbumin, GluR2, VEGF, dynein and many others. Almost surely, more crossbreedings were performed but have not been reported, because of negative or inconclusive results. These experiments are often expensive and difficult, as double transgenic animals are sometimes difficult to obtain, and the numbers obtained are often too low to allow firm statistical analysis and robust conclusions. Not surprisingly, therefore, not all results could be replicated.

This has led researchers to establish a small animal model in which multiple transgenes can be overexpressed, or which allow a non-biased genetic screen for disease-modifying genes. Both worms (*Caenorhabditis elegans*) and flies (*Drosophila melanogaster*) have been investigated as possible models, but disappointingly, were not found to be suitable. Alternatives are being actively pursued.

A large variety of potential treatments have been investigated using rodent models for ALS. Most published studies report on positive effects: it looks as if all results obtained could be translated into human therapies, and ALS patients could be cured. Almost surely, many more drugs have been tested: there is a clear bias for researchers and editors to publish only (clearly) positive results. Only a few of the treatments successful in animals have made it to human trials, and none was found to be positive. Many more disappointing results are to be expected. Why?

The above-mentioned differences between mice and humans, i.e. the inherent limitation of the mouse model, certainly may explain some of this. However, there are other factors to be invoked. Many of the animal trials were conducted in a fairly small number of animals. Only rarely, a dose–response relationship was looked for. Some of the trials were falsely positive, as the results could not be replicated. Many of the replication studies did again not make it to the peer-reviewed literature, for obvious reasons.

Most experiments in animals studied the effect of a treatment started way before onset of disease, unlike what happens in humans. In some trials, treatment started as early as day 40, which is to be compared to starting a treatment in a patient at age 25, for a disease expected to start at age 50. Few studies have tried to influence disease course of the mouse starting at disease onset. Some were started close to onset of paresis, but always, a delay of several weeks between start of treatment and onset of muscle weakness remained, and so far it was almost always obvious that the therapeutic effect of the compound of interest was smaller when initiated later.

Such trials should be considered as 'proof of concept' trials, rather than as indications for the initiation of a trial in humans. Only a (probably small) subgroup of studies with clearly positive results, obtained in a large cohort of mice, treated at disease onset, and replicated by different groups, could possibly result in a study in humans.

CONCLUSIONS

Mouse models that show selective motor neuron death and a progressive motor phenotype indicate that a number of pathogenic pathways can lead to this phenotype. Aggregation of mutated proteins, problems with axonal transport, excitotoxicity, inflammation, CNTF/VEGF shortage and defects in RNA processing can at a certain point in life compromise the survival of motor neurons. Moreover, it is highly plausible that, in at least some of these motor neuron disorders, a complicated interplay of these and other unknown mechanisms ultimately leads to motor neuron death. Therefore, it remains a challenge to find the exact contribution of and interaction between all these different mechanisms, as it will otherwise remain difficult to interfere with these multifactorial diseases, of which some are life threatening.

REFERENCES

1. Rosen DR, Siddique T, Patterson D, et al. Mutations in Cu/Zn superoxide dismutase gene are associated with familial amyotrophic lateral sclerosis. Nature 1993; 362: 59–62
2. Gurney ME, Pu H, Chiu AY, et al. Motor neuron degeneration in mice that express a human Cu,Zn superoxide dismutase mutation. Science 1994; 264: 1772–5
3. Bruijn LI, Becher MW, Lee MK, et al. ALS-linked SOD1 mutant G85R mediates damage to astrocytes and promotes rapidly progressive disease with SOD1-containing inclusions. Neuron 1997; 18: 327–38
4. Ripps ME, Huntley GW, Hof PR, et al. Transgenic mice expressing an altered murine superoxide dismutase gene provide an animal model of amyotrophic lateral sclerosis. Proc Natl Acad Sci USA 1995; 92: 689–93

5. Wong PC, Pardo CA, Borchelt DR, et al. An adverse property of a familial ALS-linked SOD1 mutation causes motor neuron disease characterized by vacuolar degeneration of mitochondria. Neuron 1995; 14: 1105–16

6. Pramatarova A, Laganiere J, Roussel J, et al. Neuron-specific expression of mutant superoxide dismutase 1 in transgenic mice does not lead to motor impairment. J Neurosci 2001; 21: 3369–74

7. Gong YH, Parsadanian AS, Andreeva A, et al. Restricted expression of G86R Cu/Zn superoxide dismutase in astrocytes results in astrocytosis but does not cause motoneuron degeneration. J Neurosci 2000; 20: 660–5

8. Clement AM, Nguyen MD, Roberts EA, et al. Wild-type nonneuronal cells extend survival of SOD1 mutant motor neurons in ALS mice. Science 2003; 302: 113–17

9. Ghadge GD, Slusher BS, Bodner A, et al. Glutamate carboxypeptidase II inhibition protects motor neurons from death in familial amyotrophic lateral sclerosis models. Proc Natl Acad Sci USA 2003; 100: 9554–9

10. Canton T, Bohme GA, Boireau A, et al. RPR 119990, a novel alpha-amino-3-hydroxy-5-methyl-4-isoxazolepropionic acid antagonist: Synthesis, pharmacological properties, and activity in an animal model of amyotrophic lateral sclerosis. J Pharmacol Exp Ther 2001; 299: 314–22

11. Gurney ME, Cutting FB, Zhai P, et al. Benefit of vitamin E, riluzole, and gabapentin in a transgenic model of familial amyotrophic lateral sclerosis. Ann Neurol 1996; 39: 147–57

12. Rothstein JD, Patel S, Regan MR, et al. Beta-lactam antibiotics offer neuroprotection by increasing glutamate transporter expression. Nature 2005; 433: 73–7

13. Van Damme P, Leyssen M, Callewaert G, et al. The AMPA receptor antagonist NBQX prolongs survival in a transgenic mouse model of amyotrophic lateral sclerosis. Neurosci Lett 2003; 343: 81–4

14. Drachman DB, Frank K, Dykes-Hoberg M, et al. Cyclooxygenase 2 inhibition protects motor neurons and prolongs survival in a transgenic mouse model of ALS. Ann Neurol 2002; 52: 771–8

15. Klivenyi P, Kiaei M, Gardian G, et al. Additive neuroprotective effects of creatine and cyclooxygenase 2 inhibitors in a transgenic mouse model of amyotrophic lateral sclerosis. J Neurochem 2004; 88: 576–82

16. Van Den Bosch L, Tilkin P, Lemmens G, Robberecht W. Minocycline delays disease onset and mortality in a transgenic model of ALS. Neuroreport 2002; 13: 1067–70

17. Zhu S, Stavrovskaya IG, Drozda M, et al. Minocycline inhibits cytochrome c release and delays progression of amyotrophic lateral sclerosis in mice. Nature 2002; 417: 74–8

18. Kaspar BK, Llado J, Sherkat N, et al. Retrograde viral delivery of IGF-1 prolongs survival in a mouse ALS model. Science 2003; 301: 839–42

19. Storkebaum E, Lambrechts D, Moreno Murciano M-P, et al. Treatment of an aggressive form of motoneuron degeneration by intracerebroventricular delivery of VEGF in a rat model of ALS. Nat Neurosci 2005; 8: 85–92

20. Azzouz M, Ralph GS, Storkebaum E, et al. VEGF delivery with retrogradely transported lentivector prolongs survival in a mouse ALS model. Nature 2004; 429: 413–17

21. Wang LJ, Lu YY, Muramatsu S, et al. Neuroprotective effects of glial cell line-derived neurotrophic factor mediated by an adeno-associated virus vector in a transgenic animal model of amyotrophic lateral sclerosis. J Neurosci 2002; 22: 6920–890

22. Klivenyi P, Ferrante RJ, Matthews RT, et al. Neuroprotective effects of creatine in a transgenic animal model of amyotrophic lateral sclerosis. Nat Med 1999; 5: 347–50

23. Kieran D, Kalmar B, Dick JR, et al. Treatment with arimoclomol, a coinducer of heat shock proteins, delays disease progression in ALS mice. Nat Med 2004; 10: 402–5

24. Li M, Ona VO, Guegan C, et al. Functional role of caspase-1 and caspase-3 in an ALS transgenic mouse model. Science 2000; 288: 335–9

25. Subramaniam JR, Lyons WE, Liu J, et al. Mutant SOD1 causes motor neuron disease independent of copper chaperone-mediated copper loading. Nat Neurosci 2002; 5: 301–7

26. Wang J, Slunt H, Gonzales V, et al. Copper-binding-site-null SOD1 causes ALS in transgenic mice: Aggregates of non-native SOD1 delineate a common feature. Hum Mol Genet 2003; 12: 2753–64

27. Bruijn LI, Houseweart MK, Kato S, et al. Aggregation and motor neuron toxicity of an ALS-linked SOD1 mutant independent from wild-type SOD1. Science 1998; 281: 1851–4

28. Durham HD, Roy J, Dong L, Figlewicz DA. Aggregation of mutant Cu/Zn superoxide dismutase proteins in a culture model of ALS. J Neuropathol Exp Neurol 1997; 56: 523–30

29. Bruening W, Roy J, Giasson B, et al. Up-regulation of protein chaperones preserves viability of cells expressing toxic Cu/Zn-superoxide dismutase mutants associated with amyotrophic lateral sclerosis. J Neurochem 1999; 72: 693–9

30. Roy J, Minotti S, Dong L, Figlewicz DA, Durham HD. Glutamate potentiates the toxicity of mutant Cu/Zn-superoxide dismutase in motor neurons by postsynaptic calcium-dependent mechanisms. J Neurosci 1998; 18: 9673–84

31. Johnston JA, Dalton MJ, Gurney ME, Kopito RR. Formation of high molecular weight complexes of mutant Cu, Zn-superoxide dismutase in a mouse model for familial amyotrophic lateral sclerosis. Proc Natl Acad Sci USA 2000; 97: 12571–6

32. Katsuno M, Adachi H, Inukai A, Sobue G. Transgenic mouse models of spinal and bulbar muscular atrophy (SBMA). Cytogenet Genome Res 2003; 100: 243–51

33. Adachi H, Katsuno M, Minamiyama M, et al. Heat shock protein 70 chaperone overexpression ameliorates phenotypes of the spinal and bulbar muscular atrophy transgenic mouse model by reducing nuclear-localized mutant androgen receptor protein. J Neurosci 2003; 23: 2203–11

34. Katsuno M, Adachi H, Kume A, et al. Testosterone reduction prevents phenotypic expression in a transgenic mouse model of spinal and bulbar muscular atrophy. Neuron 2002; 35: 843–54

35. Sopher BL, Thomas PS Jr, LaFevre-Bernt MA, et al. Androgen receptor YAC transgenic mice recapitulate SBMA motor neuronopathy and implicate VEGF164 in the motor neuron degeneration. Neuron 2004; 41: 687–99

36. Borchelt DR, Wong PC, Becher MW, et al. Axonal transport of mutant superoxide dismutase 1 and focal axonal abnormalities in the proximal axons of transgenic mice. Neurobiol Dis 1998; 5: 27–35

37. Hirano A, Donnenfeld H, Sasaki S, Nakano I. Fine structural observations of neurofilamentous changes in amyotrophic lateral sclerosis. J Neuropathol Exp Neurol 1984; 43: 461–70

38. Hirano A, Nakano I, Kurland LT, et al. Fine structural study of neurofibrillary changes in a family with amyotrophic lateral sclerosis. J Neuropathol Exp Neurol 1984; 43: 471–80

39. Rouleau GA, Clark AW, Rooke K, et al. SOD1 mutation is associated with accumulation of neurofilaments in amyotrophic lateral sclerosis. Ann Neurol 1996; 39: 128–31

40. Al-Chalabi A, Andersen PM, Nilsson P, et al. Deletions of the heavy neurofilament subunit tail in amyotrophic lateral sclerosis. Hum Mol Genet 1999; 8: 157–64

41. Julien JP. Amyotrophic lateral sclerosis. Unfolding the toxicity of the misfolded. Cell 2001; 104: 581–91

42. Robertson J, Kriz J, Nguyen MD, Julien JP. Pathways to motor neuron degeneration in transgenic mouse models. Biochimie 2002; 84: 1151–60

43. Lee MK, Marszalek JR, Cleveland DW. A mutant neurofilament subunit causes massive, selective motor neuron death: Implications for the pathogenesis of human motor neuron disease. Neuron 1994; 13: 975–88

44. De Jonghe P, Mersivanova I, Nelis E, et al. Further evidence that neurofilament light chain gene mutations can cause Charcot–Marie–Tooth disease type 2E. Ann Neurol 2001; 49: 245–9

45. Mersiyanova IV, Perepelov AV, Polyakov AV, et al. A new variant of Charcot-Marie-Tooth disease type 2 is probably the result of a mutation in the neurofilament-light gene. Am J Hum Genet 2000; 67: 37–46

46. Nie Z, Wu J, Zhai J, et al. Untranslated element in neurofilament mRNA has neuropathic effect on motor neurons of transgenic mice. J Neurosci 2002; 22: 7662–70

47. Lin H, Zhai J, Canete-Soler R, Schlaepfer WW. 3' untranslated region in a light neurofilament (NF-L) mRNA triggers aggregation of NF-L and mutant superoxide dismutase 1 proteins in neuronal cells. J Neurosci 2004; 24: 2716–26

48. Williamson TL, Bruijn LI, Zhu Q, et al. Absence of neurofilaments reduces the selective vulnerability of motor neurons and slows disease caused by a familial amyotrophic lateral sclerosis-linked superoxide dismutase 1 mutant. Proc Natl Acad Sci USA 1998; 95: 9631–6

49. Kong J, Xu Z. Overexpression of neurofilament subunit NF-L and NF-H extends survival of a mouse model for amyotrophic lateral sclerosis. Neurosci Lett 2000; 281: 72–4

50. Couillard-Despres S, Zhu Q, Wong PC, et al. Protective effect of neurofilament heavy gene overexpression in motor neuron disease induced by mutant superoxide dismutase. Proc Natl Acad Sci USA 1998; 95: 9626–30

51. Evgrafov OV, Mersiyanova I, Irobi J, et al. Mutant small heat-shock protein 27 causes axonal Charcot-

Marie-Tooth disease and distal hereditary motor neuropathy. Nat Genet 2004; 36: 602–6

52. Irobi J, Van Impe K, Seeman P, et al. Hot-spot residue in small heat-shock protein 22 causes distal motor neuropathy. Nat Genet 2004; 36: 597–601

53. Vleminckx V, Van Damme P, Goffin K, et al. Upregulation of HSP27 in a transgenic model of ALS. J Neuropathol Exp Neurol 2002; 61: 968–74

54. Beaulieu JM, Nguyen MD, Julien JP. Late onset of motor neurons in mice overexpressing wild-type peripherin. J Cell Biol 1999; 147: 531–44

55. Lariviere RC, Beaulieu JM, Nguyen MD, Julien JP. Peripherin is not a contributing factor to motor neuron disease in a mouse model of amyotrophic lateral sclerosis caused by mutant superoxide dismutase. Neurobiol Dis 2003; 13: 158–66

56. Gros-Louis F, Lariviere R, Gowing G, et al. A frameshift deletion in peripherin gene associated with amyotrophic lateral sclerosis. J Biol Chem 2004; 279: 45951–6

57. Leung CL, He CZ, Kaufmann P, et al. A pathogenic peripherin gene mutation in a patient with amyotrophic lateral sclerosis. Brain Pathol 2004; 14: 290–6

58. Martin N, Jaubert J, Gounon P, et al. A missense mutation in Tbce causes progressive motor neuronopathy in mice. Nat Genet 2002; 32: 443–7

59. Lee VM, Goedert M, Trojanowski JQ. Neurodegenerative tauopathies. Annu Rev Neurosci 2001; 24: 1121–59

60. Spittaels K, Van den Haute C, Van Dorpe J, et al. Prominent axonopathy in the brain and spinal cord of transgenic mice overexpressing four-repeat human tau protein. Am J Pathol 1999; 155: 2153–65

61. Zhang B, Higuchi M, Yoshiyama Y, et al. Retarded axonal transport of R406W mutant tau in transgenic mice with a neurodegenerative tauopathy. J Neurosci 2004; 24: 4657–67

62. Hafezparast M, Klocke R, Ruhrberg C, et al. Mutations in dynein link motor neuron degeneration to defects in retrograde transport. Science 2003; 300: 808–12

63. King SJ, Schroer TA. Dynactin increases the processivity of the cytoplasmic dynein motor. Nat Cell Biol 2000; 2: 20–4

64. LaMonte BH, Wallace KE, Holloway BA, et al. Disruption of dynein/dynactin inhibits axonal transport in motor neurons causing late-onset progressive degeneration. Neuron 2002; 34: 715–27

65. Puls I, Jonnakuty C, LaMonte BH, et al. Mutant dynactin in motor neuron disease. Nat Genet 2003; 33: 455–6

66. Kieran DM, Hafezparast M, Bohnert S, et al. A mutation in dynein rescues axonal transport defects and extends the life span of ALS mice. J Cell Biol 2005; 169: 561–7

67. Murakami T, Nagano I, Hayashi T, et al. Impaired retrograde axonal transport of adenovirus-mediated E. coli LacZ gene in the mice carrying mutant SOD1 gene. Neurosci Lett 2001; 308: 149–52

68. Bensimon G, Lacomblez L, Meininger V. A controlled trial of riluzole in amyotrophic lateral sclerosis. ALS/Riluzole Study Group. N Engl J Med 1994; 330: 585–91

69. Carriedo SG, Yin HZ, Weiss JH. Motor neurons are selectively vulnerable to AMPA/kainate receptor-mediated injury in vitro. J Neurosci 1996; 16: 4069–79

70. Rothstein JD, Bristol LA, Hosler B, et al. Chronic inhibition of superoxide dismutase produces apoptotic death of spinal neurons. Proc Natl Acad Sci USA 1994; 91: 4155–9

71. Van Den Bosch L, Van Damme P, Vleminckx V, et al. An alpha-mercaptoacrylic acid derivative (PD150606) inhibits selective motor neuron death via inhibition of kainate-induced Ca2+ influx and not via calpain inhibition. Neuropharmacology 2002; 42: 706–13

72. Van Den Bosch L, Vandenberghe W, Klaassen H, et al. Ca^{2+}-permeable AMPA receptors and selective vulnerability of motor neurons. J Neurol Sci 2000; 180: 29–34

73. Van Damme P, Callewaert G, Eggermont J, et al. Chloride influx aggravates Ca^{2+}-dependent AMPA receptor-mediated motoneuron death. J Neurosci 2003; 23: 4942–50

74. Palecek J, Lips MB, Keller BU. Calcium dynamics and buffering in motoneurones of the mouse spinal cord. J Physiol 1999; 520: 485–502

75. Van Den Bosch L, Schwaller B, Vleminckx V, et al. Protective effect of parvalbumin on excitotoxic motor neuron death. Exp Neurol 2002; 174: 150–61

76. Beers DR, Ho BK, Siklos L, et al. Parvalbumin overexpression alters immune-mediated increases in intracellular calcium, and delays disease onset in a transgenic model of familial amyotrophic lateral sclerosis. J Neurochem 2001; 79: 499–509

77. Hollmann M, Hartley M, Heinemann S. Ca2+ permeability of KA-AMPA–gated glutamate receptor

channels depends on subunit composition. Science 1991; 252: 851–3

78. Sommer B, Kohler M, Sprengel R, Seeburg PH. RNA editing in brain controls a determinant of ion flow in glutamate-gated channels. Cell 1991; 67: 11–19

79. Kawahara Y, Ito K, Sun H, et al. Glutamate receptors: RNA editing and death of motor neurons. Nature 2004; 427: 801

80. Feldmeyer D, Kask K, Brusa R, et al. Neurological dysfunctions in mice expressing different levels of the Q/R site-unedited AMPAR subunit GluR-B. Nat Neurosci 1999; 2, 57–64

81. Jia Z, Agopyan N, Miu P, et al. Enhanced LTP in mice deficient in the AMPA receptor GluR2. Neuron 1996; 17: 945–56

82. Van Damme P, Braeken D, Callewaert G, et al. GluR2 deficiency accelerates motor neuron degeneration in a mouse model of amyotrophic lateral sclerosis. J Neuropathol Exp Neurol 2005; 64: 604–12

83. Tateno M, Sadakata H, Tanaka M, et al. Calcium-permeable AMPA receptors promote misfolding of mutant SOD1 protein and development of amyotrophic lateral sclerosis in a transgenic mouse model. Hum Mol Genet 2004; 13: 2183–96

84. Howland DS, Liu J, She Y, et al. Focal loss of the glutamate transporter EAAT2 in a transgenic rat model of SOD1 mutant-mediated amyotrophic lateral sclerosis (ALS). Proc Natl Acad Sci USA 2002; 99: 1604–9

85. Guo H, Lai L, Butchbach ME, et al. Increased expression of the glial glutamate transporter EAAT2 modulates excitotoxicity and delays the onset but not the outcome of ALS in mice. Hum Mol Genet 2003; 12: 2519–32

86. Henkel JS, Engelhardt JI, Siklos L, et al. Presence of dendritic cells, MCP-1, and activated microglia/macrophages in amyotrophic lateral sclerosis spinal cord tissue. Ann Neurol 2004; 55: 221–35

87. Turner MR, Cagnin A, Turkheimer FE, et al. Evidence of widespread cerebral microglial activation in amyotrophic lateral sclerosis: an [11C](R)-PK11195 positron emission tomography study. Neurobiol Dis 2004; 15: 601–9

88. Chavany C, Vicario-Abejon C, Miller G, Jendoubi M. Transgenic mice for interleukin 3 develop motor neuron degeneration associated with autoimmune reaction against spinal cord motor neurons. Proc Natl Acad Sci USA 1998; 95: 11354–9

89. Chiang CS, Powell HC, Gold LH, et al. Macrophage/microglial-mediated primary demyelination and motor disease induced by the central nervous system production of interleukin-3 in transgenic mice. J Clin Invest 1996; 97: 1512–24

90. Dewil M, Schurmans C, Starckx, S, et al. Role of Gelatinase B/Matrix Metalloprotease-9 in a mouse model for amyotrophic lateral sclerosis. Neuroreport 2005; 16: 321–4

91. Hall ED, Oostveen JA, Gurney ME. Relationship of microglial and astrocytic activation to disease onset and progression in a transgenic model of familial ALS. Glia 1998; 23: 249–56

92. Kriz J, Nguyen MD, Julien JP. Minocycline slows disease progression in a mouse model of amyotrophic lateral sclerosis. Neurobiol Dis 2002; 10: 268–78

93. Pompl PN, Ho L, Bianchi M, et al. A therapeutic role for cyclooxygenase-2 inhibitors in a transgenic mouse model of amyotrophic lateral sclerosis. FASEB J 2003; 17: 725–7

94. Paemen L, Martens E, Norga K, et al. The gelatinase inhibitory activity of tetracyclines and chemically modified tetracycline analogues as measured by a novel microtiter assay for inhibitors. Biochem Pharmacol 1996; 52: 105–11

95. Nguyen MD, D'Aigle T, Gowing G, et al. Exacerbation of motor neuron disease by chronic stimulation of innate immunity in a mouse model of amyotrophic lateral sclerosis. J Neurosci 2004; 24: 1340–9

96. Masu Y, Wolf E, Holtmann B, et al. Disruption of the CNTF gene results in motor neuron degeneration. Nature 1993; 365: 27–32

97. Oosthuyse B, Moons L, Storkebaum E, et al. Deletion of the hypoxia-response element in the vascular endothelial growth factor promoter causes motor neuron degeneration. Nat Genet 2001; 28: 131–8

98. Lambrechts D, Storkebaum E, Morimoto M, et al. VEGF is a modifier of amyotrophic lateral sclerosis in mice and humans and protects motoneurons against ischemic death. Nat Genet 2003; 34: 383–94.

99. Van Den Bosch L, Storkebaum E, Vleminckx V, et al. Effects of vascular endothelial growth factor (VEGF) on motor neuron degeneration. Neurobiol Dis 2004; 17: 21–8

100. Ernfors P, Lee KF, Jaenisch R. Mice lacking brain-derived neurotrophic factor develop with sensory deficits. Nature 1994; 368: 147–50

101. Gao WQ, Shinsky N, Ingle G, et al. IGF-I deficient mice show reduced peripheral nerve conduction

velocities and decreased axonal diameters and respond to exogenous IGF-I treatment. J Neurobiol 1999; 39: 142–52

102. Moore MW, Klein RD, Farinas I, et al. Renal and neuronal abnormalities in mice lacking GDNF. Nature 1996; 382: 76–9

103. Anderson K, Talbot K. Spinal muscular atrophies reveal motor neuron vulnerability to defects in ribonucleoprotein handling. Curr Opin Neurol 2003; 16: 595–9

104. Schrank B, Gotz R, Gunnersen JM, Ure JM, et al. Inactivation of the survival motor neuron gene, a candidate gene for human spinal muscular atrophy, leads to massive cell death in early mouse embryos. Proc Natl Acad Sci USA 1997; 94: 9920–5

105. Jablonka S, Bandilla M, Wiese S, et al. Co-regulation of survival of motor neuron (SMN) protein and its interactor SIP1 during development and in spinal muscular atrophy. Hum Mol Genet 2001; 10: 497–505

106. McWhorter ML, Monani UR, Burghes AH, Beattie CE. Knockdown of the survival motor neuron (Smn) protein in zebrafish causes defects in motor axon outgrowth and pathfinding. J Cell Biol 2003; 162: 919–31

107. Hsieh-Li HM, Chang JG, Jong YJ, et al. A mouse model for spinal muscular atrophy. Nat Genet 2000; 24: 66–70

108. Monani UR, Sendtner M, Coovert DD, et al. The human centromeric survival motor neuron gene (SMN2) rescues embryonic lethality in Smn(-/-) mice and results in a mouse with spinal muscular atrophy. Hum Mol Genet 2000; 9: 333–9

109. Cifuentes-Diaz C, Frugier T, Tiziano FD, et al. Deletion of murine SMN exon 7 directed to skeletal muscle leads to severe muscular dystrophy. J Cell Biol 2001; 152: 1107–14

110. Frugier T, Tiziano FD, Cifuentes-Diaz C, et al. Nuclear targeting defect of SMN lacking the C-terminus in a mouse model of spinal muscular atrophy. Hum Mol Genet 2000; 9: 849–58

111. Grohmann K, Schuelke M, Diers A, et al. Mutations in the gene encoding immunoglobulin mu-binding protein 2 cause spinal muscular atrophy with respiratory distress type 1. Nat Genet 2001; 29: 75–7

112. Okuda T, Hattori H, Takeuchi S, et al. PQBP-1 transgenic mice show a late-onset motor neuron disease-like phenotype. Hum Mol Genet 2003; 12: 711–25

113. Chen YZ, Bennett CL, Huynh HM, et al. DNA/RNA helicase gene mutations in a form of juvenile amyotrophic lateral sclerosis (ALS4). Am J Hum Genet 2004; 74: 1128–35

114. Antonellis A, Ellsworth RE, Sambuughin N, et al. Glycyl tRNA synthetase mutations in Charcot–Marie–Tooth disease type 2D and distal spinal muscular atrophy type V. Am J Hum Genet 2003; 72: 1293–9

115. Jordanova A, Irobi J, Thomas FP, et al. Disrupted function and axonal distribution of mutant tyrosyl-tRNA synthetase in dominant intermediate Charcot–Marie–Tooth neuropathy. Nat Genet 2006; 38: 197–202

13

Apoptotic cell death pathways in amyotrophic lateral sclerosis: a review

Piera Pasinelli, Robert H Brown Jr

INTRODUCTION

Programmed cell death, or apoptosis, is a highly regulated form of cell death in which cells die by activating a pre-programed suicide mechanism[1]. Morphologically, it is characterized by blebbing of the plasma membrane, exposure of phosphatidylserine to the outer plasma membrane, clustering of cytoplasmic organelles and chromatin condensation[2]. It is an energy-dependent, multistep process that involves activation of both positive and negative regulatory elements such as the Bcl-2/Bax family of proteins, the p53 tumor suppressor gene, members of the tumor necrosis factor receptors (TNFR) superfamily, and cell cycle-related genes[1]. The intracellular ratio of these genes determines the fate of a given cell and may explain the selective vulnerability of some cells to death stimuli. Central components of this death mechanism are the interleukin-1β converting enzyme (ICE)-like cysteine proteases, also known as caspases. Caspases are cysteine proteases with aspartate specificity[1]. They work in a hierarchically organized manner and participate in the death of the cells either as upstream elements (e.g. caspase-8 and -9, which trigger cell death by cleaving and activating other caspases) or as downstream elements (e.g. caspase-3 and -7 that directly destroy the cells through cleavage of key components of cell viability) (Figure 13.1).

Although for years apoptosis has been recognized as the physiologic process by which developing neurons are purposefully destroyed, it is now clear that this form of cell death occurs in pathologic conditions. There is increasing evidence that apoptosis contributes to neuronal loss in many acute and chronic neurologic diseases such as stroke, Alzheimer's disease, Parkinson's disease, Huntington's disease and amyotrophic lateral sclerosis (ALS). In this chapter, we review the evidence supporting the involvement of apoptosis in motor neuron degeneration in ALS and discuss the potential implication of inhibitors of apoptosis for ALS therapy.

APOPTOSIS IN AMYOTROPHIC LATERAL SCLEROSIS: IS IT REAL?

Despite early controversies over the role of apoptosis in ALS, it is increasingly clear that key components of apoptosis are recruited to participate in the mechanisms of motor neuron degeneration[3]. Early skepticism stemmed from the difficulties in finding clear morphologic evidence of apoptosis in postmortem tissues of ALS patients. This is most likely to be due to technical difficulties rather than lack of activation of apoptosis pathways. First, cells undergoing apoptosis are phagocytosed by neighboring cells, leaving little

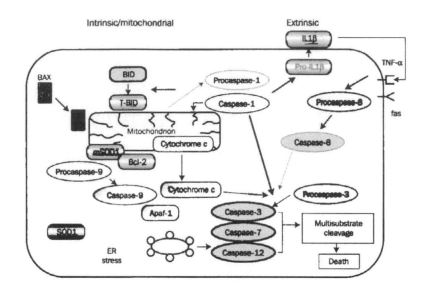

Figure 13.1   Cell death pathways in amyotrophic lateral sclerosis (ALS). This summarizes the major extrinsic and intrinsic pathways provoking apoptotic cell death. Both pathways have been implicated in mutant SOD1-related neuronal death. As indicated, in the intrinsic pathway (left) a toxic stimulus (such as mutant SOD1 protein) alters permeability of the mitochondrial membrane, release of cytochrome c, and activation of caspase-9, which is upstream of the executioner caspases 3, 7 and 12. Mitochondrial permeability changes may be triggered by multiple stimuli including caspase-1, cleavage of BID to T-BID, BAX translocation and binding of mutant SOD1 to Bcl-2 in the outer mitochondrial membrane. In the extrinsic pathway (right), stimuli exogenous to the cell (e.g. tumor necrosis factor-α or FAS ligand) bind surface receptors and thereby activate caspase-8, which is upstream of the executioner caspases. In SOD1-mediated ALS, the earliest changes are mitochondrial disruption and caspase-1 activation. This, in turn, may activate both the intrinsic pathway and, through the release of interleukin-1β, the extrinsic pathway. Death ultimately reflects both mitochondrial demise and cleavage of multiple substrates. See also Plate 10

indication that apoptosis has truly occurred. Second, apoptosis affects only relatively few cells at any given time; moreover, these may be difficult to discern because they are scattered among viable cells. Third, the rate of the process is low and, therefore, although cell death might ultimately involve a significant number of cells, at any single point in time dying cells are likely to represent less than 1% of the total cellular population. Fourth, in postmortem samples it may be that the remaining motor neurons are either healthy or are committed to die but without manifesting morphologic signs of apoptosis, either because such signs have not yet appeared or potentially because the same cells undergo non-apoptotic death. Finally, the lack of detection of apoptotic morphology does not necessarily exclude the possibility that cell death genes are nonetheless activated. For example, it has been suggested that caspase-9 activation is instrumental in paraptosis, a form of apoptosis that does not entail conventional apoptotic morphology[4].

Another argument against a central role of apoptosis in ALS pathogenesis derives from the concept that this form of cell death is very rapid and therefore cannot be involved in a chronic disease in which cells degenerate over a long period of time. Most of what we know about apoptosis derives from developmental studies wherein apoptosis is a rapid event required either to destroy cells that, if not eliminated, threaten the normal sequence of cellular and molecular development events or to remove surplus cells (e.g. eliminating neurons that form supernumerary synapses). In adult, fully differentiated neurons the timing of activation of cell death genes may be slower and, therefore, while the final events of cell death may last for only a few hours, activation of the upstream events may be much more protracted in time than apoptosis activation during development. Fortunately, the development of cellular and animal models of ALS has facilitated analysis of these events, and their chronologic relationships.

EVIDENCE FOR APOPTOSIS IN HUMAN AMYOTROPHIC LATERAL SCLEROSIS

An increasing number of reports show evidence for apoptosis in patients with ALS. Increased expression of an apoptosis-related antigen and DNA breaks have been reported in cervical spinal cord sections of ALS patients. Immunocytochemistry using an antibody to Le$^{(Y)}$, a difucosylated type-2 chain determinant characteristic of cells undergoing apoptosis, showed positive immunostaining in seven out of the ten ALS cases analyzed[5]. The same seven cases showed characteristic chromatin condensation by double staining with nick-end-labeling[5]. *In situ* fragmented DNA has been found in brain and spinal cord tissues from 12 ALS cases together with cell shrinkage and small Nissl-positive bodies[6]. While some of these changes were detected in non-neurologic controls, the extent of apoptosis was higher and more significant in the ALS cases. *In situ* hybridization was also used to analyze Bcl-2 and Bax mRNA levels in control and ALS lumbar spinal cord sections. Compared with controls, mRNA levels of the anti-apoptotic Bcl-2 were significantly lower (4.7-fold) in ALS whereas, for the pro-apoptotic Bax, the mRNA hybridization signal was significantly higher (2.8-fold) selectively in motor neurons[7]. At the protein level, strong expression of Bax was also found in muscle fibers of two ALS patients[8]. These changes were paralleled by evidence of DNA fragmentation as determined by the TUNEL method[8]. However, the interpretation of these results is somewhat controversial, because in the same study high expression of the anti-apoptotic product Bcl-2 was also found, and other

studies have later failed to replicate positive TUNEL staining in affected regions of ALS patients. Characteristic morphologic evidence of apoptosis was later found in spinal cords of ALS patients that showed signs of typical chromatolysis together with increased Bax and decreased Bcl-2 expression in the mitochondria-enriched membrane[9]. Interestingly, levels of Bcl-2, Bax and Bak were unaltered in the cytosolic compartment, indicating that the compartmental expression of members of the Bcl-2 family may be significant in ALS pathogenesis. Another member of the Bcl-2 family, Harakiri, may be involved in ALS. This is a potent pro-death molecule that is elevated in spinal cords of ALS cases; increased Harakiri expression is associated with morphologic signs of apoptosis[10].

Studies of the signal transduction pathways related to apoptosis have also been informative in ALS cases. An immunohistochemical analysis showed that the c-*Jun*-JNK/SAPK kinase pathway is dramatically overexpressed in ALS spinal cords[11]. These are stress-activated kinases that are upregulated in apoptosis. The strongest activation was found in astrocytes, while motor neurons revealed an unusually low expression of the pathway. Interestingly, while motor neurons showed morphologic changes of apoptosis, in astrocytes, JNK/SAPK overexpression was unrelated to apoptosis but was accompanied by activation of the nuclear-factor kappa B (NF-κB), a nuclear transcription factor that mediates resistance of neuronal cells against oxidative stress[12,13]. Activation of NF-κB denotes activation of a protective response to oxidative stress that was reportedly deficient in ALS motor neurons[13]. These data support the view that astrocytes are involved in the pathology of ALS via activation of an apoptotic pathway mediated by stress-activated kinases, and that motor neurons are selectively killed because of their lack of antioxidant defenses. Alterations in cyclin-dependent kinase-5 (cdk-5) pathway signal transduction pathways have also been described in human ALS[14]. Cdk-5-mediated responses have been associated with neuronal apoptosis. Intense cdk-5 immunoreactivity has been detected in degenerating ALS motor neurons[14]. How cdk-5 participates in motor neuron cell death remains speculative. Since cdk-5 phosphorylates neurofilament protein (NFP), it has been proposed to be the kinase that mediates the excessive NFP phosphorylation reported in ALS. However, Bajaj *et al.* found cdk-5 to co-localize with lipofuscin and not with NFP accumulation in motor neurons and suggested the role of cdk-5 in the pathogenesis of ALS to be associated with lipofuscin-related cell death[15].

Another interesting correlation between ALS pathogenesis and apoptosis is that dying motor neurons are ubiquitin-positive[16]. At least during development, activation of the *polyubiquitin* gene has been reported to be a marker for apoptosis. High expression of the prostate apoptosis response 4 (*PAR-4*) gene, which is induced in prostate cancer cells and in neuronal apoptosis, was reported in spinal cord sections of ALS patients[17]. In human ALS, increased p53 immunoreactivity was detected in both motor cortex and spinal cord anterior horns[18]. Although the exact role played by p53 in apoptosis is not clear, high levels of p53 have been consistently associated with neuronal apoptosis, while low levels of p53 have been shown to be neuroprotective. Sera from sporadic and familial ALS cases showed abnormally high levels of anti-Fas antibodies (25% and 22% positive, respectively). Fas is a member of the tumor necrosis factor (TNF) family and a participant in the main receptor-mediated apoptotic pathway[19].

Limited biochemical evidence has been collected so far in human samples. The first evidence of activation of an apoptotic pathway in ALS patients was the finding of increased activity of caspase-1 and caspase-9 in cerebrospinal fluid by enzyme-linked immunosorbent assay (ELISA) methods [20]. Another dataset provides evidence of aberrant protein–protein interactions between members of the Bcl-2 family. Protein–protein interactions are important in the function of Bcl-2-like proteins. Pro-death molecules such as Bax or Bad cause toxicity by interacting with, and

therefore inhibiting, anti-death molecules. Similarly, anti-death members exert their protective function by binding pro-death proteins. Co-immunoprecipitation studies in ALS patients showed subnormal Bcl-2–Bax interaction and a significantly higher Bax–Bax interaction[3], changes that are predicted to bias the cell toward an apoptotic state.

It may be argued that, these studies notwithstanding, the paucity of compelling biochemical data in human ALS weighs against an active role of cell death genes in the demise of the motor neurons. However, *in vivo* biochemical analysis can be complicated by the rarity of dying cells and thus the difficulty of detecting the biochemical markers of apoptosis. Molecular signals generated by infrequent apoptotic cells may be undetectable against the background of normal cells. Moreover, the quality of human autopsy samples is heterogeneous and often problematic (e.g. because of varying postmortem intervals); accordingly, autopsy specimens are often poorly suited for biochemical assays. At a minimum, the foregoing data allow one to conclude that late-stage motor neurons in ALS patients clearly reveal some characteristic features of apoptosis.

APOPTOSIS IN CELLULAR AND ANIMAL MODELS OF AMYOTROPHIC LATERAL SCLEROSIS: LESSONS FROM THE MUTANT SOD1-MEDIATED TOXICITY

The most compelling data implicating apoptosis in motor neuron death in ALS have been generated in studies examining the cytotoxicity of mutant SOD1[3] (see also Table 13.1). That mutations in the gene encoding SOD1 cause ALS in a subset of familial cases[21] has provided the first molecular basis for studying the mechanism of neurodegeneration in ALS. Central to these mechanistic studies has been the generation of both cell-based and transgenic animal models of mutant SOD1-mediated ALS[22]. (A detailed

Table 13.1   SOD1-mediated toxicity in apoptosis

Observation	References
Human ALS autopsy studies	
Le(y)(+) cells; chromatin condensation	5
Fragmented DNA in brain and spinal cord	6
Decreased Bcl-2 mRNA, increased Bax mRNA	7
Increased Bax protein	8
Decreased Bcl-2, increased Bax in mitochondrial membranes	9
Increased Harakiri in spinal cord	10
Increased c-Jun-JNK/SAPK in astrocytes	11
Elevated CDK5 immunoreactivity	14
Increased CSF caspases-1 and -9	20
Elevated expression of PAR-4 and p53 in motor cortex and spinal cord	17, 18
Aberrant interaction between Bcl-2-like protein	3
Studies in transgenic SOD1-G93A ALS mice	
DNA fragmentation, altered expression of Bcl-2 family proteins	3, 23, 24
Overexpression of Bcl-2 delays onset and prolongs survival	25
Sequential activation of caspases-1 and -3	3, 26–28
Mitochondrial swelling and cytochrome c release	3
Caspase-1-mediated Bid cleavage	3
mSOD1/Bcl-2 complex in spinal cord mitochondria	29
Inhibition of apoptosis prolongs survival	3, 28, 30–32
Cell culture models of mutant SOD1-induced neuronal death	
ALS-related mutations convert SOD1 from anti- to pro-apoptotic	33, 34
Mutant SOD1-expressing cells undergo PCD	26, 35 37
Activation of multiple caspases	26–28, 38
Bcl-2 expression protects cells from mutant SOD1 toxicity	36
Decreased Bag-1, increased Bak and Bnip3	39
Enhanced expression of PAR-4	40
Activation of p53	41
Aberrant interaction of Bcl-2 and SOD1	29
FAS-mediated activation of Daxx, ASK1 and p38	38
Mutant SOD1 binds Hsp70	42

description of the animal models is provided in Chapter 12.) Transgenic mice expressing mutant SOD1 protein develop a slowly progressive motor neuron disorder with clinical and pathologic hallmarks of human ALS[22]. Because of the remarkable clinical, pathologic and molecular similarities between SOD1-mediated and other forms of human ALS, it is widely assumed that understanding the molecular basis of cell death mechanisms underlying mutant SOD1-mediated death will illuminate all forms of ALS. Whether this assumption is valid remains to be confirmed. Interest in the study of apoptosis in mutant SOD1-mediated ALS was fueled by early reports suggesting that ALS-related SOD1 mutations transform SOD1, which in its wild-type form is anti-apoptotic in cultures, into a pro-death protein[33,34,43]. Indeed, cultured neuronal cells either transfected or microinjected with mutant SOD1 cDNAs die by apoptosis[26,35–37]. In different cellular systems, ranging from neuronal cell lines to cultured primary motor neurons, forced expression of the mutant SOD1 protein either increases the predisposition of the cells to apoptosis or causes apoptosis by activating several upstream and/or downstream caspases[26,37]. Mutant SOD1-mediated toxicity is blocked by overexpression of Bcl-2 in several neural cell lines[36]. Gene expression profiling of apoptosis-related genes has shown that, in motor neuronal cell lines transfected with the SOD1-G93A mutant, expression of *Bag-1* (a Bcl-2-associated gene that enhances Bcl-2 anti-apoptotic function) is decreased, while Bak and Bnip3 (another pro-death molecule of the large Bcl-2 family) expression is increased[39]. Interestingly, Bak is selectively increased in the mitochondrial fraction[40]. In agreement with the human data showing elevated Par-4 in spinal cords of ALS patients, *in vitro* studies have shown that Par-4 induces death of cultured primary motor neurons and that oxidative stress induces increases in Par-4 expression prior to apoptosis in a neuronal cell line[44,45].

The pro-apoptotic influence of the mutant SOD1 protein is not confined to neurons in culture. Signs of apoptosis have been detected in spinal cord and cortex of the three major lines of ALS mutant SOD1 mice and in ALS rats. These include DNA fragmentation, altered expression of members of the Bcl-2 family and caspase activation[3,39]. DNA laddering was found in the spinal cord of two lines of mice expressing low (approximately 12) or high (approximately 24) copies of the human *SOD1-G93A* gene[46]. This was visible in symptomatic animals only just before or at end-stage. Altered expression of Bcl-2 and Bcl-x proteins and of the Bad protein have also been detected in the SOD1-G93A mice[23,24]. In asymptomatic mice, expression of these proteins does not differ from control mice. However, in symptomatic mice Bcl-2 and Bcl-x expression is significantly decreased, while Bad expression is dramatically increased[23]. Accordingly, overexpression of the Bcl-2 transgene delays disease onset and prolongs survival for about 1 month in the same mice[25]. The pro-death molecule Bid is also highly expressed in SOD1-G93A compared to control

non-transgenic mice[3]. The mutant SOD1 protein can also activate p53, a nuclear phosphoprotein that is directly involved in activating apoptosis[41]. However, targeted disruption of p53 does not affect disease progression in the SOD1-G93A mice[47].

It is well established that expression of mutant SOD1 in mice triggers activation of several caspases specifically in affected tissues. Activation of caspase-1, one of the early events in mutant SOD1-mediated toxicity and the earliest molecular abnormality detected so far in the SOD1-G85R mice, occurs very early in the course of the disease, months before signs of motor neuron death and clinical onset[26-28]. Caspase-1 activation is followed months later by activation of caspase-3, which is likely to be one of the key components responsible for the death of the motor neurons. In three different lines of ALS mice, caspase-3 activation occurs immediately before or at the time of disease onset and coincides with loss of large motor axons and appearance of apoptotic morphology[26,27]. In the spinal cord of the mice, activated caspase-3 is found in both astrocytes and motor neurons[26]. The same sequential activation of caspase-1 and -3 has been found in a line of ALS rats carrying the G93A mutation[48]. In addition to caspase-3, another downstream caspase, caspase-7, may be involved in motor neuron death. At least in the SOD1-G93A mice, activation of caspase-7 coincides with disease onset[3]. In agreement with the established organization of apoptotic events and with the hierarchical order of caspase activation, in the SOD1-G93A mouse cytochrome c translocation to the cytosol and concomitant caspase-9 activation follows caspase-1 activation and precedes activation of caspase-3 and -7[49,50]. Supporting these observations is the finding that either expression of a dominant inhibitory form of caspase-1 or intraventricular administration of a pan-caspase inhibitor slows disease progression in the SOD1-G93A mice[28,30]. Moreover, prevention of cytochrome c release extends survival in the same mice supporting the concept that, at least in mutant SOD1-mediated

ALS, apoptosis occurs through activation of the mitochondrial pathway[3]. Elevated expression of two additional caspases has been shown in the SOD1-G93A mice. The inflammatory caspase-11 is upregulated in the spinal cord of these mice before disease onset[51]. However, despite elevated levels of caspase-11 protein, no increase in caspase-11 activity has been reported[51]. This, together with the report that deletion of caspase-11 in the ALS mice does not prolong survival and does not reduce motor neuron death, argues against the involvemement of caspase-11 in apoptosis of the motor neurons[52]. High levels of caspase-11 may represent activation of an inflammatory pathway that causes the astrocytosis that is commonly observed in the mice. Increased expression and activity of caspase-12 (a caspase linked to the endoplasmatic reticulum-associated cell death pathway) have been reported[3]. However, the involvement of caspase-12 in motor neuron death may be questioned in view of another study in which evidence of active caspase-12 was also found at baseline in control, non-transgenic, mice[51].

Like caspase-11, caspase-1 is involved in both apoptosis and inflammation. Therefore, it is possible that the prolonged caspase-1 activation in the ALS mice might either contribute to or be a consequence of the inflammatory pathway. However, experimental evidence favors a participation of caspase-1 in apoptosis in this model. First, expression of a dominant negative form of caspase-1 delays disease onset in the SOD1-G93A mice[30]. Second, in an independent study, a dominant negative mutant of caspase-1 blocked Bid cleavage, mitochondrial release of cytochrome c and subsequent activation of caspase-9 and -3[3]. Further, caspase-1 plays a key role in the truncation of Bid[3]. Upon cleavage, Bid is transformed into a potent pro-death molecule. Thus, in the ALS mice, caspase-1 could function as an early, initiating step in the apoptosis process by cleaving Bid.

As indicated above, the prolonged activation of caspase-1 and the gradual increase in activation of apoptosis genes over disease progression is, at first consideration, at odds with the rapid nature of apoptosis. However, as discussed above, adult neuronal apoptosis may differ from the form of apoptosis that is essential during development. Indeed, data from the systematic analysis of activation of cell death genes in the ALS mice argue that neuronal, degenerative apoptosis is not a rapid, secondary phenomenon responsible for the final demise of the motor neurons, but rather is a slowly progressive process that, over months and years, impairs and ultimately kills motor neurons and surrounding cells. A critical question is how this process is initiated, and whether it is directly triggered by mutant SOD1.

MUTANT SOD1 PROTEIN AS AN INITIATOR OF CELL DEATH

The gradual activation of an apoptotic pathway in mutant SOD1-mediated ALS, together with the striking finding that wild-type SOD1 protein is anti-apoptotic, suggest that SOD1 is directly involved in the regulation of cell death. Thus, wild-type SOD1 may protect the cells directly or indirectly by interacting with proteins that mediate apoptosis, including members of the Bcl-2 family. The corollary prediction is that mutant SOD1 proteins acquire one or more pro-apoptotic properties by altering this interaction and therefore become pro-death molecules. Consistent with this hypothesis, we recently reported that both wild-type and mutant SOD1 bind Bcl-2 and, more importantly, that mutations in SOD1 alter this binding and entrap Bcl-2 into detergent-resistant aggregates[29] (Figure 13.2). The Bcl-2 family of pro- and anti-apoptotic proteins are the check-point of the mitochondrial apoptotic pathway. Altering and/or decreasing the function of anti-apoptotic members such as Bcl-2 represents the point of no return for the cells that become committed to die[53]. Thus, a possible consequence of the entrapment of Bcl-2 into mutant SOD1 aggregates may be loss of Bcl-2 expression and function: a signal for the cells to die.

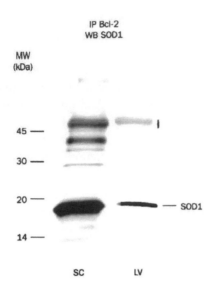

IP Bcl-2
WB SOD1

Figure 13.2 Mutant SOD1 protein forms insoluble SOD1–Bcl-2 complexes. Mitochondria isolated from the spinal cord and liver of SOD1-G93A mice were immunoprecipitated with an anti-Bcl-2 antibody. Proteins thus isolated were separated on the illustrated Western immunoblot and immunostained for SOD1 proteins. In addition to a band corresponding to monomeric SOD1, there is evidence of a higher molecular weight, Bcl-2–SOD1 protein complex (asterisks) specifically in spinal cord but not liver mitochondria. SC, spinal cord, LV, liver. (Modified from reference 29)

Because motor neurons at baseline show reduced expression of Bcl-2 compared to other cells, including sensory and sympathetic neurons[54], they may be more sensitive to the loss of Bcl-2. Another possible consequence of the binding between mutant SOD1 and Bcl-2 is that Bcl-2 itself is rendered non-functional. To the extent that Bcl-2 functions by binding other pro- and anti-apoptotic proteins[53], segregation into mutant SOD1 aggregates may block Bcl-2 function. Alternatively, upon binding to mutant SOD1, Bcl-2 could undergo conformational modification and become toxic. Entrapment and depletion of Bcl-2 is in agreement with the studies mentioned above that show reduced levels of Bcl-2 in SOD1 mice and ALS patients. A caveat is that these mechanisms are pertinent only to mutant SOD1 and do not explain the observed changes in Bcl-2 expression and function in non-SOD1 ALS cases.

Once the death signal has been initiated, many secondary abnormalities develop in the spinal cord of the ALS mice that probably contribute to disease amplification and propagation. Early caspase-1 activation may amplify the death signal through cleavage of Bid[3] and render the cells even more vulnerable to various insults. In parallel, caspase-1-derived release of inflammatory factors and cytokines such as interleukin (IL)-1β and TNF-α may further amplify the death process. TNF-α activates caspase-8[38], which is activated late in life in the ALS mice[38]. TNF-α and its receptor are part of a large family of a superfamily of related proteins that include Fas. The finding that cultured embryonic motor neurons are selectively sensitive to Fas-induced apoptosis has suggested that these inflammatory/pro-apoptotic molecules may represent the key mediators of a motor neuron apoptotic pathway (involving Daxx, ASK1 and p38) and therefore explain the selective death of motor neurons in ALS[38].

MITOCHONDRIA AND APOPTOSIS

Apoptosis occurs through activation of two major pathways: the intracellular (mitochondrial) or the extracellular (death receptor) pathway. The two pathways are independent and involve activation of distinct upstream elements[53]. They converge at the level of downstream, effector caspases. Mitochondria tightly regulate the intracellular pathway in which an intracellular apoptotic stimulus directly or indirectly acts on the mitochondria. Damaged mitochondria release pro-apoptotic factors such as cytochrome c and trigger a cascade of events that ultimately lead to cell death[53].

As discussed in great detail in Chapter 18, an increasing body of evidence implicates the mitochondria in ALS pathogenesis. Both morphologic and biochemical mitochondrial abnormalities are observed in human and murine ALS. In the ALS mice, changes in mitochondrial function and morphology precede disease onset[55–57], suggesting a primary role of the mitochondria in triggering the disease. The mechanisms underlying these abnormalities and their origin are not understood.

At least for the mutant SOD1 protein, one possible mechanism is the presence of the mutant SOD1 in the mitochondria. Recent studies from different groups have shown that a small fraction of SOD1 protein, usually considered to be a cytosolic protein, localizes to the mitochondria[42,58,59]. Despite arguments regarding the intramitochondrial localization of the SOD1 protein and regarding the mutant-specific mitochondrial localization[29,59–61], the general agreement is that mutant SOD1 forms insoluble, detergent-resistant aggregates in the mitochondria[29,59,61]. It is speculated that these aggregates represent the toxic killer that causes mitochondrial dysfunction and motor neuron degeneration[60]. Within the mitochondria, mutant SOD1 could directly activate the mitochondrial apoptotic pathway. In line with this hypothesis, mutant SOD1 that is linked to the mitochondria triggers apoptosis more strongly than the cytosolic mutant protein[62]. Moreover, mutant SOD1-mediated toxicity entails activation of the mitochondrial apoptotic pathway[49]. Finally, mitochondrial aggregates of mutant SOD1 form aberrant interactions with mitochondrial regulators of apoptosis like the heat shock protein 27 (HSP27) and Bcl-2[42].

THERAPIES THAT BLOCK APOPTOSIS AND THEIR EFFECT IN AMYOTROPHIC LATERAL SCLEROSIS

Several treatments that target apoptosis have been tested in the mutant SOD1 ALS mice. These include the use of genetically modified mice, gene therapy and pharmacologic interventions.

Transgenic expression of Bcl-2 delays disease onset (30–35 days) and extends the lifespan of SOD1-G93A mice[25]. However, intraspinal injection of recombinant adeno-associated virus (AAV) coding for Bcl-2 did not show any effect in the same SOD1-G93A mice[63]. Inhibition of caspase-1, via a dominant negative caspase-1 protein,

moderately extended the lifespan of the same mice[30]. Inhibiting a large number of caspases rather than just one achieved a more robust effect. Administration of the pan-caspase inhibitor ZVAD-FMK delayed disease onset by about 20% (20 days) and prolonged survival by about 22% (27 days)[28]. Transgenic expression of either an X-linked inhibitor of apoptosis (XIAP) or the baculoviral p35 protein, a pan-caspase inhibitor, ameliorated the disease in the SOD1-G93A mice[31]. Two additional pharmacologic treatments thought to interfere with the apoptosis machinery have been tested in the mice and have been shown to prolong survival. Minocycline, a second generation of tetracyclines, delays disease progression, and extends survival of the SOD1-G93A mice when given alone[32,64,65] or in combination with creatine (to enhance energy storage capacity of the mitochondria) or both nimodipine and riluzole. In the spinal cord of the mice, minocycline blocks cytochrome c release from the mitochondria and caspase-3 activation[32]. Whether inhibition of apoptosis is the mode of action of minocycline is not completely known. It has also been suggested that minocycline reduces the inflammatory responses observed in the ALS mice[64]. Despite the described positive results, other laboratories failed to reproduce the effect of minocycline. Currently, a phase III clinical trial is under way in ALS patients. Another possible anti-apoptotic drug is cyclosporine, which marginally increases survival of the SOD1-G93A mice[66]. However, whether cyclosporine blocked the opening of the mitochondrial transition pore, therefore inducing apoptosis, or exerted an immunosuppressant effect in the ALS mice is not clear.

Therapeutic manipulation of apoptosis may represent only one way to treat ALS. ALS pathogenesis involves activation of different pathways of cell death that include oxidative stress, deposition of abnormal proteins, axonal strangulation due to neurofilament misaccumulation, excitotoxicty and mitochondrial dysfunction. Thus, the best therapy for ALS may come in a combination of treatments that simultaneously blocks different pathways.

CONCLUSIONS

Despite early skepticism, there is now clear evidence that apoptosis participates in ALS pathogenesis. Morphologic and biochemical changes characteristic of apoptosis have been found in human ALS cases, and studies in ALS mice and cell culture models of ALS have identified apoptosis pathways that are activated in the presence of the mutant SOD1 protein. The similarities between the findings in the mutant SOD1 mice and in postmortem tissues from ALS patients suggest that a common pathway of apoptosis underlies the pathogenesis of all forms of the disease. Therapeutic manipulation of the apoptosis pathways may represent a possible way to slow disease progression. However, concern has been expressed about the timing of intervention. If apoptosis is a late phenomenon that ultimately kills the motor neurons, then inhibition of apoptosis may not be successful, as it targets severely injured and already dysfunctional motor neurons. A combination of therapies that, together with anti-apoptotic drugs, targets multiple pathways of motor neuron death may represent the best therapeutic approach.

ACKNOWLEDGMENTS

We thank the National Institutes for Aging (NIA) and for Neurological Disease and Stroke (NINDS), the Muscular Dystrophy Association, the ALS Association, Project ALS, The Pierre L de Bourgknecht ALS Foundation, the Al-Athel ALS Foundation and the ALS Therapy Alliance and the Delaney Fund for their financial support.

REFERENCES

1. Danial NN, Korsmeyer SJ. Cell death: critical control points. Cell 2004; 116: 205–19
2. Kerr JF, Wyllie AH, Currie AR. Apoptosis: a basic biological phenomenon with wide-ranging implications in tissue kinetics. Br J Cancer 1972; 26: 239–57
3. Guegan C, Przedborski S. Programmed cell death in amyotrophic lateral sclerosis. J Clin Invest 2003; 111: 153–61
4. Sperandio S, Poksay K, de Belle I, et al. Paraptosis: Mediation by MAP kinases and inhibition by AIP-1/Alix. Cell Death Differ 2004; 11: 1066–75
5. Yoshiyama Y, Yamada T, Asanuma K, Asahi T. Apoptosis related antigen, Le(Y) and nick-end labeling are positive in spinal motor neurons in amyotrophic lateral sclerosis. Acta Neuropathol (Berl) 1994; 88: 207–11
6. Troost D, Aten J, Morsink F, Jong JD. Apoptosis is not resctricted to motoneurons: Bcl-2 expression is increased in post-central cortex, adjacent to affected motor cortex. J Neurol Sci 1995; 129 (Suppl): 79–80
7. Mu X, He J, Anderson D, et al. Altered expression of bcl-2 and bax mRNA in amyotrophic lateral sclerosis spinal cord motor neurons. Ann Neurol 1996; 40: 379–86
8. Tews D, Goebel H, Meinck H. DNA-fragmentation and apoptosis-related proteins of muscle cells in motor neuron disorders. Acta Neurol Scand 1997; 96: 380–6
9. Martin LJ. Neuronal death in amyotrophic lateral sclerosis is apoptosis: Possible contribution of a programmed cell death mechanism. J Neuropathol Exp Neurol 1999; 58: 459–71
10. Shinoe T, Wanaka A, Nikaido T, et al. Upregulation of the pro-apoptotic BH3-only peptide harakiri in spinal neurons of amyotrophic lateral sclerosis patients. Neurosci Lett 2001; 313: 153–7
11. Migheli A, Piva R, Atzori C, et al. c-Jun, JNK/SAPK kinases and transcription factor NF-kappa B are selectively activated in astrocytes, but not motor neurons, in amyotrophic lateral sclerosis. J Neuropathol Exp Neurol 1997; 56: 1314–22
12. Goto S, Radak Z, Nyakas C, et al. Regular exercise: an effective means to reduce oxidative stress in old rats. Ann NY Acad Sci 2004; 1019: 471–4
13. Taylor JM, Crack PJ. Impact of oxidative stress on neuronal survival. Clin Exp Pharmacol Physiol 2004; 31: 397–406
14. Nakamura S, Kawamoto Y, Nakano S, et al. Cyclin-dependent kinase 5 and mitogen-activated protein kinase in glial cytoplasmic inclusions in multiple system atrophy. J Neuropathol Exp Neurol 1998; 57: 690–8
15. Bajaj NP, Al-Sarraj ST, Anderson V, et al. Cyclin-dependent kinase-5 is associated with lipofuscin in motor neurones in amyotrophic lateral sclerosis. Neurosci Lett 1998; 245: 45–8

16. Migheli A, Attanasio A, Schiffer D. Ubiquitinated fila-mentous inclusions in spinal cord of patients with motor neuron disease. Neurosci Lett 1990; 114: 5–10

17. Pedersen WA, Luo H, Kruman I, et al. The prostate apoptosis response-4 protein participates in motor neuron degeneration in amyotrophic lateral sclerosis. FASEB J 2000; 14: 913–24

18. Martin LJ. p53 is abnormally elevated and active in the CNS of patients with amyotrophic lateral sclero-sis. Neurobiol Dis 2000; 7: 613–22

19. Sengun IS, Appel SH. Serum anti-Fas antibody levels in amyotrophic lateral sclerosis. J Neuroimmunol 2003; 142: 137–40

20. Ilzecka J, Stelmasiak Z, Dobosz B. Interleukin-1beta converting enzyme/Caspase-1 (ICE/Caspase-1) and soluble APO-1/Fas/CD 95 receptor in amyotrophic lateral sclerosis patients. Acta Neurol Scand 2001; 103: 255–8

21. Rosen DR. Mutations in Cu/Zn superoxide dismu-tase gene are associated with familial amyotrophic lat-eral sclerosis. Nature 1993; 362: 59–62

22. Gurney M. Mutant mice, Cu,Zn superoxide dismu-tase, and motor neuron degeneration: Response. Sci-ence 1994; 266: 1586

23. Gonzalez de Aguilar JL, Gordon JW, Rene F, et al. Alteration of the Bcl-x/Bax ratio in a transgenic mouse model of amyotrophic lateral sclerosis: Evi-dence for the implication of the p53 signaling path-way. Neurobiol Dis 2000; 7: 406–15

24. Vukosavic S, Dubois-Dauphin M, Romero N, Przed-borski S. Bax and Bcl-2 interaction in a transgenic mouse model of familial amyotrophic lateral sclerosis. J Neurochem 1999; 73: 2460–8

25. Kostic V, Jackson-Lewis V, Bilbao FD, et al. Bcl-2: prolonging life in a transgenic mouse model of famil-ial amyotrophic lateral sclerosis. Science 1997; 277: 559–62

26. Pasinelli P, Houseweart MK, Brown RH Jr, Cleveland DW. Caspase-1 and -3 are sequentially activated in motor neuron death in Cu,Zn superoxide dismutase-mediated familial amyotrophic lateral sclerosis. Proc Natl Acad Sci USA 2000; 97: 13901–6

27. Vukosavic S, Stefanis L, Jackson-Lewis V, et al. Delay-ing caspase activation by Bcl-2: A clue to disease retardation in a transgenic mouse model of amy-otrophic lateral sclerosis. J Neurosci 2000; 20; 9119–25

28. Li M, Ona VO, Guegan C, et al. Functional role of caspase-1 and caspase-3 in an ALS transgenic mouse model. Science 2000; 288: 335–9

29. Pasinelli P, Belford ME, Lennon N, et al. Amy-otrophic lateral sclerosis-associated SOD1 mutant

30. Friedlander RM, Brown RH, Gagliardini V, et al. Inhibition of ICE slows ALS in mice. Nature 1997; 388: 31

31. Inoue H, Tsukita K, Iwasato T, et al. The crucial role of caspase-9 in the disease progression of a transgenic ALS mouse model. EMBO J 2003; 22: 6665–74

32. Zhu S, Stavrovskaya IG, Drozda M, et al. Minocy-cline inhibits cytochrome c release and delays pro-gression of amyotrophic lateral sclerosis in mice. Nature 2002; 417: 74–8

33. Greenlund L, Deckwerth T, Johnson E. Superoxide dismutase delays neuronal apoptosis: A role for reac-tive oxygen species in programmed neuronal death. Neuron 1995; 14: 303–15

34. Jordan J, Ghadge GD, Prehn JH, et al. Expression of human copper/zinc superoxide dismutase inhibits the death of rat sympathetic neurons caused by with-drawal of nerve growth factor. Mol Pharmacol 1995; 47: 1095–100

35. Durham H, Roy J, Dong L, Figlewicz D. Aggregation of mutant Cu/Zn superoxide dismutase proteins in a culture model of ALS. J Neuropathol Exp Neurol 1997; 56: 523–30

36. Ghadge G, Lee JP, Bindokas VP, et al. Mutant super-oxide dismutase-1-linked familial amyotrophic lateral sclerosis: Molecular mechanisms of neuronal death and protection. J Neurosci 1997; 17: 8756–66

37. Pasinelli P, Borchelt DR, Houseweart MK, et al. Cas-pase-1 is activated in neural cells and tissue with amy-otrophic lateral sclerosis-associated mutations in cop-per–zinc superoxide dismutase. Proc Natl Acad Sci USA 1998; 95: 15763–8

38. Raoul C, Estevez AG, Nishimune H, et al. Motoneu-ron death triggered by a specific pathway downstream of Fas. Potentiation by ALS-linked SOD1 mutations. Neuron 2002; 35: 1067–83

39. Sathasivam S, Ince PG, Shaw PJ. Apoptosis in amy-otrophic lateral sclerosis: A review of the evidence. Neuropathol Appl Neurobiol 2001; 27: 257–74

40. Menzies FM, Ince PG, Shaw PJ. Mitochondrial involvement in amyotrophic lateral sclerosis. Neu-rochem Int 2002; 40: 543–51

41. Cho KJ, Chung YH, Shin C, et al. Reactive astrocytes express p53 in the spinal cord of transgenic mice expressing a human Cu/Zn SOD mutation. Neurore-port 1999; 10: 3939–43

42. Okado-Matsumoto A, Fridovich I. Amyotrophic lat-eral sclerosis: A proposed mechanism. Proc Natl Acad Sci USA 2002; 99: 9010–4

proteins bind and aggregate with Bcl-2 in spinal cord mitochondria. Neuron 2004; 43: 19–30

43. Rabizadeh S, Gralla EB, Borchelt DR, et al. Mutations associated with amyotrophic lateral sclerosis convert superoxide dismutase from an antiapoptotic gene to a proapoptotic gene: Studies in yeast and neural cells. Proc Natl Acad Sci 1995; 92: 3024–8

44. Xie J, Awad KS, Guo Q. RNAi knockdown of Par-4 inhibits neurosynaptic degeneration in ALS-linked mice. J Neurochem 2005; 92: 59–71

45. Mattson MP, Duan W, Chan SL, Camandola S. Par-4: an emerging pivotal player in neuronal apoptosis and neurodegenerative disorders. J Mol Neurosci 1999; 13: 17–30

46. Spooren WP, Hengerer B. DNA laddering and caspase 3-like activity in the spinal cord of a mouse model of familial amyotrophic lateral sclerosis. Cell Mol Biol (Noisy-le-grand) 2000; 46: 63–9

47. Kuntz CT, Kinoshita Y, Beal MF, et al. Absence of p53: No effect in a transgenic mouse model of familial amyotrophic lateral sclerosis. Exp Neurol 2000; 165; 184–90

48. Nagai M, Aoki M, Miyoshi I, et al. Rats expressing human cytosolic copper–zinc superoxide dismutase transgenes with amyotrophic lateral sclerosis: Associated mutations develop motor neuron disease. J Neurosci 2001; 21: 9246–54

49. Guegan C, Vila M, Rosoklija G, et al. Recruitment of the mitochondrial-dependent apoptotic pathway in amyotrophic lateral sclerosis. J Neurosci 2001; 21: 6569–76

50. Kirkinezos IG, Bacman SR, Hernandez D, et al. Cytochrome c association with the inner mitochondrial membrane is impaired in the CNS of G93A-SOD1 mice. J Neurosci 2005; 25: 164–72

51. Yoshihara T, Ishigaki S, Yamamoto M, et al. Differential expression of inflammation- and apoptosis-related genes in spinal cords of a mutant SOD1 transgenic mouse model of familial amyotrophic lateral sclerosis. J Neurochem 2002; 80: 158–67

52. Kang SJ, Sanchez I, Jing N, Yuan J. Dissociation between neurodegeneration and caspase-11-mediated activation of caspase-1 and caspase-3 in a mouse model of amyotrophic lateral sclerosis. J Neurosci 2003; 23: 5455–60

53. Danial NN, Korsmeyer SJ. Cell death. Critical control points. Cell 2004; 116: 205–19

54. Yachnis AT, Giovanini MA, Eskin TA, et al. Developmental patterns of BCL-2 and BCL-X polypeptide expression in the human spinal cord. Exp Neurol 1998; 150: 82–97

55. Dal Canto M, Gurney M. Neuropathological changes in two lines of mice carrying a transgene for mutant human Cu, Zn SOD, and in mice overexpressing wild type human SOD: A model of familial amyotrophic lateral sclerosis. Brain Res 1995; 676: 25–40

56. Wong P, Pardo CA, Borchelt DR, et al. An adverse property of a familial ALS-linked SOD1 mutation causes motor neuron disease characterized by vacuolar degeneration of mitochondria. Neuron 1995; 14: 1105–16

57. Kong J, Xu Z. Massive mitochondrial degeneration in motor neurons triggers the onset of amyotrophic lateral sclerosis in mice expressing a mutant SOD1. J Neurosci 1998; 18: 3241–50

58. Higgins CM, Jung C, Ding H, Xu Z. Mutant Cu, Zn superoxide dismutase that causes motoneuron degeneration is present in mitochondria in the CNS. J Neurosci 2002; 22, RC215

59. Mattiazzi M, D'Aurelio M, Gajewski CD, et al. Mutated human SOD1 causes dysfunction of oxidative phosphorylation in mitochondria of transgenic mice. J Biol Chem 2002; 277: 29626–33

60. Liu J, Lillo C, Jonasson PA, et al. Toxicity of familial ALS-linked SOD1 mutants from selective recruitment to spinal mitochondria. Neuron 2004; 43: 5–17

61. Vijayvergiya C, Beal MF, Buck J, Manfredi G. Mutant superoxide dismutase 1 forms aggregates in the brain mitochondrial matrix of amyotrophic lateral sclerosis mice. J Neurosci 2005; 25: 2463–70

62. Takeuchi H, Kobayashi Y, Ishigaki S, et al. Mitochondrial localization of mutant superoxide dismutase 1 triggers caspase-dependent cell death in a cellular model of familial amyotrophic lateral sclerosis. J Biol Chem 2002; 277: 50966–72

63. Houseweart MK, Cleveland DW. Bcl-2 overexpression does not protect neurons from mutant neurofilament-mediated motor neuron degeneration. J Neurosci 1999; 19: 6446–56

64. Van Den Bosch L, Tilkin P, Lemmens G, Robberecht W. Minocycline delays disease onset and mortality in a transgenic model of ALS. Neuroreport 2002; 13: 1067–70

65. Kriz J, Nguyen MD, Julien JP. Minocycline slows disease progression in a mouse model of amyotrophic lateral sclerosis. Neurobiol Dis 2002; 10: 268–78

66. Kirkinezos IG, Hernandez D, Bradley WG, Moraes CT. An ALS mouse model with a permeable blood–brain barrier benefits from systemic cyclosporine A treatment. J Neurochem 2004; 88: 821–6

14

Amyotrophic lateral sclerosis and neurodegeneration: possible insights from the molecular biology of aging

Anne-Marie A Wills, Robert H Brown Jr

INTRODUCTION

Like virtually all of the neurodegenerative disorders, amyotrophic lateral sclerosis (ALS) is age-dependent. Even when germline mutations in the *SOD1* gene and protein are present from conception, it is rare to encounter ALS cases that begin before mid-adulthood. Thus, the events that are permissive for the development of neurodegeneration in general, and ALS in particular, must be understood in the context of the molecular physiology of aging. Aging events establish the molecular and cellular contexts required for the development of motor neuron degeneration in ALS. The critical question that arises is whether new insights into ALS can be garnered from the rapidly emerging description of the molecular and cellular basis of normal aging, as summarized below. While a definitive answer is not yet available, several points of intersection between the biology of normal aging and the pathophysiology of ALS and related brain disorders suggest that this will be a fruitful line of inquiry.

OVERVIEW OF AMYOTROPHIC LATERAL SCLEROSIS

ALS is a neurodegenerative disorder that affects upper and lower motor neurons with an incidence of 0.6–2.6/100 000; males are affected somewhat more frequently[1,2]. As noted, like most other neurodegenerative conditions (e.g. Alzheimer's, Parkinson's and Huntington's diseases), susceptibility to ALS is highly dependent on the aging process. The mean age at onset of ALS is 55 years; cases before the age of 30 are distinctly unusual. The incidence rate of ALS increases from < 0.1 per 100 000 in people aged less than 50, to 1.5 per 100 000 annually between the ages of 60 and 70[3]. Survival in ALS is typically 3–5 years.

ALS is predominantly sporadic (SALS) but 10% of cases are familial (FALS), usually segregating in an autosomal dominant fashion. Mutations in cytosolic, copper–zinc superoxide dismutase 1 (*SOD1*) account for ~25% of autosomal dominant FALS cases[4]. Several hypotheses have been proposed to explain the etiology of ALS in the 90% of cases that are not inherited. These include: atypical enteroviral or retroviral infections[5,6]; autoantibody-provoked calcium influxes[7]; motor neuron excitotoxicity mediated in part by progressive decline in glutamate transport by the glutamate transporter GLT1/EAAT2[8]; microglial inflammation; and elevated levels of cyclooxygenase (COX)-2[9] or environmental toxins such as lead[10] or, in the Western Pacific, cycad seed toxicity[11,12].

Cytosolic Cu/Zn superoxide dismutase

The concept that Mendelian genetics might elucidate ALS pathogenesis was partially realized in 1993 when it was reported that mutations in the gene encoding cytosolic SOD1 account for about a quarter of cases of FALS or 2–3% of all cases. None of the 110 different SOD1 mutations reported to date[13] are predicted to ablate production of an SOD1 protein. This is compatible with the prediction based on the dominant inheritance of this disorder that the disease is mediated by one or more acquired, adverse or toxic properties of the mutant protein. That the mutant protein is toxic is further indicated by the finding that forced expression of high levels of a mutant SOD1 transgene ($SOD1^{G93A}$) causes a progressive motor neuron disease in mice that recapitulates the major features of FALS in humans[14]. This was subsequently confirmed using diverse mutant alleles (e.g. $SOD1^{G37R}$, $SOD1^{G85R}$, $SOD1^{G86R}$ and $SOD1^{D90A}$). More recently, we and others have developed transgenic rat models of ALS[15,16] that recapitulate the features of motor neuron death in humans and transgenic murine ALS models. Expression of the mutant SOD1 alleles in various cell culture models produces cell death in both neuronal and non-neuronal cells. In these mouse and culture models, dismutation activities are normal or elevated, consistent with the hypothesis that the mutations kill cells not by loss of activity but through an acquired form of toxicity. This conclusion is underscored by the finding that mice with targeted inactivation of the SOD1 gene do not develop motor neuron disease[17].

Studies in the past 5 years have addressed the molecular mechanisms whereby mutations in the SOD1 gene trigger cell death, and have provided insights into possible ALS therapies (Figure 14.1). It is likely that the fundamental pathology involves both oxidative pathology arising from aberrant copper catalysis and conformational instability of the mutant SOD1 protein. Studies in mice chimeric for wild-type and mutant SOD1 indicate that the status of non-neuronal cells is an important determinant of viability of spinal cord motor neurons[18]. Recent reports have also highlighted a role for programed cell death in at least the terminal process of motor neuron death in ALS[19–21].

Other Mendelian ALS genes (ALS2/alsin, dynactin, senataxin and VAPB) and loci

Other Mendelian gene defects have been reported and identified as ALS genes. Of these, the only gene whose mutations lead to a true ALS phenotype is the novel vesicle trafficking protein VAPB[22]. Loss of function mutations in the gene encoding alsin result in a slowly progressive, predominantly corticospinal and corticobulbar degenerative disorder that closely resembles childhood-onset hereditary spastic paraparesis[23,24]. The alsin protein shows homology to motifs in guanine-nucleotide exchange factors for GTPases that function in axonal outgrowth, signaling cascades and vesicular trafficking. An adult-onset, dominantly inherited, slowly progressive, predominantly lower motor neuron disorder with early bulbar features is caused by mutations in the gene encoding the motor protein dynactin[25]. Another adult-onset, slowly progressive ALS-like disease is caused by mutations in the senataxin gene, which encodes a DNA helicase[26].

OVERVIEW OF AGING MECHANISMS

Aging is a universal and inevitable biological process whose implications for human mortality have long fascinated biologists and artists alike. Aging can be defined as a process whereby cells and tissues of somatic lineage deteriorate with time, becoming progressively more vulnerable to environmental insults, eventually resulting in disease and death. It is axiomatic that all cells that are not germline undergo aging[27].

Multiple theories exist as to why and how organisms age. For this review we focus on those

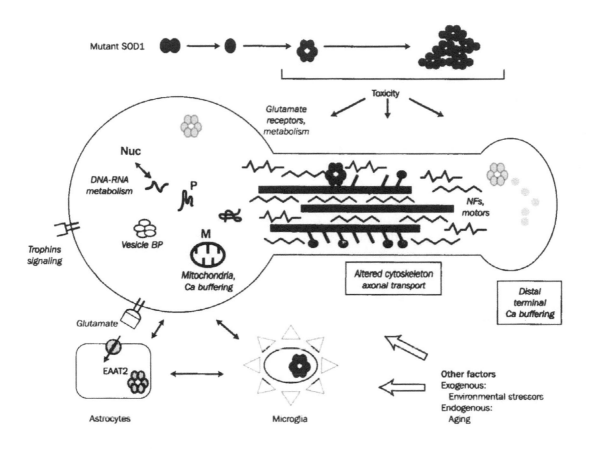

Figure 14.1 The toxicity of mutant SOD1 protein is multifactorial. The mutant SOD1 is conformationally unstable and potentially prone both to aberrant catalytic reactions of copper and misfolding. Either as microaggregates or larger misfolded superstructures, the mutant SOD1 compromises viability of the motor neuron by perturbing several normal processes including glutamate trafficking, metabolism of DNA and RNA, trophic factor signaling, mitochondrial generation of ATP, axonal transport and calcium metabolism. The toxicity is multifactorial in two other senses: (1) the mutant protein impairs critical astroglial functions (such as transport of glutamate by EAAT2) and probably activates microglial; and (2) exogenous stimuli and endogenous events (e.g. aging) are presumed to alter the threshold for initiation of cell death by mutant SOD1 protein

theories that propose molecular mechanisms of aging. The *oxidative damage theory* proposed by Harman in 1981[28] proposes that reactive oxygen species (ROS) including superoxide, hydrogen peroxide and hydroxyl radicals generated primarily by the mitochondria react with and damage macromolecules including nucleic acids, proteins and lipids (reviewed in reference 29). This leads to damage of both nuclear and mitochondrial DNA and modification of proteins, potentially leading to protein aggregates such as amyloid (in

Alzheimer's disease), synuclein (in Parkinson's disease) and ubiquitin (in ALS). This concept, a recurring theme in aging studies over the past quarter century, has been significantly challenged by a recent finding that mice with mutations in a mitochondrial polymerase have accelerated accumulation of mutations in mitochondrial DNA without evidence of an increased burden of reactive oxygen[30].

Closely related to the theory of oxidative damage is the concept that over time the accumulation of DNA damage can overwhelm a cell's repair mechanisms, leading to cellular senescence. This concept has been described as the *somatic mutation theory* of aging[31]. In some instances, senescence is presumed to be protective, preventing aberrant cell division and cancer formation. That there is a progressive accumulation of defective DNA is well documented in many species, including humans. For example, Lu *et al.* found progressively greater amounts of oxidatively damaged DNA with increasing age in postmortem brains from individuals aged 26–106[32].

Also thought to be important in aging is *replicative senescense*: non-germline cells are limited in the number of times they are able to divide and thereby repair injured tissues. One explanation for the limited proliferative capacity of somatic cells is telomere loss. With each replication, the telomeres that cap the ends of chromosomes shorten, eventually preventing cell division[33]. Germline cells are not limited in their ability to divide, because the enzyme telomerase lengthens the telomere with each cell division. Pathologic states, such as oxidative stress, may increase rates of telomere loss. Because neurons are post-mitotic, it can be argued that replicative senescense is not relevant to neurodegenerative disorders. Moreover, accumulation of DNA damage should have less of an effect on neurons than on highly mitotic tissues such as skin and intestinal lining. However, several lines of investigation define an important role for glia in maintaining neuronal viability; it may therefore be that age-dependent loss of glial function via both accumulation of oxidative stress and replicative senescence may secondarily impair neuronal viability.

Genetic factors are also related to the aging process. Although aging is clearly influenced by environmental factors, there appears to be a strong genetic component to aging within and between different species. Thus, it is now well established that longevity may run in families. One epidemiologic analysis has reported that siblings of centenarians have a 17-fold higher likelihood of surviving to 100[34]. Because it probably entails many

convergent mechanisms, aging is commonly described as a complex trait. Nonetheless, single genes with profound effects on longevity have been identified in the past 10 years in lower organisms such as yeast, worms and flies. These genes can be grouped into several evolutionarily conserved pathways that modulate rates of aging and encompass energy metabolism, mitochondrial respiration, DNA repair and apoptotic pathways. That there is a genetic influence on longevity is also documented by the reciprocal observation that various forms of premature aging arise as Mendelian disorders (e.g. several progeroid syndromes), typically involving defects in proteins such as helicases that are essential for maintaining the integrity of genomic DNA[35,36].

Caloric restriction and longevity pathways

That environmental factors also importantly modulate aging is demonstrated by studies of aging and calorie restriction (CR); CR is the best-studied and most consistent method of increasing lifespan in lower organisms. McCay *et al.* in 1935 first reported that underfeeding rats by 40% (feeding only on alternate days) increased lifespan by 30–40%[37]. These findings have since been extended to yeast, worms, flies and fish but still await validation in primates[38]. In humans it is impossible to perform a prospective randomized study of CR on lifespan given the length of human lives. However, a randomized study of 20–30% calorie restriction over 2–3 years in humans is under way (CALERIE – Comprehensive Assessment of Long-term Effects of Restricted Intake of Energy). One goal of this investigation is to study the effects of CR on markers of age-related disease. A recent study of individuals who voluntarily engaged in CR found remarkably beneficial effects on blood pressure, lipid levels and carotid artery intimal thickness[39]. CR in mice and rats decreases the incidence of nephropathy, diabetes, atherosclerotic lesions and neoplasms[40]. There is also some evidence that CR may reduce or prevent the development of neurodegenerative diseases including Alzheimer's disease[41].

There are several proposed physiologic mechanisms by which CR improves longevity. During CR, animals are more resistant to heat and oxidative stress and show decreased lipid peroxidation and reduced deletion frequency of mtDNA[40]. Calorie restriction also appears to reduce the production of ROS and has been reported to increase expression of SOD1 in rat liver[42]. However, no prolongation in lifespan was seen following dietary restriction in the transgenic SOD1^{G93A} mouse model of ALS[43].

Over the past decade, the molecular mechanisms underlying the effects of CR on longevity have begun to be delineated. These entail genes and pathways that are evolutionarily conserved (Figure 14.2). Perhaps the most important pathway is the insulin/insulin-like growth factor (IGF)

signaling pathway. In the worm, *Caenorhabditis elegans*, the presence of glucose and growth hormone (i.e. with a normocaloric diet) leads to the production of insulin or IGFs. Binding of these to the worm homolog of IGF-I receptors (the daf-2 protein) triggers a cascade that involves phosphorylation and activation of phosphoinositide-3-OH kinase (PI3K, encoded by the *age-1* gene). In turn, this phosphorylates and activates protein kinase B (PKB, expressed from the *akt* gene), which then phosphorylates the transcription factor daf-16. Because it cannot diffuse into the nucleus, phospho-daf-16 is inactive. However, when calories are restricted, daf-2 signaling is reduced and, because it is unphosphorylated, the daf-16 protein can diffuse into the nucleus where it upregulates expression of a wide range of stress defense genes, including antioxidant genes such as manganese superoxide dismutase (*SOD2*) and catalase, heat

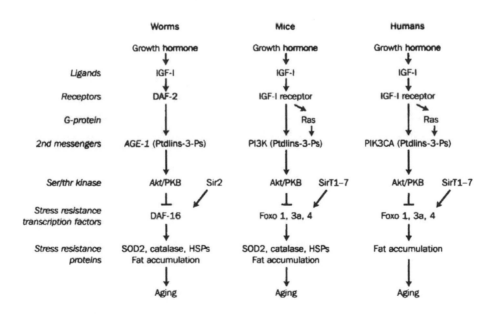

Figure 14.2 Insulin/insulin-like growth factor-I (IGF-I) signaling pathways influence longevity in multiple species. Ligands responsive to the metabolic status of these organisms (e.g. insulin and insulin-like growth factors such as IGF-I) trigger a cascade that entails binding to IGF-I receptors or their homologs, followed by activation of phosphoinositide-3-OH kinase (PI3K) and then protein kinase B (PKB), which subsequently phosphorylates the transcription factors daf-16 or forkhead (Foxo). In their phosphorylated forms, these factors are inactive because they are confined to the cytosol. G proteins (e.g. Ras) modulate activity of PI3K, while selected sirtuins modify the activity of daf-16 and the forkhead proteins. (Modified from reference 45)

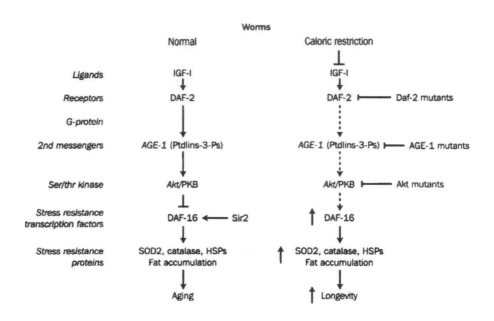

Figure 14.3   With caloric restriction or loss-of-function mutations, the insulin/insulin-like growth factor-I (IGF-I) signaling pathway activates stress response genes. With either caloric restriction or mutations that inactivate the IGF-I receptor, PI3K or protein kinase B (PKB), the daf-2/Foxo transcription factors are not phosphorylated and thus can diffuse into the nucleus to up-regulate expression of stress defense genes, including antioxidant genes such as manganese superoxide dismutase (SOD2) and catalase, heat shock proteins (HSPs) and DNA repair genes

shock proteins and DNA repair genes (Figure 14.3)[44,45]. In yeast and *C. elegans*, activity of daf-16 (and its yeast homologs Msn2 and Msn4) are increased by interactions with sir2, a nicotin-amide-adenine dinucleotide (NAD)-dependent histone deacetylase (see below). Importantly, activity of this insulin signaling pathway is diminished not only by CR, but also by mutations that ablate the function of the insulin receptor gene *daf-2*, *age-1* or *akt*. *Daf-2* and *age-1* mutant worms have significantly increased longevity, and are resistant to many forms of stress including hypoxia, heat shock, ultraviolet light, hydrogen peroxide and paraquat (reviewed in reference 27). *Age-1* mutants have also been shown to have increased levels of SOD1 and catalase activity[46].

In addition to the above mutants, other gene mutations and variants that affect longevity in mice may be related to the insulin signaling pathway. Dwarf mice including the Snell mouse (which has a spontaneous point mutation in *Pit1*, a pituitary specific transcription factor 1 gene) and the Ames mouse (which has a point mutation in the *Prop-1* gene, immediately upstream of Pit1) weigh only one-third of the weight of a normal mouse and have severely impaired reproduction (reviewed in reference 45). These mutations lead to defective pituitary development and lack of growth hormone (GH), thyroid-stimulating hormone (TSH) and prolactin (PRL). Their longevity is postulated to be due to abnormal IGF and insulin signaling; these mice also have elevated levels of SOD1 and catalase.

As suggested in Figure 14.2, highly analogous insulin-longevity pathways exist in virtually all eukaryotes from yeast to flies, mice and higher mammals. Thus, in *Drosophila*, inactivating mutations in the insulin-like receptor (InR) increase lifespan by 85%[45,47] while ablation of CHICO, an insulin receptor substrate-like signaling protein, increases lifespan by 48% (reviewed in reference 48). The same pathway exists in primates but is less completely characterized. In mammals, the homolog of daf-16 is the Forkhead (Foxo) family of transcription factors. Foxo3a is a daf-16 homolog that, like daf-16, increases manganese SOD2 expression in response to ROS[49].

That this insulin/longevity pathway is likely to be important in mammalian aging is suggested by studies of IGF-I receptor inactivation in mice. Heterozygous *Igf1r+/-* knockout mouse females lived a mean of 33% longer than their wild-type littermates (males lived 16% longer but this was not statistically significant)[50]. The heterozygous *Igf1r+/-* mice are more resistant to paraquat and hydrogen peroxide than are *Igf1r+/+* littermates. In humans, polymorphisms in the *IGFIR* gene may also affect lifespan. A recent study suggested a possible relation between the insulin-like growth factor I gene (*IGFI*) and human aging, reporting that a variant (A rather than G at codon 1013) in the gene for the IGF-I receptor is associated with lower plasma IGF-I levels and longer survival[51].

The sirtuins and histone deacetylation

As noted above, in yeast, the chromosomal silencing element *sir2* (*silent information regulator 2*) is an important regulator of lifespan that interacts in some manner with the daf-2/daf-16 (Msn2/Msn4) pathway. In yeast and *C. elegans*, deletion mutations of Sir2 shorten lifespan, while extra copies of this gene prolong lifespan (measured in yeast as increased budding)[27,52]. Sir2 functions as an NAD[+]-dependent histone deacetylase, and thus may be responsive to the metabolic status of the cell, which determines levels of NAD[+]/NADH[53]. NADH is produced in yeast by fermentation when glucose is abundant and inhibits Sir2, while NAD[+], whose levels are higher during caloric restriction, activates Sir2. Sir2 mutations abrogated the effect of CR on longevity in yeast and the fruitfly *Drosophila*, supporting the theory that Sir2 mediates the effects of CR[54].

Sir2 is likely to regulate longevity via more than one mechanism. Thus, while it regulates levels of daf-16-related transcription factors, at least in yeast, it also exerts other effects that extend longevity, including reduction in levels of toxic forms of extrachromosomal circular rRNA[55,56]. Further confounding the situation is the observation that there are yeast strains that do not require Sir2 for lifespan extension after CR[57]. In addition to Sir2, a related pathway mediates the effects of caloric restriction via the *PNC1* gene (pyrazinamidase/nicotinamidase 1). Deletion of *PNC1* attenuated the effects of CR on yeast longevity, while yeast with extra copies of *PNC1* lived 70% longer than their wild-type counterparts[58]. The PNC1 protein degrades nicotinamide into nicotinic acid (NA) and then synthesizes NAD[+] from NA and ADP-ribose in a salvage pathway for NAD[+] synthesis[58]. Because nicotinamide is a competitive inhibitor of Sir2, while NAD activates Sir2, it is anticipated that PNC1 may upregulate Sir2 in strains in which both proteins are present. Thus, PNC1 may affect Sir2 activity by regulating nicotinamide/NAD[+] levels. Thus, it appears that this NAD[+] salvage pathway is another important mechanism by which CR increases lifespan.

In yeast, sir2 increases activity of the yeast transcription factors Msn2 and Msn4. In humans, the situation is considerably more complex. Sir2 has seven mammalian homologs in mice and humans (SIRT1-7); CR induces SIRT1 expression in mammalian cells[59]. The sirtuins have multiple functions including deacetylation of the p53 and Foxo proteins[60]. SIRT1 complexes with and subsequently deacetylates Foxo3a in response to stresses such as H_2O_2, ultraviolet radiation and heat shock. This deacetylation represses Foxo3a expression but nonetheless improves the efficiency with which Foxo3a induces a cellular stress response, possibly because it specifically decreases the pro-apoptotic properties of acetylated Foxo3a[61,62]. Interestingly, Bellizzi *et al.* found that a polymorphism that is predicted to decrease activity of SIRT3, a mitochondrial sirtuin, was significantly underrepresented in older Italian males[63].

As noted, the Sir2 and SIRT1 are NAD-dependent histone deacetylases whose effect on prolonging longevity probably reflects, at least partially, the ability of these proteins to regulate expression of critical genes involved in aging. Histone deacetylases maintain chromatin condensed in nucleosomes in a silent, inaccessible state. One thus might anticipate that Sir2 and SIRT1 repress transcription of selected genes that promote the aging process, although in reality altered acetylation both reduces and enhances transcription of diverse genes. In addition to the sirtuins, other histone deacetylases are also implicated in the control of aging. Another deacetylase in yeast is the *rpd3* gene, whose deletion results in increased acetylation of histones and increased lifespan[65]. It initially appears paradoxical that normal and enhanced levels of sirtuins (predicted to reduce acetylation and gene expression) and deletion of *rpd3* (predicted to enhance acetylation and gene expression) should both enhance longevity. This may be explained by the observation that *rpd3* and *sir2* silence very different regions of chromatin[66]. Phenylbutyrate, a broad inhibitor of histone deacetylases, was observed to increase lifespan in *Drosophila* concomitantly with both augmented and reduced expression of diverse genes. Those whose expression was increased included superoxide dismutase, glutathione S-transferase and hsp60[67].

Mitochondrial genes

Mitochondria are extremely important to aging, as these organelles are critical in energy generation, metabolism and the formation of some ROS such as superoxide anion. The importance of the mitochondria was demonstrated in a systematic RNAi screen of genes affecting lifespan in *C. elegans* in which mitochondrial genes emerged as the largest group (almost 15%)[68]. Mitochondrial genes thus far identified in mutagenesis studies include *hpd-1*, *nuo-1*, *isp-1* (a component of complex III of the respiratory chain) and the clock gene *clk-1*, homologous to mammalian coenzyme Q7. In

C. elegans, clk-1/daf-2 double mutants have a five-fold increase in lifespan[69]. Interestingly, *clk-1* mutants have increased levels of demethoxy-ubiquinone (DMQ), a precursor of ubiquinone (coenzyme Q10), which has been extensively studied as an antioxidant.

Several mitochondrial mutations have been identified that accelerate aging, including loss-of-function mutations in mitochondrial superoxide dismutase (SOD2) and Mev-1 (a subunit of the mitochondrial enzyme succinate dehydrogenase[29]). In *C. elegans*, loss-of-function mutations in the *catalase* gene also shorten survival. These observations are consonant with the view that oxidative damage is implicated in aging because these mutants generate increased ROS and demonstrate increased evidence of nuclear DNA damage. Also relevant is the reciprocal observation that overexpression of several antioxidant genes prolongs lifespan in *Drosophila*. Thus, *Drosophila* with forced expression of high levels of cytosolic copper/zinc SOD jointly with catalase have a 30% increase in lifespan[70]. Additional protective antioxidant genes include methionine sulfoxide reductase A in *Drosophila* and thioredoxin in mice (reviewed in reference 71). Melov *et al.* increased the lifespan of *C. elegans* by 44% using synthetic SOD1 and catalase mimetics EUK-8 and EUK-134[72]. These pharmacologic agents rescued the shortened lifespan of *mev-1* mutants[70].

Human linkage studies

The importance of these aging pathways in human disease is only beginning to be explored. In addition to the variations in known genes discussed above, genome-wide linkage studies point to a strong genetic component in human longevity. Candidate aging genes in humans have recently been reported. Perls *et al.* reported that siblings of centenarians had a significant reduction in mortality at all ages in life as compared to age-matched controls; correspondingly, they had a substantially increased likelihood of survival to age 100 (17-fold for males, eight-fold for females)[73].

Additional linkage studies of centenarians and their siblings have identified several genes related to lipid metabolism. A locus for enhanced survival on chromosome 4 was found to contain variants within the microsomal triglyceride transfer protein (MTP) which was associated with extreme longevity in a large US cohort (although not in a French cohort)[74]. MTP functions in the rate-limiting step in lipoprotein assembly. The variant associated with prolonged survival (-493G) lies in the MTP promoter and diminishes expression (50% reduced) of the MTP protein. In turn, this correlates with data showing that targeted inactivation of this gene, and pharmacologic inhibition of the MTP protein, improve lipid profiles (e.g. reduce triglycerides) and decrease serum glucose and insulin levels. The implication of these studies is that a genetic variant that favorably alters lipid metabolism enhances aging by diminishing the occurrence of lipid-related disorders. Prolonged lifespan in humans also correlates with a variant (I405V) of the cholesteryl ester transfer protein (CETP) which regulates high-density (HDL) and low-density lipoprotein (LDL) particle sizes[75]. How these lipid-related genes might relate to neurodegenerative diseases is unknown at this time.

AGING, AMYOTROPHIC LATERAL SCLEROSIS AND NEURODEGENERATION

In the most general sense, it is tempting to speculate that upregulation of stress-activated defense systems (such as heat shock proteins and families of multiple antioxidant proteins) will be beneficial, at least in SOD1-mediated ALS, insofar as two components of this disease are proposed to be protein misfolding and oxidative pathology. In this context, it is intriguing that SOD1 itself has been implicated in aging, as its overexpression jointly with catalase extends longevity in flies (above). Analogously, if inadequate ATP synthesis and generation of aberrant radical oxygen species is another element in ALS, then it is anticipated

that therapy with agents such as coenzyme Q10 may be beneficial in human ALS, as indeed they are reported to be when administered early in transgenic murine ALS[76]. On the other hand, coenzyme Q10 supplementation of normal C57B6 mice begun at 14 months did not increase lifespan[77]. These considerations have prompted a current multicenter study of coenzyme Q10 in ALS, whose rationale is underscored by reports that coenzyme Q10 at high doses was beneficial in animal models and possibly beneficial in a human study of Parkinson's diseases[78].

As described above, histone deacetylases are implicated in the regulation of aging. Here it is relevant that, in perhaps the broadest category of neurodegenerative disorders, the polyglutamine tract diseases (arising from expanded triplets of coding CAG repeats) there is evidence of subnormal histone acetylation. Reversal of this hypoacetylation by overexpression of CREB-binding protein (CBP) or administration of deacetylase inhibitors reduced cell death in an *in vitro* model of polyglutamine cytotoxicity[79]. Also of note here is a recent report that sodium phenylbutyrate improved survival in a mouse model of Huntington's disease (with a transgene expressing expanded polyglutamine) and also in the SOD1[G93A] transgenic ALS mice. As noted above, one of the primary targets of action of sodium phenylbutyrate is inhibition of histone deacetylases[80,81].

Another line of inquiry has suggested a direct molecular intersection between aging and neurodegeneration pathways. These studies focus on a remarkable mouse mutant with a heritable resistance to axonal degeneration that is transmitted as a Mendelian trait[82]. In young mice with this genetic defect, Wallerian degeneration after axonal injury is slowed, and accordingly the mice are designated slow Wallerian degeneration or *WLD^S*. The *WLD^S* trait also entails slowed axonal degeneration in neurons cultured from these animals. In mature *WLD^S* mice, the capacity of this mutation to ameliorate Wallerian degeneration is less pronounced. It is striking that the introduction of the *WLD^S* mutation into selected, early-onset mouse neurodegenerative disorders (e.g. the *pmn* mouse with defects in tubulin chaperone function) slows the degenerative process[83]. By contrast, this mutation slows the course of transgenic SOD1[G93A] murine ALS only minimally[84] or not at all[85], possibly because the motor neuron degenerative process in that model begins later than does the *pmn* neuronal death process.

The genetic defect in the *WLD^S* mice is a fusion of two genes: Ufd2a E4B, a protein active in ubiquitin-dependent protein degradation, and nicotinamide mononucleotide adenylyl-transferase 1 (Nmnat), which generates NAD, thereby increasing activities of NAD-dependent enzymes such as PARP and the sirtuin proteins. Recently Araki and colleagues have shown that the effects of the *WLD^S* mutation *in vitro* can be mimicked by addition of NAD or resveratrol, a small-molecule sirtuin activator[86]. Reciprocally, reduction in the activity of SIRT1 (but not the other sirtuins) by RNAi silencing ablates the effect of the *WLD^S* mutation on axonal degeneration *in vitro*. On the other hand, it remains unclear how fully these findings from studies *in vitro* will apply *in vivo*. A cautionary note is the preliminary finding that transgenic expression of NMNAT1 in mice does not slow Wallerian degeneration (discussed in reference 87). Nonetheless, the implication of these observations is that *SIRT1*, a critical aging gene in mammals, is a determinant of axonal viability in response to injury. This raises the hypothesis that one component of augmented aging may be enhanced axonal viability; reciprocally, if sirtuin expression and regulation are abnormal, it is conceivable that axonal degeneration might be one consequence, representing a form of focal, accelerated aging.

CONCLUDING COMMENTS

Aging research has made remarkable discoveries in the past 10 years. Whether these discoveries will lead to new insights into age-related diseases, including neurodegenerative diseases such as ALS,

remains to be seen. However, despite these uncertainties, there are at least three reasons why it will continue to be instructive to use the power of contemporary genetics and molecular biology to define molecular events that determine human longevity.

First, as in small animal models, insight into these events will provide further understanding of the biology of normal aging of both cells and tissues in humans. With the exception of germline cells, the normal fate of any cell is to differentiate and age; a genetic analysis of this process should disclose parameters that determine the rate of aging, its cell-type specificity and how such parameters are altered by genetic variants and exogenous variables such as environmental factors.

Second, successful aging can, in part, be construed as a state of avoidance of common disorders such as atherosclerotic cardiovascular disease, cancer, diabetes, osteoporosis and age-dependent neurodegenerative conditions such as Alzheimer's and Parkinson's diseases. Identification of genetic alleles that are under-represented in populations of aged individuals should reveal putative risk factors for those disorders. Conversely, alleles that are over-represented in the aged may confer protection against those diseases. This point is epitomized in the aforementioned studies that have identified two genes (*MTP, CETP*) whose variants appear to decrease the risk of lipid-related disorders (above). Analogously, it is striking that the allele of apolipoprotein E (E4) that predisposes to Alzheimer's disease is under-represented in centenarians[88].

Finally, research into the basic biologic processes of normal aging should contribute to our understanding of neurodegenerative disorders such as ALS, which are characterized by age-dependent cell death and features of accelerated aging, even if these disorders are not commonplace (by comparison with atherosclerosis, cancer and diabetes). This genetic approach may be particularly powerful in disorders such as ALS, for which insights into pathogenesis and associated therapies have otherwise been elusive.

Ultimately, a practical hope for these inquiries is that they will eventually provide insight into new treatments for age-dependent disorders. It is already apparent that there are small molecules that can, in small organisms, retard aging and prolong longevity (e.g. resveratrol in yeast[64] or antioxidants such as EUK-134 in worms[72]). Conceivably such reagents may, alone or in combination, prove beneficial in neurodegenerative disorders, particularly if the occurrence of those disorders is contingent on aging processes. In this context, the aforementioned benefits of coenzyme Q10 are noted, as is the slight but statistically significant extension of lifespan in the SOD1^{G93A} mice following therapy EUK-134 (244 vs. 221 days)[89].

ACKNOWLEDGMENTS

RHB is supported by the NINDS, the NIA, the ALS Association, Project ALS, the Angel Fund, the Delaney Fund, the Al-Athel ALS Research Foundation and the Pierre L. de Bourghknecht ALS Research Foundation. A-MW is supported by the American Parkinson Disease Association, the MGH/MIT Morris Udall Center of Excellence in Parkinson Disease Research (NIH, NINDS), and the Francis and Heide Schumann Fellowship in Parkinsons Disease Research at the Massachusetts General Hospital.

REFERENCES

1. Nelson LM, Epidemiology of ALS. Clin Neurosci 1995; 3: 327–31
2. Traynor BJ, Codd MB, Corr B, et al. Incidence and prevalence of ALS in Ireland, 1995–1997: A population-based study. Neurology 1999; 52: 504–9
3. Chancellor AM, Warlow CP, Adult onset motor neuron disease: Worldwide mortality, incidence and distribution since 1950. J Neurol Neurosurg Psychiatry 1992; 55: 1106–15
4. Rosen DR. Mutations in Cu/Zn superoxide dismutase gene are associated with familial amyotrophic lateral sclerosis. Nature 1993; 362: 59–62
5. Andrews WD, Tuke PW, Al-Chalabi A, et al. Detection of reverse transcriptase activity in the serum of patients with motor neurone disease. J Med Virol 2000; 61: 527–32
6. Steele AJ, Al-Chalabi A, Ferrante K, et al. Detection of serum reverse transcriptase activity in patients with ALS and unaffected blood relatives. Neurology 2005; 64: 454–8
7. Kimura F, Smith RG, Delbono O, et al. Amyotrophic lateral sclerosis patient antibodies label Ca2+ channel alpha 1 subunit [see comments]. Ann Neurol 1994; 35: 164–71
8. Rothstein JD, Martin LJ, Kuncl RW. Decreased glutamate transport by the brain and spinal cord in amyotrophic lateral sclerosis [see comments]. N Engl J Med 1992; 326: 1464–8
9. Drachman DB, Rothstein JD. Inhibition of cyclooxygenase-2 protects motor neurons in an organotypic model of amyotrophic lateral sclerosis. Ann Neurol 2000; 48: 792–5
10. Conradi S, Ronnevi LO, Vesterberg O. Abnormal tissue distribution of lead in amyotrophic lateral sclerosis. J Neurol Sci 1976; 29: 259–65
11. Spencer PS, Ludolph AC, Kisby GE. Neurologic diseases associated with use of plant components with toxic potential. Environ Res 1993; 62: 106–13
12. Cox PA, Sacks OW, Cycad neurotoxins, consumption of flying foxes, and ALS-PDC disease in Guam. Neurology 2002; 58: 956–9
13. Andersen PM, Sims KB, Xin WW, et al. Sixteen novel mutations in the Cu/Zn superoxide dismutase gene in amyotrophic lateral sclerosis: A decade of discoveries, defects and disputes. Amyotroph Lateral Scler Other Motor Neuron Disord 2003; 4: 62–73
14. Gurney ME, Pu H, Chiu AY, et al. Motor neuron degeneration in mice that express a human Cu,Zn superoxide dismutase mutation. Science 1994; 264: 1772–5
15. Nagai M, Aoki M, Miyoshi I, et al. Rats expressing human cytosolic copper–zinc superoxide dismutase transgenes with amyotrophic lateral sclerosis: Associated mutations develop motor neuron disease. J Neurosci 2001; 21: 9246–54
16. Howland DS, Liu J, She Y, et al. Focal loss of the glutamate transporter EAAT2 in a transgenic rat model of SOD1 mutant-mediated amyotrophic lateral sclerosis (ALS). Proc Natl Acad Sci USA 2002; 99: 1604–9
17. Reaume AG, Elliott JL, Hoffman EK, et al. Motor neurons in Cu/Zn superoxide dismutase-deficient mice develop normally but exhibit enhanced cell death after axonal injury. Nat Genet 1996; 13: 43–47

18. Clement AM, Nguyen MD, Roberts EA, et al. Wild-type nonneuronal cells extend survival of SOD1 mutant motor neurons in ALS mice. Science 2003; 302: 113–17

19. Friedlander RM. Apoptosis and caspases in neurode-generative diseases. N Engl J Med 2003; 348: 1365–75

20. Guegan C, Przedborski S. Programmed cell death in amyotrophic lateral sclerosis. J Clin Invest 2003; 111: 153–61

21. Pasinelli P, Belford ME, Lennon N, et al. Amy-otrophic lateral sclerosis-associated SOD1 mutant proteins bind and aggregate with Bcl-2 in spinal cord mitochondria. Neuron 2004; 43: 19–30

22. Nishimura AL, Mitue-Neto M, Silva HC, et al. A mutation in the vesicle-trafficking protein VAPB causes late-onset spinal muscular atrophy and amy-otrophic lateral sclerosis. Am J Hum Genet 2004; 75: 822–31

23. Yang Y, Hentati A, Deng HX, et al. The gene encod-ing alsin, a protein with three guanine-nucleotide exchange factor domains, is mutated in a form of recessive amyotrophic lateral sclerosis. Nat Genet 2001; 29: 160–5

24. Hadano S, Hand CK, Osuga H, et al. A gene encod-ing a putative GTPase regulator is mutated in famil-ial amyotrophic lateral sclerosis 2. Nat Genet 2001; 29: 166–73

25. Puls I, Jonnakuty C, La Monte BH, et al. Mutant dynactin in motor neuron disease. Nat Genet 2003; 33: 455–6

26. Chen YZ, et al. DNA/RNA helicase gene mutations in a form of juvenile amyotrophic lateral sclerosis (ALS4). Am J Hum Genet 2004; 74: 1128–35

27. Guarente L, Kenyon C. Genetic pathways that regu-late ageing in model organisms. Nature 2000; 408: 255–62

28. Harman D. The aging process. Proc Natl Acad Sci USA 1981; 78: 7124–8

29. Balaban RS, Nemoto S, Finkel T. Mitochondria, oxi-dants, and aging. Cell 2005; 120: 483–95

30. Trifunovic A, Hausson A, Wredenberg A, et al. Somatic mtDNA mutations cause aging phenotypes without affecting reactive oxygen species production. Proc Natl Acad Sci USA 2005; 102: 17993–8

31. Kirkwood TB. Understanding the odd science of aging. Cell 2005; 120: 437–47

32. Lu T, Pan Y, Kao SY, et al. Gene regulation and DNA damage in the ageing human brain. Nature 2004; 429: 883–91

33. Blasco MA. Telomeres and human disease: ageing, cancer and beyond. Nat Rev Genet 2005; 6: 611–22

34. Perls T, Kunkel L, Puca A. The genetics of aging. Curr Opin Genet Dev 2002; 12: 362–9

35. Martin GM. Genetic modulation of senescent phe-notypes in Homo sapiens. Cell 2005; 120: 523–32

36. Puzianowska-Kuznicka M, Kuznicki J. Genetic alter-ations in accelerated ageing syndromes. Do they play a role in natural ageing? Int J Biochem Cell Biol 2005; 37: 947–60

37. McCay CM, Cromwell MF, Marynard LA. The effect of retarded growth upon the length of life span and ultimate body size. J Nutrition 1935; 10: 63–79

38. Roth GS, Mattison JA, Ottinger MA, et al. Aging in rhesus monkeys: Relevance to human health inter-ventions. Science 2004; 305: 1423–6

39. Fontana L, Meyer TE, Klein S, et al. Long-term calo-rie restriction is highly effective in reducing the risk for atherosclerosis in humans. Proc Natl Acad Sci USA 2004; 101: 6659–63

40. Koubova J, Guarente L. How does calorie restriction work? Genes Dev 2003; 17: 313–21

41. Zhu H, Guo Q, Mattson MP. Dietary restriction pro-tects hippocampal neurons against the death-promot-ing action of a presenilin-1 mutation. Brain Res 1999; 842: 224–9

42. Semsei I, Rao G, Richardson A. Changes in the expression of superoxide dismutase and catalase as a function of age and dietary restriction. Biochem Bio-phys Res Commun 1989; 164: 620–5

43. Pedersen WA, Mattson MP. No benefit of dietary restriction on disease onset or progression in amy-otrophic lateral sclerosis Cu/Zn-superoxide dismutase mutant mice. Brain Res 1999; 833: 117–20

44. Murphy CT, McCarroll SA, Bargmann CI, et al. Genes that act downstream of DAF-16 to influence the lifespan of Caenorhabditis elegans. Nature 2003; 424: 277–83

45. Longo VD, Finch CE. Evolutionary medicine: From dwarf model systems to healthy centenarians? Science 2003; 299: 1342–6

46. Larsen PL. Aging and resistance to oxidative damage in Caenorhabditis elegans. Proc Natl Acad Sci USA 1993; 90: 8905–9

47. Hekimi S, Guarente L. Genetics and the specificity of the aging process. Science 2003; 299: 1351–4

48. Kenyon C. The plasticity of aging: Insights from long-lived mutants. Cell 2005; 120: 449–60

49. Kops GJ, Dansen TB, Polderman PE, et al. Fork-head transcription factor FOXO3a protects quies-cent cells from oxidative stress. Nature 2002; 419: 316–21

50. Holzenberger M, Dupont J, Ducos B, et al. IGF-1 receptor regulates lifespan and resistance to oxidative stress in mice. Nature 2003; 421: 182–7

51. Bonafe M, Barbieri M, Marchegiani F, et al. Polymorphic variants of insulin-like growth factor I (IGF-I) receptor and phosphoinositide 3-kinase genes affect IGF-I plasma levels and human longevity: Cues for an evolutionarily conserved mechanism of life span control. J Clin Endocrinol Metab 2003; 88: 3299–304

52. Tissenbaum HA, Guarente L. Increased dosage of a sir-2 gene extends lifespan in Caenorhabditis elegans. Nature 2001; 410: 227–30

53. Guarente L, Picard F. Calorie restriction – the SIR2 connection. Cell 2005; 120: 473–82

54. Lin SJ, Defossez PA, Guarente L. Requirement of NAD and SIR2 for life-span extension by calorie restriction in Saccharomyces cerevisiae. Science 2000; 289: 2126–8

55. Sinclair DA, Guarente L. Extrachromosomal rDNA circles – a cause of aging in yeast. Cell 1997; 91: 1033–42

56. Kaeberlein M, McVey M, Guarente L. The SIR2/3/4 complex and SIR2 alone promote longevity in Saccharomyces cerevisiae by two different mechanisms. Genes Dev 1999; 13: 2570–80

57. Kaeberlein M, Kirkland KT, Fields S, et al. Sir2-independent life span extension by calorie restriction in yeast. PLoS Biol 2004; 2: E296

58. Anderson RM, Bitterman KJ, Wood JG, et al. Nicotinamide and PNC1 govern lifespan extension by calorie restriction in Saccharomyces cerevisiae. Nature 2003; 423: 181–5

59. Cohen HY, Miller C, Bitterman KJ, et al. Calorie restriction promotes mammalian cell survival by inducing the SIRT1 deacetylase. Science 2004; 305: 390–2

60. Luo J, Nikolaev AY, Imai S, et al. Negative control of p53 by Sir2alpha promotes cell survival under stress. Cell 2001; 107: 137–48

61. Brunet A, Sweeney LB, Sturgill JF, et al. Stress-dependent regulation of FOXO transcription factors by the SIRT1 deacetylase. Science 2004; 303: 2011–5

62. Motta MC, Divecha N, Lemieux M, et al. Mammalian SIRT1 represses forkhead transcription factors. Cell 2004; 116: 551–63

63. Bellizzi D, Ross G, Cavalcante P, et al. A novel VNTR enhancer within the SIRT3 gene, a human homologue of SIR2, is associated with survival at oldest ages. Genomics 2005; 85: 258–63

64. Howitz KT, Bitterman KJ, Cohen HY, et al. Small molecule activators of sirtuins extend Saccharomyces cerevisiae lifespan. Nature 2003; 425: 191–6

65. Kim S, Benguria A, Lai CY, et al. Modulation of lifespan by histone deacetylase genes in Saccharomyces cerevisiae. Mol Biol Cell 1999; 10: 3125–36

66. Robyr D, Suka Y, Xenarios I, et al. Microarray deacetylation maps determine genome-wide functions for yeast histone deacetylases. Cell 2002; 109: 437–46

67. Kang HL, Benzer S, Min KT. Life extension in Drosophila by feeding a drug. Proc Natl Acad Sci USA 2002; 99: 838–43

68. Lee SS, Lee RY, Fraser AG, et al. A systematic RNAi screen identifies a critical role for mitochondria in C. elegans longevity. Nat Genet 2003; 33: 40–8

69. Lakowski B, Hekimi S. Determination of life-span in Caenorhabditis elegans by four clock genes. Science 1996; 272: 1010–3

70. Orr WC, Sohal RS. Extension of life-span by overexpression of superoxide dismutase and catalase in Drosophila melanogaster. Science 1994; 263: 1128–30

71. Hadley EC, Lakatta EG, Morrison-Bogorad N, et al. The future of aging therapies. Cell 2005; 120: 557–67

72. Melov S, Ravenscroft J, Malik S, et al. Extension of life-span with superoxide dismutase/catalase mimetics. Science 2000; 289: 1567–9

73. Perls TT, Wilmoth J, Levenson R, et al. Life-long sustained mortality advantage of siblings of centenarians. Proc Natl Acad Sci USA 2002; 99: 8442–7

74. Geesaman BJ, Benson E, Brewster SJ, et al. Haplotype-based identification of a microsomal transfer protein marker associated with the human lifespan. Proc Natl Acad Sci USA 2003; 100: 14115–20

75. Barzilai N, Atzmon G, Schechter C, et al. Unique lipoprotein phenotype and genotype associated with exceptional longevity. JAMA 2003; 290: 2030–40

76. Matthews RT, Yang L, Browne S, et al. Coenzyme Q10 administration increases brain mitochondrial concentrations and exerts neuroprotective effects. Proc Natl Acad Sci USA 1998; 95: 8892–7

77. Lee CK, Pugh TD, Klopp RG, et al. The impact of alpha-lipoic acid, coenzyme Q10 and caloric restriction on life span and gene expression patterns in mice. Free Radic Biol Med 2004; 36: 1043–57

78. Shults CW, Oakes D, Kieburtz K, et al. Effects of coenzyme Q10 in early Parkinson disease: Evidence of slowing of the functional decline. Arch Neurol 2002; 59: 1541–50

79. McCampbell A, Taye AA, Whitty L, et al. Histone deacetylase inhibitors reduce polyglutamine toxicity. Proc Natl Acad Sci USA 2001; 98: 15179–84

80. Gardian G, Browne SE, Choi DK, et al. Neuroprotective effects of phenylbutyrate in the N171-82Q transgenic mouse model of Huntington's disease. J Biol Chem 2005; 280: 556–63

81. Ryu H, Smith K, Camelo SI, et al. Sodium phenylbutyrate prolongs survival and regulates expression of anti-apoptotic genes in transgenic amyotrophic lateral sclerosis mice. J Neurochem 2005; 93: 1087–98

82. Lunn ER, Perry VH, Gordon S. Absence of Wallerian degeneration does not hinder regeneration in peripheral nerve. Eur J Neurol 1989; 1: 27–33

83. Ferri A, Sanes JR, Coleman MP, et al. Inhibiting axon degeneration and synapse loss attenuates apoptosis and disease progression in a mouse model of motoneuron disease. Curr Biol 2003; 13: 669–73

84. Fischer LR, Culver DG, Davis AA, et al. The WldS gene modestly prolongs survival in the SOD1G93A fALS mouse. Neurobiol Dis 2005; 19: 293–300

85. Vande Velde C, et al. The neuroprotective factor Wlds does not attenuate mutant SOD1-mediated motor neuron disease. Neuromolecular Med 2004; 5: 193–203

86. Araki T, Sasaki Y, Milbrandt J. Increased nuclear NAD biosynthesis and SIRT1 activation prevent axonal degeneration. Science 2004; 305: 1010–13

87. Coleman M. Axon degeneration mechanisms: Commonality amid diversity. Nat Rev Neurosci 2005; 6: 889–98

88. Schachter F, Faure-Delanef L, Guenot F, et al. Genetic associations with human longevity at the APOE and ACE loci. Nat Genet 1994; 6: 29–32

89. Jung C, Rong Y, Doctrow S, et al. Synthetic superoxide dismutase/catalase mimetics reduce oxidative stress and prolong survival in a mouse amyotrophic lateral sclerosis model. Neurosci Lett 2001; 304: 157–60

15

Neurotrophic factors

Michael Sendtner

DEVELOPMENTAL MOTONEURON CELL DEATH AND NEUROTROPHIC FACTORS

In higher vertebrates, spinal and brainstem motor neurons are generated in excess during embryonic development. After these cells have grown out axons and made functional contacts to skeletal muscle, a significant proportion of these cells degenerate. For example, from about 6000 motor neurons in the lumbar spinal cord of rat embryos at embryonic day 15, about 50% are lost at postnatal day 3[1,2]. This process, which is called 'physiologic motor neuron cell death', is widely used as a model for understanding the mechanisms underlying the degeneration of motor neurons in various forms of human motor neuron disease.

Experiments by Victor Hamburger[3,4] and others in the first half of the 20th century have shown that the developmental cell death of motor neurons is guided by influences from the target tissue. Removal of a limb bud in chick embryos massively enhances developmental motor neuron loss, and transplantation of an additional limb reduces the number of dying motor neurons. Thus, individual organisms have the capacity to react to deviations from genetically determined developmental programs, and this kind of plasticity might have contributed to the generation of the highly complex nervous system in higher vertebrates during

evolution. On the other hand, the higher complexity offers many possibilities for disturbances such as gene mutations and dysregulation of gene expression which can be a cause of disease.

Since the discovery of nerve growth factor (NGF) as a prototypic target-derived neurotrophic molecule that regulates survival of paravertebral sympathetic neurons and subpopulations of sensory neurons, a variety of neurotrophic factors which belong to distinct gene families have been identified (Table 15.1) and characterized on a molecular level. In particular, many factors have been found which support motor neuron survival, and it is to be expected that, despite the completion of the human and mouse genome projects, not all neurotrophic factors that play a role in maintenance of developing and postnatal motor neurons have yet been identified. This indicates that the regulation of motor neuron survival, the growth and maintence of axons, and the development and function of motor endplates are highly complex processes that are influenced by more than one neurotrophic factor. Moreover, many of these molecules are only expressed postnatally, indicating that postnatal survival is also controlled by neurotrophic factors, and that these factors serve additional functions for motor neurons (e.g. the regulation of functional properties such as transmitter synthesis, sprouting, synaptic stability and activity).

Table 15.1 Neurotrophic factors for motor neurons and their receptors

	Receptor on motor neurons
Neurotrophins	
Brain-derived neurotrophic factor (BDNF)	p75^{NTR}, trk-B
Neurotrophin-3 (NT-3)	p75^{NTR}, trk-C
Neurotrophin-4/5 (NT-4/5)	p75^{NTR}, trk-B
CNTF/LIF family	
Ciliary neurotrophic factor (CNTF)	CNTFRα, LIFRβ, gp130
Leukemia inhibitory factor (LIF)	LIFRβ, gp130
Cardiotrophin-1 (CT-1)	?, LIFRβ, gp130
Cardiotrophin-1-like cytokine (CLC)	CNTFRα, LIFRβ, gp130
Hepatocyte growth factor/scatter factor	
(HGF/SF)	c-met
Insulin-like growth factors	
IGF-I	IGFR-1
IGF-II	IGFR-1, mannose-6P receptor
Glia-derived neurotrophic factor and related factors	
Glia-derived neurotrophic factor (GDNF)	c-ret, GFRα
Neurturin (NTR)	c-ret, GFRα-2
Persephin	c-ret, GFRα-3
Artemin	c-ret, GFRα-4
Vascular endothelial growth factors	
VEGF	VEGFR-1 (Flt), VEGFR-2 (Flk/KDR)
PlGF	VEGFR-1 (Flt)
VEGF-B	VEGFR-1 (Flt)
VEGF-C	VEGFR-2 (Flk/KDR), VEGFR-3(Flt4)
VEGF-D	VEGFR-2 (Flk/KDR), VEGFR-3(Flt4)
VEGF$_{165}$	NP-1, NP-2
VEGF$_{145}$	NP-2

The hypothesis that factors from developing muscle play a central role in regulation of motor neuron survival during development has recently been challenged by observations that other types of cell, in particular Schwann cells, are also important in this context. For example, mice with a severe deficit of developing Schwann cells, such as erbB3 knockout mice, exhibit a significant reduction (79%) in motor neurons[5]. These data indicate that developing Schwann cells are at least as important for providing trophic support for motor neurons as skeletal muscle. However, the data do not rule out the possibility that the motor neurons first become dependent on muscle-derived neurotrophic support and then on Schwann cell-derived support. In the context of motor neuron disease, such influences which come into play late during development or even in the adult might be even more important. However, the network of trophic signaling between muscle, Schwann cells and motor neurons appears complex. Neuregulin/glial growth factor (GGF) is also synthesized and secreted from developing motor neurons[6,7] and regulates the expression of acetylcholine receptor subunits at the motor end-plate. The same receptor, erbB3, which mediates the effects of GGF in Schwann cells, is also expressed in skeletal muscle[8–10] and could be responsible for proper development of neuromuscular synapses, possibly a prerequisite for the production and secretion of neurotrophic factors from muscle. Axonal neuregulin, which is produced in motor neurons, also regulates myelination and the thickness of the myelin sheet in Schwann cells[11]. Therefore, final conclusions on the relative importance of muscle- and Schwann cell-derived neurotrophic support for developing motor neurons and on how motor neuron-derived factors such as neuregulin contribute to this network of mutual signaling and trophic support cannot be drawn at the moment. Rather, we have to assume that neurotrophic support from various sources is necessary for proper function of motor neurons, and that disturbances in such processes could represent pathomechanisms which underlie or propagate neuronal dysfunction and cell death in human motor neuron disease.

PATHOMECHANISMS OF HUMAN MOTOR NEURON DISEASE AND NEUROTROPHIC FACTORS

A variety of gene defects, in particular mutations in the superoxide dismutase (*SOD1*), *alsin, senataxin* and vesicle-associated membrane protein (*VAPB*) genes, have been identified and characterized, and underlie the inherited forms of amyotrophic lateral sclerosis (ALS) (see Chapters 9 and 10) and other forms of motor neuron disease in the adult. However, in contrast to spinal muscular atrophy in children and young adults, most forms of ALS are sporadic. This does not necessarily mean that they are not genetically determined. It is possible that at least a proportion of these disorders have a multigenetic origin. Thus, the disease becomes apparent only when several gene defects come together. Such cases will not follow Mendelian rules of inheritance and could appear as sporadic cases. Moreover, such genetic predispositions together with epigenetic (e.g. toxic) influences could be responsible for ALS. Not much is known about such genetic predispositions. Alterations in the genes for neurotrophic factors, both in coding and non-coding regions, could be candidates for such genetic predispositions:

(1) Many neurotrophic factors share their receptors or receptor components with other members of the same gene families. Thus, in case of genetic defects leading to reduced expression or lack of expression of one factor, other members of the same gene family could compensate for this deficiency, and significant functional deficits only occur when more than one factor is lacking. Mice lacking cilary neurotrophic factor (CNTF), leukemia inhibitory factor (LIF) and cardiotrophin-1 (CT-1) (Figure 15.1) provide an example for such conditions[12,13].

(2) Most motor neurons express several receptors and are thus responsive to a variety of neurotrophic molecules. The signaling pathways downstream from these receptors show a high degree of overlap. Therefore, motoneurons could receive support from other gene families of neurotrophic factors (for example glia-derived neurotrophic factor, insulin-like growth factor (IGF), vascular endothelial growth factor (VEGF)) in case of lack of signaling from other neurotrophic factors (for example neurotrophins).

(3) The anti-apoptotic signaling by neurotrophic factors interferes with various pathomechanisms which could be responsible for motor neuron disease, in particular the induction of neuronal cell death through glutamate, free radicals and other SOD mutations associated with familial ALS[14–21].

Thus, a lack of neurotrophic factors, even if it does not lead to motor neuron disease on its own,

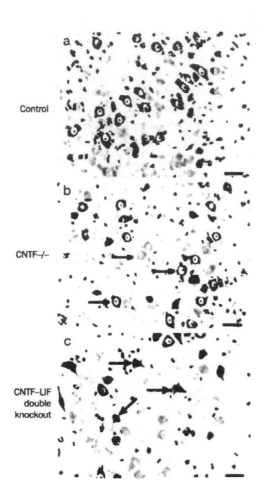

Figure 15.1 Morphology of facial motor neurons in mouse mutants that lack CNTF or LIF, or both. (a) Morphology of motor neurons in a 6-week-old control mouse. (b) Morphology of motor neurons in a 6-week-old CNTF–/– mouse. The arrows point to atrophic cells; the relative size of the cytoplasm in comparison to the nucleus has significantly decreased. (c) Morphology of motor neurons in a 6-week-old CNTF–LIF double knockout mouse. A significant number of motor neurons are lost in these mice, and other motor neurons show morphologic signs of atrophy and degeneration (arrows), in particular the loss of Nissl structure and decentralized nuclei. (Reproduced from reference 12 with permission)

the splice acceptor site of the second exon of the human CNTF gene was identified which leads to a shift of the reading frame and thus to a truncated, biologically inactive CNTF protein[22]. This mutation is abundant in the Asian and European populations. About one-third of these populations is heterozygous for this gene mutation. The number of *CNTF*-deficient individuals is in the range of 1–3%[22,23]. Because the percentage of individuals with a *CNTF*–/– genotype was similar in healthy controls and patients with neurologic disorders, it was concluded that deficiency of *CNTF* is not responsible for the development of neurologic disorders. However, the average age of persons in the healthy control group in this study[22] was much lower than, for example, in the group of patients with motor neuron disorders.

The best evidence for a potential role of *CNTF* deficiency on ALS disease severity comes from experiments in which G93A SOD mutant mice were crossbred with *CNTF* gene knockout mice. Disease onset shifted from 37 weeks to 27 weeks in the SOD mutant mice when CNTF was deficient[24]. Also in a family of patients where a V148G SOD mutation was coupled with the *CNTF* gene defect, patients with combined mutation showed very early disease onset at 25 years in comparison to 55 years for a patient with V148G SOD mutation but an intact *CNTF* allele. The question whether *CNTF* mutations are also associated with earlier disease onset in patients with sporadic ALS is controversial. In a study with more than 800 sporadic ALS patients, those patients with homozygous mutations for the *CNTF* gene showed earlier onset (48 ± 15 years) than ALS patients without the mutation (58 ± 9 years). In another study with 400 ALS patients, this effect of the *CNTF* mutation was not observed. Given that the number of homozygous *CNTF* mutant individuals is only around 2% in both the normal and the diseased population, large-scale studies with several thousands of patients allowing the analysis of at least 50–100 patients and controls with the homozygous *CNTF* mutation are necessary to find a reliable

could be a component in the development of motor neuron disease if coinciding with other pathogenic processes. A series of observations support this concept.

Mutations in the genes for some neurotrophic factors are abundant. In 1995, a mutation close to answer to this question. As long as these studies are not feasible, studies with mouse models appear more suitable to address the question on a modifier role of this and other neurotrophic factor genes in motor neuron disease.

Targeted mutation of the *CNTF* gene has been introduced in mice in order to determine the physiologic role of this factor for motor neurons. Homozygous mutant mice show a loss of about 20% of their motor neurons during the first 6 postnatal months, corresponding to a small reduction (10%) in muscle strength at the same age[25]. Of course, the same scenario in humans would not be considered pathologic. It is believed that at least 50% of the motor neurons should be lost until motor neuron disease develops in humans[26]. Therefore, the findings in mice and in humans do not contradict each other.

Not much is known about other gene defects in sporadic ALS. Polymorphisms in the gene for leukemia inhibitory factor which lead to loss of biologic function of the LIF protein are found more frequently in patients with ALS[27]. This corresponds to findings that LIF deficiency in combination with other gene defects has profound effects on motor endplate size, motor neuron survival and motor performance in double and triple knockout mice[13]. Recently, polymorphisms that reduce the expression of VEGF have been found to be associated with a higher incidence of ALS[28]. These data have received confirmation by the finding that mouse models that lack the HIF response element in the *VEGF* gene promoter also develop motor neuron disease[29]. Nothing is known so far about mutations in the genes for CT-1, glial-derived neurotrophic factor (GDNF), neurturin or persephin in ALS patients.

Such gene defects need not necessarily mimic the effects of homozygous gene knockout in mice. For most of these factors, transcription of the mRNA is driven from various promoters, or the primary transcripts are processed in a tissue-specific manner. Thus, many possibilities exist which could lead to dysregulation or lack of function of individual neurotrophic factors in ALS.

CILIARY NEUROTROPHIC FACTOR AND RELATED MOLECULES

CNTF was originally identified and characterized as a component of chick eye extracts, and found to share many biologic activities with a protein that was purified from rat sciatic nerve. After cloning and recombinant expression of this factor[30,31], it became apparent that this protein was a potent survival factor for developing motor neurons[32,33]. Surprisingly, CNTF expression during embryonic development is low and not found in regions such as peripheral nerves or muscle which are expected to be important sources of survival-promoting activity. *CNTF* differs from neurotrophins and other members of the same gene family such as *LIF* by lack of a hydrophobic signal peptide and thus is not released via the conventional secretory pathway.

CNTF acts through a tripartite receptor complex which is composed of a low-affinity binding subunit (CNTF-receptor-α; CNTFRα) and two transmembrane proteins (gp130 and LIF-receptor-β; LIFRβ)[34]. The CNTFRα exists both in a membrane-bound form which is linked via a glycosylphosphatidylinositol (GPI) anchor to the cell membrane, and in a soluble form which apparently is shed from synthesizing cells, most probably skeletal muscle[35]. The two transmembrane components, gp130 and LIFRβ, show significant homologies in particular in their intracellular domains[36]. Gp130 has originally been identified as a signal-transducing component of the interleukin (IL)-6-receptor, and LIFRβ as a low-affinity receptor for LIF. LIFRβ and gp130 are also involved in the receptor complexes for oncostatin-M (OSM), CT-1 and cardiotrophin-like cytokine (CLC)[37–40], a cytokine that mediates its trophic actions as a heterodimer with cytokine-like factor (CLF) or CNTFRα[41]. This appears as the structural basis for the overlapping effects of CNTF, LIF, CT-1 and other members of this family, in particular motor neurons.

CNTF is not expressed during embryonic development, but is produced in very high quantities in differentiated myelinating Schwann cells. This protein as well as CT-1[40] lack a hydrophobic leader sequence and thus are not released via the classical secretory pathway from producing cells. Very little CNTF is released from myelinating Schwann cells[42]. However, after nerve lesion or other conditions leading to leakage of the Schwann cell membrane, CNTF could be released and act locally on neurons via receptors on axons. In contrast to CNTF, which is constitutively expressed at high levels in myelinating Schwann cells, LIF mRNA levels are very low under physiologic conditions, but they rapidly increase after peripheral nerve lesion[43], so that significant quantities of this factor become available to lesioned motor neurons.

Mice with homozygous targeted disruption of the CNTF gene show a loss of about 20% of motor neurons. Mice lacking endogenous LIF do not exhibit any pathologic signs in motor neurons[12]. However, mice that are double-deficient for CNTF and LIF show a more severe loss of motor neurons (more than 30%) (Figure 15.1), which corresponds to a significant reduction in muscle strength (about 30% in comparison to controls). In contrast to CNTF- and/or LIF-deficient mice, *CT-1* gene knockout mice show a significant reduction of motor neurons at birth, but there is no further postnatal loss[44], indicating that deficiency of this factor is compensated by other members of this family. When all three factors are deleted in combination, severe loss of muscle strength occurs, and it becomes apparent that the loss of LIF particularly affects motor endplate size[13]. After peripheral nerve lesion in the adult, lack of CNTF has only a very small effect on motor neuron survival, whereas lack of both CNTF and LIF leads to reduced survival of axotomized motor neurons (66% survival at 2 weeks after lesion)[12]. These data indicate that CNTF and probably also other members of this ligand family for gp130 and LIFRβ act together and at least partially compensate each other in case of deficiency due to gene mutations.

In contrast to mice lacking the individual ligands for this receptor complex, mice with targeted disruption of the genes for LIFRβ[45], CNTFRα[46] or gp130[47] show severe defects in the nervous system which are not compatible with life after birth. All these mouse mutants show enhanced cell death during the developmental period of physiologic motor neuron cell death, indicating that at least one member of the CNTF/LIF gene family is involved in regulating motor neuron survival during this period. Likely candidates are CT-1 and the composite ligand CLC/CLF[37–40], which are expressed in skeletal muscle, in contrast to CNTF and LIF, which are made available to motor neurons from Schwann cells[48].

CNTF has been tested in a variety of mouse mutants for experimental treatment of motor neuron disease. Systemic administration of CNTF to pmn[49–51], wobbler[52,53] and mnd[54] mice shows significant effects on the course of the disease (Figure 15.1), although the mechanisms for how CNTF interferes with the pathogenic processes underlying these mouse mutants may be quite different. The endogenous expression of CNTF is normal in these mouse mutants, at least in pmn and wobbler mice. The gene defect in pmn mice has been identified: a single nucleotide exchange encodes a single amino acid exchange in the tubulin-specific chaperone E protein[55,56]. Motor neurons isolated from these mice survive normally in cell culture but exhibit shorter axons with prominent swellings, suggesting that axonal microtubule synthesis is the primary pathomechanism and that reduced survival is a consequence of this primary defect.

At least in the case of the pmn mouse, the levels of endogenous CNTF in peripheral nerves are much higher than the levels of CNTF that can be measured in the blood after pharmacologic application[42]. These data again suggest that very little CNTF becomes available under physiologic conditions to motor neurons from myelinating Schwann cells. However, when a peripheral nerve is transected in pmn mice, significantly improved survival of the lesioned motor neurons can be observed. In contrast, pmn mice lacking endogenous CNTF do not show this significant improvement of motor neuron survival after nerve lesion, indicating that endogenous CNTF is indeed a lesion factor which can rescue motor neurons after release from lesioned Schwann cells.

NEUROTROPHINS

The neurotrophins constitute a family of five proteins which are related to NGF. NGF is the prototypic target-derived trophic factor (reviewed by reference 57). Its biologic activities are limited to specific populations of peripheral and central neurons. The biologic effects of NGF on responsive neurons are mediated by a low-affinity receptor which is common to all neurotrophins (p75[NTR]) and through a specific high-affinity receptor, tropomyosin receptor kinase (trk-A)[58]. The p75[NTR] receptor is highly expressed in motor neurons during embryonic development. Expression drops to undetectable levels after birth, and it is re-expressed only after nerve lesion or motor neuron disease, in particular ALS[59,60]. For some time, it was thought that the biologic functions of NGF on survival and neurite outgrowth were exclusively mediated though the trk-A transmembrane tyrosine kinase receptor. Only recent years have seen clear evidence for an involvement of the p75[NTR] receptor in signal transduction[61,62]. The p75[NTR] receptor also mediates pro-apoptotic signaling responses[63,64], and it forms a high-affinity receptor for pro-NGF and other precursor proteins of neurotrophins[65-67].

However, reports on this function in transgenic mouse models that lack p75[NTR] have been confusing. The first reports on enhanced survival of cholinergic neurons in the basal forebrain in p75[NTR] knockout mice had to be revisited[68], and other data which are based on experiments with p75[NTR] gene knockout mice and neuronal cultures derived from these mice showed that p75[NTR] cooperates with trk receptors in mediating pro-survival effects[69]. The observation that p75[NTR] preferentially binds to proforms of neurotrophins[65] which have not yet been cleaved to the shorter mature neurotrophins has led to the hypothesis that cleavage of neurotrophin precursor protein decides on pro- versus anti-apoptotic effects of these molecules, and that neurotrophin precursor proteins mediate cell death via p75[NTR] and mature neurotrophins mediate survival through trk receptors or complexes of trk and p75[NTR] subunits. This appears to be confirmed by recent data[70] indicating that tissue plasminogen activator plays a role in the processing of pro-neurotrophins, in particular proBDNF, to mature neurotrophins which bind to trk receptors. This leads to interesting questions whether alterations in expression and activity of such extracellular proteases contribute to the development of motor neuron disease.

Reports on pro-apoptotic functions of neurotrophins through p75[NTR] correspond to pro-apoptotic effects of NGF on various types of neuron. For example, in newborn rats, the application of NGF increases the number of degenerating motor neurons after sciatic nerve lesion[71] and after facial nerve lesion[72]. During embryonic development, endogenous NGF promotes cell death of retinal ganglion cells through p75[NTR] [73]. This scenario could also be relevant when p75[NTR] is re-expressed in motor neurons, such as in neurodegenerative disorders like ALS.

The p75[NTR] receptor is also involved in functions other than mediating cell death and survival signals. These functions have been observed long before neurotrophin receptors were identified on a molecular level. For example, trk-A is not expressed in motor neurons, whereas relatively high levels of p75[NTR] are observed during development or after nerve lesion. The high expression of p75 explains why NGF can be taken up and retrogradely transported in embryonic motor neurons of newborn, but not adult, rats[74,75]. Some effects of NGF have been observed in motor neurons, among them hypertrophy of a subpopulation of NGF-receptor-positive lumbar motor neurons[76] or a short-term effect on neurite outgrowth in cultured embryonic motor neurons[77-79]. These effects are caused by activation of rhoA by direct interaction with p75[NTR] [80].

In 1989, the gene for BDNF was cloned[81]. BDNF is the second member of the neurotrophin family. Its discovery paved the way to identification of neurotrophin-3[82,83] and neurotrophin-4/5[84,85]. BDNF and NT-4/5 specifically interact with trk-B, and NT-3 preferentially binds to trk-C receptors. All neurotrophins bind to the p75[NTR] with similar affinity. The expression of the trk receptors defines the specificity for actions on various populations of neurons.

For example, motor neurons express full-length trk-B but not trk-A and therefore do not rely for their survival on NGF. A subpopulation of motor neurons also expresses trk-C, which is a specific cellular receptor for NT-3[86,87]. The positive effects of BDNF and NT-3 were discovered when these proteins were applied to lesioned motor neurons in newborn rats[72,88] or to the allantoic membrane of developing chick embryos[89]. Although virtually all of the motor neurons express trk-B, only a subpopulation of about 50–60% of the motor neurons survive after BDNF administration in vivo[72,88] or in vitro[86,90]. The reason for this apparent discrepancy is still not clear. As this effect is observed both in cultured motor neurons from different embryonic stages as well as in vivo in postnatal motor neurons, it has to be assumed that the responsiveness of motor neurons to BDNF through trk-B does not simply increase during embryonic development, but is regulated by other cellular or extracellular signals.

The genes for BDNF and NT-3 as well as the genes for the corresponding receptors trk-B and trk-C have been knocked out in mice. Mice without BDNF survive after birth, but feed poorly and usually die within 4 weeks. Histologic examination has shown loss of sensory neurons in the dorsal root ganglia and in particular the vestibular and nodose ganglia (reviewed in reference 91). Interestingly, developmental motor neuron cell death is not enhanced in BDNF-deficient mice. It was speculated that this could be due to the presence of NT-4 in muscle and a compensatory effect of this neurotrophin through trk-B which is

shared as a receptor. However, mice in which both BDNF and NT-4 were deleted also did not show enhanced motor neuron loss[92,93]. Similarly, and in contrast to original reports[94], mice with inactivated trk-B also did not show enhanced motor neuron cell death[46]. The loss of sensory neurons was slightly higher in the trigeminal ganglia in trk-B knockout mice[94] than in BDNF-deficient mice[92]. The highest loss of neurons in BDNF-deficient mice was observed in the vestibular ganglion (90–96% reduction) and in the nodose–petrosal ganglion complex (60% loss). This result indicates that NT-4 does not compensate for lack of BDNF in this neuronal population. Altogether, these analyses revealed that the physiologic requirement of these different populations of neurons for individual factors of the neurotrophin family vary, and that compensatory effects between various members of the neurotrophin family exist, but they are not of major relevance for survival during development.

Many types of neuron also express trk-C, the specific receptor for NT-3, often in combination with trk-B. In particular spinal motor neurons express relatively high levels of this receptor. This appears to be relevant, as NT-3 is the most abundantly expressed neurotrophin in skeletal muscle, both during development and in the adult. For comparison, levels of BDNF expression in muscle are very low[87]. From trk-C and NT-3 knockout mice, there is good evidence that the γ-motor neurons innervating the muscle spindles are dependent on NT-3 for their physiologic development[95,96]. However, NT-3 also supports survival of facial motor neurons after nerve lesion, a population of motor neurons which does not contain γ-motor neurons[72]. Therefore, subpopulations of α-motor neurons should also be responsive to NT-3. This is also suggested by the observation that trk-C mRNA is highly expressed in spinal and brainstem motor neurons. During embryonic development, the spinal motor neurons express NT-3 at relatively high levels[97]. This suggested that NT-3 could function as an autocrine factor during this period. However, gene ablation of

NT-3 did not lead to reduced numbers of α-motor neurons. It appears that the NT-3 produced in motor neurons serves as a neurotrophic factor and axon-attractant for proprioceptive neurons which invade the spinal cord through the dorsal horn and make contacts with the ventral motor neurons. In addition, NT-3 from motor neurons could function on upper motor neurons, which have been shown to respond to this factor[98].

NT-4/5 can also bind to trk-B and support motor neurons, most probably through this receptor. Therefore, redundancy of these two ligands in their functional motor neurons has been suggested[90,92,93]. However, this is not necessarily the case. Splice variants of trk-B have been identified with increased specificity for BDNF[99], and it is not clear so far whether such splice variants with increased specificity for each of these ligands are expressed on motor neurons. This could be relevant for consideration of the therapeutic potential of these two ligands for treatment of neurodegenerative diseases.

NT-3 expression is detectable in skeletal muscle both during development and in the adult. After muscle denervation either by nerve transection or by transient blockade of neuronal transmission by injection of tetrodotoxin into the sciatic nerve, NT-4 expression is rapidly down-regulated in adult rats[87]. Electrical stimulation of motor nerves leads to the opposite effect, a significant upregulation of NT-4 expression[100]. These data suggest that neuronal activity at the neuromuscular endplate has a significant influence on NT-4 expression in skeletal muscle, and NT-4 could be involved in regulating the efficacy of neuromuscular transmission, as has been shown in co-cultures of *Xenopus* motor neurons and skeletal muscle after addition of NT-3 or BDNF[101].

GLIA-DERIVED NEUROTROPHIC FACTOR AND RELATED MOLECULES

GDNF was identified in 1993 as a potent survival factor for midbrain dopaminergic neurons[102].

Very soon it became apparent that this protein, which shares distant structural homologies with members of the transforming growth factor (TGF)β gene family, is also an effective survival factor for other populations of neurons, in particular motor neurons. In cell cultures of embryonic rat motor neurons, 0.2 pg/ml corresponding to 7 fM supported half-maximal survival[103]. Thus GDNF appears to be several orders of magnitude more potent than brain-derived neurotrophic factor (BDNF), CNTF or LIF. The same report showed no effect of GDNF on sensory, trigeminal or sympathetic neurons derived from embryonic or perinatal rats[104]. GDNF is expressed in skeletal muscle of 13-day-old rat embryos, but expression in this tissue is not detectable in adult rats. However, GDNF mRNA is found in Schwann cell lines, and nerve lesion increases GDNF mRNA expression within 2 days to maximal levels. Therefore, a function of GDNF as an endogenous lesion factor for axotomized motor neurons (and probably other types of neuron) was proposed, closely resembling the function of LIF and CNTF.

An effect of GDNF on peripheral sympathetic and sensory neurons was observed in studies with chick embryos[105]. The application of GDNF to the chorioallantoic membrane led to increased motor neuron survival during the critical period of physiologic cell death, but also increased the number of surviving sympathetic and sensory neurons.

Mice in which the GDNF gene was inactivated showed renal agenesis and a complete lack of neurons in the autonomic ganglia of the gut which form the myenteric plexus[106–108]. Analysis of the nervous system identified deficits in several populations of sensory neurons, in particular from dorsal root, sympathetic and nodose ganglia. A small reduction in trigeminal and spinal lumbar motor neurons in the range of 20% was found, but not in facial motor neurons. Therefore GDNF does not play a key role in regulating survival of motor neurons during embryonic development.

The GDNF receptor complex involves a low-affinity binding component (GFRα1)[109], which is linked to the membrane via a GPI anchor in a similar manner to CNTFRα. In contrast to the CNTF/LIF-receptor complex, signal transduction of GDNF and related molecules is mediated by a tyrosine kinase (c-ret), which associates with the GFRα receptors after ligand binding and transmits the ligand-induced signal to the cell[110–112]. Thus, Ret-deficient mice show similar severe defects in kidney development and in the enteric nervous system[113,114].

The GDNF gene family now comprises three additional factors which also activate the Ret tyrosine kinase receptor which is shared by all these ligands. These molecules have been named neurturin, persephin and artemin. They seem to bind with some preference to one of the four α receptors, named GFRα1, GFRα2, GFRα3 and GFRα4. GDNF preferentially binds to GFRα1, neurturin to GFRα2, artemin to GFRα3 and persephin to GFRα4. However, neurturin and artemin also bind to GFRα1, so that there is a structural basis for functional overlap between these ligands. The genes for the Ret tyrosine kinase, the GFRα receptors, GDNF and other ligands have been inactivated in mice by standard techniques. Mice with deficiency in Ret[115], GFRα1[116] and GDNF[106–108] die during development. GDNF- and GFRα1-deficient mice fail to develop kidneys and enteric neurons and die around birth. Ret and GFRα1 are expressed in the embryonic ureteric bud, and GDNF is found in the metanephrogenic mesenchyme to which the ureteric buds grow during development. In ret-deficient mice, in addition to the lack of kidneys, many apoptotic cells are found in the foregut, and these mice show a massive loss of sympathetic neurons in the superior cervical ganglia. In this respect, they differ from GDNF-deficient mice. Significant loss of neurons in the GDNF-/- mice is also observed in nodose and sensory dorsal root ganglia, whereas loss of motor neurons is in the range of 20–30%, thus resembling CT-1-/- mice.

Neurturin binds preferentially to GFRα2, and gene knockout for this ligand or its corresponding α receptor does not lead to severe developmental defects. The mice are born, and they develop and breed normally, without any major organ defects[117,118]. A decrease in density of the myenteric plexus was observed which correlates with the relatively high expression of the GFRα2 receptor in autonomic neurons within the gut and bowel after birth. Also, some reduction of GFRα2-expressing sensory neurons in the dorsal root ganglia of neurturin-deficient mice have been observed, in particular in a population of neurons conferring heat sensitivity. However, it is not yet clear whether this reflects a loss of this subpopulation or simply the fact that expression of GFRα2 is reduced and function is disturbed when the ligand is lacking.

Mice with gene knockout of GFRα3 have been generated[119], and the phenotype of these mice indicates that artemin/GFRα3 signaling plays a major role for migration and differentation of sympathetic neurons in the superior cervical ganglion. GFRα3-deficient mice show ptosis, which is due to lack of lacrimal gland innervation. Interestingly, no major defect was observed in paravertebral sympathetic and sensory ganglia. Mice with deficiency of GFRα4 have been generated; they seem to be viable and fertile, and no gross abnormalities have been observed to date[120].

Altogether, a significant overlap of defects between the GDNF and the neurotrophin families was observed, indicating that these two families of neurotrophic factors act together in promoting migration, differentiation, survival and function of specific populations of neurons. Currently, many efforts are being made to investigate these functional co-operations in more detail, and mouse models, in particular mice in which individual gene defects are combined in double and triple mutants, play a major role in these studies. So far, there is no evidence that gene defects in any member of the GDNF family or in the receptor genes is associated with motor neuron disease. Based on the high potency of GDNF in supporting survival of motor neurons, this factor has been used in clinical trials with ALS patients, but these have not demonstrated any efficacy. Interestingly, the application of GDNF to pmn mutant mice led to a significant effect on the survival of the motor neurons, but there was no clinical effect because the factor did not inhibit or delay axonal degeneration[121]. It is possible that the same effect occurred in patients. However, no data are available from the clinical trials on whether GDNF could prevent the cell death of motor neuron cell bodies in the spinal cord. If this were the case, then combinations of GDNF with drugs that specifically block axonal degeneration would be worth reconsidering for further clinical development.

HEPATOCYTE GROWTH FACTOR/SCATTER FACTOR

The hepatocyte growth factor (HGF) and its specific receptor, the c-*met*-receptor tyrosine kinase, regulate growth, motility and morphogenesis of many cell types and organs. Originally, HGF was identified as a mitogen for developing hepatocytes. Its effect on the motility of cultured cells led to its independent discovery under the name 'scatter factor (SF)'. In addition, the factor was shown to promote survival of serum-deprived PC-12 rat pheochromocytoma cells[122] and thus was brought in context with neuronal survival factors. The effect on motor neurons first became apparent when researchers investigated its role in axon outgrowth[123]. It was found that HGF could attract motor axons and function as a chemoattractant from limb-mesenchyme for the developing and growing motor axons. Mice in which the receptor for HGF/SF was inactivated showed a severe defect in the migration of muscle precursor cells into the developing limb[124]. As a consequence, skeletal muscle did not form in limb and the diaphragm. Thus, the HGF/SF produced in limb-mesenchyme could serve as a chemoattractant both for migrating muscle precursor cells and growing motor axons. At later stages, when the myoblasts have migrated into the developing limbs and formed skeletal muscle, expression of

this factor can be identified directly in skeletal muscle. Moreover, isolated motor neurons from 15-day-old rat embryos showed enhanced survival in the presence of HGF/SF which was in the same range as with other neurotrophic factors such as CNTF, BDNF or GDNF[125]. These results were confirmed by other groups[126]. Interestingly, the effect of HGF/SF on motor neuron survival was shown to be synergistic with CNTF, and co-treatment with CNTF and HGF could protect cultured motor neurons from at least some of the toxic effects of vincristine.

However, HGF/SF acts only on a subpopulation (40%) of isolated motor neurons[126] corresponding to a restricted expression of c-*met* in subgroups of motor neurons, in particular those innervating the upper and lower limbs. Around birth, c-*met* expression is markedly reduced in motor neurons, indicating that motor neurons respond to HGF/SF only during this developmental period. However, two recent studies have demonstrated that both HGF/SF and c-*met* expression is upregulated in motor neurons under pathophysiological conditions in ALS[127]. The upregulation of HGF was also observed in a gene expression screen from the spinal cord of ALS patients[128]. In light of these data, reports that HGF/SF overexpression leads to a robust beneficial effect in the mutant SOD mouse model of familial ALS are of great interest[20]. Future studies have to show how HGF interferes with the disease process, and whether endogenous HGF/SF expression plays a modulatory role in the disease.

INSULIN-LIKE GROWTH FACTORS

The IGFs (IGF-I and IGF-II) are members of a family that also includes insulin and relaxins[129]. In contrast to most other neurotrophic factors, IGFs are found in significant quantities in the circulation and act as hormones. For example, IGF-I has been shown to be the effector of growth hormone actions in various tissues. Indeed, most cells express receptors for IGF-I and -II and the actions of these factors are not specific to motor neurons. The IGF-I-receptor which mediates the cellular effects of IGF-I and IGF-II is highly expressed in developing brain, but downregulated after birth. In contrast, most motor neurons maintain relatively high levels of IGF-I-receptor expression throughout life. What the specific functions of IGF-I and IGF-II for survival and functional maintenance of developing and postnatal motor neurons are, is not yet clear. The actions of IGFs are modulated by several binding proteins, and at least one of these binding proteins (IGF-BP-5) is strongly expressed in Schwann cells[130] and skeletal muscle. It is highly likely that the actions of glia- and muscle-derived IGFs on motoneurons are modulated by such IGF-binding proteins. These findings have consequences for the potential therapeutic functions of IGFs in patients with ALS, as such binding proteins influence the pharmacokinetics and availability of systemically injected IGFs.

Mice that lack either IGF-I, IGF-II or IGFR expression[131–133] were not helpful in defining the specific role of these molecules for developing motor neurons. These mice showed retarded growth and defects in many organs, so that a putative reduction in motor neuron survival could have many reasons, such as dysgenesis of Schwann cells and skeletal muscle. On the other hand, IGFs are potent survival factors for cultured motor neurons[90], and injection of IGF into skeletal muscle or lesioned nerve stump shows distinct effects on motor neurons, in particular terminal sprouting at the motor endplates and enhanced survival of motor neuron cell bodies[134–136]. Clinical trials with IGF-I in patients with ALS have led to controversial conclusions (Table 15.2) and it is not yet clear so far whether this factor can be used for therapy. However, recent data showing robust effects of IGF-I gene therapy in SOD mutant mice[137] rise hopes again that this factor could be further developed for therapy, at least for sub-populations of ALS patients.

VASCULAR ENDOTHELIAL GROWTH FACTOR AND ITS HOMOLOGS

VEGF was discovered in 1983 as a molecule which increases vascular permeability, hence it was originally named 'vascular permeability factor'[138]. VEGF has many effects on endothelial cells: it regulates their proliferation, migration and survival. The protein forms a homodimer and binds to three types of tyrosine kinase receptor, which are called VEGFR-1 (Flt1), VEGFR-2 (KDR/Flk1) and VEGFR-3. Ligand-binding induces receptor dimerization, tyrosine phosphorylation and activation of down-stream signaling pathways which are similar to those activated by trk-receptors or c-*ret* and other transmembrane tyrosine kinase receptors with neurotrophic activity.

VEGF belongs to a family of growth factors that includes placenta growth factor (PlGF), VEGF-B, VEGF-C and VEGF-D. These ligands differ in their preference for binding to VEGFR-1, VEGFR-2 and VEGFR-3. VEGF binds both to VEGFR-1 and -2. PlGF and VEGF-B bind to VEGFR-1, whereas VEGF-C and VEGF-D bind to VEGFR-2 and VEGFR-3, which is also named Flt4. Gene knockout studies in mice revealed that VEGFR-2 signaling plays a major role for angiogenesis in response to VEGF[139], whereas VEGFR-1 modulates the VEGF/VEGFR-2 response. Interestingly, there are two additional VEGF receptors which are named neuropilin-1 and neuropilin-2, which specifically bind two splice variants of VEGF named VEGF165 and VEGF155 in the case of neuropilin-2[140,141]. These receptors are not tyrosine kinase receptors, and they have initially been identified as receptors for semaphorin 3A and semaphorin 3C and 3F[142].

The first evidence that VEGF also has neurotrophic activity came from experiments with explant cultures of dorsal root ganglia. In these explants, VEGF stimulated axon outgrowth and neuronal survival. This effect was mediated through the VEGFR-2 receptor[143,144]. Similar neurotrophic effects were also observed for dopaminergic neurons of the ventral mesencephalon[145]

				BW, 3 injections per week	indications for efficacy	loss	
CNTF	ALS	Phase 1, placebo-controlled 4 weeks	43 patients in treatment and placebo groups	Subcutaneous, 2–200 µg/kg BW daily	Safe, tolerated within acceptable limits	Fever, HSV-1 stomatitis, diarrhea, fatigue, cough, weight loss	148
CNTF	ALS	Phase 2–3, placebo-controlled 6 months	570 patients	Subcutaneous, 0.5–5µg/kg BW daily	No beneficial effects, increased adverse events in the 5 µg/kg group and increased deaths	Injection-site reactions, cough, asthenia, nausea, anorexia, weight loss, increased salivation	149
CNTF	ALS	Phase 2–3, Placebo-controlled 9 months	730 patients	Subcutaneous, 15–30 µg/kg BW, 3 times a week	No beneficial effects	Anorexia, weight loss, cough	150
CNTF	ALS	Phase 1, open label	6 patients	Cell capsules, intrathecal, approximately 0.5 µg/day	Safe, motor performance did not improve	Headache radicular pain	151
CNTF	ALS	Phase 1, open label, 48 h per week, 2-week cycles	4 patients	Intrathecal delivery with pumps, 0.4–8 µg/h	Tolerable side-effects	Rise in lymphocyte numbers and protein levels in CSF, headache. radicular pain	152
NGF	Diabetic neuropathy	Phase 1–2, placebo controlled 6 months	250 patients	Subcutaneous, 0.3µg/kg BW, 3 times a week	Preliminary evidence for efficacy, well tolerated	Injection site pain	153
NGF	Diabetic neuropathy	Phase 3, placebo-controlled, double-blind 48 weeks	1019 patients, 505 NGF treated, 515 placebo group	Subcutaneous 0.1 µg/kg, 3 times a week	No clinical benefit	Minor side-effects, injection site pain	154
NGF	HIV neuropathy	Phase 2, placebo-controlled 18 weeks	270 patients	Subcutaneous, 0.1–0.3 µg/kgm BW, twice a week	Significant improvements in neuro-pathic pain	Injection-site pain	155
NGF	HIV neuropathy	Phase 2, open label follow-up study 48 weeks	200 patients	Subcutaneous, 0.1–0.3 µg/kg BW Twice a week	Well tolerated, improvement in pain symptoms, no improvement of neuropathy severity	Injection-site pain	156
BDNF	ALS	Phase 1–2 6 months	224 patients with BDNF 59 patients with placebo	Subcutaneous, 10–300 µg/kg BW, daily	Safe, tolerable, less deterioration in forced vital capacity and walking speed	Injection-site reactions, bowel urgency, diarrhea	157

Continue

Table 15.2 Continued...

	Disease	Type of trial	n	Application, dose	Result	Side-effects	Reference
BDNF	ALS	Phase 2–3, placebo-controlled 9 months	748 patients with BDNF, 387 patients with placebo	Subcutaneous, 25–100 μg/kg BW	No significant effect, subgroup of patients with early respiratory impairment and those developing altered bowel function showed statistically significant benefit	Injection-site reactions, diarrhea, bowel urgency, generally mild or moderate	158
BDNF	ALS	Phase 1–2, placebo-controlled, double-blind 12 weeks	25 patients	Intrathecal, continuous pump delivery, 25–1000 μg/day	Well tolerated at 150 μg/day or lower	Paresthesias, sleep disturbance, dry mouth, agitation at higher doses	159
BDNF	ALS	Phase 2–3, placebo-controlled, double-blind	250 patients	Intrathecal	No clinical benefit	Paresthesias, sleep disturbance	Unpublished
BDNF	Diabetic neuropathy	Phase 1–2, placebo-controlled, double-blind 3 months	30 patients, 21 with BDNF treatment, 9 patients with placebo	Subcutaneous, daily 100 μg/kg BW	No measurable beneficial effect; safe, tolerable	Non-painful injection-site reactions	160
NT-3	Healthy subjects Diabetic neuropathy Chemotherapy-induced neuropathy	Phase 1, placebo-controlled, double-blind, 7 days and unpublished	70 healthy subjects, 49 treated with NT-3 and 21 with placebo No published report on patient studies	Subcutaneous, daily, 3–500 μg/kg/day, and unpublished	Tolerable side-effects, patient studies discontinued in 1997	Diarrhea, injection-site pain, rise in SGOT and SGPT	161 and unpublished
IGF-I	ALS	Phase 2–3, placebo-controlled, double-blind 9 months	266 patients, 176 with IGF-I, 90 placebo	Subcutaneous, 50 or 100 μg/kg/day	Trend to functional improvement	Injection-site pain, no major side-effects	162
IGF-I	ALS	Phase 2–3, placebo-controlled, double-blind 9 months	124 patients with IGF-I, 59 patients with placebo	Subcutaneous, 100 μg/kg/day	No significant clinical improvement	Injection-site pain	163

and in cortical neuronal culture after hypoxia[164,165]. The functions in the nervous system are not restricted to neurons. VEGF also affects glial cells. For example, it stimulates mitosis of astrocytes[145,166] and this effect seems to be mediated by VEGFR-1, which is predominantly expressed in glial cells of the nervous system. Also, Schwann cells of the peripheral nervous system react to VEGF; these cells express VEGFR-1, VEGFR-2 and NP-1. VEGF stimulates Schwann cell migration via VEGFR-2[167].

In general, VEGF expression is induced by tissue hypoxia. This then leads to angiogenesis and increased supply of oxygen to ischemic tissues. There is a specific domain in the promoter region of the VEGF gene, the hypoxia response element (HRE), which specifically binds the hypoxia-inducible transcription factor-1 (HIF-1)[168,169]. HIF-1 is composed of two subunits called HIF-1α and HIF-1β. HIF-1α is strongly upregulated by hypoxia and rapidly degraded under non-toxic conditions.

An important first indication that VEGF also plays a role in the pathogenesis of motor neuron disease came from experiments with mice in which the HRE in the VEGF promoter was inactivated. These so-called VEGF$^{\delta/\delta}$ mice express lower levels of VEGF under normal conditions, and the upregulation of VEGF expression after hypoxia does not occur in the nervous system. About half of these mice die around birth, and the others develop motor neuron disease at an age of about 6 months[29]. Interestingly, sensory defects were not observed. Signs of motor neuron degeneration were seen both on the histopathological level and in many behavioral tests. The relevance of these findings for development of motor neuron disease in humans became clear by genetic testing in sporadic ALS patients. It appeared that polymorphisms in the VEGF promoter region which led to lower levels of VEGF were more common in ALS patients than in controls[28]. However, a significant difference was not found in another study with 96 ALS patients and 188 controls[170]. On the other hand, mouse models for spinal and bulbar muscular atrophy (Kennedy's disease) also showed reduced levels of VEGF, and this reduction was observed even at a presymptomatic stage[171]. These findings raise the question of whether vascular defects contribute to the pathogenesis of motor neuron disease, or whether insufficiency to respond to hypoxic conditions such as under reduced levels of HIF-1 or reduced expression of VEGF is involved in the pathogenesis of motor neuron disease. Interestingly, in the VEGF$^{\delta/\delta}$ mice, no signs of microangiopathy were observed. However, reduced blood flow was detectable, and it could well be that chronic ischemia contributes to development of motor neuron degeneration, at least in this mouse model[29]. Alternatively, it could be that VEGF plays a direct role in motor neuron survival and functional maintenance. This is supported by findings that VEGF also promotes survival and axon growth of isolated embryonic motor neurons[29]. Both neuropilin-1 and VEGFR-2 play a role as receptors to mediate this effect. Treatment of SOD G93A mutant rats with VEGF led to a significant delay of disease onset and ameliorated the deterioration in motor performance[172]. These effects were observed both after direct intracerebroventricular infusion of the VEGF protein in rats and in mice after intramuscular injection of lentivirus, which could be taken up by motor neurons and led to VEGF production in the neurons after retrograde transport[173].

These findings raise high hopes that VEGF could be used for therapy of ALS. However, VEGF also stimulates astrocytes and microglia. Moreover, VEGF leads to enhanced vascular permeability, so that activation of glial cells as well as alterations in the blood–brain barrier are to be expected as side-effects. It needs to be clarified whether such side-effects preclude the suitability of this protein for therapy, and whether it is possible to develop either special modes of administration or, alternatively, isoforms of VEGF that do not show such side-effects.

PREVIOUS CLINICAL TRIALS AND THERAPEUTIC POTENTIAL OF NEUROTROPHIC FACTORS FOR TREATMENT OF AMYOTROPHIC LATERAL SCLEROSIS

A series of studies have been performed during recent years in order to assess the therapeutic potential of neurotrophic factors in ALS patients (Table 15.2). In general, the results of these clinical trials were not encouraging[174]. The effects on disease progression were generally low or not significant, and side-effects became apparent, in particular in the case of CNTF. In general, these observations are not very surprising. Neurotrophic factors are normally produced in cells that are in direct contact with motor neurons and reach the motor neurons within a microenvironment determined by the contact sites of these two cells. In this sense, the situation differs completely from other recombinant proteins which are successfully introduced as therapeutic agents, such as erythropoietin, a hormone that is secreted into the circulation and then enhances the generation of erythrocytes or, as a second example, interferons, which are produced in a variety of tissues, released into the blood and other body fluids, and thus influence cells of the immune system. Nevertheless, the positive effects of neurotrophic factors in mouse mutants serving as animal models for human motor neuron disease (Figure 15.2) demonstrate that these molecules can interfere with apoptotic mechanisms which underlie the degeneration of motor neurons in human ALS[175]. Therefore, improved techniques for administration of these neurotrophic factors at sites where they can be taken up and retrogradely transported in motor neurons should be helpful in providing adequate conditions under which these factors might interfere with pathogenic processes in ALS.

At the moment, there are no clinically established means of administering neurotrophic factors in a way resembling the physiological availability from Schwann cells or muscle cells. Viral gene transfer in Schwann cells and skeletal muscle[176–178]

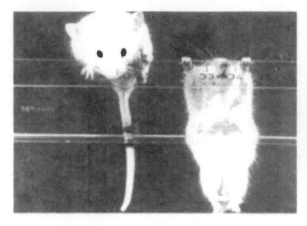

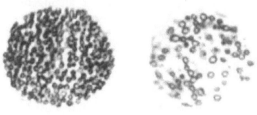

Figure 15.2 The effect of CNTF treatment in pmn mice. Two homozygous pmn mice were treated either with CNTF-secreting D3 cells (left) or with untransfected control cells (right). The cells were injected intraperitoneally after the first symptoms could be detected in these mice at postnatal day 20. The mice shown are 36 days old. The CNTF-treated mice survived longer and showed improved motor performance. Morphology of the phrenic nerve of the CNTF-treated and untreated pmn mouse: in CNTF-treated pmn mice, more myelinated axons could be detected in the phrenic nerve, suggesting that the CNTF treatment did not only maintain motor neuron cell bodies, but led to axonal preservation and regeneration. (Reproduced with permission from reference 49. © Macmillan Magazines Ltd)

has shown promising results in pmn mice and in newborn rats after peripheral nerve lesion. In particular, survival in the presence of BDNF could be prolonged in comparison to experimental setups in which the factor was given systemically or repeatedly at high concentrations[179–181].

Intrathecal administration, which is an established method to administer Baclofen to spinal neurons, appears as a promising technique to make these factors continuously available to ventral roots, where they can be taken up and retrogradely transported the short distance to the cell bodies of

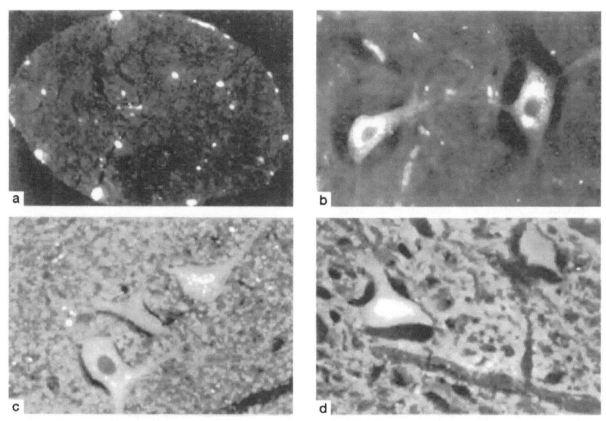

Figure 15.3 Distribution and effect of intrathecally administrated brain-derived neurotrophic factor (BDNF) in adult sheep. After chronic intrathecal infusion of BDNF, BDNF is (a) taken up in axons within the ventral root and (b) retrogradely transported to the motor neuron cell bodies, where it can be detected in vesicle-like structures around the nucleus. C-*fos* immunoreactivity in spinal motor neurons of (c) a control saline-treated sheep, and (d) a sheep that was treated with BDNF for 7 weeks. Chronic infusion of BDNF led to an increase of c-*fos* immunoreactivity and a translocation to cellular compartments in or close to the nucleus. (Reproduced with permission from reference 182)

motor neurons[182] and lead to celluar effects (Figure 15.3). Alternatively, the implantation of encapsulated cells continuously releasing such neurotrophic factors in low, but physiologically relevant concentrations also appears straightforward[151] for therapeutic administration of neurotrophic molecules. Also, recombinant viruses have been developed which are specifically taken up by motor neurons and retrogradely transported, and which are thought to lead to specific expression of therapeutic genes only in motor neurons. Using such viruses for gene transfer of IGF-I[137], robust therapeutic effects can be observed in SOD mutant mice, the model for familial ALS type I.

Not much is known on how the availability and kinetics of pharmacologically administered neurotrophic factors is modified *in vivo*. In the case of IGF-I and IGF-II, several binding proteins exist which influence the biologic functions of these molecules *in vivo*. This could explain why the systemic delivery of the factor in patients (Table 15.2) or in mouse models of ALS[183,184] leads to less robust effects than delivery with recombinant lentiviruses which are specifically taken up by motor neurons[137]. IGF-I differs from other neurotrophic factors by its capability of crossing the blood–brain barrier[185]. Endogenous IGF-I is present in relatively high quantities in blood, but apparently this endogenous resource of IGF-I does not become available to the degenerating motor neurons in ALS patients. Similarly, BDNF is found at high concentrations in human platelets[186], and again, one has to assume that the degenerating motor neurons do not have access to BDNF from this circulating source. The physiologic function of BDNF in platelets is not clear. Therefore, systemic BDNF administration could interfere with such unknown functions and cause side-effects. Side-effects are also expected when specific receptors for neurotrophic factors are expressed in many organs. For example, liver cells express the receptors for hepatocyte growth factor and leukemia-inhibitory factor, so that side-effects are likely in members of the CNTF family[187] or hepatocyte growth factors are administered systemically. In addition, receptors for neurotrophins (p75[NTR], trk-C, trk-B) are widely expressed in the peripheral nervous system, and specific side-effects are to be expected even when these molecules are administered more locally, for example into the subarachnoidal space.

Experiments with isolated motor neurons in cell culture as well as data from *in vivo* experiments have shown that neurotrophic factors cooperate in supporting motor neuron survival. Some combinations even appear supra-additive. The combination of CNTF and IGF-I, for example, enhances survival of embryonic chick motor neurons in culture at a rate that is higher than the addition of the survival effects of each factor alone[33,90]. Such potentiating effects by combinations of neurotrophic molecules have been observed in many studies. It is to be expected that studies with intercrosses of different gene knockout mice[13] will lead to a better understanding of the individual function of each neurotrophic factor both on motor neuron survival and on distinct functional parameters such as axon regeneration, dendrite growth, motor endplate function and synaptic activity. A better understanding of these functions, which meets a more detailed knowledge about the pathogenic processes underlying human ALS and spinal muscular atrophy, will help to redefine the therapeutic potential of these factors for treatment of this form of human motor neuron disease.

REFERENCES

1. Oppenheim RW. The absence of significant postnatal motoneuron death in the brachial and lumbar spinal cord of the rat. J Comp Neurol 1986; 246: 281–6

2. Oppenheim RW. Naturally occuring cell death during neural development. TINS 1985; 8: 487–93

3. Hamburger V. The effects of wing bud extirpation on the development of the central nervous system in chick embryos. J Exp Zool 1934; 68: 449–94

4. Hamburger V. Regression versus peripheral control of differentiation in motor hyperplasia. Am J Anat 1958; 102: 365–410

5. Riethmacher D, Sonnenberg-Riethmacher E, Brinkmann V, et al. Severe neuropathies in mice with targeted mutations in the ErbB3 receptor. Nature 1997; 389: 725–30

6. Falls DL, Rosen KM, Corfas G, et al. ARIA, a protein that stimulates acetylcholine receptor synthesis, is a member of the neu ligand family. Cell 1993; 72: 801–15

7. Marchionni MA, Goodearl ADJ, Chen MS, et al. Glial growth factors are alternatively spliced erbB2 ligands expressed in the nervous system. Nature 1993; 263: 312–18

8. Altiok N, Bessereau JL, Changeux JP. ErbB3 and ErbB2/neu mediate the effect of heregulin on acetylcholine receptor gene expression in muscle: Differential expression at the endplate. EMBO J 1995; 15: 4258–66

9. Jo SA, Zhu X, Marchionni MA, Burden SJ. Neuregulins are concentrated at nerve–muscle synapses and activate ACh-receptor gene expression. Nature 1995; 373: 158–61

10. Tansey MG, Chu GC, Merlie JP. ARIA/HRG regulates AChR epsilon subunit gene expression at the neuromuscular synapse via activation of phosphatidylinositol 3- kinase and Ras/MAPK pathway. J Cell Biol 1996; 134: 465–76

11. Michailov GV, Sereda MW, Brinkmann BG, et al. Axonal neuregulin-1 regulates myelin sheath thickness. Science 2004; 304: 700–3

12. Sendtner M, Götz R, Holtmann B, et al. Cryptic physiological trophic support of motoneurons by

LIF disclosed by double gene targeting of CNTF and LIF. Curr Biol 1996; 6: 686–94

13. Holtmann B, Wiese S, Samsam M, et al. Triple knock-out of CNTF, LIF, and CT-1 defines cooperative and distinct roles of these neurotrophic factors for motoneuron maintenance and function. J Neurosci 2005; 25: 1778–87

14. Skaper SD, Negro A, Dal Toso R, Facci L. Recombinant human ciliary neurotrophic factor alters the threshold of hippocampal pyramidal neuron sensitivity to excitotoxin damage: Synergistic effects of monosialogangliosides. J Neurosci Res 1992; 33: 330–7

15. Scala S, Wosikowski K, Giannakakou P, et al. Brain-derived neurotrophic factor protects neuroblastoma cells from vinblastine toxicity. Cancer Res 1996; 56: 3737–42

16. Benigni F, Villa P, Demitri MT, et al. Ciliary neurotrophic factor inhibits brain and peripheral tumor necrosis factor production and, when coadministered with its soluble receptor, protects mice from lipopolysaccharide toxicity. Mol Med 1995; 1: 568–75

17. Ho TW, Bristol LA, Coccia C, et al. TGFbeta trophic factors differentially modulate motor axon outgrowth and protection from excitotoxicity. Exp Neurol 2000; 161: 664–75

18. Iwasaki Y, Ikeda K. Prevention by insulin-like growth factor-I and riluzole in motor neuron death after neonatal axotomy. J Neurol Sci 1999; 169: 148–55

19. Corse AM, Bilak MM, Bilak SR, et al. Preclinical testing of neuroprotective neurotrophic factors in a model of chronic motor neuron degeneration. Neurobiol Dis 1999; 6: 335–46

20. Sun W, Funakoshi H, Nakamura T. Overexpression of HGF retards disease progression and prolongs life span in a transgenic mouse model of ALS. J Neurosci 2002; 22: 6537–48

21. Vincent AM, Mobley BC, Hiller A, Feldman EL. IGF-I prevents glutamate-induced motor neuron programmed cell death. Neurobiol Dis 2004; 16: 407–16

22. Takahashi R, Yokoji H, Misawa H, et al. A null mutation in the human CNTF gene is not causally related to neurological diseases. Nat Genet 1994; 7: 79–84

23. Giess R, Götz R, Schrank B, et al. Potential implications of a ciliary neurotrophic factor gene mutation in a German population of patients with motor neuron disease. Muscle Nerve 1998; 21: 236–8

24. Giess R, Holtmann B, Braga M, et al. Early onset of severe familial amyotrophic lateral sclerosis with a SOD-1 mutation: Potential impact of CNTF as a candidate modifier gene. Am J Hum Genet 2002; 70: 1277–86

25. Masu Y, Wolf E, Holtmann B, et al. Disruption of the CNTF gene results in motor neuron degeneration. Nature 1993; 365: 27–32

26. Munsat TL, Andres PL, Finison L, et al. The natural-history of motoneuron loss in amyotrophic lateral sclerosis. Neurology 1988; 38: 409–13

27. Giess R, Beck M, Goetz R, et al. Potential role of LIF as a modifier gene in the pathogenesis of amyotrophic lateral sclerosis. Neurology 2000; 54: 1003–5

28. Lambrechts D, Storkebaum E, Morimoto M, et al. VEGF is a modifier of amyotrophic lateral sclerosis in mice and humans and protects motoneurons against ischemic death. Nat Genet 2003; 34: 383–94

29. Oosthuyse B, Moons L, Storkebaum E, et al. Deletion of the hypoxia-response element in the vascular endothelial growth factor promoter causes motor neuron degeneration. Nat Genet 2001; 28: 131–8

30. Stöckli KA, Lottspeich F, Sendtner M, et al. Molecular cloning, expression and regional distribution of rat ciliary neurotrophic factor. Nature 1989; 342: 920–3

31. Lin L-F, Mismer D, Lile JD, et al. Purification, cloning, and expression of ciliary neurotrophic factor (CNTF). Science 1989; 246: 1023–5

32. Sendtner M, Kreutzberg GW, Thoenen H. Ciliary neurotrophic factor prevents the degeneration of motor neurons after axotomy. Nature 1990; 345: 440–1

33. Arakawa Y, Sendtner M, Thoenen H. Survival effect of ciliary neurotrophic factor (CNTF) on chick embryonic motoneurons in culture: Comparison with other neurotrophic factors and cytokines. J Neurosci 1990; 10: 3507–15

34. Stahl N, Yancopoulos GD. The tripartite CNTF receptor complex: Activation and signaling involves components shared with other cytokines. J Neurobiol 1994; 25: 1454–66

35. Davis S, Aldrich TH, Ip NY, et al. Released form of cntf receptor-alpha component as a soluble mediator of cntf responses. Science 1993; 259: 1736–9

36. Gearing DP, Thut CJ, VandeBos T, et al. Leukemia inhibitory factor receptor is structurally related to the IL-6 signal transducer, gp130. EMBO J 1991; 10: 2839–48

37. Guillet C, Lelievre E, Plun-Favreau H, et al. Functionally active fusion protein of the novel composite cytokine CLC/soluble CNTF receptor. Eur J Biochem 2002; 269: 1932–41

38. Senaldi G, Varnum BC, Sarmiento U, et al. Novel neurotrophin-1/B cell-stimulating factor-3: A cytokine of the IL-6 family. Proc Natl Acad Sci USA 1999; 96: 11458–63

39. Gearing DP, Comeau MR, Friend DJ, et al. The IL-6 signal transducer, gp130: an oncostatin M receptor and affinity converter for the LIF receptor. Science 1992; 255: 1434–7

40. Pennica D, Shaw KJ, Swanson TA, et al. Cardiotrophin-1. Biological activities and binding to the leukemia inhibitory factor receptor/gp130 signaling complex. J Biol Chem 1995; 270: 10915–22

41. Elson GC, Lelievre E, Guillet C, et al. CLF associates with CLC to form a functional heteromeric ligand for the CNTF receptor complex. Nat Neurosci 2000; 3: 867–72

42. Sendtner M, Götz R, Holtmann B, Thoenen H. Endogenous ciliary neurotrophic factor is a lesion factor for axotomized motoneurons in adult mice. J Neurosci 1997; 17: 6999–7006

43. Banner LR, Patterson PH. Major changes in the expression of the mRNAs for cholinergic differentiation factor/leukemia inhibitory factor and its receptor after injury to adult peripheral nerves and ganglia. Proc Natl Acad Sci USA 1994; 91: 7109–13

44. Oppenheim RW, Wiese S, Prevette D, et al. Cardiotrophin-1, a muscle-derived cytokine, is required for the survival of subpopulations of developing motoneurons. J Neurosci 2001; 21: 1283–91

45. Li M, Sendtner M, Smith A. Essential function of LIF receptor in motor neurons. Nature 1995; 378: 724–7

46. DeChiara TM, Vejsada R, Poueymirou WT, et al. Mice lacking the CNTF receptor, unlike mice lacking CNTF, exhibit profound motor neuron deficits at birth. Cell 1995; 83: 313–22

47. Yoshida K, Taga T, Saito M, et al. Targeted disruption of gp130, a common signal transducer for the interleukin 6 family of cytokines, leads to myocardial and hematological disorders. Proc Natl Acad Sci USA 1996; 93: 407–11

48. Sendtner M, Stöckli KA, Thoenen H. Synthesis and location of ciliary neurotrophic factor in the rat sciatic nerve of the adult rat after lesion and during regeneration. J Cell Biol 1992; 118: 139–48

49. Sendtner M, Schmalbruch H, Stöckli KA, et al. Ciliary neurotrophic factor prevents degeneration of motor neurons in mouse mutant progressive motor neuronopathy. Nature 1992; 358: 502–4

50. Sagot Y, Tan SA, Baetge E, et al. Polymer encapsulated cell lines genetically engineered to release ciliary neurotrophic factor can slow down progressive motor neuronopathy in the mouse. Eur J Neurosci 1995; 7: 1313–22

51. Ikeda K, Klinkosz B, Greene T, et al. Effects of brain-derived neurotrophic factor on motor dysfunction in wobbler mouse motor neuron disease. Ann Neurol 1995; 37: 505–11

52. Mitsumoto H, Ikeda K, Klinkosz B, et al. Arrest of motor neuron disease in wobbler mice cotreated with CNTF and BDNF. Science 1994; 265: 1107–10

53. Mitsumoto H, Ikeda K, Holmlund T, et al. The effects of ciliary neurotrophic factor on motor dysfunction in wobbler mouse motor neuron disease. Ann Neurol 1994; 36: 142–8

54. Helgren ME, Friedman B, Kennedy M, et al. Ciliary neurotrophic factor (CNTF) delays motor impairments in the mnd mouse, a genetic model of motor neuron disease. Neurosci Abstr 1992; 267.11: 618

55. Martin N, Jaubert J, Gounon P, et al. A missense mutation in Tbce causes progressive motor neuronopathy in mice. Nat Genet 2002; 32: 443–7

56. Bommel H, Xie G, Rossoll W, et al. Missense mutation in the tubulin-specific chaperone E (Tbce) gene in the mouse mutant progressive motor neuronopathy, a model of human motoneuron disease. J Cell Biol 2002; 159: 563–9

57. Barde Y-A. The nerve growth factor family. Prog Growth Factor Res 1990; 2: 237–48

58. Eide FF, Lowenstein DH, Reichardt LF. Neurotrophins and their receptors – Current concepts and implications for neurologic disease. Exp Neurol 1993; 121: 200–14

59. Kerkhoff H, Troost D, Louwerse ES, et al. Inflammatory cells in the peripheral nervous system in motor neuron disease. Acta Neuropathol (Berl) 1993; 85: 560–5

60. Seeburger JL, Tarras S, Natter H, Springer JE. Spinal cord motoneurons express p75[NGFR] and p145[trkB] mRNA in amyotrophic lateral sclerosis. Brain Res 1993; 621: 111–15

61. Kaplan DR, Miller FD. Neurotrophin signal transduction in the nervous system. Curr Opin Neurobiol 2000; 10: 381–91

62. Dechant G, Barde YA. Signalling through the neurotrophin receptor p75NTR. Curr Opin Neurobiol 1997; 7: 413–18

63. Bothwell M. p75NTR: A receptor after all. Science 1996; 272: 506–7

64. Rabizadeh S, Oh J, Zhong L, et al. Induction of apoptosis by the low-affinity NGF receptor. Science 1993; 261: 345–8

65. Lee R, Kermani P, Teng KK, Hempstead BL. Regulation of cell survival by secreted proneurotrophins. Science 2001; 294: 1945–8

66. Nykjaer A, Lee R, Teng KK, et al. Sortilin is essential for proNGF-induced neuronal cell death. Nature 2004; 427: 843–8

67. Kim H, Li Q, Hempstead BL, Madri JA. Paracrine and autocrine functions of brain-derived neurotrophic factor (BDNF) and nerve growth factor (NGF) in brain-derived endothelial cells. J Biol Chem 2004; 279: 33538–46

68. Van der Zee CE, Ross GM, Riopelle RJ, Hagg T. Survival of cholinergic forebrain neurons in developing p75NGFR-deficient mice [see comments] [retracted by Hagg T. In: Science 1999; 285: 340]. Science 1996; 274: 1729–32

69. Wiese S, Metzger F, Holtmann B, Sendtner M. The role of p75NTR in modulating neurotrophin survival effects in developing motoneurons. Eur J Neurosci 1999; 11: 1668–76

70. Pang PT, Teng HK, Zaitsev E, et al. Cleavage of proBDNF by tPA/plasmin is essential for long-term hippocampal plasticity. Science 2004; 306: 487–91

71. Miyata Y, Kashihara Y, Homma S, Kuno M. Effects of nerve growth factor on the survival and synaptic function of Ia sensory neurons axotomized in neonatal rats. J Neurosci 1986; 6: 2012–18

72. Sendtner M, Holtmann B, Kolbeck R, et al. Brain-derived neurotrophic factor prevents the death of motoneurons in newborn rats after nerve section. Nature 1992; 360: 757–8

73. Frade JM, Rodriguez Tebar A, Barde YA. Induction of cell death by endogenous nerve growth factor through its p75 receptor. Nature 1996; 383: 166–8

74. Yan Q, Snider WD, Pinzone JJ, Johnson EM Jr. Retrograde transport of nerve growth factor (NGF) in motoneurons of developing rats: Assessment of potential neurotrophic effects. Neuron 1988; 1: 335–43

75. Stoeckel K, Schwab M, Thoenen H. Specificity of retrograde transport of nerve growth factor (NGF) in sensory neurons: A biochemical and morphological study. Brain Res 1975; 81: 1–14

76. Koliatsos VE, Shelton DL, Mobley WC, Price DL. A novel group of nerve growth factor receptor-immunoreactive neurons in the ventral horn of the lumbar spinal cord. Brain Res 1991; 541: 121–8

77. Wayne DB, Heaton MB. Retrograde transport of NGF by early chick embryo spinal cord motoneurons. Dev Biol 1988; 127: 220–3

78. Wayne DB, Heaton MB. The response of cultured trigeminal and spinal cord motoneurons to nerve growth factor. Dev Biol 1990; 138: 473–83

79. Wayne DB, Heaton MB. The ontogeny of specific retrograde transport of nerve growth factor by motoneurons of the brainstem and spinal cord. Dev Biol 1990; 138: 484–98

80. Yamashita T, Tucker KL, Barde YA. Neurotrophin binding to the p75 receptor modulates Rho activity and axonal outgrowth. Neuron 1999; 24: 585–93

81. Leibrock J, Lottspeich F, Hohn A, et al. Molecular cloning and expression of brain-derived neurotrophic factor. Nature 1989; 341: 149–52

82. Maisonpierre PC, Belluscio L, Squinto SP, et al. Neurotrophin-3: A neurotrophic factor related to NGF and BDNF. Science 1990; 247: 1446–51

83. Hohn A, Leibrock J, Bailey K, Barde Y-A. Identification and characterzation of a novel member of the nerve growth factor/brain-derived neurotrophic factor family. Nature 1990; 344: 339–41

84. Hallböök F, Ibáñez CF, Persson H. Evolutionary studies of the nerve growth factor family reveal a novel member abundantly expressed in Xenopus ovary. Neuron 1991; 6: 845–58

85. Berkemeier LR, Winslow JW, Kaplan DR, et al. Neurotrophin-5: A novel neurotrophic factor that activates trk and trkB. Neuron 1991; 7: 857–66

86. Henderson CE, Camu W, Mettling C, et al. Neurotrophins promote motor neuron survival and are present in embryonic limb bud. Nature 1993; 363: 266–70

87. Griesbeck O, Parsadanian AS, Sendtner M, Thoenen H. Expression of neurotrophins in skeletal muscle: Quantitative comparison and significance for motoneuron survival and maintenance of function. J Neurosci Res 1995; 42: 21–33

88. Yan Q, Elliott J, Snider WD. Brain-derived neurotrophic factor rescues spinal motorneurons from axotomy-induced cell death. Nature 1992; 360: 753–5

89. Oppenheim RW, Qin-Wei Y, Prevette D, Yan Q. Brain-derived neurotrophic factor rescues develop-

ing avian motoneurons from cell death. Nature 1992; 360: 755–7

90. Hughes RA, Sendtner M, Thoenen H. Members of several gene families influence survival of rat motoneurons in vitro and in vivo. J Neurosci Res 1993; 36: 663–71

91. Snider WD. Functions of the neurotrophins during nervous system development: What the knockouts are teaching us. Cell 1994; 77: 627–38

92. Conover JC, Erickson JT, Katz DM, et al. Neuronal deficits, not involving motor neurons, in mice lacking BDNF and/or NT4. Nature 1995; 375: 235–8

93. Liu X, Ernfors P, Wu H, Jaenisch R. Sensory but not motor neuron deficits in mice lacking NT4 and BDNF. Nature 1995; 375: 238–40

94. Klein R, Smeyne RJ, Wurst W, et al. Targeted disruption of the trkB neurotrophin receptor results in nervous system lesions and neonatal death. Cell 1993; 75: 113–122

95. Ernfors P, Kucera J, Lee KF, et al. Studies on the physiological role of brain-derived neurotrophic factor and neurotrophin-3 in knockout mice. Int J Dev Biol 1995; 39: 799–807

96. Kucera J, Ernfors P, Jaenisch R. Reduction in the number of spinal motor neurons in neurotrophin-3-deficient mice. Neuroscience 1995; 69: 312–30

97. Ernfors P, Persson H. Developmentally regulated expression of NDNF/NT-3 mRNA in rat spinal cord motoneurons and expression of BDNF mRNA in embryonic dorsal root ganglion. Eur J Neurosci 1991; 3: 953–61

98. Schnell L, Schneider R, Kolbeck R, et al. Neurotrophin-3 enhances sprouting of corticospinal tract during development and after spinal cord lesion. Nature 1994; 367: 170–3

99. Strohmaier C, Carter BD, Urfer R, et al. A splice variant of the neurotrophin receptor trkB with increased specificity for brain-derived neurotrophic factor. EMBO J 1996; 15: 3332–7

100. Funakoshi H, Belluasdo N, Arenas E, et al. Muscle-derived neurotrophin-4 as an activity-dependent trophic signal for adult motor neurons. Science 1995; 268: 1495–9

101. Lohof AM, Ip NY, Poo M. Potentiation of developing neuromuscular synapses by the neurotrophins NT-3 and BDNF. Nature 1993; 363: 350–3

102. Lin L-FH, Doherty DH, Lile JD, et al. GDNF: A glial cell line-derived neurotrophic factor for midbrain dopaminergic neurons. Science 1993; 260: 1130–2

103. Henderson CE, Phillips HS, Pollock RA, et al. GDNF: a potent survival factor for motoneurons present in peripheral nerve and muscle. Science 1994; 266: 1062–4

104. Henderson CE, Phillips HS, Pollock RA, et al. GDNF: a potent survival factor for motoneurons present in peripheral nerve and muscle [see comments]. Science 1994; 266: 1062–4

105. Oppenheim RW, Houenou LJ, Johnson JE, et al. Developing motor neurons rescued from programmed and axotomy-induced cell death by GDNF. Nature 1995; 373: 344–6

106. Moore MW, Klein RD, Farinas I, et al. Renal and neuronal abnormalities in mice lacking GDNF. Nature 1996; 382: 76–9

107. Pichel JG, Shen L, Sheng HZ, et al. Defects in enteric innervation and kidney development in mice lacking GDNF. Nature 1996; 382: 73–6

108. Sanchez MP, Silos Santiago I, Frisen J, et al. Renal agenesis and the absence of enteric neurons in mice lacking GDNF. Nature 1996; 382: 70–3

109. Jing S, Wen D, Yu Y, et al. GDNF-induced activation of the ret protein tyrosine kinase is mediated by GDNFR-alpha, a novel receptor for GDNF. Cell 1996; 85: 1113–24

110. Durbec P, Marcos Gutierrez CV, Kilkenny C, et al. GDNF signalling through the Ret receptor tyrosine kinase. Nature 1996; 381: 789–93

111. Trupp M, Arenas E, Fainzilber M, et al. Functional receptor for GDNF encoded by the c-ret proto-oncogene. Nature 1996; 381: 785–8

112. Treanor JJ, Goodman L, de Sauvage F, et al. Characterization of a multicomponent receptor for GDNF. Nature 1996; 382: 80–3

113. Taraviras S, Marcos-Gutierrez CV, Durbec P, et al. Signalling by the RET receptor tyrosine kinase and its role in the development of the mammalian enteric nervous system. Development 1999; 126: 2785–97

114. Baloh RH, Enomoto H, Johnson EM Jr, Milbrandt J. The GDNF family ligands and receptors. Curr Opin Neurobiol 2000; 10: 103–10

115. Schuchardt A, D'Agati V, Larsson-Blomberg L, et al. Defects in the kidney and enteric nervous system of mice lacking the tyrosine kinase receptor Ret. Nature 1994; 367: 380–3

116. Enomoto H, Araki T, Jackman A, et al. GFR alpha1-deficient mice have deficits in the enteric nervous system and kidneys. Neuron 1998; 21: 317–24

117. Rossi J, Luukko K, Poteryaev D, et al. Retarded growth and deficits in the enteric and parasympathetic nervous system in mice lacking GFR alpha2, a functional neurturin receptor. Neuron 1999; 22: 243–52

118. Heuckeroth RO, Enomoto H, Grider JR, et al. Gene targeting reveals a critical role for neurturin in the development and maintenance of enteric, sensory, and parasympathetic neurons [see comments]. Neuron 1999; 22: 253–63

119. Nishino J, Mochida K, Ohfuji Y, et al. GFR alpha3, a component of the artemin receptor, is required for migration and survival of the superior cervical ganglion. Neuron 1999; 23: 725–36

120. Airaksinen MS, Saarma M. The GDNF family: signalling, biological functions and therapeutic value. Nat Rev Neurosci 2002; 3: 383–94

121. Sagot Y, Tan SA, Hammang JP, et al. GDNF slows loss of motoneurons but not axonal degeneration or premature death of pmn/pmn mice. J Neurosci 1996; 16: 2335–41

122. Matsumoto K, Kagoshima M, Nakamura T. Hepatocyte growth factor as a potent survival factor for rat pheochromocytoma PC12 cells. Exp Cell Res 1995; 220: 71–78

123. Ebens A, Brose K, Leonardo ED, et al. Hepatocyte growth factor/scatter factor is an axonal chemoattractant and a neurotrophic factor for spinal motor neurons. Neuron 1996; 17: 1157–72

124. Bladt F, Riethmacher D, Isenmann S, et al. Essential role for the c-met receptor in the migration of myogenic precursor cells into the limb bud. Nature 1995; 376: 768–71

125. Wong V, Glass DJ, Arriaga R, et al. Hepatocyte growth factor promotes motor neuron survival and synergizes with ciliary neurotrophic factor. J Biol Chem 1997; 272: 5187–91

126. Yamamoto Y, Livet J, Pollock RA, et al. Hepatocyte growth factor (HGF/SF) is a muscle-derived survival factor for a subpopulation of embryonic motoneurons. Development 1997; 124: 2903–13

127. Kato S, Funakoshi H, Nakamura T, et al. Expression of hepatocyte growth factor and c-Met in the anterior horn cells of the spinal cord in the patients with amyotrophic lateral sclerosis (ALS): Immunohistochemical studies on sporadic ALS and familial ALS with superoxide dismutase 1 gene mutation. Acta Neuropathol (Berl) 2003; 106: 112–20

128. Jiang YM, Yamamoto M, Kobayashi Y, et al. Gene expression profile of spinal motor neurons in sporadic amyotrophic lateral sclerosis. Ann Neurol 2005; 57: 236–51

129. LeRoith D, Roberts CT Jr. Insulin-like growth factors. Ann NY Acad Sci 1993; 692: 1–9

130. Cheng HL, Randolph A, Yee D, et al. Characterization of insulin-like growth factor-I and its receptor and binding proteins in transected nerves and cultured Schwann cells. J Neurochem 1996; 66: 525–36

131. Liu J-P, Baker J, Perkins AS, et al. Mice carrying null mutations of the genes encoding insulin-like growth factor I (Igf-1) and type 1 IGF receptor (Igf1r). Cell 1993; 75: 59–72

132. Beck KD, Powell Braxton L, Widmer HR, et al. Igf1 gene disruption results in reduced brain size, CNS hypomyelination, and loss of hippocampal granule and striatal parvalbumin-containing neurons. Neuron 1995; 14: 717–30

133. DeChiara TM, Robertson EJ, Efstratiadis A. Parental imprinting of the mouse insulin-like growth factor II gene. Cell 1991; 64: 849–59

134. Caroni P, Schneider C. Signaling by insulin-like growth factors in paralyzed skeletal muscle: Rapid induction of IGF1 expression in muscle fibers and prevention of interstitial cell proliferation by IGF-BP5 and IGF-BP4. J Neurosci 1994; 14: 3378–88

135. Caroni P, Schneider C, Kiefer MC, Zapf J. Role of muscle insulin-like growth factors in nerve sprouting: Suppression of terminal sprouting in paralyzed muscle by IGF-binding protein 4. J Cell Biol 1994; 125: 893–902

136. Caroni P, Grandes P. Nerve sprouting in innervated skeletal muscle induced by exposure to elevated levels of insulin-like growth factors. J Cell Biol 1990; 110: 1307–17

137. Kaspar BK, Llado J, Sherkat N, et al. Retrograde viral delivery of IGF-1 prolongs survival in a mouse ALS model. Science 2003; 301: 839–42

138. Senger DR, Galli SJ, Dvorak AM, et al. Tumor cells secrete a vascular permeability factor that promotes accumulation of ascites fluid. Science 1983; 219: 983–5

139. Ferrara N. Role of vascular endothelial growth factor in regulation of physiological angiogenesis. Am J Physiol Cell Physiol 2001; 280: C1358–C1366

140. Soker S, Takashima S, Miao HQ, et al. Neuropilin-1 is expressed by endothelial and tumor cells as an isoform-specific receptor for vascular endothelial growth factor. Cell 1998; 92: 735–45

141. Miao HQ, Soker S, Feiner L, et al. Neuropilin-1 mediates collapsin-1/semaphorin III inhibition of

endothelial cell motility: Functional competition of collapsin-1 and vascular endothelial growth factor-165. J Cell Biol 1999; 146: 233–42

142. Chen H, Chedotal A, He Z, et al. Neuropilin-2, a novel member of the neuropilin family, is a high affinity receptor for the semaphorins Sema E and Sema IV but not Sema III. Neuron 1997; 19: 547–59

143. Sondell M, Lundborg G, Kanje M. Vascular endothelial growth factor has neurotrophic activity and stimulates axonal outgrowth, enhancing cell survival and Schwann cell proliferation in the peripheral nervous system. J Neurosci 1999; 19: 5731–40

144. Sondell M, Sundler F, Kanje M. Vascular endothelial growth factor is a neurotrophic factor which stimulates axonal outgrowth through the flk-1 receptor. Eur J Neurosci 2000; 12: 4243–54

145. Silverman WF, Krum JM, Mani N, Rosenstein JM. Vascular, glial and neuronal effects of vascular endothelial growth factor in mesencephalic explant cultures. Neuroscience 1999; 90: 1529–41

146. ALS CNTF Treatment Study (ACTS) Group. Recombinant human ciliary neurotrophic factor (rhCNTF) in amyotrophic lateral sclerosis: Phase I-II safety, tolerability and pharmakokinetic studies (abstract). Neurology 1993; 43: A416

147. ALS CNTF Treatment Study (ACTS) Phase I-II Group. The pharmacokinetics of subcutaneously adminstered recombinant human ciliary neurotrophic factor (rHCNTF) in patients with amyotrophic lateral scerosis. Clin Neuropharm 1995; 18: 500–18

148. Miller RG, Bryan WW, Dietz M, et al. Safety, tolerability and pharmakokinetics of recombinant human ciliary neurotrophic factor (rhCNTF) in patients with amyotrophic lateral sclerosis. Ann Neurol 1993; 34: 304

149. Miller RG, Petajan JH, Bryan WW, et al. A placebo-controlled trial of recombinant human ciliary neurotrophic (rhCNTF) factor in amyotrophic lateral sclerosis. Ann Neurol 1996; 39: 256–60

150. The ALS CNTF Study Group. A double-blind placebo-controlled clinical trial of subcutaneous recombinant human ciliary neurotrophic factor (rHCNTF) in amyotrophic lateral sclerosis. ALS CNTF Treatment Study Group. Neurology 1996; 46: 1244–9

151. Aebischer P, Schluep M, Deglon N, et al. Intrathecal delivery of CNTF using encapsulated genetically modified xenogeneic cells in amyotrophic lateral sclerosis patients. Nat Med 1996; 2: 696–9

152. Penn RD, Kroin JS, York MM, Cedarbaum JM. Intrathecal ciliary neurotrophic factor delivery for treatment of amyotrophic lateral sclerosis. Neurosurgery 1997; 40: 94–100

153. Apfel SC, Kessler JA, Adornato BT, et al. Recombinant human nerve growth factor in the treatment of diabetic polyneuropathy. NGF Study Group. Neurology 1998; 51: 695–702

154. Apfel SC, Schwartz S, Adornato BT, et al. Efficacy and safety of recombinant human nerve growth factor in patients with diabetic polyneuropathy: A randomized controlled trial. rhNGF Clinical Investigator Group. J Am Med Assoc 2000; 284: 2215–21

155. McArthur JC, Yiannoutsos C, Simpson DM, et al. A phase II trial of nerve growth factor for sensory neuropathy associated with HIV infection. AIDS Clinical Trials Group Team 291. Neurology 2000; 54: 1080–8

156. Schifitto G, Yiannoutsos C, Simpson DM, et al. Long-term treatment with recombinant nerve growth factor for HIV-associated sensory neuropathy. Neurology 2001; 57: 1313–16

157. Bradley WG, The BDNF Study Group. A phase I/II study of recombinant human brain-derived neurotrophic factor in patients with amyotrophic lateral sclerosis. Ann Neurol 1995; 38: 971

158. A controlled trial of recombinant methionyl human BDNF in ALS: The BDNF Study Group (Phase III). Neurology 1999; 52: 1427–33

159. Ochs G, Penn RD, York M, et al. A phase I/II trial of recombinant methionyl human brain derived neurotrophic factor administered by intrathecal infusion to patients with amyotrophic lateral sclerosis. Amyotroph Lateral Scler Other Motor Neuron Disord 2000; 1: 201–6

160. Wellmer A, Misra VP, Sharief MK, et al. A double-blind placebo-controlled clinical trial of recombinant human brain-derived neurotrophic factor (rhBDNF) in diabetic polyneuropathy. J Peripher Nerv Syst 2001; 6: 204–10

161. Chaudhry V, Giuliani M, Petty BG, et al. Tolerability of recombinant-methionyl human neurotrophin-3 (r-metHuNT3) in healthy subjects. Muscle Nerve 2000; 23: 189–92

162. Lai EC, Felice KJ, Festoff BW, et al. Effect of recombinant human insulin-like growth factor-I on progression of ALS. A placebo-controlled study. The North America ALS/IGF-I Study Group. Neurology 1997; 49: 1621–30

163. Borasio GD, Robberecht W, Leigh PN, et al. A placebo-controlled trial of insulin like growth factor-I in amyotrophic lateral sclerosis. European ALS/IGF-I Study Group. Neurology 1998; 51: 583–6

164. Jin K, Mao XO, Batteur SP, et al. Caspase-3 and the regulation of hypoxic neuronal death by vascular endothelial growth factor. Neuroscience 2001; 108: 351–8

165. Ogunshola OO, Antic A, Donoghue MJ, et al. Paracrine and autocrine functions of neuronal vascular endothelial growth factor (VEGF) in the central nervous system. J Biol Chem 2002; 277: 11410–15

166. Krum JM, Mani N, Rosenstein JM. Angiogenic and astroglial responses to vascular endothelial growth factor administration in adult rat brain. Neuroscience 2002; 110: 589–604

167. Schratzberger P, Schratzberger G, Silver M, et al. Favorable effect of VEGF gene transfer on ischemic peripheral neuropathy. Nat Med 2000; 6: 405–13

168. Forsythe JA, Jiang BH, Iyer NV, et al. Activation of vascular endothelial growth factor gene transcription by hypoxia-inducible factor 1. Mol Cell Biol 1996; 16: 4604–13

169. Liu Y, Cox SR, Morita T, Kourembanas S. Hypoxia regulates vascular endothelial growth factor gene expression in endothelial cells. Identification of a 5' enhancer. Circ Res 1995; 77: 638–43

170. Gros-Louis F, Laurent S, Lopes AA, et al. Absence of mutations in the hypoxia response element of VEGF in ALS. Muscle Nerve 2003; 28: 774–5

171. Sopher BL, Thomas PS Jr, LaFevre-Bernt MA, et al. Androgen receptor YAC transgenic mice recapitulate SBMA motor neuronopathy and implicate VEGF164 in the motor neuron degeneration. Neuron 2004; 41: 687–99

172. Storkebaum E, Lambrechts D, Dewerchin M, et al. Treatment of motoneuron degeneration by intracerebroventricular delivery of VEGF in a rat model of ALS. Nat Neurosci 2005; 8: 85–92

173. Azzouz M, Ralph GS, Storkebaum E, et al. VEGF delivery with retrogradely transported lentivector prolongs survival in a mouse ALS model. Nature 2004; 429: 413–17

174. Thoenen H, Sendtner M. Neurotrophins: From enthusiastic expectations through sobering experiences to rational therapeutic approaches. Nat Neurosci 2002; 5 (Suppl): 1046–50

175. Troost D, Aten J, Morsink F, de Jong JM. Apoptosis in amyotrophic lateral sclerosis is not restricted to motor neurons. Bcl-2 expression is increased in unaffected post-central gyrus. Neuropathol Appl Neurobiol 1995; 21: 498–504

176. Haase G, Kennel P, Pettmann B, et al. Gene therapy of murine motor neuron disease using adenoviral vectors for neurotrophic factors. Nat Med 1997; 3: 429–36

177. Haase G, Pettmann B, Bordet T, et al. Therapeutic benefit of ciliary neurotrophic factor in progressive motor neuronopathy depends on the route of delivery. Ann Neurol 1999; 45: 296–304

178. Gravel C, Götz R, Lorrain A, Sendtner M. Adenoviral gene transfer of ciliary neurotrophic factor and brain-derived neurotrophic factor leads to longterm survival of axotomized motoneurons. Nat Med 1997; 3: 765–70

179. Eriksson NP, Lindsay RM, Aldskogius H. BDNF and NT-3 rescue sensory but not motoneurones following axotomy in the neonate. Neuroreport 1994; 5: 1445–8

180. Vejsada R, Sagot Y, Kato AC. BDNF-mediated rescue of axotomized motor neurones decreases with increasing dose. Neuroreport 1994; 5: 1889–92

181. Vejsada R, Sagot Y, Kato AC. Quantitative comparison of the transient rescue effects of neurotrophic factors on axotomized motoneurons in vivo. Eur J Neurosci 1995; 7: 108–15

182. Dittrich F, Ochs G, Grobe-Wilde A, et al. Pharmakokinetics of intrathecally applied BDNF and effects on spinal motoneurons. Exp Neurol 1996; 141: 225–39

183. Festoff BW, Yang SX, Vaught J, et al. The insulin-like growth factor signaling system and ALS neurotrophic factor treatment strategies. J Neurol Sci 1995; 129: 114–21

184. Hantai D, Akaaboune M, Lagord C, et al. Beneficial effects of insulin-like growth factor-I on wobbler mouse motoneuron disease. J Neurol Sci 1995; 129: 122–6

185. Reinhardt RR, Bondy CA. Insulin-like growth factors cross the blood–brain barrier. Endocrinology 1994; 135:1753–61

186. Yamamoto H, Gurney ME. Human platelets contain brain-derived neurotrophic factor. J Neurosci 1990; 10: 3469–78

187. Dittrich F, Thoenen H, Sendtner M. Ciliary neurotrophic factor: Pharmakokinetics and acute phase response. Ann Neurol 1994; 35: 151–63

16

Axonal transport and amyotrophic lateral sclerosis

Andy Grierson, Chris Miller

INTRODUCTION

Amyotrophic lateral sclerosis (ALS) is an adult-onset neurodegenerative disease affecting large motor neurons in the brain and spinal cord. Although we only know the genetic defects underlying a few per cent of all ALS cases, a number of common mechanisms have been suggested that apply to both sporadic and familial forms of the disease. In particular, the accumulation of specific proteins in the perikarya and axons of motor neurons are pathologic hallmarks of ALS. While the precise mechanisms leading to this pathology are unclear, in this chapter we review the evidence that links this phenomenon with defective axonal transport of essential cargoes in ALS. First, the molecular basis for axonal transport of cargoes by molecular motor proteins, and experimental approaches employed to investigate transport in the laboratory are described. Second, we critically appraise the evidence for axonal transport defects in ALS, highlighting studies in cultured cells, vertebrate disease models and human ALS patients. Finally, we speculate on the potential to use novel therapeutic agents to regulate axonal transport, and also to utilize molecular motors to deliver drugs via the axon.

AXONAL TRANSPORT

Transport of molecules and organelles is a fundamental process in all cells, including neurons. Transport is central to neuronal development, survival, intracellular signaling and trafficking. Essentially all components of the axon are synthesized in the cell body, and must therefore be transported over great distances (1 m or more). Directional transport is also essential to maintain the highly polarized and distinct axonal and dendritic compartments within neurons. The molecular basis for transport has been investigated using genetic and cell biology approaches; this has led to the identification of families of molecular motor proteins, and several distinct modes of transport within cells. It appears that the bulk of long-distance transport in neurons occurs on microtubules, and involves kinesin motors in the anterograde direction (towards the axonal terminus), and dynein motors in the retrograde direction (towards the cell body). In order to understand the underlying molecular mechanisms responsible for transport in healthy and diseased neurons, several experimental systems have been developed for analysis of transport *in vitro* and *in vivo*. Microscopic observation of live neurons

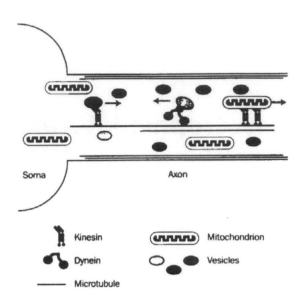

Soma   Axon

Kinesin   Mitochondrion

Dynein   Vesicles

—— Microtubule

Figure 16.1   Simplified scheme of axonal motors and cargoes

reveals the dynamic and complex system of cargo transport. Within this continuous 'rush hour' of intracellular traffic, distinct cargoes must be delivered to precise subcellular locations in a temporally defined manner; this process must be regulated in some way, therefore, structural and molecular mechanisms are likely to be important (Figure 16.1).

Molecular motor proteins

Microtubules are polarized within axons, such that their plus-ends are directed towards the synapse, and their minus-ends towards the cell body[1,2]. Therefore, in order to deliver cargoes to and from the synapse, directional molecular motors are needed. The kinesin family of molecular motors transports cargoes towards the plus-end of microtubules[3,4], while the dynein molecular motor retrogradely transports cargoes toward the minus-end of microtubules[5,6]. Motor proteins share a common structural organization, and comprise a motor domain, which binds to microtubules, and a cargo-binding domain.

The motor domain hydrolyses adenosine triphosphate (ATP) in order to move along microtubules. Motor domains of kinesin are highly evolutionarily conserved, but the non-motor domains and kinesin accessory proteins are not so well conserved. Indeed, amongst the members of the kinesin family of molecular motors, the cargo-binding domains are divergent, and this is thought to be the basis for the recognition of a wide range of different cargoes, and the transport of specific cargoes by specific motors[7]. It is proposed that certain motor–cargo interactions are mediated by adaptor proteins, which act as cargo receptors.

Kinesins are a large superfamily of motor proteins, and more than 40 different kinesin molecules have been identified[7], classified by homology into 14 kinesin families (kinesin 1 to kinesin 14)[8]. A number of orphan kinesins exist; these have no identified cargo, nor phylogenetic evidence for membership of an existing kinesin family. Now that the majority of kinesins have been identified, several key questions remain: (1) Why are there so many different kinesins, are they divergent or overlapping with respect to cargo binding or cell/tissue expression? (2) What is the level of redundancy amongst kinesins? Although some motors are essential for viability e.g. kinesin heavy chain KIF5B, others are not, e.g. kinesin heavy chain KIF5C[9,10]. Any functional redundancy may have implications for dysfunction of anterograde transport in disease. (3) What are the mechanisms that regulate kinesin function, i.e. binding to cargo, transport rate, release of cargo? Basic research into these areas is critical to our understanding of axonal transport in healthy and diseased states.

Dynein is thought to be the major retrograde transport motor in neurons. There are many dynein isoforms in humans, but most are thought to be axonemal, and function in ciliary and flagellar movement. Two isoforms are referred to as 'cytoplasmic': cytoplasmic dynein heavy chain 1 (DNCH1) and DNCH1b (the latter is sometimes called dynein 2)[11–13]. DNCH1 is widely expressed and well studied, whereas DNCH1b is only expressed in a few ciliated cells. The heavy chain (HC) of dynein is associated with a number of smaller subunits: intermediate (IC), light intermediate (LIC) and light chains (LCs), but the motor domain for this complex is encoded by the HC. The dynein motor is much larger than that of kinesin, and is a member of the AAA family of ATPases (ATPases Associated with diverse cellular Activities). A subunit of dynein is thought to include two HCs, two ICs, two LICs and a small, variable number of LCs[14]. The smaller subunits interact with the N-terminal (non-motor) domain of the HCs. This complex makes contact with a second complex, termed dynactin, via association with the p150[Glued] protein[15,16]. Dynactin is thought to function as either an activator of dynein-mediated transport, or as a cargo-receptor[17,18]. Numerous other interactions between dynein complex subunits have been reported, mostly associations of retrogradely transported cargoes with the LCs.

There is increasing evidence that kinesin and dynein bind to cargoes via interactions with cargo-receptors. Kinectin was identified as a putative receptor for kinesin, but this molecule is not conserved in evolutionarily distant species, nor is it present in axons[19,20]. Other proteins have recently been identified as transport intermediaries, linking motors to cargoes. These can be classified as transmembrane proteins, vesicle adaptor and coat proteins and signaling proteins. Two transmembrane proteins (amyloid precursor protein (APP) and rhodopsin) are known to interact with Kinesin-1 and dynein, respectively. APP has been shown to regulate transport rates in Drosophila, and mice lacking APP have decreased rates of Kinesin-1 transport[21,22]. The vesicles transported via APP have been shown to contain β-site APP converting enzyme (BACE), presenilin-1, GAP-43 and TrkA[22].

Signaling molecules are known to be regulators of biologic processes, and since they are needed in axons, they are also cargoes for motor proteins. Small GTPases including Rab and Ran are known to regulate vesicle trafficking and endocytosis:

Rab6 interacts with Kinesin-X, RanBP2 interacts with KIF5A and KIF5C, Rab4 associates with dynein LIC1[23–25]. Since these GTPases interact with motors they may also regulate transport during trafficking and endocytosis. Another signaling-related molecule that may be a kinesin receptor is a scaffolding protein called JIP (c-jun N-terminal kinase (JNK) interacting protein). This molecule is thought to link JNK signaling complexes with the transmembrane receptor ApoER2, and kinesin-1, and the pathway seems to be conserved in Drosophila[26,27].

Vesicle coat proteins including clathrin and coatomer proteins (COPs) recruit cargoes to the cytoplasmic surface of vesicles. Spectrin is one such protein, and has been demonstrated to link dynein–dynactin complexes to vesicles[28]. Fodrin is a neuronal isoform of spectrin which binds to kinesin-associated protein 3 (KAP3), part of the Kinesin-2 motor complex[29]. AP-1, the clathrin-associated adaptor complex mediates KIF13A-dependent transport from the trans-Golgi to the plasma membrane[30]. mLin-10 (also called X11 or Mint) has been shown to link the kinesin KIF17 to vesicles containing NMDA receptors[31], while GRIP-1 (GluR2-interacting protein) enables kinesin heavy chain transport of AMPA receptors[32].

Transport rates

Transport of cargoes by the molecular motor proteins described above proceeds at fast rates. The kinesin and dynein motors are capable of transporting cargoes at speeds of up to $20\,\mu m/s$ in vitro and in vivo (see following section for methodology)[33]. These speeds are required for timely delivery of cargoes within typically sized cells, such as fibroblasts, but are they sufficient for constant delivery of axonal cargoes towards the synapse or cell body? For example, the velocity of the KIF1A/UNC104 motor has been analyzed in vitro and in vivo in mammals and Caenorhabditis elegans. These experiments showed that the purified motor moved at $1.2–1.7\,\mu m/s$ in vitro, and

1.00–1.02 µm/s *in vivo* in live *C. elegans* and transfected rat hippocampal neurons[34-37]. In a long motor neuron axon, e.g. of 1 m in length, a cargo transported at 1 µm/s would take over 11 days to travel from cell body to the synapse. This is probably not fast enough for a 'just in time' delivery system, so it is likely that there is an alternative means of supplying cargoes. It is possible that cargoes are maintained at particular concentrations along the length of the axon, such that they have to move over a far shorter distance when needed. In this way, regulated movement of cargoes over a relatively short distance would be required. However, this does not seem to be compatible with the 'signaling endosome' model of retrograde signaling[38]. These recently discovered pathways are proposed to be the mechanisms by which neurons receive signals from their target tissues or synapses, and signal to the nucleus to transcribe new messenger RNA. The paradigm most frequently studied involves the TrkA nerve growth factor (NGF) receptor, which, once it binds to NGF at the cell surface, becomes internalized and then transported retrogradely at rates of 1.75 µm/s. At this speed, in a 1-m axon it would take nearly a week to deliver a signaling endosome to the cell body. In this case it seems likely that multiple pathways are activated by NGF binding, some of which signal at a very fast rate to the nucleus, perhaps involving serial phosphorylation cascades or propagation of ionic fluxes, others that utilize retrograde transport by dynein (reviewed in references 38 and 39).

The cytoskeleton and its associated proteins are transported at slow rates (mm/day) compared to the fast cargoes described in this chapter. The slow rate is divided into two slow components (SCs), SCa and SCb, which move at 0.3–3 mm/day and 2–8 mm/day, respectively. The microtubule and intermediate filament cytoskeleton, as well as some microtubule-associated proteins such as Tau, move in SCa, while other associated proteins, e.g. dynein and dynactin, and the microfilaments, move in SCb (reviewed in reference 40). This is important, as the major function

of the cytoskeleton is to provide a rigid support for the cell. If the cytoskeleton was so dynamic that it was permanently moving, it would compromise this property. However, over the past few years it has been demonstrated that a small proportion of cytoskeletal components such as neurofilaments and tubulin, actually move at fast rates of up to 3 µm/s in some experimental systems[41,42]. This suggests that neurofilaments and tubulin are transported through axons by 'fast' motors such as kinesin and dynein, but that only a small fraction is transported at any given time, providing the rigid cytoskeleton which is essential, and allowing dynamic movements to occur to drive the overall slow rates of transport.

Experimental approaches to the study of axonal transport

Several approaches have been used to study axonal transport and motor protein function *in vitro* and *in vivo*. *In vitro* it is possible to study motor function using microtubule-gliding assays[43,44]. In these experiments motor proteins are immobilized on glass coverslips, at a solution containing fluorescently labeled microtubules, and ATP is added. The immobilized motors 'walk' along the microtubules, displacing them. The microtubule movement can be imaged using fluorescence microscopy, and information about the velocity of the motor determined. Since microtubules are polarized, and have a plus-end and a minus-end, if they are specifically labeled on one end, information about the direction of the motor can be obtained. An improved method has been developed to enable single-molecule recordings *in vitro*. Recombinant motors are labeled with fluorophores, and incubated with purified fluorescently labeled sea urchin axonemal preparations[45]. Using total internal reflection microscopy it is possible to record kinesin motility along the axonemal microtubules (Figure 16.2).

In cultured cells and neurons, several approaches have been used to study motor function. The most straightforward assays rely on

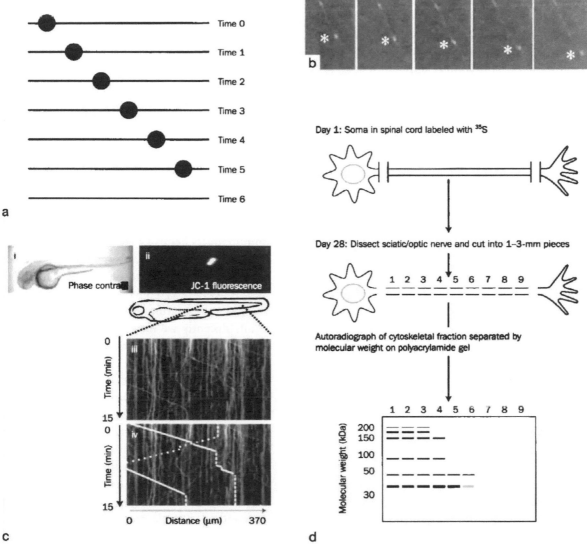

Figure 16.2 (a) Model of axonemal transport assay. Fluorescently labeled motors are incubated with sea urchin axoneme preparations, and are imaged by time-lapse microscopy. Precise motor velocities can be measured. (b) Axonal transport of green fluorescent protein (GFP)-tagged neurofilament proteins in transfected neurons. GFP-tagged NFM was transfected into 5-day-old cortical neurons using the calcium phosphate method; 48 h later, fluorescently labeled neurofilaments are recorded by time-lapse microscopy (one image every 5 s). A small number of neurofilaments move at any given time (asterisk); the majority are stationary. (c) Quantifying axonal transport *in vivo* in a live zebrafish embryo. (i and ii) Low-magnification phase contrast and fluorescent images of JC-1-injected 48-h zebrafish embryo. (iii and iv) High-power magnification kymograph of the annotated region of the same zebrafish. To create the kymograph the frames constituting the original time-lapse sequence were converted into a single montage with successive frames beneath one another. Along the x-axis of the montage is distance along the peripheral lateral line nerve; along the y-axis is time. The montage was then compressed along the y-axis so each individual frame was represented as a 1-pixel high line. In this way, the position of individual mitochondria can be shown on a two-dimensional image. Mitochondria that move towards the cell body (retrograde, dotted lines) or growth cone (anterograde, solid lines) and stationary mitochondria (dashed lines) can be distinguished. Examples of mitochondria with anterograde, retrograde, or no net displacement are shown in (iv). (See also Plate 11). (d) Radiolabeled amino acids are injected into the eye (to label proteins transported in the optic nerve), or the ventral region of the spinal cord (to label proteins in the sciatic nerve). Newly synthesized proteins are labeled and transported into the axons of the optic or sciatic nerve. Rates of transport can be calculated by sectioning the nerve into 1–2-mm proximal–distal segments, and separating the different-sized proteins on an acrylamide gel

phase contrast or differential interference contrast (DIC) microscopy. In these assays many subcellular cargoes are observed simultaneously, so it is a suitable method for determining global effects on transport rates. It is more difficult to analyze subsets of vesicle cargoes using this approach; however, some organelles, such as mitochondria, are easier to identify[46]. An alternative strategy is to utilize cell-permeable fluorescent probes, which label organelles specifically, or according to their pH or membrane potential. Many of these have been developed, and it is possible to study mitochondrial, Golgi, endosomal and lysosomal compartments in live neurons (see Figure 16.2). Another approach is to utilize fusion proteins that are targeted to specific subcellular domains. The most widely used approach for live cell imaging uses green fluorescent protein (GFP) fusion proteins. This technology now enables visualization of microfilaments, intermediate filaments and neurofilaments (see Figure 16.2), nuclei, mitochondria, endoplasmic reticulum, Golgi apparatus, peroxisomes, endosomes and motor proteins themselves (for example, see references 36 and 37). The same approach could potentially be employed to study the transport of any protein, so long as care is taken to ensure that the GFP-fusion protein functions normally, and behaves in the same manner as the non-tagged protein. These methods have now largely superseded existing transport assays, where fluorescently labeled protein was injected into cells, an area of the axon bleached with a laser, and the fluorescence recovery after photobleaching (FRAP) recorded as an indirect measurement of the transport rate[47] of the labeled protein.

Measuring transport *in vivo* is a major challenge; the majority of studies have used indirect approaches, most suitable for studying the slow component of axonal transport. In these experiments, radiolabeled amino acids are injected into a suitable location in a rodent, typically the eye, to label proteins transported in the optic nerve, or the ventral region of the spinal cord to label proteins in the sciatic nerve. The label is incorporated into newly synthesized proteins, which are transported into the axons of the optic or sciatic nerve[48]. Fast cargoes will rapidly enter the nerve process, and their movement can be inferred by sectioning the nerve into 1–2-mm proximal–distal segments, and separating the different-sized proteins on an acrylamide gel. In the same manner, to study slow transport, it is possible to dissect the nerve segments several weeks after the injection. After a cytoskeletal extract has been prepared, radiolabeled cytoskeletal proteins can be separated on an acrylamide gel (as in Figure 16.2). Another, less direct approach suitable for studying transport *in vivo*, involved ligating a nerve and looking with immunohistochemistry at which proteins accumulated proximally and distally of the ligature[49]. Although it is possible to obtain quantitative data in this way, it is conceivable that the damage caused by the ligature may affect the experimental result. Recently we have utilized a new approach to study transport *in vivo*, using transparent zebrafish embryos (see Figure 16.2). Since zebrafish develop quickly, it is possible to study fast and slow axonal transport of fluorescently labeled cargoes over distances of 1–2 mm in 72-h embryos, using conventional fluorescence microscopy.

However one measures the transport of motors and cargoes in the above experiments, analysis of the data remains a major hurdle. A completely freestanding particle tracking and analysis program would be a significant advance, although a number of investigators have devised semi-automated approaches using freely available software such as ImageJ[50]. Several laboratories use kymographs as a rapid method of analysing data[36,51] and (see Figure 16.2), although this only reveals substantial effects on motility.

TRANSPORT DEFECTS IN AMYOTROPHIC LATERAL SCLEROSIS

Evidence for an axonal transport defect in ALS was first reported several years ago, and recently new data have emerged to support this mechanism. Within motor neuron axons, vital cargoes must be transported over long distances along microtubule tracks to maintain neuronal viability. The bulk of axonal transport is mediated by the molecular motors, kinesin (anterograde transport towards the growth cone) and cytoplasmic dynein (retrograde transport towards the cell body). Several findings indicate that defects in axonal transport contribute to the initiation or progression of ALS:

(1) Mice overexpressing G37R and G85R mutant SOD1 have decreased rates of slow axonal transport prior to the onset of clinical signs of disease[52]. The transport of neurofilaments and tubulin is slowed months before the onset of clinical symptoms of disease in these mice, suggesting that it is an early feature of the toxicity associated with mutant SOD1. The mechanism by which this occurs is not known, as disruption of the motor proteins, their cargoes or the microtubules may be the primary defect. Indeed, it is possible that all these may be affected at some stage during the development of ALS.

(2) Postmortem studies have demonstrated accumulations of neurofilaments, mutant SOD1 and ubiquitin-positive inclusions in the surviving motor neurons of ALS patients[53,54] (Figure 16.3). Such pathology may be associated with the disruption of intracellular transport, especially since transport rates have been shown to slow prior to the onset of pathology in mutant SOD1 mice[52]. Additionally, there is evidence for other mechanisms affecting intermediate filament protein transport in ALS. First, it is known that neurofilaments are phosphoproteins. The C-terminus of the neurofilament heavy chain (NFH) in particular is heavily phosphorylated *in vivo*, and this phosphorylation correlates with subcellular localization of neurofilaments. For instance, more heavily phosphorylated neurofilaments are enriched

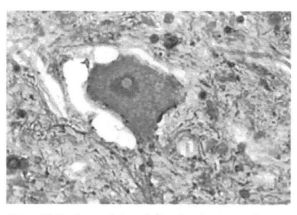

Figure 16.3 Accumulation of phosphorylated neurofilament proteins in a spinal motor neuron from a sporadic amyotrophic lateral sclerosis patient. Immunocytochemistry using the SMI31 antibody to detect phosphorylated neurofilaments. See also Plate 12

in the distal axon compared to more proximal regions, and there is evidence that increased phosphorylation of the C-terminus of the neurofilament medium chain (NFM) and NFH is associated with decreased rates of neurofilament transport[42,55]. Since neurofilament kinase activity may also be elevated in ALS[56-60], this may be a direct mechanism that results in the slowing of neurofilament transport in disease. Genetic evidence also links neurofilaments to ALS, since insertion and deletion mutations affecting the C-terminal phosphorylation domain of NFH are found in about 1% of sporadic ALS patients[61-63]. How these mutations may relate to ALS pathogenesis is unclear, but since the phosphorylation domain is preferentially affected, it is conceivable that neurofilament transport is disturbed. Finally, mutations in peripherin, another intermediate filament protein expressed in motor neurons have been reported in ALS[64,65]. These mutations are predicted to disrupt intermediate filament assembly and, consistent with this, protein aggregates that contain intermediate filament proteins are reported in the pathology of at least one of these cases[65].

(3) Accumulations of proteins and organelles in motor neurons have been shown to underlie the neuromuscular phenotype observed in *Drosophila* harboring mutations in kinesin-1[66]. This indicates that mutation of the broadly expressed motor, kinesin-1, can generate ALS-like pathology in a fly, suggesting that generically interfering with transport may specifically effect long axons.

(4) The upregulation of KIF3-associated protein (KAP3) and KIF1A have been reported in pre-symptomatic mice expressing mutant SOD1[67]. This suggests that a complex alteration in the transport machinery may occur during the development of ALS (Figure 16.4). Since we know that slow transport is compromised in the mice at this early stage in the pathogenesis of disease in this model, it is unclear whether this upregulation of the transport machinery is a compensatory pathway, or perhaps an early response to damage in the axon.

In agreement with a role of deregulation of axonal transport in ALS, several recent studies have shown that mutations in molecular motors themselves can cause motor neuron disorders with similarities to ALS.

Mutations in conventional kinesin (KIF5A) have been reported in a large family with hereditary spastic paraplegia, a disease similar to ALS with progressive lower extremity spasticity, resulting from axonal degeneration[68]. This mutation may behave in a similar manner to the *Drosophila* kinesin-1 mutants described above, and although the pathology in these patients is not yet known, it seems consistent with the finding that kinesin mutations will preferentially affect the longest axons.

Functional disruption of the dynactin complex that links cytoplasmic dynein to its cargo and to microtubules, by mutation of the p150/Glued subunit, have been found in families and sporadic ALS patients. A range of clinical phenotypes are seen, and the disease may show variable genetic

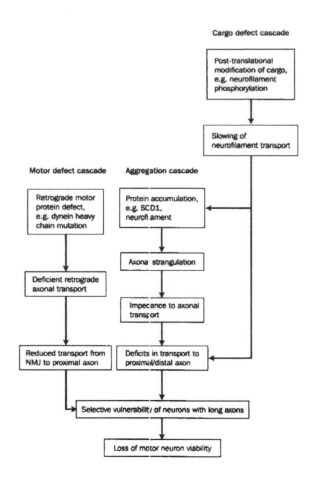

Figure 16.4 Putative axonal transport-related cascades implicated in the degeneration of motor neurons in amyotrophic lateral sclerosis. NMJ, neuromuscular junction

penetrance in families[69,70]. These mutations seem to act dominantly, and it has been speculated that the disease results from haploinsufficiency of the p150 subunit of the dynactin complex. This is likely to disrupt retrograde transport of certain cargoes, perhaps resulting in a deficient supply of neurotrophic factors, or an unknown factor, to the cell body[69].

Disruption of the dynactin complex in transgenic mice that overexpress the p50/dynamitin subunit resulted in late-onset ALS[71]. The rationale behind these experiments was that p50 overexpression acts to disassemble the dynactin complex; therefore, overexpressing p50 with a neuron-specific promoter indirectly tests the function of the dynein/dynactin complex in neurons. The Thy-1 promoter that was used to drive p50 expression is expressed only in postnatal neurons, which precluded any developmental abnormalities that may otherwise have complicated the interpretation of results.

Finally, mutations in the dynein heavy chain have been found in two lines of mutant mice – *legs at odd angles* (*loa*) and *cramping 1* – both of which develop an age-related progressive loss of muscle tone and locomotor ability with motor neuron pathology resembling that of ALS, e.g. SOD1/neurofilament/CDK5-positive inclusions[72]. The precise way in which these mutations affect transport is not yet clear, but experiments in cultured motor neurons homozygous for the *loa* mutation revealed a deficit in retrograde transport of a fluorescently labeled tetanus toxin reporter[72].

Although it is likely that motor protein mutations are rare in ALS patients, taken together the evidence suggests that the deregulation of axonal transport is a common theme in the initiation, progression and pathology of ALS, and it is possible that the pathology associated with mutant SOD1 arises as a result of decreased transport rates. However, this is not yet established as a mechanism of disease in ALS, and a number of significant gaps exist in our understanding. First, we do not understand the mechanisms responsible for the slowing of transport. The assays that are traditionally used to measure transport *in vivo* require radioactive labeling of cargoes, and dissection of nerve processes at a much later time point. Transport rates are then inferred by calculating the distance traveled over time. Although informative, these assays at best give an estimate of the net effect on transport, and offer no insight into the underlying mechanism. Second we do not know whether the mechanisms are specific to certain cargoes, or if they affect transport in general. Evidence from previous *in vivo* experiments suggests some specificity, but these experiments measured the transport only of cargoes that moved in the slow components, i.e. the cytoskeleton (0.3–3 mm/day)[52]. The bulk of axonal transport occurs at fast rates (200–400 mm/day), so this must be investigated to gain full understanding of the transport defect in ALS. Third, it is not known whether slowing of transport is important for the development of pathology and disease in ALS. In support of this, similar pathology is observed in experimental models where transport in motor neurons is directly disrupted by knockout, mutation or overexpression of motor proteins, e.g. KIF5A, *Drosophila* kinesin and dynactin[66,71,73]. These observations support the hypothesis that deregulation of axonal transport is a common theme in the initiation, progression and pathology of ALS.

FUTURE PERSPECTIVES

Technical advances may soon allow a thorough examination of axonal transport in living experimental models of ALS. For instance, we may utilize zebrafish embryos carrying ALS-causing mutations. The potential to image transport in patients using magnetic resonance imaging and affiliated technologies may soon become a possibility. This could be a valuable diagnostic tool, and allow us to investigate if clinical interventions that target transport are useful to perturb the development of ALS. Which therapeutic agents may be relevant to treating an axonal transport defect in ALS? One could either try to modulate the regulation of the motors, by regulating their expression, or by manipulating post-translational modifications that regulate motor activity (e.g. phosphorylation[74]). Another approach may be to utilize axonal transport as a therapeutic aid. This is in fact an integral part of the retrograde delivery of viral particles from muscle to the spinal cord recently used by Azzouz and co-workers[75]. In this respect it is interesting to note the success of the approach in the mutant SOD1 mouse model, which has a presymptomatic transport effect[52]. However, in this model the defect seems to affect anterograde transport, which would not affect the retrograde delivery of the viral particle to the spinal cord. The fact that several mouse models of ALS, and some human patients, have been shown to have mutations in the retrograde transport machinery may have implications for the usefulness of drug delivery via this route in at least a subset of patients. An attractive alternative approach may be to couple the viral entry route into motor neuron nerve terminals with a self-propelled retrograde motor, which would circumvent problems with the endogenous machinery.

SUMMARY

In conclusion, the evidence for a transport defect in ALS is growing. We now know that the axonal blockages found in pathological specimens may actually be caused by mutations in motors in a small percentage of patients. In other cases it is likely that indirect damage to motors and cargoes underlies the observed pathology. It is essential that we understand the regulation of motor function and cargo transport better to understand the mechanisms that are responsible for defective transport in ALS.

REFERENCES

1. Burton PR, Paige JL. Polarity of axoplasmic microtubules in the olfactory nerve of the frog. Proc Natl Acad Sci USA 1981; 78: 3269–73
2. Heidemann SR, Landers JM, Hamborg MA. Polarity orientation of axonal microtubules. J Cell Biol 1981; 91: 661–5
3. Vale RD, Schnapp BJ, Mitchison T, et al. Different axoplasmic proteins generate movement in opposite directions along microtubules in vitro. Cell 1985; 43: 623–32
4. Vale RD, Reese TS, Sheetz MP. Identification of a novel force-generating protein, kinesin, involved in microtubule-based motility. Cell 1985; 42: 39–50
5. Schroer TA, Steuer ER, Sheetz MP. Cytoplasmic dynein is a minus end-directed motor for membranous organelles. Cell 1989; 56: 937–46

6. Schnapp BJ, Reese TS. Dynein is the motor for retrograde axonal transport of organelles. Proc Natl Acad Sci USA 1989; 86: 1548–52
7. Miki H, Setou M, Kaneshiro K, Hirokawa N. All kinesin superfamily protein, KIF, genes in mouse and human. Proc Natl Acad Sci USA 2001; 98: 7004–11
8. Lawrence CJ, Dawe RK, Christie KR, et al. A standardized kinesin nomenclature. J Cell Biol 2004; 167: 19–22
9. Tanaka Y, Kanai Y, Okada Y, et al. Targeted disruption of mouse conventional kinesin heavy chain, kif5B, results in abnormal perinuclear clustering of mitochondria. Cell 1998; 93: 1147–58
10. Kanai Y, Okada Y, Tanaka Y, et al. KIF5C, a novel neuronal kinesin enriched in motor neurons. J Neurosci 2000; 20: 6374–84
11. Paschal BM, Vallee RB. Retrograde transport by the microtubule-associated protein MAP 1C. Nature 1987; 330: 181–3
12. Pazour GJ, Dickert BL, Witman GB. The DHC1b (DHC2) isoform of cytoplasmic dynein is required for flagellar assembly. J Cell Biol 1999; 144: 473–81
13. Porter ME, Bower R, Knott JA, et al. Cytoplasmic dynein heavy chain 1b is required for flagellar assembly in Chlamydomonas. Mol Biol Cell 1999; 10: 693–712
14. Vallee RB, Wall JS, Paschal BM, Shpetner HS. Microtubule-associated protein 1C from brain is a two-headed cytosolic dynein. Nature 1988; 332: 561–3
15. Vaughan KT, Vallee RB. Cytoplasmic dynein binds dynactin through a direct interaction between the intermediate chains and p150Glued. J Cell Biol 1995; 131: 1507–16
16. Karki S, Holzbaur EL. Affinity chromatography demonstrates a direct binding between cytoplasmic dynein and the dynactin complex. J Biol Chem 1995; 270: 28806–11
17. King SJ, Schroer TA. Dynactin increases the processivity of the cytoplasmic dynein motor. Nat Cell Biol 2000; 2: 20–4
18. Holleran EA, Ligon LA, Tokito M, et al. Beta III spectrin binds to the Arp1 subunit of dynactin. J Biol Chem 2001; 276: 36598–605
19. Goldstein LS, Gunawardena S. Flying through the drosophila cytoskeletal genome. J Cell Biol 2000; 150: F63–8
20. Toyoshima I, Sheetz MP. Kinectin distribution in chicken nervous system. Neurosci Lett 1996; 211: 171–4

21. Gunawardena S, Goldstein LS. Disruption of axonal transport and neuronal viability by amyloid precursor protein mutations in Drosophila. Neuron 2001; 32: 389–401

22. Kamal A, Almenar-Queralt A, LeBlanc JF, et al. Kinesin-mediated axonal transport of a membrane compartment containing beta-secretase and presenilin-1 requires APP. Nature 2001; 414: 643–8

23. Echard A, Jollivet F, Martinez O, et al. Interaction of a Golgi-associated kinesin-like protein with Rab6. Science 1998; 279: 580–5

24. Cai Y, Singh BB, Aslanukov A, et al. The docking of kinesins, KIF5B and KIF5C, to RanBP2 is mediated via a novel RanBP2 domain. J Biol Chem 2001; 11: 11

25. Bielli A, Thornqvist PO, Hendrick AG, et al. The small GTPase Rab4A interacts with the central region of cytoplasmic dynein light intermediate chain-1. Biochem Biophys Res Commun 2001; 281: 1141–53

26. Bowman AB, Kamal A, Ritchings BW, et al. Kinesin-dependent axonal transport is mediated by the sunday driver (SYD) protein. Cell 2000; 103: 583–94

27. Verhey KJ, Meyer D, Deehan R, et al. Cargo of kinesin identified as JIP scaffolding proteins and associated signaling molecules. J Cell Biol 2001; 152: 959–70

28. Muresan V, Stankewich MC, Steffen W, et al. Dynactin-dependent, dynein-driven vesicle transport in the absence of membrane proteins: A role for spectrin and acidic phospholipids. Mol Cell 2001; 7: 173–83

29. Takeda S, Yamazaki H, Seog DH, et al. Kinesin superfamily protein 3 (KIF3) motor transports fodrin-associating vesicles important for neurite building. J Cell Biol 2000; 148: 1255–65

30. Nakagawa T, Setou M, Seog D, et al. A novel motor, KIF13A, transports mannose-6-phosphate receptor to plasma membrane through direct interaction with AP-1 complex. Cell 2000; 103: 569–81

31. Setou M, Nakagawa T, Seog DH, Hirokawa N. Kinesin superfamily motor protein KIF17 and mLin-10 in NMDA receptor-containing vesicle transport. Science 2000; 288: 1796–802

32. Setou M, Seog DH, Tanaka Y, et al. Glutamate-receptor-interacting protein GRIP1 directly steers kinesin to dendrites. Nature 2002; 417: 83–7

33. Oiwa K, Takahashi K. The force–velocity relationship for microtubule sliding in demembranated sperm flagella of the sea urchin. Cell Struct Funct 1988; 13: 193–205

34. Okada Y, Yamazaki H, Sekine-Aizawa Y, Hirokawa N. The neuron-specific kinesin superfamily protein KIF1A is a unique monomeric motor for anterograde axonal transport of synaptic vesicle precursors. Cell 1995; 81: 769–80

35. Pierce DW, Hom-Booher N, Otsuka AJ, Vale RD. Single-molecule behavior of monomeric and heteromeric kinesins. Biochemistry 1999; 38: 5412–21

36. Zhou HM, Brust-Mascher I, Scholey JM. Direct visualization of the movement of the monomeric axonal transport motor UNC-104 along neuronal processes in living Caenorhabditis elegans. J Neurosci 2001; 21: 3749–55

37. Lee JR, Shin H, Ko J, et al. Characterization of the movement of the kinesin motor KIF1A in living cultured neurons. J Biol Chem 2003; 278: 2624–9

38. Campenot RB, MacInnis BL. Retrograde transport of neurotrophins: Fact and function. J Neurobiol 2004; 58: 217–29

39. Howe CL, Mobley WC. Signaling endosome hypothesis: A cellular mechanism for long distance communication. J Neurobiol 2004; 58: 207–16

40. Brown A. Slow axonal transport: Stop and go traffic in the axon. Nat Rev Mol Cell Biol 2000; 1: 153–6

41. Wang L, Brown A. Rapid movement of microtubules in axons. Curr Biol 2002; 12: 1496–501

42. Ackerley S, Thornhill P, Grierson AJ, et al. Neurofilament heavy chain side arm phosphorylation regulates axonal transport of neurofilaments. J Cell Biol 2003; 161: 489–95

43. Vale RD, Schnapp BJ, Reese TS, Sheetz MP. Organelle, bead, and microtubule translocations promoted by soluble factors from the squid giant axon. Cell 1985; 40: 559–69

44. Allen RD, Weiss DG, Hayden JH, et al. Gliding movement of and bidirectional transport along single native microtubules from squid axoplasm: Evidence for an active role of microtubules in cytoplasmic transport. J Cell Biol 1985; 100: 1736–52

45. Friedman DS, Vale RD. Single-molecule analysis of kinesin motility reveals regulation by the cargo-binding tail domain. Nat Cell Biol 1999; 1: 293–7

46. Brady ST, Lasek RJ, Allen RD. Fast axonal transport in extruded axoplasm from squid giant axon. Science 1982; 218: 1129–31

47. Takeda S, Funakoshi T, Hirokawa N. Tubulin dynamics in neuronal axons of living zebrafish embryos. Neuron 1995; 14: 1257–64

48. Ochs S, Sabri MI, Johnson J. Fast transport system of materials in mammalian nerve fibers. Science 1969; 163: 686–7

49. Warita H, Itoyama Y, Abe K. Selective impairment of fast anterograde axonal transport in the peripheral

nerves of asymptomatic transgenic mice with a G93A mutant SOD1 gene. Brain Res 1999; 819: 120–31

50. De Vos K, Sable J, Miller K, Sheetz MP. Expression of phosphatidylinositol (4,5) bisphosphate-specific pleckstrin homology domains alters direction but not the level of axonal transport of mitochondria. Mol Biol Cell 2003; 14: 3639–49

51. Miller KE, Sheetz MP. Axonal mitochondrial transport and potential are correlated. J Cell Sci 2004; 117: 2791–804

52. Williamson TL, Cleveland DW. Slowing of axonal transport is a very early event in the toxicity of ALS-linked SOD1 mutants to motor neurons. Nat Neurosci 1999; 2: 50–6

53. Ince PG, Tomkins J, Slade JY, et al. Amyotrophic lateral sclerosis associated with genetic abnormalities in the gene encoding Cu/Zn superoxide dismutase: Molecular pathology of five new cases, and comparison with previous reports and 73 sporadic cases of ALS. J Neuropathol Exp Neurol 1998; 57: 895–904

54. Shibata N, Hirano A, Kobayashi M, et al. Intense superoxide dismutase-1 immunoreactivity in intracytoplasmic hyaline inclusions of familial amyotrophic lateral sclerosis with posterior column involvement. J Neuropathol Exp Neurol 1996; 55: 481–90

55. Ackerley S, Grierson AJ, Brownlees J, et al. Glutamate slows axonal transport of neurofilaments in transfected neurons. J Cell Biol 2000; 150: 165–76

56. Hu JH, Zhang H, Wagey R, et al. Protein kinase and protein phosphatase expression in amyotrophic lateral sclerosis spinal cord. J Neurochem 2003; 85: 432–42

57. Hu JH, Chernoff K, Pelech S, Krieger C. Protein kinase and protein phosphatase expression in the central nervous system of G93A mSOD over-expressing mice. J Neurochem 2003; 85: 422–31

58. Ackerley S, Grierson AJ, Banner S, et al. p38alpha stress-activated protein kinase phosphorylates neurofilaments and is associated with neurofilament pathology in amyotrophic lateral sclerosis. Mol Cell Neurosci 2004; 26: 354–64

59. Tortarolo M, Veglianese P, Calvaresi N, et al. Persistent activation of p38 mitogen-activated protein kinase in a mouse model of familial amyotrophic lateral sclerosis correlates with disease progression. Mol Cell Neurosci 2003; 23: 180–92

60. Bendotti C, Atzori C, Piva R, et al. Activated p38MAPK is a novel component of the intracellular inclusions found in human amyotrophic lateral sclerosis and mutant SOD1 transgenic mice. J Neuropathol Exp Neurol 2004; 63: 113–19

61. Tomkins J, Usher P, Slade JY, et al. Novel insertion in the KSP region of the neurofilament heavy gene in amyotrophic lateral sclerosis (ALS). Neuroreport 1998; 9: 3967–70

62. Al-Chalabi A, Andersen PM, Nilsson P, et al. Deletions of the heavy neurofilament subunit tail in amyotrophic lateral sclerosis. Hum Mol Genet 1999; 8: 157–64

63. Figlewicz DA, Krizus A, Martinoli MG, et al. Variants of the heavy neurofilament subunit are associated with the development of amyotrophic lateral sclerosis. Hum Mol Genet 1994; 3: 1757–61

64. Gros-Louis F, Lariviere R, Gowing G, et al. A frameshift deletion in peripherin gene associated with amyotrophic lateral sclerosis. J Biol Chem 2004; 279: 45951–6

65. Leung CL, He CZ, Kaufmann P, et al. A pathogenic peripherin gene mutation in a patient with amyotrophic lateral sclerosis. Brain Pathol 2004; 14: 290–6

66. Hurd DD, Saxton WM. Kinesin mutations cause motor neuron disease phenotypes by disrupting fast axonal transport in Drosophila. Genetics 1996; 144: 1075–85

67. Dupuis L, de Tapia M, Rene F, et al. Differential screening of mutated SOD1 transgenic mice reveals early up-regulation of a fast axonal transport component in spinal cord motor neurons. Neurobiol Dis 2000; 7: 274–85

68. Reid E, Kloos M, Ashley-Koch A, et al. A kinesin heavy chain (KIF5A) mutation in hereditary spastic paraplegia (SPG10). Am J Hum Genet 2002; 71: 1189–94

69. Puls I, Jonnakuty C, LaMonte BH, et al. Mutant dynactin in motor neuron disease. Nat Genet 2003; 33: 455–6

70. Munch C, Sedlmeier R, Meyer T, et al. Point mutations of the p150 subunit of dynactin (DCTN1) gene in ALS. Neurology 2004; 63: 724–6

71. LaMonte BH, Wallace KE, Holloway BA, et al. Disruption of dynein/dynactin inhibits axonal transport in motor neurons causing late-onset progressive degeneration. Neuron 2002; 34: 715–27

72. Hafezparast M, Klocke R, Ruhrberg C, et al. Mutations in dynein link motor neuron degeneration to defects in retrograde transport. Science 2003; 300: 808–12

73. Xia CH, Roberts EA, Her LS, et al. Abnormal neurofilament transport caused by targeted disruption of neuronal kinesin heavy chain KIF5A. J Cell Biol 2003; 161: 55–66

74. Morfini G, Szebenyi G, Elluru R, et al. Glycogen synthase kinase 3 phosphorylates kinesin light chains and
negatively regulates kinesin-based motility. EMBO J
2002; 21: 281–93

75. Azzouz M, Ralph GS, Storkebaum E, et al. VEGF
delivery with retrogradely transported lentivector
prolongs survival in a mouse ALS model. Nature
2004; 429: 413–17

17

Mitochondrial dysfunction and energy metabolism in amyotrophic lateral sclerosis

Giovanni Manfredi, M Flint Beal

INTRODUCTION

In recent years, research has increasingly focused on the role of mitochondrial defects in the pathogenesis of neurodegenerative disorders. This is not surprising if considering of the fundamental role that mitochondria play in modulating the life and death of a cell. Traditionally considered to be the 'powerhouse' of the cell because of their ability to convert nutrients into ATP, mitochondria are likely to be implicated in the neuronal demise occurring in various neurodegenerative diseases, particularly because of their contribution to the process of programed cell death or apoptosis.

Mitochondrial dysfunction has been directly or indirectly implicated in the pathogenesis of a number of relatively common neurodegenerative disorders including Parkinson's disease and Alzheimer's disease[1], and recently it has emerged as a potentially important contributing factor in the pathogenesis of amyotrophic lateral sclerosis (ALS). In this chapter we review the current evidence supporting the involvement of mitochondria in ALS and discuss the potential implications in the pathogenesis of this neurodegenerative disease.

MITOCHONDRIAL INVOLVEMENT IN AMYOTROPHIC LATERAL SCLEROSIS

Similarly to other neurodegenerative disorders with still undefined etiology, such as Alzheimer's disease and Parkinson's disease, ALS is probably a syndrome, which can have diverse causes (see Chapters 1 and 2). ALS is predominantly a sporadic disorder (SALS), but approximately 10% of cases are familial (FALS). Although several interesting observations suggest that mitochondrial dysfunction may be occurring in SALS, they are, by their very nature, circumstantial. Because human studies on human tissues are performed well after disease onset or even postmortem, it is difficult to assess whether mitochondrial abnormalities at such late stages are causally involved in the disease process or simply an epiphenomenon. As discussed below, an important advancement in the field that promises to shed light on the role of mitochondrial dysfunction in ALS derives from mutant superoxide dismutase-1 (SOD1) transgenic animal models, which have provided an excellent platform to investigate the biochemical and molecular mechanisms involved in the pathogenesis of FALS. In the past decade, we have benefited from valuable transgenic animal and cellular models of FALS that recapitulate the main clinical and pathologic hallmarks of the disease. Such models have provided crucial tools, not only for studying the pathogenesis of FALS, but also for testing a wide number of therapeutic approaches. Thus, researchers have resorted to working mostly with these transgenic models to investigate the potential role of mitochondrial dysfunction in ALS. Thus, we first briefly analyze the more circumstantial evidence for mitochondrial dysfunction in SALS, and then discuss more in depth the substantial body of evidence supporting mitochondrial involvement in FALS models associated with mutations in SOD1. Clearly, whether or not the findings obtained in FALS can be generalized and extended to the more common forms of SALS is still an important question to be answered.

Evidence for mitochondrial involvement in sporadic amyotrophic lateral sclerosis

Morphologic and ultrastructural abnormalities of mitochondria have been observed in autopsies of patients with SALS. Aggregates of abnormal mitochondria were found both in skeletal muscle and in intramuscular nerves[2,3]. Mitochondrial morphologic abnormalities were also detected in proximal axons[4] and in the anterior horns of the spinal cord[5]. Since these initial observations, evidence of mitochondrial dysfunction in various tissues of SALS patients has accumulated. Increased mitochondrial volume and elevated calcium levels within the mitochondria were found in muscle biopsies of ALS patients[6]. Furthermore, defects in the activities of mitochondrial respiratory chain complex I[7] and IV[8] have been identified in muscle and spinal cord of SALS patients[9,10], suggesting that an impairment of the mitochondrial respiratory chain might be of importance in the pathogenesis of SALS. The mitochondrial respiratory chain is constituted by a series of enzymatic complexes, whose primary function is to provide the

energy necessary for ATP synthesis. The mitochondrial respiratory chain is controlled by two genomes, and, although most mitochondrial constituents are encoded by nuclear DNA, mutations in the mitochondrial DNA (mtDNA) are associated with impairment of the respiratory chain function and with heterogeneous diseases in humans, including neurodegenerative disorders[11]. It has been proposed that mtDNA mutations, either inherited maternally or acquired in the course of life, may be associated with mitochondrial dysfunction and SALS. For example, a single mtDNA frameshift mutation in the gene for subunit I of complex IV of the mitochondrial respiratory chain has been shown to cause a form of SALS[12]. A role for mutations in the mtDNA has also been postulated based on studies of cybrids (mtDNA-less cells repopulated with mtDNA from a donor source) obtained from mitochondria of SALS patients. These cybrid cells have a defective respiratory chain, increased free radical production and impaired calcium homeostasis[13]. These findings were obtained in cybrids derived from neuroblastoma (as mtDNA acceptor cells) cells but were not replicated in non-neuronal cell types[14], suggesting that the effect of SALS-related mtDNA abnormalities may be detectable only in cells that express neuronal phenotypes.

Evidence for mitochondrial involvement in SOD1 familial amyotrophic lateral sclerosis

Approximately 20% of FALS cases are due to mutations in the gene encoding SOD1 (Cu,Zn dismutase, MIM 147450[15]). In eukaryotic cells, superoxide is a normal byproduct of aerobic respiration and it is produced by oxidative phosphorylation in the mitochondria[16]. SOD1 is a ubiquitous metalloprotein that prevents damage by oxygen-mediated free radicals by catalyzing the dismutation of superoxide into molecular oxygen and hydrogen peroxide[17]. The symptoms and pathology of FALS patients with SOD1 mutations closely resemble those of patients with SALS, and pathologic alterations in motor neurons from mice expressing mutant SOD1 are strikingly similar to those found in ALS patients, suggesting that the mechanisms of neurodegeneration for SALS and FALS share common components.

Since the initial report of mutated SOD1, more than 100 different mutated forms of the *SOD1* gene, most of which are missense mutations, have been identified in FALS patients. Because several pathogenic mutations do not affect SOD1 activity significantly[18], a toxic gain of function of the mutated protein, rather than a lack of antioxidant function, has been postulated. A number of toxic effects of mutated SOD1 have been proposed, including impairment of mitochondrial energy metabolism and apoptosis.

A striking pathologic feature observed in SOD1 transgenic mice is the presence of membrane-bound vacuoles observed in the motor neurons of mice carrying the G93A[19] and the G37R mutations[20], which appear to derive from massive mitochondrial degeneration. It was shown that, at the onset of the disease, characterized by rapid loss of muscle strength but with still very little motor neuron death, there is an explosive increase in degenerating, vacuolated mitochondria in the spinal cord of G93A SOD1 mutant mice[21]. The vacuoles are most abundant in neuronal processes, including axons and dendrites. This observation suggests that mitochondrial alterations may represent an early event triggering the onset of the disease, rather than simply a byproduct of cell degeneration. Ultrastructural studies of these mitochondrial vacuoles suggest that they may derive from expansion of the mitochondrial outer membrane[22,23]. In a further development, Higgins and colleagues demonstrated that mitochondrial vacuolization in G93A SOD1 mutant mice resulted from a progressive detachment of the outer membrane from the inner membrane. Eventually, the inner membrane disintegrated and a large vacuole containing remnants of the membranes were formed[24].

Several lines of evidence obtained in cellular models indicate that expression of mutant SOD1 is not only associated with mitochondrial morphologic changes but also with mitochondrial dysfunction. Mitochondrial depolarization, one of the markers of bioenergetic dysfunction, has been detected in human neuroblastoma cells expressing mutant SOD1. These mutant cells also show an impairment of mitochondrial calcium handling, causing an increase of cytoplasmic calcium[25]. Decreased mitochondrial membrane potential and impaired mitochondrial calcium homeostasis have also been reported in cultured primary motor neurons from G93A transgenic mice[26], whereas defective respiratory chain enzymes and reduced cellular ATP content were found in cultured motor neuron-like cells expressing mutant SOD1[27].

In vivo studies in the G93A mutant SOD1 mouse have also shown that mitochondrial bioenergetics is impaired. With different techniques, it was demonstrated that in the nervous tissue of these transgenic mice there is an impairment of the mitochondrial respiratory chain [28,29]. Respiratory chain dysfunction was also reported in spinal cord from FALS patients[30]. These respiratory defects became more severe with the progression of the disease and they affected the spinal cord more that other tissues. Furthermore, brain and spinal cord of G93A mice display bioenergetic defects as shown by decreased oxygen consumption and mitochondrial ATP synthesis[29]. Recently, we have found that the bioenergetic failure in the SOD1 mutant mice results in an impairment of mitochondrial calcium uptake both in the spinal cord and in the brain[31]. Calcium capacity defects in SOD1 mutant mitochondria may provide a functional link between mitochondrial dysfunction and glutamate excitotoxicity, which has been proposed as one of the potential mechanisms of the tissue specificity of SOD1 toxicity[32]. In support of this hypothesis, it was shown that a G93A SOD1 mutant transgenic mouse, which expresses high levels of the calcium-impermeable gluR2 subunit in motor neurons, displays improved motor functions and lifespan[33]. Since mitochondria are a major short-term buffering system of intracellular calcium[34], defective mitochondrial calcium buffering may potentially cause excito-toxic damage in glutamatergic cells, such as motor neurons. Elevation of cytosolic calcium levels in neurons may compromise mitochondrial integrity and functions, for example by inducing enhanced production of free radicals from mitochondria. Although the functional link between intracellular calcium and free radical production has not been conclusively defined, there is compelling evidence that free radicals play an important role in several forms of neurodegeneration[35]. It has been proposed that aberrant copper chemistry by mutant SOD1 may cause oxidative damage and apoptosis in neuronal cells[36].

Causes of mitochondrial dysfunction in SOD1 familial amyotrophic lateral sclerosis

The mechanisms underlying the morphological changes and the biochemical abnormalities observed in mice expressing mutant SOD1 are still being investigated. A development in the field that has helped in shedding some light on the mechanisms of mitochondrial dysfunction caused by mutant SOD1 is the finding that a proportion of SOD1 is localized in the mitochondria. SOD1 activity was first detected in rat liver mitochondria by Weisiger and Fridovich in 1973[37]. The exis-tence of SOD1 in mitochondria of eukaryotic cells was then confirmed by different groups using different techniques. Using immuno-gold electron microscopy, Higgins and Jaarsma and their col-leagues have shown that SOD1 localized in the mitochondria of motor neurons in the spinal cord of transgenic mice[22,38]. Using cell fractionation and mitochondrial purification, SOD1 was also detected in the mitochondria of the yeast *Saccha-romyces cerevisiae*[39], of rat liver[40], and of mouse brain and spinal cord[29]. These studies have shown that both wild-type and mutant SOD1 are local-ized in mitochondria, but Okado-Matsumoto and Fridovich have proposed that the mitochondrial import of mutant SOD1 is partly impeded by its interaction with cytosolic heat shock proteins[41]. Field and colleagues showed that the retention of SOD1 inside yeast mitochondria was dependent upon the interaction with its copper chaperone CCS, because SOD1 mutants that interact poorly with CCS 'escape' from mitochondria[42]. Based on mitochondrial fractionation, it has been proposed that SOD1 concentrates in the intermembrane space (IMS) of mitochondria[29,39,40]. However, recent evidence suggests that, in mice expressing high levels of transgenic human SOD1, a portion of this transgenic SOD1 also localizes in the matrix space of mitochondria, where it forms large aggregates containing SOD1 and possibly other mitochondrial matrix proteins[43].

Although the mechanism by which mutant SOD1 in mitochondria results in mitochondrial dysfunction is still unclear, there are several non-mutually exclusive possibilities (Figure 17.1). Hig-gins and colleagues[38] observed that SOD1 and cytochrome c, a resident protein of the IMS, co-localized at the early stages of mitochondrial vac-uolization in mutant SOD1 transgenic mice. In some cases, they observed very large aggregates containing SOD1 within the vacuoles.

Peroxisomes are associated with mitochondrial vacuoles, suggesting that one mechanism for the expansion of the mitochondrial outer membrane resulting in vacuolization may be fusion of mito-chondria with peroxisomes. The expanded outer membrane could become exceedingly porous and allow for leakage of cytochrome c in the cytosol, potentially triggering the apoptotic cascade[24,44].

Liu and colleagues recently reported that, in transgenic mice, mutant SOD1, but not wild-type SOD1, associated preferentially with mitochon-dria of the spinal cord They hypothesized that mutant SOD1, which progressively accumulates and aggregates in the outer membrane, may cause 'clogging' of the protein translocation machinery of mitochondria (TOM), which eventually would result in loss of protein import and mitochondrial dysfunction[45]. This is an intriguing hypothesis. Since the spinal cord is the site where most of the pathologic changes develop in these mouse models

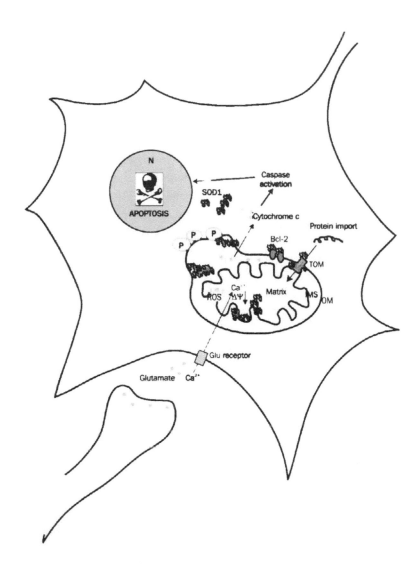

Figure 17.1   Diagram of potential pathways of mitochondrial involvement in SOD1-related amyotrophic lateral sclerosis. Mutant SOD1 has been proposed to affect mitochondrial functions in several ways. All these mechanisms of mitochondrial involvement are not mutually exclusive and may interact and co-operate in establishing a vicious cycle, ultimately resulting in mitochondrial dysfunction and cell death. Mutant SOD1 may affect mitochondria directly within the organelles or indirectly from the cytoplasm in a yet undisclosed manner. Within mitochondria, mutant SOD1 may interfere with the anti-apoptotic function of Bcl-2[46], affect mitochondrial import by interfering with the translocation machinery (TOM/TIM)[45], generate toxic reactive oxygen species (ROS) via aberrant superoxide chemistry[36], accumulate and aggregate in the intermembrane space (IMS) and in the matrix, promote outer membrane (OM) expansion and mitochondrial vacuolization[24]. These changes may then result in abnormal mitochondrial energy metabolism[29], Ca^{2+} handling[31] and release of pro-apoptotic factors[50]. See also Plate 13

of FALS, it suggests that mitochondrial localization of mutant SOD1 resulting in protein import impairment may be an important factor in determining the tissue specificity of the disease process.

The observations by Liu and colleagues are in partial disagreement with those mentioned above, where both wild-type and mutant SOD1 were detected in the IMS of mitochondria of various tissues including brain and liver. It is likely that some of these discrepancies can be explained by differences in the strategies for mitochondrial purification and detection systems. Although more work needs to be done to clarify the exact intramitochondrial localization of SOD1, there is a consensus in the field that mutant SOD1 forms aggregates in mitochondria. The next challenges will be to characterize the molecular structure and the composition of these aggregates, and to establish whether or not they are directly involved in mitochondrial dysfunction. In particular, it will be interesting to assess whether mutant SOD1 forms abnormal interactions with other mitochondrial proteins that may result in mitochondrial dysfunction. An interesting example of potentially harmful protein–protein interaction has already been identified between Bcl-2 and mutant SOD1[46], and it is possible that several other proteins involved in different processes, such as mitochondrial bioenergetics and biogenesis, may also be involved.

Mitochondria as modulators of apoptotic cell death in SOD1 familial amyotrophic lateral sclerosis

Mitochondria are the site of initiation of the intrinsic apoptotic pathway, which is activated by the release of pro-apoptotic factors from mitochondria and can be either caspase-dependent or caspase-independent[47]. Several lines of evidence suggest that the mitochondrial apoptotic pathway may play an important role in SOD1-mediated neuronal degeneration. Mutant SOD1 predisposes neuronal cells to apoptosis in response to various challenges. Oxidative stress causes the sequential activation of the executioner caspases 1 and 3 in differentiated neuroblastoma cells expressing mutant SOD1[48,49]. *In vivo*, in G93A SOD1 mutant spinal cord motor neurons, cytochrome c is released from mitochondria, resulting in caspase-9 activation[50]. Pasinelli *et al.* have shown that SOD1 interacts with the anti-

apoptotic protein Bcl-2 both *in vitro* and *in vivo* in the transgenic SOD1 mouse[46]. These authors found that mutant SOD1 binds to Bcl-2 on the outer mitochondrial membrane. This finding suggests that the interaction with mutant SOD1 may result in defective Bcl-2 anti-apoptotic functions and predispose neurons to apoptosis.

Consistent with the suggestion that caspase-mediated apoptosis contributes to the pathogenesis of FALS, it was also shown that both pharmacologic inhibition of caspase activation[51] and overexpression of the mitochondrial anti-apoptotic protein Bcl-2[52] resulted in life extension in G93A SOD1 mutant mice.

Despite the evidence that apoptosis may be involved in neuronal death in ALS, there are some contradictory observations that need to be mentioned. For example, mutant SOD1 mice genetically devoid of caspase-11, an upstream regulator of the executioner caspase-1 and -3, showed no improvement of the ALS disease phenotype[53]. Furthermore, morphologic and biochemical markers of apoptotic cell death, such as positive TUNEL staining, are difficult to detect both in ALS patients and in transgenic animals. These considerations suggest that, if intrinsic apoptosis is initiated by the mitochondria of ALS motor neurons, it may follow an atypical course, where the process may be initiated in some cells but not necessarily completed. Mitochondrial dysfunction in certain ALS motor neurons may be limited to distal neuronal processes and result in quantal release of pro-apoptotic factors, for example in response to calcium-mediated toxicity. However, it is possible that the pro-apoptotic stimulus is too localized or quantitatively insufficient to cause a downstream effect resulting in cell death. These motor neurons may linger in a twilight zone between life and death, until they are hit by another wave of toxic events and eventually degenerate and die. According to this model, only a small number of cells are actually displaying detectable apoptosis at any given time in the course of the disease.

Is mitochondrial dysfunction a necessary step in amyotrophic lateral sclerosis pathogenesis?

Answering the question of whether or not mitochondrial dysfunction is a necessary step in the development of ALS is going to be a difficult task. The first problem is that, although mitochondrial morphological abnormalities are prominent pathologic features in the G93A and the G37R SOD1 transgenic mice, other mouse models, such as the G85R, do not share these features[54,55]. This is puzzling, because both G85R and G37R mutant SOD1 have been found to localize and aggregate in spinal cord mitochondria from transgenic mice[45]. It is possible that SOD1 may affect mitochondrial functions in these mouse models without causing major morphologic changes such as large vacuoles. In the future, it will be important to determine whether the findings of mitochondrial dysfunction obtained from the G93A mouse may be extended to other mouse models, in order to determine whether mitochondrial dysfunction is a general outcome of the disease.

The second problem is that, since SOD1 is expressed both in the cytosol and in mitochondria, it is virtually impossible to ascribe mitochondrial dysfunction definitely to a direct noxious effect of mitochondrial SOD1. It is difficult to exclude that mitochondrial dysfunction may arise as an indirect consequence of mutant SOD1 'toxic gain of function' in other cell compartments, where SOD1 is abundant. For example, cytosolic mutant SOD1 could promote aberrant production of reactive oxygen species[36], which secondarily damage mitochondrial components, or it could sequester protective factors such as the heat shock proteins that are involved in anti-apoptotic defense mechanisms[41]. A theoretical approach to address this issue could be to generate cellular and animal models where mutant SOD1 is selectively targeted to the mitochondria. Conversely, the identification of protein domains in SOD1 crucial for its mitochondrial import could allow for the generation of SOD1 mutant models, where the

mitochondrial content of mutant SOD1 is reduced or eliminated. The comparison of these models with those where mutant SOD1 is expressed in both the cytosolic and mitochondrial compartments would help us in defining the role that mitochondrial mutant SOD1 plays in mitochondrial dysfunction and in the pathogenesis of the disease.

The third problem is to determine whether therapeutic approaches aimed at improving mitochondrial functions and protecting mitochondria from mitochondrial apoptosis can affect the progression of the disease. As mentioned above, it was shown that genetic[52] or pharmacologic[51,56] manipulations of the mitochondrial apoptotic pathway resulted in an extension in the lifespan of mutant SOD1 transgenic mice. Furthermore, dietary supplementation with creatine[57], an important component of the energy buffering system in the cell, or with free radical scavenging agents[58,59] have been shown to prolong the lifespan of mutant SOD1 transgenic mice. Clearly, more work needs to be done in this direction. There is a need in the future to identify efficient approaches that directly target the pathogenic processes taking place in mitochondria of ALS patients.

SUMMARY AND CONCLUSIONS

Mitochondria play a pivotal role in many metabolic and apoptotic pathways that regulate the life and death of cells, and multiple lines of evidence are accumulating, suggesting that mitochondrial dysfunction is involved in ALS pathogenesis. Several investigators are studying the mechanisms underlying mitochondria impairment in ALS. Morphologic and biochemical mitochondrial abnormalities have been described in sporadic human ALS cases, but the implications of these findings in terminally ill individuals or in postmortem tissues are difficult to decipher. However, remarkable mitochondrial abnormalities have also been identified in the transgenic mouse models of familial ALS expressing mutant SOD1. Detailed studies conducted in these mouse models indicate that mitochondrial abnormalities begin prior to the clinical and pathologic onset of the disease, suggesting that mitochondrial dysfunction may be causally involved in the pathogenesis of ALS. Mitochondrial dysfunction may cause motor neuron death in a number of ways: by enhancing calcium-mediated excitotoxicity, by increasing generation of reactive oxygen species, or by initiating the intrinsic apoptotic pathway. Although the mechanisms whereby mitochondria are damaged by mutant SOD1 still remain to be fully understood, the finding that a portion of mutant SOD1 is localized in mitochondria, where it forms aberrant aggregates and protein interactions, opened many avenues of investigation. The future challenges are to devise models to gain better understanding of the effects of mutant SOD1 in mitochondria, and the relative contribution of mitochondrial dysfunction to the pathogenesis of ALS, as well as to identify therapeutic approaches that target mitochondrial dysfunction and its consequences.

ACKNOWLEDGMENTS

We thank NIH/NINDS, the Robert Packard ALS Research Center at Johns Hopkins, ALSA, and the Muscular Dystrophy Association for their financial support.

REFERENCES

1. Schon EA, Manfredi G. Neuronal degeneration and mitochondrial dysfunction. J Clin Invest 2003; 111: 303–12

2. Atsumi T. The ultrastructure of intramuscular nerves in amyotrophic lateral sclerosis. Acta Neuropathol (Berl) 1981; 55: 193–8

3. Afifi AK, Aleu FP, Goodgold J, MacKay B. Ultrastructure of atrophic muscle in amyotrophic lateral sclerosis. Neurology 1966; 16: 475–81

4. Hirano A, Donnenfeld H, Sasaki S, Nakano I. Fine structural observations of neurofilamentous changes in amyotrophic lateral sclerosis. J Neuropathol Exp Neurol 1984; 43: 461–70

5. Sasaki S, Iwata M. Impairment of fast axonal transport in the proximal axons of anterior horn neurons in amyotrophic lateral sclerosis. Neurology 1996; 47: 535–40

6. Siklos L, Engelhardt J, Harati Y, et al. Ultrastructural evidence for altered calcium in motor nerve terminals in amyotropic lateral sclerosis. Ann Neurol 1996; 39: 203–16

7. Wiedemann FR, Winkler K, Kuznetsov AV, et al. Impairment of mitochondrial function in skeletal muscle of patients with amyotrophic lateral sclerosis. J Neurol Sci 1998; 156: 65–72

8. Vielhaber S, Kunz D, Winkler K, et al. Mitochondrial DNA abnormalities in skeletal muscle of patients with sporadic amyotrophic lateral sclerosis. Brain 2000; 123: 1339–48

9. Borthwick GM, Johnson MA, Ince PG, et al. Mitochondrial enzyme activity in amyotrophic lateral sclerosis: Implications for the role of mitochondria in neuronal cell death. Ann Neurol 1999; 46: 787–90

10. Wiedemann FR, Manfredi G, Mawrin C, et al. Mitochondrial DNA and respiratory chain function in spinal cords of ALS patients. J Neurochem 2002; 80: 616–25

11. DiMauro S. Mitochondrial diseases. Biochim Biophys Acta 2004; 1658: 80–8

12. Comi GP, Bordoni A, Salani S, et al. Cytochrome c oxidase subunit I microdeletion in a patient with motor neuron disease. Ann Neurol 1998; 43: 110–16

13. Swerdlow RH, Parks JK, Cassarino DS, et al. Mitochondria in sporadic amyotrophic lateral sclerosis. Exp Neurol 1998; 153: 135–42

14. Gajewski CD, Lin MT, Cudkowicz ME, et al. Mitochondrial DNA from platelets of sporadic ALS patients restores normal respiratory functions in rho(0) cells. Exp Neurol 2003; 179: 229–35

15. Rosen DR, Siddique T, Patterson D, et al. Mutations in Cu/Zn superoxide dismutase gene are associated with familial amyotrophic lateral sclerosis. Nature 1993; 362: 59–62

16. Lenaz G. Role of mitochondria in oxidative stress and ageing. Biochim Biophys Acta 1998; 1366: 53–67

17. Klug D, Rabani J, Fridovich I. A direct demonstration of the catalytic action of superoxide dismutase through the use of pulse radiolysis. J Biol Chem 1972; 247: 4839–42

18. Borchelt DR, Lee MK, Slunt HS, et al. Superoxide dismutase 1 with mutations linked to familial amyotrophic lateral sclerosis possesses significant activity. Proc Natl Acad Sci USA 1994; 91: 8292–6

19. Dal Canto MC, Gurney ME. Neuropathological changes in two lines of mice carrying a transgene for mutant human Cu,Zn SOD, and in mice overexpressing wild type human SOD: A model of familial amyotrophic lateral sclerosis (FALS). Brain Res 1995; 676: 25–40

20. Wong PC, Pardo CA, Borchelt DR, et al. An adverse property of a familial ALS-linked SOD1 mutation causes motor neuron disease characterized by vacuolar degeneration of mitochondria. Neuron 1995; 14: 1105–16

21. Kong J, Xu Z. Massive mitochondrial degeneration in motor neurons triggers the onset of amyotrophic lateral sclerosis in mice expressing a mutant SOD1. J Neurosci 1998; 18: 3241–50

22. Jaarsma D, Rognoni F, van Duijn W, et al. CuZn superoxide dismutase (SOD1) accumulates in vacuolated mitochondria in transgenic mice expressing amyotrophic lateral sclerosis-linked SOD1 mutations. Acta Neuropathol (Berl) 2001; 102: 293–305

23. Bendotti C, Calvaresi N, Chiveri L, et al. Early vacuolization and mitochondrial damage in motor neurons of FALS mice are not associated with apoptosis or with changes in cytochrome oxidase histochemical reactivity. J Neurol Sci 2001; 191: 25–33

24. Higgins CM, Jung C, Xu Z. ALS-associated mutant SOD1G93A causes mitochondrial vacuolation by expansion of the intermembrane space and by involvement of SOD1 aggregation and peroxisomes. BMC Neurosci 2003; 4: 16

25. Carri MT, Ferri A, Battistoni A, et al. Expression of a Cu,Zn superoxide dismutase typical of familial amyotrophic lateral sclerosis induces mitochondrial alteration and increase of cytosolic Ca2+ concentration in transfected neuroblastoma SH-SY5Y cells. FEBS Lett 1997; 414: 365–8

26. Kruman II, Pedersen WA, Springer JE, Mattson MP. ALS-linked Cu/Zn-SOD mutation increases vulnerability of motor neurons to excitotoxicity by a mechanism involving increased oxidative stress and perturbed calcium homeostasis. Exp Neurol 1999; 160: 28–39

27. Menzies FM, Cookson MR, Taylor RW, et al. Mitochondrial dysfunction in a cell culture model of familial amyotrophic lateral sclerosis. Brain 2002; 125: 1522–33

28. Jung C, Higgins CM, Xu Z. A quantitative histochemical assay for activities of mitochondrial electron transport chain complexes in mouse spinal cord sections. J Neurosci Meth 2002; 114: 165–72

29. Mattiazzi M, D'Aurelio M, Gajewski CD, et al. Mutated human SOD1 causes dysfunction of oxidative phosphorylation in mitochondria of transgenic mice. J Biol Chem 2002; 277: 29626–33

30. Browne SE, Bowling AC, Baik MJ, et al. Metabolic dysfunction in familial, but not sporadic, amyotrophic lateral sclerosis. J Neurochem 1998; 71: 281–7

31. Damiano M, Starkov AA, Petri S, et al. Neural mitochondrial Ca^{2+} capacity impairment precedes the onset of motor symptoms in G93A Cu/Zn-superoxide dismutase mutant mice. J Neurochem 2006; 96: 1349–61

32. Rothstein JD. Excitotoxicity hypothesis. Neurology 1996; 47 (4 Suppl 2): S19–25

33. Tateno M, Sadakata H, Tanaka M, et al. Calcium-permeable AMPA receptors promote misfolding of mutant SOD1 protein and development of amyotrophic lateral sclerosis in a transgenic mouse model. Hum Mol Genet 2004; 13: 2183–96

34. Reynolds IJ. Mitochondrial membrane potential and the permeability transition in excitotoxicity. Ann NY Acad Sci 1999; 893: 33–41

35. Beal MF. Mitochondrial dysfunction and oxidative damage in Alzheimer's and Parkinson's diseases and coenzyme Q10 as a potential treatment. J Bioenerg Biomembr 2004; 36: 381–6

36. Estevez AG, Crow JP, Sampson JB, et al. Induction of nitric oxide-dependent apoptosis in motor neurons by zinc-deficient superoxide dismutase. Science 1999; 286: 2498–500

37. Weisiger RA, Fridovich I. Superoxide dismutase. Organelle specificity. J Biol Chem 1973; 248: 3582–92

38. Higgins CM, Jung C, Ding H, Xu Z. Mutant Cu, Zn superoxide dismutase that causes motoneuron degeneration is present in mitochondria in the CNS. J Neurosci 2002; 22: RC215

39. Sturtz LA, Diekert K, Jensen LT, et al. A fraction of yeast Cu,Zn-superoxide dismutase and its metallochaperone, CCS, localize to the intermembrane space of mitochondria. A physiological role for SOD1 in guarding against mitochondrial oxidative damage. J Biol Chem 2001; 276: 38084–9

40. Okado-Matsumoto A, Fridovich I. Subcellular distribution of superoxide dismutases (SOD) in rat liver: Cu,Zn-SOD in mitochondria. J Biol Chem 2001; 276: 38388–93

41. Okado-Matsumoto A, Fridovich I. Amyotrophic lateral sclerosis: A proposed mechanism. Proc Natl Acad Sci USA 2002; 99: 9010–14

42. Field LS, Furukawa Y, O'Halloran TV, Culotta VC. Factors controlling the uptake of yeast copper/zinc superoxide dismutase into mitochondria. J Biol Chem 2003; 278: 28052–9

43. Vijayvergiya C, Beal MF, Buck J, Manfredi G. Mutant superoxide dismutase 1 forms aggregates in the brain mitochondrial matrix of amyotrophic lateral sclerosis mice. J Neurosci 2005; 25: 2463–70

44. Xu Z, Jung C, Higgins C, Levine J, Kong J. Mitochondrial degeneration in amyotrophic lateral sclerosis. J Bioenerg Biomembr 2004; 36: 395–9

45. Liu J, Lillo C, Jonsson PA, et al. Toxicity of familial ALS-linked SOD1 mutants from selective recruitment to spinal mitochondria. Neuron 2004; 43: 5–17

46. Pasinelli P, Belford ME, Lennon N, et al. Amyotrophic lateral sclerosis-associated SOD1 mutant proteins bind and aggregate with Bcl-2 in spinal cord mitochondria. Neuron 2004; 43: 19–30

47. Green DR, Kroemer G. The pathophysiology of mitochondrial cell death. Science 2004; 305: 626–9

48. Pasinelli P, Borchelt DR, Houseweart MK, et al. Caspase-1 is activated in neural cells and tissue with amyotrophic lateral sclerosis-associated mutations in copper–zinc superoxide dismutase. Proc Natl Acad Sci USA 1998; 95: 15763–8

49. Pasinelli P, Houseweart MK, Brown RH Jr, Cleveland DW. Caspase-1 and -3 are sequentially activated in motor neuron death in Cu,Zn superoxide dismutase-mediated familial amyotrophic lateral sclerosis. Proc Natl Acad Sci USA 2000; 97: 13901–6

50. Guegan C, Vila M, Rosoklija G, et al. Recruitment of the mitochondrial-dependent apoptotic pathway in amyotrophic lateral sclerosis. J Neurosci 2001; 21: 6569–76

51. Li M, Ona VO, Guegan C, et al. Functional role of caspase-1 and caspase-3 in an ALS transgenic mouse model. Science 2000; 288: 335–9

52. Kostic V, Jackson-Lewis V, de Bilbao F, et al. Bcl-2: Prolonging life in a transgenic mouse model of familial amyotrophic lateral sclerosis. Science 1997; 277: 559–62

53. Kang SJ, Sanchez I, Jing N, Yuan J. Dissociation between neurodegeneration and caspase-11-mediated activation of caspase-1 and caspase-3 in a mouse model of amyotrophic lateral sclerosis. J Neurosci 2003; 23: 5455–60

54. Ripps ME, Huntley GW, Hof PR, et al. Transgenic mice expressing an altered murine superoxide dismutase gene provide an animal model of amyotrophic lateral sclerosis. Proc Natl Acad Sci USA 1995; 92: 689–93

55. Bruijn LI, Houseweart MK, Kato S, et al. Aggregation and motor neuron toxicity of an ALS-linked SOD1 mutant independent from wild-type SOD1. Science 1998; 281: 1851–4

56. Zhu S, Stavrovskaya IG, Drozda M, et al. Minocycline inhibits cytochrome c release and delays progression of amyotrophic lateral sclerosis in mice. Nature 2002; 417: 74–8

57. Klivenyi P, Ferrante RJ, Matthews RT, et al. Neuroprotective effects of creatine in a transgenic animal model of amyotrophic lateral sclerosis. Nat Med 1999; 5: 347–50

58. Jung C, Rong Y, Doctrow S, et al. Synthetic superoxide dismutase/catalase mimetics reduce oxidative stress and prolong survival in a mouse amyotrophic lateral sclerosis model. Neurosci Lett 2001; 304: 157–60

59. Wu AS, Kiaei M, Aguirre N, et al. Iron porphyrin treatment extends survival in a transgenic animal model of amyotrophic lateral sclerosis. J Neurochem 2003; 85: 142–50

Section 5

Therapy of amyotrophic lateral sclerosis and related disorders

18

Therapeutic trials in amyotrophic lateral sclerosis: past, present and future

Jacqueline Lau, Robin Conwit, Robert Miller, Merit Cudkowicz

INTRODUCTION

Approximately 20 clinical trials have been completed in patients with amyotrophic lateral sclerosis (ALS) in the past decade. Only one drug, riluzole, slows the disease course. Nonetheless, results of past trials contribute to our understanding of ALS, and provide direction for future investigations. The process through which drugs are selected for clinical testing, therapeutic trials and the lessons learned from these studies are presented.

DRUG SCREENING METHODS

Recent studies provide new insights into the molecular and cellular processes leading to selective motor neuron death in ALS. Proposed mechanisms of pathogenesis include glutamate toxicity, oxidative stress, apoptosis, cytotoxicity, protein aggregation and neuroinflammation[1]. Based on these putative pathways, numerous pharmaceutical agents have been identified for testing in patients with ALS.

Several laboratory-based models are used to understand the biology of the illness and to facilitate drug screening. Models of disease initially consisted of pure motor neurons cultured *in vitro*, and organotypic slices of the spinal cord[2]. The discovery of mutations in the Cu/Zn superoxide dismutase (*SOD1*) gene in familial ALS led to the development of *in vitro* models of cell death based on SOD1 dysfunction[3,4]. *In vitro* models of SOD1-mediated toxicity have been developed in mouse neuroblastoma cultures[3], SHSY5Y human neuroblastoma cells[5] and PC12 cell lines[6].

Transgenic mice and rats expressing mutant forms of SOD1 provide a valuable animal model of ALS for understanding pathways that can lead to motor neuron cell death[7-9]. Expression of human SOD1 containing the mutations G93A, G37R, or G85R at sufficient levels in transgenic mice causes a progressive paralytic disease that essentially resembles human ALS. Disease course varies with transgene dosage and mutation. The most commonly used model for drug screening is the SOD1-G93A high expressing line, which has an average survival of 5 months[10]. Clinical features in these mice become evident at 3 months, at which time they develop a subtle shaking in their limbs and a progressive decline in wheel running. By 4 months, progressive paralysis mainly affecting the rear legs is evident. The similarity of symptom progression to human ALS has made these mouse models useful in studying the biology of the disease and in the screening of therapeutic approaches for human ALS.

Three additional ALS genes have been found. The *ALS2* gene codes for alsin, a novel protein with homology to guanine-nucleotide exchange factors for GTPases[11,12]. Loss-of-function of ALS2 leads to denervation beginning in the first decade, with predominant corticobulbar and corticospinal signs, and very slow progression. Mutations in a dynactin gene have been shown to be responsible for a slowly progressive, bulbar-predominant form of lower motor neuropathy[13]. Finally, a third gene encoding the senataxin protein has been associated with a rare, slowly progressive, early-onset form of ALS, known as ALS4[14]. As these newly identified genes are further studied, additional models for drug screening should become available.

In an effort to accelerate *in vitro* drug screening, the National Institute of Neurological Disorders and Stroke (NINDS) initiated the Neurodegeneration Drug Screening Consortium (NDSC) to use high throughput screening technology for drug identification. Under the NDSC, a collaboration of investigators from 26 academic laboratories carried out blind tests on 1040 Food and Drug Administration (FDA)-approved drugs, using 29 different assays designed to emulate some aspects of neurodegeneration. Each assay examined a target relevant to neuropathogenesis, including protein aggregation, protein toxicity, excitotoxicity and apoptosis. The preliminary findings found seven compounds that were active in several ALS-related assays, once of which is being prepared for human studies (see Ceftriaxone, p. 343).

CLINICAL TRIALS IN AMYOTROPHIC LATERAL SCLEROSIS

Completed trials

Anti-excitotoxic agents

The excitotoxicity theory was first proposed in the early 1970s to describe neurodegeneration resulting from excessive exposure to excitatory amino acids[15]. That glutamate excitotoxicity might be involved in ALS was first supported by the discovery of increased glutamate levels in plasma[16] and cerebrospinal fluid (CSF)[17] from patients with ALS. *In vitro* studies confirmed that, in spinal motor neuron cultures, glutamate causes a dose-dependent induction of programed cell death[18]. Subsequently, it was reported that, in the majority of patients with ALS, there was a selective defect in the astrocyte glutamate transporter, excitatory amino acid transporter 2 (EAAT2), in motor control areas of the brain and spinal cord[19]. Anti-excitotoxic drugs have been tested in several clinical trials in patients with ALS.

Riluzole was originally developed as an anticonvulsant. The drug inhibits the pre-synaptic release of glutamate and reduces neuronal damage in several experimental models[20]. Besides its effects on glutamate release, riluzole blocks voltage-gated sodium channels[21], interacts with potassium channels[22] and inhibits calcium currents[23]. Although the influence on glutamatergic transmission is currently favored as an explanation of neuroprotection, the blockage of sodium and other ion channels may also contribute to its neuroprotective properties.

Two randomized, double-blind, placebo-controlled trials have been conducted in patients with ALS and both indicate a survival benefit of riluzole. In the first trial, 155 patients with probable or definite ALS were randomized to receive either 100 mg riluzole or placebo daily[24]. Randomization was stratified according to the site of disease onset (limb vs. bulbar). The two primary outcome measures were survival (determined by death or tracheostomy) and rates of change in functional status as determined by a four-point rating composed of scores for bulbar and limb function. Secondary outcome measures were muscle function according to the five-grade scale of the Medical Research Council (MRC), respiratory function as measured by the forced vital capacity (FVC), scores on the Clinical Global Impression of Change scale (CGIC), and the patient's subjective evaluations of fasciculations, cramps, stiffness and tiredness, expressed on four 100-mm visual-analog scales (VAS).

Riluzole had a significant effect on rates of survival and muscle strength deterioration. At 12 months, 58% of patients in the placebo group remained alive compared with 74% in the riluzole group ($p = 0.014$). The bulbar-onset group showed a greater treatment effect with 1-year survival rates of 35% with placebo and 73% with riluzole ($p = 0.014$), compared with the limb-onset patients who had 1-year survival rates of 64% with placebo and 74% with riluzole ($p = 0.017$). The survival advantage with riluzole was smaller at the end of the placebo-controlled period (37% with placebo vs. 49% with riluzole), but remained significant in the overall population ($p = 0.046$) as well as in the patients with bulbar-onset disease ($p = 0.013$). With respect to the secondary outcome measures, only the deterioration of limb strength at 12 months was significantly slower in the treated group ($p = 0.028$). Asthenia, stiffness and increased aminotransferase levels in the blood were among the notable side-effects.

Although results indicated a favorable effect of riluzole on survival and muscle function, criticisms of the study arose surrounding the disproportionate contribution of the bulbar-onset subgroup to the observed effect of the whole, and the observation that a more favorable baseline distribution of prognostic variables existed in theriluzole-treated bulbar-onset group[25,26]. The use of tracheostomy as a surrogate for death was questioned, as practice variations in ventilatory support among the participating centers may have introduced bias[27].

A second, larger, dose-ranging trial was conducted in 1996 and it confirmed the therapeutic effect of riluzole[28]. This study involved 959 patients receiving 50, 100, 200 mg riluzole or placebo for up to 18 months. The design of the study was similar to the first, but included additional statistical analyses to validate the relevance of the prognostic factors identified in the initial study. After a median follow-up of 18 months,

50% of the placebo-treated patients and 57% of those who received 100 mg/day riluzole were alive without tracheostomy (adjusted risk 0.65 $p = 0.002$). There was no apparent added benefit at a higher dosage. Unlike the first study, no significant difference was present according to site of symptom onset and there was no observed effect of treatment on functional outcomes. The authors concluded that riluzole conferred a dose-dependent benefit to tracheostomy-free survival and that the 100-mg dose provided the optimal risk/benefit ratio.

Although quality of life measurements have not been examined directly in past riluzole trials, a retrospective analysis of the second trial suggests that patients who took riluzole remained for a longer period of time in a milder health state compared to those patients taking placebo[29]. These data suggest an advantage to taking the drug in earlier stages of the disease compared to late stages.

Studies by Groeneveld and colleagues found a high interindividual variability of riluzole serum concentrations at the standard prescribed dose of 100 mg a day[30]. In a follow-up study, the same authors sought to determine whether a serum concentration–effect relationship exists by measuring serum riluzole concentrations in 162 ALS patients taking riluzole 50 mg bid, and relating these data with disease progression and survival[31]. Riluzole trough and peak serum concentrations were determined; the area under the serum concentration–time curve per kg body weight (AUC/kg) was calculated and used as a measure for total riluzole exposure. Linear regression analysis showed a trend of an effect of the AUC/kg on the slope of the arm megascore. Subgroup analysis revealed a slower rate of deterioration of arm muscle strength among patients with the highest AUC/kg levels; survival in this group was also higher than among the rest of the patients, but this difference failed to reach statistical significance ($p = 0.13$). These findings suggest that patients with high riluzole serum levels may benefit more than those with lower levels. Individualization of riluzole dosing may be called for if these findings can be confirmed. However, serum levels of riluzole are not widely available.

The safety concerns for riluzole are relatively few, with side-effects mainly confined to fatigue, nausea or vomiting, and very occasionally elevated liver enzymes, renal function impairment (see Physician Desk Reference (PDR)), vertigo or somnolence. Neutropenia and interstitial pneumonitis have been described[32]. It is, at present, the only drug of documented efficacy and the only drug approved for ALS by the FDA in the USA. The drug was the subject of a practice advisory published by the American Academy of Neurology[33] and a systematic review by the Cochrane Collaboration[34].

Gabapentin Studies suggest that the anticonvulsant gabapentin may reduce glutamate activity, but its exact mechanism of action upon the glutamatergic system has not been fully elucidated. The drug has a modest neuroprotective effect against glutamate toxicity[2] and prolongs survival slightly in the SOD1 transgenic mouse model[35]. In a randomized, placebo-controlled phase II trial, 152 patients with ALS were enrolled at eight sites in the USA to receive gabapentin 800 mg tid or placebo for 6 months[36]. The primary endpoint was the slope of the arm megascore as measured by maximum voluntary isometric contraction (MVIC) and the secondary endpoint was the rate of decline of FVC (per cent predicted). Data analysis revealed a trend ($p = 0.057$) toward slower decline of arm strength in patients taking gabapentin compared with those taking placebo (mean difference 24%), with no observed effect on FVC.

These results prompted the undertaking of a second placebo-controlled trial using a higher dose of gabapentin, a larger sample size, and a longer period of follow-up[37]. A total of 204 patients were randomly assigned to receive oral gabapentin 1200 mg tid or placebo daily for 9 months. Outcome measures were similar to those in the phase II trial. There was no beneficial effect of the drug on the primary or secondary outcome

measures. Analysis of the combined data from the two trials revealed a more rapid decline of FVC in patients treated with gabapentin than those treated with placebo. The authors concluded that there was no evidence of any beneficial effect of gabapentin on disease progression or symptoms in patients with ALS.

Topiramate is an FDA-approved agent for epilepsy. In cultured neurons, topiramate reduces glutamate release from neurons and blocks kainate activation of the α-amino-3-hydroxy-5-methyl-isoxazole-4-propionic (AMPA) receptor[38]. In an *in vitro* model of chronic glutamate toxicity, topiramate protected motor neurons in a dose-dependent fashion[39]. Topiramate did not affect disease course in the G93A mutant SOD1 mouse model[39]. A NINDS funded double-blind, placebo-controlled multicenter randomized trial was conducted by the North Eastern ALS (NEALS) Consortium to determine the safety and efficacy of the drug in slowing disease progression in ALS patients[40]. A total of 296 patients were randomized in a 2:1 scheme to receive 800 mg/day topiramate or placebo, for 12 months. The primary endpoint was the rate of change in upper limb motor function as measured by MVIC. Secondary outcome measures included safety and the rate of decline of FVC, grip strength, ALS Functional Rating Scale (ALSFRS) and survival. At the dose studied, patients treated with topiramate showed a faster decrease in arm strength. Topiramate did not significantly affect survival, nor did it alter the decline in FVC or ALSFRS. Patients treated with topiramate had an increased frequency of anorexia, depression, diarrhea, ecchymosis, nausea, kidney calculus, paresthesia, taste perversion, thinking abnormalities, weight loss and abnormal blood clotting, with deep venous thrombosis and pulmonary emboli. Authors concluded that further studies of topiramate at this dosage were not warranted.

Other anti-excitotoxic therapies Clinical studies of dextromethorphan[41,42], lamotrigine[43] and verapamil[44] have been conducted in ALS. All studies were small and underpowered, with indeterminate results.

Summary   The anti-excitotoxic drug strategy has yielded the first and currently only drug approved to modify the course of ALS. Riluzole as an active drug has largely contributed to stimulate research into the possible role of glutamate-induced excitotoxicity in the pathogenesis of ALS. Unfortunately, though many other anti-excitotoxic drugs have been tested in ALS, none have yet had a significant impact on survival or disease progression.

Neurotrophic factors

In preclinical experiments, neurotrophic factors have shown substantial promise in their potential to protect motor neurons from degeneration[45,46]. Using recombinant protein, these treatment strategies have been evaluated in human trials of ALS, but have not found success. Recent efforts have focused on improving CNS penetration using different drug delivery methods, including viral vectors.

Brain-derived neurotrophic factor (BDNF) promotes motor neuron survival in a number of animal models of motor neuron and peripheral nerve damage[47,48]. It has been tested in humans, in whom it has been administered by subcutaneous injection and by intrathecal delivery. In a placebo-controlled phase III trial, 1135 ALS patients were randomized to placebo, 25 or 100 μg/kg subcutaneous recombinant human BDNF (rhBDNF) for 9 months[49,50]. Primary endpoints were survival and change from baseline in the 6-month FVC. The study failed to show any significant benefit of rhBDNF treatment for the primary endpoints, though there was a trend toward increased survival in the 100 μg/kg group ($p = 0.15$). For those patients who reported diarrhea, perhaps indicating a biologic effect of the drug, 9-month survival was significantly better than with placebo (97.5% vs. 85%).

These data prompted two further multicenter placebo-controlled trials. In the first study, 350 trial participants were randomized to receive either placebo or 300 μg/kg per day rhBDNF by subcutaneous injection for 12 months. The second study enrolled 270 patients into three groups receiving either rhBDNF (25 or 150 mg/day) or placebo by continuous intrathecal infusion for up to 18 months. Both trials were terminated early for lack of efficacy.

Ciliary neurotrophic factor (CNTF) is a Schwann cell-derived protein that promotes motor neuron survival *in vitro*[50] and delays motor dysfunction in animal models of motor neuron injury[51]. Two trials have been conducted in patients with ALS using subcutaneous injections of recombinant human CNTF (rhCNTF).

In one study, 570 ALS patients were randomized to receive either placebo or subcutaneous rhCNTF in doses of 0.5, 2 or 5 μg/kg per day for 6 months[52]. The primary outcome measure was the change from baseline to the last on-treatment value of a combination megascore for limb strength (MVIC) and pulmonary function. Secondary endpoints included arm and leg megascores, FVC, quality of life and survival. At all doses tested, rhCNTF had no beneficial effect on the primary or secondary endpoints. Certain adverse events appeared to be dose related (injection site reactions, cough, asthenia, nausea, anorexia, weight loss, increased salivation), and an increased number of deaths occurred at the highest dose level.

In a concurrent clinical trial 730 patients with ALS were randomized to receive 30 μg/kg or 15 μg/kg rhCNTF or placebo subcutaneously three times a week for 9 months[53]. The primary outcome measure was the rate of decline of isometric muscle strength, while secondary endpoints were the rate of loss of pulmonary function, timed functional tests and functional scales. There was no statistically significant difference in primary or secondary endpoints between rhCNTF- and placebo-treated patients. Mortality was similar in all three study arms. As in the other rhCNTF study, dose-related adverse effects were common.

Based on these results, it is unlikely that subcutaneously administered rhCNTF will be of clinical use in the treatment of patients with ALS. It has been postulated that the direct delivery of the drug into the central nervous system (CNS) might provide improved efficacy and fewer toxic effects[54]. Based on this rationale, a phase I study was undertaken to determine the safety of intrathecal delivery of CNTF in four ALS patients[55]. The drug was well distributed along the spinal canal, and the systemic side-effects that were observed with subcutaneous rhCNTF did not occur.

Insulin-like growth factor-I (IGF-I) promotes motor neuron survival in cell culture studies and reduces apoptotic motor neuron death during development in animal models[56]. There have been two double-blind, placebo-controlled trials investigating the efficacy of recombinant human IGF-I (rhIGF-I) in the treatment of ALS.

The first study, conducted at eight centers in North America, enrolled 266 patients who were randomized to receive either 0.05 or 0.1 mg/kg per day rhIGF-I or placebo, for 9 months[57]. The primary outcome measure was disease symptom progression, as determined by the rate of change (per patient slope) in the Appel ALS (AALS) rating scale total score. Secondary outcome analyses were conducted on the following variables: changes from baseline by month in the AALS total score, time to attainment of protocol-specified termination criteria (AALS ≥115 or FVC <39%), time to 20-point progression of the AALS total score, the change from baseline to the last value of the sickness impact profile, and the slope of post-randomization FVC measurements.

Primary outcome analysis demonstrated smaller slopes of the AALS total score in the rhIGF-I-treated patients (both dose groups combined) than in the placebo patients (3.4 vs. 4.2 points per month). A dose–response relationship was observed in that the AALS slope in the low-dose group (3.8 ± 0.3) was greater than in the high-dose group (3.1 ± 0.3 points/month).

Among the secondary outcome measures, lower monthly AALS scores were observed consistently from months 1–9. The change in AALS total score from randomization to last value was greater in the placebo (mean 23.5 ± 1.8) than in the high-dose group (mean 17.5 ± 1.8, $p = 0.01$). The percentages of patients who met either protocol-specified criterion for early termination (AALS total score ≥115 or FVC <39%) were as follows: 36% of the placebo, 39% of the low-dose and 23% of the high-dose treatment groups. The relative risk (RR) of a protocol-specific early termination was 0.56 (95% CI 0.32, 0.97) for the high-dose group compared with the placebo group ($p = 0.04$), indicating that high-dose patients had a 44% lower risk of these events. The RR of 20-point progression in the high-dose group was half that of the placebo group (RR 0.50; 95% CI 0.33, 0.76; $p = 0.001$). A comparison of the changes in SIP scores from baseline to last value among the three treatment groups demonstrated dose-related and significant differences between the placebo and the high-dose rhIGF-I-treated groups for the overall ($p = 0.01$) and psychosocial dimension ($p = 0.02$) scores.

A second clinical trial involving 183 ALS patients was conducted at eight European centers[58]. Patients were randomized in a 2:1 ratio to receive rhIGF-I 0.1 mg/kg per day or placebo subcutaneously for 9 months. The primary efficacy variable was the change in AALS total score from baseline to study endpoint for each individual patient. The secondary endpoint was the SIP. At study completion, there was no significant beneficial effect of rhIGF-I on the progression of ALS.

A recent Cochrane review found the methodological quality of the two trials unsatisfactory, with unequal baseline status of patients, and recommended further trials to determine whether IGF-I shows efficacy in ALS[59]. The 2:1 randomization scheme used in the European study resulted in too low a number of controls (59 patients), which might have biased the trial toward a negative result and overemphasized side-effects. There was also concern about the reliance on an endpoint very sensitive to missing data. In both trials a large number of patients withdrew from the study for various reasons (death, protocol-specific terminations, adverse experience, patient request, non-compliance), and it is quite possible that patients with missing data were more seriously affected, and their omission biased the results. Blinding of both trials was also unsatisfactory, as many patients receiving IGF-I experienced drug-related adverse effects, notably injection site inflammation. Based on these and other observations, the reviewers found that the opportunity to evaluate the potential efficacy of IGF-I in ALS was compromised by faulty trial design.

A third trial in North America was initiated in June 2003, and enrolled 330 patients in 16 centers. Patients are followed for 2 years and results are expected in 2007. The primary endpoint is the rate of change in manual muscle testing, and secondary endpoints will include tracheostomy-free survival and change in ALSFRS. A study to evaluate the efficacy of retrograde viral delivery of IGF-I is in the planning stage (see Drugs in development).

Xaliproden (SR 57746A) is a non-peptide compound that is able to cross the blood–brain barrier and exhibits neurotrophic activity in several cell culture systems[60]. It has affinity for 5-HT1A receptors, but it is unclear whether this is related to its observed neurotrophic actions. Though not tested in preclinical ALS animal models, the drug showed promise in phase II trials, appearing to slow the decline in all measured functional ratings in patients receiving 2 mg daily of SR57746A, compared with placebo[61]. Phase III trials were initiated by the manufacturer, Sanofi Recherche, to evaluate the effectiveness, safety and tolerability of 1 mg and 2 mg doses of xaliproden in patients with ALS[62]. One study included 1210 patients concurrently taking riluzole 50 mg bid, and the other study included 867 patients not taking this drug. The two primary endpoints were time to death, tracheostomy or permanent assisted ventilation, and time to vital capacity (VC) < 50%.

Secondary endpoints were rates of change of various functional measures. All patients were studied for a period of 18 months. Neither study reached statistical significance, but there was a trend in favor of 1 mg xaliproden as an add-on to riluzole for time to vital capacity < 50% predicted. The results were not convincing enough to apply for regulatory approval.

Summary The lack of efficacy of subcutaneously administered neurotrophic factors in clinical ALS therapy can be attributed to several factors. Pharmacokinetics, dosage, bioavailability and systemic toxic effects are among the most obvious. Trials of intrathecal administration of factors such as BDNF and CNTF proved the feasibility of this mode of delivery, if not efficacy. Recent studies have explored the use of viral vectors in the delivery of growth factors, but their effect in human ALS is not yet known. Neurotrophic strategies remain promising therapeutic agents for ALS and clearly merit further consideration, perhaps with alternative methods of delivery, or in combination with other agents in a drug cocktail.

Antioxidants

Oxidative stress may be involved in the pathogenesis of various neurodegenerative diseases including ALS[63]. Many patients take antioxidant supplements. It is important to determine whether antioxidants are effective therapies in ALS.

Vitamin E The antioxidant vitamin E (α-tocopherol) delays the onset and progression of paralysis in transgenic mice expressing a mutation in SOD1[64]. In 1987, a small trial open-label study of α-tocopherol in patients with ALS indicated a possibility of lessening of fatigue, fasciculations and cramps[65]. Recently, a randomized controlled trial was carried out in Europe in which 289 ALS patients, concurrently taking riluzole, were randomized to receive either α-tocopherol 500 mg bid or placebo daily for one year[66]. The primary outcome measure was the rate of deterioration of function as assessed by the modified Norris limb scale; survival was also recorded. Biomarkers of oxidative stress were assessed in a subset of patients at trial entry and at 3 months. After 12 months of treatment, there was no significant effect of α-tocopherol on the primary outcome measure or overall survival. However, among secondary outcome measures, there was a slower progression from the milder health state A to a more severe health state B of the ALS Health State scale among patients taking vitamin E. After 3 months, there was an increase in glutathione activity in plasma and a decrease in lipid peroxidation activity in the treatment group, indicating some beneficial change in biochemical markers of oxidative stress.

N-Acetylcysteine (NAC) is a free radical scavenger that improves survival and preserves motor performance in the SOD1 G93 transgenic mouse model when administered subcutaneously at a dose of 2.0 mg/kg per day[67]. It was tested in a double-blind placebo-controlled study in 111 patients with ALS at the dose of 50 mg/kg[68]. The primary outcome measure was survival free of tracheostomy, long-term assisted ventilation or positive-pressure breathing. Secondary measures of efficacy were the rates of disease progression as expressed by manual muscle strength testing, myometry, FVC, ability to perform activities of daily living, the degree of independence, and bulbar function. *N-Acetylcysteine* did not induce a significant increase in survival or slowing of the disease in the overall study population; however, there were beneficial trends in survival in the patients with limb-onset disease ($p = 0.06$).

Summary Results from human ALS trials of antioxidants have been largely inconclusive. It is possible that a combination of antioxidants may be more beneficial than a single agent, but further studies are required.

Bioenergetics agents

The role of mitochondrial dysfunction in ALS has been investigated in several preclinical models, and it appears likely that abnormalities in mitochondria occur early in the disease course. Morphologic studies have demonstrated mitochondrial abnormalities in both neural and non-neural tissue from patients with ALS[69–72]. Mitochondrial swelling and vacuolization are seen prior to symptom onset in two strains of familial ALS mice[7,9,73,74]. A highly preferential association of mutant SOD1 with spinal cord mitochondria has been demonstrated, implicating the recruitment of mutant SOD1 to spinal mitochondria as the basis for their selective toxicity in ALS[75,76].

Creatine plays an important role in mitochondrial ATP production and serves as an energy shuttle in neurons[77]. In the SOD1-G93A transgenic mouse model of ALS, creatine monohydrate protected motor neurons and prolonged survival by 26 days, twice the effect of riluzole[78]. Two human clinical trials have been conducted to assess the effect of creatine in ALS. In a double-blind, placebo-controlled trial in the Netherlands, 175 patients with probable or definite ALS were randomly assigned to receive either 10 g creatine monohydrate or placebo daily[79]. Primary outcome measures were death, persistent assisted ventilation, or tracheostomy, while secondary outcome measures were rate of decline of isometric arm muscle strength, FVC, functional status and quality of life. Results at both 12 and 16 months indicated that creatine did not have a beneficial effect on survival or disease progression, and the trial was terminated. This study used a novel futility design that may improve efficiency of future ALS trials, although early stopping may lead to erroneous results[80].

In a clinical trial carried out by the NEALS Consortium, 104 patients were enrolled and randomized to receive either placebo or creatine at a dose of 20 g daily for 5 days, followed by a daily dose of 5 g for 6 months. The primary outcome measure was the MVIC of eight upper extremity muscles; secondary outcome measures included grip strength, ALSFRS and motor unit number estimation. No benefit was demonstrated in the group taking creatine. However, the study was powered only to detect a 50% or greater change in the rate of progression of ALS. As such, the failure to show a significant positive effect of treatment might have missed a more modest benefit[81]. One additional trial of creatine at 5 g/day was also negative. It is not clear in any of the trials of creatine, that sufficient CNS levels were achieved to have the desired neuroprotective effect.

Drugs in development

Anti-excitotoxic agents

Cyclo-oxygenase-2 (COX-2) inhibitors COX-2 may play a key role in glutamate-mediated excitotoxicity by producing prostaglandins that trigger neuronal and astrocytic glutamate release and free radical formation[82]. COX-2 expression is elevated at the protein and mRNA levels in the mutant SOD1 mouse model of ALS. Reflecting the activity of the increased COX-2 levels, the concentration of its product, prostaglandin (PG)E_2, was significantly increased in spinal cords of transgenic ALS mice at clinical onset and endstage compared to non-transgenic control mice[83]. Elevated levels of PGE_2 have been demonstrated in spinal cords of humans who died of ALS, as compared with autopsy control spinal cords[84]. Inhibition of COX-2 may therefore offer a neuroprotective benefit in ALS. There are several COX-2 inhibitors, many of which are approved by the FDA for their anti-inflammatory, analgesic and antipyretic effects. Celecoxib (Celebrex) is a COX-2 inhibitor approved for the treatment of osteoarthritis.

To evaluate the potential therapeutic effect of COX-2 inhibition, an analog of Celebrex (SC236) was tested in an *in vitro* model of glutamate excitotoxicity[85]. SC236 protected against motor neuron death from chronic glutamate toxicity. Celecoxib was subsequently tested in the SOD1-G93A transgenic mouse. Treatment markedly inhibited production of PGE_2 and significantly delayed the onset of weakness and weight loss, and prolonged survival by 25%. In another preclinical study with the SOD1-G93A mouse model, dietary supplementation with the COX-2 inhibitor nimesulide resulted in a significant delay in the onset of

motor impairment[86]. In a third study, oral administration of either celecoxib or rofecoxib, another COX-2 inhibitor, significantly improved motor performance, attenuated weight loss and extended survival by 21% in the SOD1-G93A mouse model[87].

A double-blind, placebo-controlled trial of Celebrex in ALS patients was initiated by the NEALS Consortium. Enrolled subjects were randomized in a 2:1 ratio to receive either Celebrex or placebo over 12 months. Three hundred subjects were enrolled across 27 participating sites. No efficacy was found.

Ceftriaxone is a third-generation cephalosporin antibiotic typically used for the treatment of septicemia, pneumonia, meningitis and urinary tract infections. Ceftriaxone was identified by the NDSC as an agent with neuroprotective properties relevant to ALS. The cephalosporin antibiotics were the only class of compounds identified to be active in the majority of ALS-relevant assays, and showed strong activity in assays measuring EAAT2 expression and protection from SOD1 toxicity. Ceftriaxone has been reported to have protective properties against radiation-induced neurodegeneration in *in vitro* models[88]. It is able to penetrate the blood–brain barrier under normal conditions; this is enhanced in meningitis[89].

A human clinical trial, funded by the NINDS and initiated by the NEALS Consortium is in initial planning stages. The objective of the study is to determine the pharmacokinetics, safety and efficacy of long-term ceftriaxone treatment in subjects with ALS.

Neurotrophic factors

Insulin-like growth factor-I gene therapy Naturally occurring trophic factors that promote neuronal growth have been attractive candidates for therapy in neurodegenerative disease, but thus far, none have shown success in ALS trials. Recent efforts have shown that survival in a mouse model of SOD1 mutant-mediated ALS could be prolonged by delivering IGF-I with a gene therapy approach[90]. The authors used the retrograde transport ability of adeno-associated virus (AAV) in a mouse model by injecting AAV into respiratory and motor limb muscles to directly target the affected motor neurons. When injected before disease onset, AAV delivery of IGF-I was found to delay disease onset by 31 days when compared to controls. Of additional interest was the therapeutic benefit received when the vector was delivered at the time of disease onset: IGF-I treatment extended median lifespan by 22 days compared to the control group in these experiments. The AAV–IGF-I-mediated survival extension was accompanied by retention of hind-limb strength, slowed loss of spinal motor neurons, decreased astrocytic proliferation and modest slowing of forelimb paralysis. A human phase I trial is being planned.

Vascular endothelial growth factor (VEGF) gene therapy   VEGF is essential in angiogenesis and has also been implicated in neuroprotection[91,92]. Expression of the *VEGF* gene is induced by hypoxia through response elements that become bound by oxygen-sensitive transcription factors. In mice lacking these response elements, limb dysfunction and muscle atrophy are observed, with many neuropathologic and clinical signs reminiscent of human ALS[93]. The involvement of VEGF in human ALS was recently implicated in a European study that showed that individuals carrying any one of three variations in the VEGF gene had a 1.8 times greater risk of developing ALS[94]. The investigators also found that treatment of wild-type mice with VEGF salvaged motor neurons at risk of irreversible damage after spinal cord ischemia reperfusion.

A novel method of VEGF delivery has recently been developed using a retrogradely transported lentivector, and has been tested in SOD1-G93A mice[95]. In these studies, a single injection of a VEGF-expressing lentiviral vector into various muscles delayed onset and slowed progression of ALS even when the treatment was initiated only at the onset of paralysis. VEGF treatment also increased the life expectancy of ALS mice by 30% without causing toxic side-effects. The therapeutic potential of VEGF gene therapy in human ALS is still unknown, but clinical trials are likely to start soon.

Although promising gene therapy results from mouse studies raise hope for an ALS treatment, there are both practical and safety concerns. Experience with the use of viral vectors in human subjects has been limited, and its potential for complications largely remains unknown. Potential problems include the development of antibodies to the virus, the possible need for repeat injections at a later time and inability to turn off protein production[96]. There are many questions that need to be answered before gene therapy can become a viable therapeutic option in ALS, but steady advancements in this field bring us close to testing this real possibility.

Antioxidants

AEOL 10150 (manganese (III) meso-tetrakis (di-N-ethylimidazole) porphyrin) is a catalytic antioxidant compound that has demonstrated efficacy in an animal model of ALS. In recent experiments with the SOD1-G93A mouse model, the survival time period after symptom onset for the AEOL 10150-treated group was 2.5 times the survival time period of the control group[97]. A phase 1 single-dose study has been completed and a mutidose study is currently enrolling subjects.

Bioenergetics agents

Coenzyme Q10 (CoQ10) is an essential cofactor of the electron transport chain and a potent antioxidant in lipid and mitochondrial membranes. In preclinical studies using the SOD1-G93A mouse model, oral administration of CoQ10 increased lifespan modestly[98,99]. CoQ10 has also been studied in other human trials of neurodegenerative disorders whose pathogenesis involves mitochondrial dysfunction. At a dosage of 600 mg/day, CoQ10 slowed the rate of functional decline in Huntington's disease patients by 15%[100], and at

1200 mg/day, slowed the rate of Parkinson's disease worsening by 40%[101]. To investigate the therapeutic benefit of CoQ10 in ALS patients, a small open-label pilot study was initiated at Columbia University using a single dose of 600 mg/day of powdered CoQ10. Because only ten of 16 patients completed the study, the benefit of CoQ10 was difficult to determine. A second pilot study was conducted to assess the safety and tolerability of high-dose, solubilized CoQ10. Thirty-five patients received a liquid preparation of either 1000 mg solubilized CoQ10 or placebo for 4 weeks, followed by open-label 1000 mg CoQ10 daily for up to 6 months. The researchers concluded that the liquid, solubilized CoQ10 preparation used in this pilot study had excellent bioavailability. The NEALS Consortium conducted an open-label dose escalation study of CoQ10. Thirty patients received CoQ10 for up to 8 months. The highest tested dose was 3000 mg/day. Administration of CoQ10 was found to be safe and well tolerated up to 3000 mg/day[102].

A NINDS-funded randomized, placebo-controlled, double-blind, clinical trial of CoQ10 is scheduled to begin recruitment. The first stage of the trial will identify which of two doses of CoQ10 is preferred, using a selection procedure (1000 mg or 2000 mg daily). The second stage will compare the selected dose against placebo to assess whether there is sufficient early evidence of its efficacy to justify continuing this comparison in a future phase III trial. The primary outcome measure is the change in ALSFRS-R over 9 months for CoQ10 treatment compared to placebo. Secondary efficacy measures are the changes in FVC, fatigue severity, health-related quality of life and serum oxidative stress markers.

Anti-apoptotic drugs

Minocycline, a tetracycline antibiotic, has anti-inflammatory and neuroprotective properties and is known to penetrate the blood–brain barrier readily. It has neuroprotective effects in animal models of stroke/ischemic injury and neurodegenerative disorders and was found to extend survival and delay disease onset in ALS mouse models. To determine the effects of the drug in human ALS patients, two double-blind, randomized, placebo-controlled phase I/II trials were conducted[103]. The primary aim of the trials was to determine whether treatment with minocycline was safe and well tolerated in conjunction with riluzole (Trial 1), and whether patients with ALS could tolerate doses of up to 400 mg (Trial 2). In the first trial, the 19 subjects enrolled tolerated the drug combination over 6 months with no significant difference in adverse events between the two groups. In the second trial, 23 subjects received up to 400 mg/day in an 8-month crossover trial; the mean tolerated dose was 387 mg/day. Using these data, the authors designed a phase III trial to determine whether minocycline delays disease progression in ALS patients. Enrollment opened in the fall of 2003, and is expected to include 400 patients at completion. The total study length will be 48 months: 24 months for patient recruitment, 4 months of serial monthly evaluations to determine baseline slopes of progression for each patient followed by 9 months of intervention (minocycline or placebo), and 11 additional months of survival follow-up, data analysis and preparation of publications.

TCH346 (dibenz[b,f]oxepin-10-ylmethyl-prop-2-ynyl-amine, hydrogen maleate salt) is a novel compound that interacts with the glycolytic enzyme glyceraldehyde 3-phosphate dehydrogenase (GAPDH) in a way that may block programed cell death. TCH346 prevented the degeneration of neurons in a variety of *in vitro* models of apoptosis[101], but had no significant effects on survival in the G93A mice[103]. In a phase IIa study in patients with ALS, TCH346 was safe and well tolerated in oral daily doses of 0.5, 2.5 or 10 mg. A phase IIb trial was initiated with the primary objectives of exploring the dose–response relationship of TCH346, and identifying at least one dose of TCH346 that will be superior to placebo for use in future phase III trials. The clinical effects of four oral doses of TCH346 (1.0, 2.5, 7.5, 15 mg qd) were evaluated in 500 patients with ALS for at least 24 weeks. The primary efficacy variable that was evaluated assessed the rate of functional decline as defined by the slope in the ALSFRS-revised scores over time. There was no benefit of TCH346 in ALS.

Other

Pentoxifylline (Ikomio) ExonHit Therapeutics recently identified pentoxifylline as a potential ALS treatment candidate through a patented screening technique called differential analysis of transcripts with alternative splicing (DATAS), which the company developed to detect altered genetic sequences that could lead to ALS-related chemical changes. Although its precise role in ALS is not known, researchers have speculated that its ability to block phosphodiesterases might be involved. A double-blind and randomized trial was initiated in October 2002 to evaluate the compound as an add-on therapy to riluzole, with the primary endpoint being survival[104]. Four hundred patients were enrolled at 12 European centers. The study was reported as ineffective.

LESSONS LEARNED

Only one therapy tested to date has shown efficacy in patients with ALS. Several other studies have definitively demonstrated that a compound at a given dosage does not work in ALS (e.g. gabapentin, topiramate, subcutaneous BDNF and CNTF). Other studies unfortunately did not provide clear answers (IGF-I, creatine). The design and implementation of past clinical trials in ALS has been reviewed in the hope of learning better ways to effectively test therapies.

Use of preclinical models

An analysis of the major clinical trials conducted in ALS in the past decade indicates that all drugs were tested in an *in vitro* model to have neuroprotective effects before entering human trials (Table 18.1). With the exception of xaliproden, all drugs were also investigated in animal models of motor neuron injury. For every drug tested in patients with ALS, it appears that preclinical investigations were conducted.

Reconciling preclinical studies and human clinical trials

The predictive value of the mutant SOD1 transgenic mouse models with regard to the identification of drugs that are efficacious in human ALS is not yet known[1]. In the case of riluzole, the rationale for using the drug in human studies was reinforced by its positive effects in three preclinical models. Riluzole was found to prevent neuronal degeneration of cultured cells induced by the CSF from ALS patients[20]. Another study reported that this drug was a potent neuroprotectant in a model of chronic glutamate-mediated motor neuron toxicity using organotypic spinal cord cultures[35]. Results of human trials in ALS have demonstrated a positive effect of riluzole on survival[24,28]. These findings correlate closely with those in SOD1-G93A transgenic mice, in which the drug increased survival by 11%[64]. There are several therapies that have failed both in humans and in the mouse model (topiramate, BDNF and CNTF).

On the other hand, creatine chronically administered to the transgenic ALS mouse before clinical evidence of disease substantially delayed onset and prolonged survival by 18% in mice[105]. However, two independent clinical trials of creatine at different doses[79,106] failed to demonstrate a clinical benefit. Questions about dosage and CNS penetration of creatine remain.

The data from creatine studies, however, demonstrate an important point: all preclinical models have inherent limitations. Dose equivalency is one area in which the relationship between effects seen in the transgenic mouse are not necessarily predictive of a similar effect in

Drug	pathway	ence	Neuroprotective effect	ence	model	Symptom progression	Survival %	onset
Riluzole	Excitotoxicity	2	Organotypic spinal cord cultures	64	SOD1-G93A	n/a	11	No
Gabapentin	Excitotoxicity	2	Organotypic spinal cord cultures	64	SOD1-G93A	n/a	9	No
Topiramate	Excitotoxicity	39	Organotypic spinal cord cultures	39	SOD1-G93A	n/a	0	n/a
BDNF – sc	Neurotrophic	107	Rat spinal motor neurons	108	Wobbler	Retarded motor dysfunction	n/a	n/a
CNTF – sc	Neurotrophic	109	Chick embryonic motoneurons	45	Pmn/pmn	Improved motor function	Prolonged	n/a
IGF-I – sc	Neurotrophic	110	Rat spinal cord cultures	111	Wobbler	Increased muscle strength, fiber size	0	n/a
Xaliproden	Neurotrophic	112 113	PC12 co-treated with nerve growth factor Embryonic purified mouse motoneurons	60	Rat model of neurodegeneration (not ALS model)			
α-Tocopherol	Antioxidant	114	Mouse clonal hippocampal HT22 cells	64	SOD1-G93A	Prolonged normal wheel activity	0	14
Creatine	Bioenergetic agent	115	Rat hippocampal neurons	105	SOD1-G93A	Delayed decline in rotorod	15	No effe
				116	Rat hippocampal and striatal neurons			
				117	Wobbler	Grip strength, biceps weight	0	No effe
				118	SOD1-G93A	Delayed decline in rotorod, weight loss	15	11%
Celebrex	Excitotoxicity	85	Organotypic spinal cord culture	119	SOD1-G93A	Delayed decline in rotorod, weight loss	25	14
Ceftriaxone	Excitotoxicity	88	Primary cortical cultures	120	SOD1-G93A	n/a	Prolonged	n/a
		121	Active in multiple ALS screening assays (NDSC)					
IGF-I gene therapy	Neurotrophin	See IGF-I – sc above		90	SOD1-G93A	Delayed decline in rotorod, weight loss	30[1]	14[1] 18[2]
VEGF gene therapy	Neurotrophin	91	Hippocampal neuronal cell line	95	SOD1-G93A	n/a	30	29
AEOL 10150	Antioxidant	None		97	SOD1-G93A	n/a	16[3] 26[4]	0
Coenzyme Q10	Bioenergetic agent	122	Cultured cerebellar granule cells	98	SOD1-G93A	n/a	4	n/a
Minocycline	Apoptosis	123	Mixed spinal cord cultures	124	SOD1-G93A	n/a	8.9	21
				125	SOD1-G37R	Grip strength	6.4	Yes
TCH346	Apoptosis	126	PC12 culture	127	SOD1-G93A	n/a	0	n/a

[1]Vector delivery at 60 days of age (before disease onset); [2]Vector delivery at 90 days of age (at disease onset); [3]part I of study; [4]part II of study

human disease. The transgenic mouse was engineered to have early disease onset and rapid course by greatly overexpressing the human mutant *SOD1* gene. Therapeutic efficacy in this model may therefore not directly translate to human disease, where the mutant gene product is not artificially overexpressed. In addition, although familial ALS is similar to sporadic ALS with regard to a wide range of cytotoxic events, including evidence for excitotoxicity (e.g. loss of glutamate transport protein), oxidative injury, markers/genes reflecting programed cell death, and neuroinflammation, complete equivalency between sporadic and familial disease has not been demonstrated. In the next few years, results from several human studies with agents that have shown efficacy in the transgenic mutant SOD1 mouse model will be available. This information will be extremely helpful in answering the questions about the therapeutic predictive capabilities of this mouse model.

Should every drug considered for human trial first be evaluated in the available mouse models? The predictive power of the multiple pathway assays performed in the NINDS neurodegeneration screen described earlier may have equal or greater predictive power than a single mouse study. Most drugs that come from the pharmaceutical industry are derived and decided upon through multiple *in vitro* assays. A review of previous and currently planned studies in ALS by large pharmaceutical companies show that few rely on the transgenic ALS mice to make decisions regarding clinical trials (e.g. xaliproden, Novartis TCH346, Ikomio, IGF-I) but instead rely on preclinical assays for trial decisions.

Pharmacokinetic testing and drug dosing

An analysis of all major trials conducted in the past decade has demonstrated considerable variation in dose selection methods and the extent to which dose-ranging is employed. Of nine drugs studied in humans in the past decade, five were tested at more than one dose. Among these,

riluzole demonstrated an inverse dose response in risk of death, while rhBDNF, rhIGF-I and xaliproden offered some positive dose-ranging trends in therapeutic benefit. The argument in favor of dose-ranging in ALS clinical trials is strengthened by the dose correlations observed in these studies. Although this method requires greater resources in terms of subject recruitment, study length and finances, it may improve the efficiency of trial process as a whole. In the case of gabapentin, phase II studies of 2400 mg/day indicated a trend toward slower decline of arm strength compared to placebo. The subsequent higher dosage study at 3600 mg/day, however, showed no evidence of beneficial effect on disease progression. The authors acknowledged that the higher dose might in fact have been less effective than the smaller dose used in the prior trial, and offered this as an explanation for the contrasting results. Had more than one dose been tested in the second study, more comprehensive findings might have been obtained.

As with all clinical trials, ALS trials are organized such that phase I studies are conducted to determine the pharmacokinetics of the drug in humans, while phase II trials are performed for dose finding and safety profiles. However, phase III efficacy studies are not always preceded by this paradigm, as alternative methods of proving safety and dose selection are sometimes employed. Doses may be determined directly from animal studies or previously established pharmacokinetic profiles if the drug has been proved safe in other applications. For example, in the study of topiramate in ALS, 800 mg/day was selected as the upper limit dose based on preclinical *in vitro* studies of therapeutic plasma levels[40]. In previous studies of topiramate in epilepsy, 800 mg/day was found to be well within the approved dose, and was therefore accepted to be safe in the ALS study. However, high-dose topiramate was found to accelerate the decline in arm strength in ALS patients, and it was suggested that this might have been due to some adverse effect of the drug. Based on these results, and findings in mice that high-dose topiramate might reverse any neuroprotective effects of the drug, the authors concluded that lower doses of topiramate may be worth studying further in ALS.

Of nine drugs tested in trials, riluzole, CNTF and BDNF were tested in phase I and II studies before phase III efficacy trials were conducted. The phase I and II studies were used to determine dosage. Subcutaneous IGF-I and creatine were studied in mouse models for dose selection, and topiramate in *in vitro* models. The remaining trials with gabapentin, α-tocopherol, and xaliproden did not disclose their method of dose selection. Failure to identify an optimal dose may compromise the success of a drug and may lead to certain drugs being inappropriately discarded. It is critical to carry out adequate dose-finding studies and to recognize situations in which multiple dosages should be investigated.

Surrogate endpoints and selection of outcome measures

Surrogate endpoints can be defined as laboratory measures or other tests that have no direct or obvious relationship to any clinical symptom, but on which a beneficial effect of a drug is presumed to predict a desired beneficial effect[128]. Validated surrogate endpoints are those tests for which there is adequate evidence that a drug effect on the measure predicts the clinical benefit desired. They hold considerable value in many potential applications, including diagnosis, prognosis, disease progression and response to therapy. In terms of clinical research, trials that rely on surrogate endpoints can be shorter and smaller than those that rely on more traditional outcomes.

In ALS, direct evidence of motor neuronal degeneration would ideally be used as the primary marker in studies, but since brain or spinal cord biopsies cannot be obtained, surrogates must be used as substitutes. There is currently no validated surrogate endpoint identified for ALS clinical trials. Instead, a number of unvalidated surrogates are commonly used as outcome measures to track patient progress in clinical trials.

Survival is generally regarded as the 'gold standard' for measuring outcome in ALS. However, while having the advantage of being clearly defined, it is limited by the requirement for adequate length of study to achieve significance against placebo, and the natural variation in disease progression may make this endpoint less representative. The ALSFRS is a ten-item functional inventory that assesses patients' level of self-sufficiency in areas of feeding, grooming, ambulation and communication. The ALSFRS has been shown to be a predictor of patient survival[129], and is commonly used as an outcome measure in ALS clinical trials. However, one if its weaknesses is its disproportionate weighting of limb and bulbar, as compared to respiratory, dysfunction. A revised version of the ALSFRS (ALSFRS-R) incorporates additional assessments of dyspnea, orthopnea and the need for ventilatory support[130]. Respiratory function, as measured by the FVC has also been shown to correlate with survival[131]. Innovative clinical trial designs using ALSFRS as a surrogate marker are currently in use. This includes futility designs and use of a lead-in phase. These designs decrease the sample size requirements for the studies.

Other outcome measures are being developed; these include magnetic resonance spectroscopy, motor unit number estimation, transcranial magnetic stimulation, functional magnetic resonance imaging, and blood and CSF proteomics and metabolomics biomarkers.

Enrollment and study retention

ALS is a relatively rare disease with a mean survival of approximately 3.5 years from first symptoms, and both a low incidence and prevalence. Clinical trials testing drugs that are available by prescription have had slow enrollment. Other studies of experimental agents that are not available outside clinical trials often complete enrollment quickly. Study dropout is an important problem in current ALS clinical trials. Among major past clinical

Table 18.2   Withdrawal rates in major completed clinical trials (1994–2004)

Drug	Reference	Study length	Enrolled	Deaths (%)	Withdrawal rate %			Reasons
					Total	Drug	Placebo	
Riluzole	24	12 mos	155	34.2[1]	28.4	35.1	21.8	Serious adverse events, withdrawal of consent
	28	12 mos	959	44.9[1]	21.5	20.7	21.8	Serious adverse events, withdrawal of consent
Gabapentin	36	6 mos	152	2.6	20.4	20.2	21.4	Adverse events, non-compliance, inappropriate enrollment, loss to follow-up
	37	9 mos	204	6.4	21.6	22.5	20.6	Adverse events, non-compliance, loss to follow-up
Topiramate	40	12 mos	296[2]	14.2	30.4	32.5	26.8	Adverse events, subject choice
BDNF	49	9 mos	1135[2]	9.2	12.9	14.8	9.3	Not provided
SC		12 mos	350	27				Not provided
IT		18 mos	281	35	12	13	11	Not provided
CNTF	53	9 mos	730	20.1	15.3	17.9	10.2	Not provided
	52	6 mos	570	7.4	8.4	9	8	Not provided
IGF-I[3]	57	9 mos	266	9.8	12.0	13.3	11.4	Adverse events, intercurrent illness, patient request, non-compliance, unable to travel
	58	9 mos	183	12.6	10.4	12.9	5.1	Adverse events, intercurrent illness, patient request, non-compliance
Xaliproden	61	32–46 weeks	78	17.9	11.5	6.4	5.1	Lack of efficacy, elevated liver function tests
	62	18 mos	867 (I)	37.8	32.1	31.8	32.5	
			1210 (II)	34.5	25.6	48	24.9	
α-Tocopherol	66	12 mos	289	23.9[1]	26.6	Not provided	Not provided	Withdrawal of consent, adverse events
Creatine	79	16 mos	175	33.1	8.6	5.1	3.4	Adverse events, other serious illness, use of commercial creatine, other
	106	6 mos	104	8	11	4	7	Adverse events, subject choice

[1]Death rates include patients with tracheostomy; [2]patients randomized in 2:1 drug:placebo ratio; [3]withdrawal rates do not include protocol-specified terminations of Appel amyotrophic lateral sclerosis (AALS) total score $\geq$ 115 and forced vital capacity < 39% predicted value; SC, subcutaneous; IT, intrathecal

trials, the average rate of withdrawal due to death was 1.75% of the enrolled subjects per month (range: 0.43–3.74% per month) while withdrawals due to reasons other than death averaged 1.74% per month of enrolled subjects (range: 0.53–3.4% per month) (Table 18.2). In some clinical trials, more than one quarter of the enrolled subjects terminated study participation early for reasons other than death. Common reasons for withdrawal included the occurrence of adverse experiences, non-compliance, inability to continue to come to the center and intercurrent illness. High dropout rates make recruitment of a sufficient number of patients to enter into clinical trials a challenge to researchers. The need for such a large number of patients has necessitated the involvement of multicenter and multinational trials, bringing new logistical and financial challenges. However, the successful execution of trials with riluzole demonstrates that it is possible to carry out such large trials with sufficient statistical power.

Many ALS trials in the past have been insufficiently powered in terms of patient numbers to achieve statistical significance. In these studies, the intervention being studied would have to have had an enormous impact on disease course to reject the null hypothesis, given that often only small patient numbers were used. Since such a huge difference seems unrealistic in ALS, it is possible that some drug treatments will have been perhaps erroneously rejected along with the scientific hypotheses behind their use.

Design issues in placebo-controlled trials

In phase II trials involving a fatal illness such as ALS, various authors have argued that the use of placebo controls may be inappropriate. Furthermore, many patients continue to take supplements of vitamin E or creatine, for example, and problems arise in controlling for such polypharmacy. The use of natural history controls has been explored in the past using a pre-trial 'lead-in' period, with the implication that trials might be designed to compare an active treatment group with a database from patients in an observational, natural history study. This type of study might be feasible for a phase II trial, as it would not only eliminate the need for a placebo arm, but would also greatly reduce the cost of the trial. Muscle strength, ALSFRS and FVC decrease linearly[132,133] and appear unchanged over time and different ALS cohorts. This suggests that natural history controls might be useful in exploratory trials to screen out ineffective treatments. Other innovative approaches include use of futility designs (CoQ10 ALS trial) and Christmas tree design (creatine ALS study). Several trials have used a 2:1 randomization process to increase the chance of treatment for patients with ALS.

CONCLUSIONS

The lessons learned from clinical trials have contributed to our understanding of the underlying disease mechanisms and have helped clinical researchers find more efficient and innovative clinical trial design methods. Advances in understanding the biology of the disease will no doubt continue to generate new ideas of therapeutic approaches. Advances in imaging modalities and biochemical technologies hold promise for improved surrogate markers of disease progression and monitoring during therapy. Current investigations in stem cell research and gene therapy offer much hope for novel therapeutic approaches to reverse or impede motor neuron loss.

REFERENCES

1. Cleveland D, Rothstein J. From Charcot to Lou Gehrig: Deciphering selective motor neuron death in ALS. Nat Rev Neurosci 2001; 2: 806–19
2. Rothstein J, Kuncl R. Neuroprotective strategies in a model of chronic glutamate-mediated motor neuron toxicity. J Neurochem 1995; 65: 643–51
3. Pasinelli P, Borchelt D, Houseweart M, et al. Caspase-1 is activated in neural cells and tissue with amyotrophic lateral sclerosis-associated mutations in copper-zinc superoxide dismutase. Proc Natl Acad Sci USA 1998; 95: 15763–8
4. Pasinelli P, Houseweart M, Brown R, Cleveland D. Caspase-1 and -3 are sequentially activated in motor neuron death in Cu/Zn superoxide dismutase

mediated familial amyotrophic lateral sclerosis. Proc Natl Acad Sci USA 2000; 97: 13901–6

5. Flanagan S, Anderson R, Ross M, Oberley L. Over-expression of manganese superoxide dismutase attenuates neuronal death in human cells expressing mutant (G37R) Cu/Zn-superoxide dismutase. J Neurochem 2002; 81: 170–7

6. Ghadge G, Lee J, Bindokas V, et al. Mutant superoxide dismutase-1-linked familial amyotrophic lateral sclerosis: Molecular mechanisms of neuronal death and protection. J Neurosci 1997; 17: 8756–66

7. Gurney ME, Pu H, Chiu AY, et al. Motor neuron degeneration in mice that express a human Cu/Zn superoxide dismutase mutation. Science 1994; 264: 1772–5

8. Ripps ME, Huntley GW, Hof PR, et al. Transgenic mice expressing an altered murine superoxide dismutase gene provide an animal model of amyotrophic lateral sclerosis. Proc Natl Acad Sci USA 1995; 92: 689–93

9. Wong P, Pardo C, Borchelt D, et al. An adverse property of a familial ALS-linked SOD1 mutation causes motor neuron disease characterized by vacuolar degeneration of mitochondria. Neuron 1995; 14: 1105–16

10. Chiu AY, Zhai P, Dal Canto MC, et al. Age-dependent penetrance of disease in a transgenic mouse model of familial amyotrophic lateral sclerosis. Mol Cell Neurosci 1995; 6: 349–62

11. Yang Y, Hentati A, Deng H, et al. The gene encoding alsin, a protein with three guanine–nucleotide exchange factor domains, is mutated in a form of recessive amyotrophic lateral sclerosis. Nat Genet 2001; 29: 160–5

12. Hadano S, Hand C, Osuga H, et al. A gene encoding a putative GTPase regulator is mutated in familial amyotrophic lateral sclerosis 2. Nat Genet 2001; 29: 166–73

13. Puls I, Jonnakuty C, LaMonte B, et al. Mutant dynactin in motor neuron disease. Nat Genet 2003; 33: 455–6

14. Chen YZ, Bennett CL, Huynh HM, et al. DNA/RNA helicase gene mutations in a form of juvenile amyotrophic lateral sclerosis (ALS4). Am J Hum Genet 2004; 74: 1128–35

15. Olney JW, Sharpe LG, Feigin RD. Glutamate-induced brain damage in infant primates. J Neuropathol Exp Neurol 1972; 31: 464–88

16. Plaitakis A, Caroscio JT. Abnormal glutamate metabolism in amyotrophic lateral sclerosis. Ann Neurol 1987; 22: 575–9

17. Rothstein J, Tsai G, Kuncl R, et al. Abnormal excitatory amino acid metabolism in amyotrophic lateral sclerosis. Ann Neurol 1990; 28: 18–25

18. Vincent AM, Mobley BC, Hiller A, Feldman EL. IGF-I prevents glutamate-induced motor neuron programmed cell death. Neurobiol Dis 2004; 16: 407–16

19. Lin C, Bristol L, Jin L, et al. Aberrrant RNA processing in a neurodegenerative disease: The cause for absent EAAT2, a glutamate transporter, in amyotrophic lateral sclerosis. Neuron 1998; 20: 589–602

20. Couratier P, Sindou P, Esclaire F, et al. Neuroprotective effects of riluzole in ALS CSF toxicity. Neuroreport 1994; 5: 1012–14

21. Benoit E, Escande D. Riluzole specifically blocks inactivated Na channels in myelinated nerve fibre. Pflugers Arch 1991; 419: 603–9

22. Zona C, Siniscalchi A, Mercuri, NB, et al. Riluzole interacts with voltage-activated sodium and potassium currents in cultured rat cortical neurons. Neuroscience 1998; 85: 931–8

23. Stefani A, Spadoni F, Bernardi G. Differential inhibition by riluzole, lamotrigine, and phenytoin of sodium and calcium currents in cortical neurons: Implications for neuroprotective strategies. Exp Neurol 1997; 147: 115–22

24. Bensimon G, Lacomblez L, Meininger V. A controlled trial of riluzole in amyotrophic lateral sclerosis. N Engl J Med 1994; 330: 585–91

25. MacRae K. Riluzole in amyotrophic lateral sclerosis [letter]. N Engl J Med 1994; 331: 272–3

26. Murphy J. Riluzole in amyotrophic lateral sclerosis [letter]. N Engl J Med 1994; 331: 273

27. Rowland L. Riluzole for the treatment of amyotrophic lateral sclerosis – Too soon to tell? N Engl J Med 1994; 330: 636–7

28. Lacomblez L, Bensimon G, Leigh P, et al. Dose-ranging study of riluzole in amyotrophic lateral sclerosis. Lancet 1996; 347: 1425–31

29. Riviere M, Meininger V, Zeisser P, Munsat T. An analysis of extended survival in patients with amyotrophic lateral sclerosis treated with riluzole. Arch Neurol 1998; 55: 526–8

30. Groeneveld GJ, van Kan HJ, Torano JS, et al. Inter- and intraindividual variability of riluzole serum concentrations in patients with ALS. J Neurol Sci 2001; 191: 121–5

31. Groeneveld GJ, Van Kan HJ, Kalmijn S, et al. Riluzole exposure in patients with ALS: Association with disease progression and survival. Amyotroph

Lateral Scler Other Motor Neuron Disord 2003; 4 (Suppl 1): 77

32. North W, Khan A, Yamase H, Sporn J. Reversible granulocytopenia in association with riluzole therapy. Ann Pharmacother 2000; 34: 322–4

33. Practice advisory on the treatment of amyotrophic lateral sclerosis with riluzole: Report of the Quality Standards Subcommittee of the American Academy of Neurology. Neurology 1997; 49: 657–9

34. Miller R, Mitchell J, Lyon M, Moore D. Riluzole for amyotrophic lateral sclerosis (ALS)/motor neuron disease (MND). Cochrane Neuromuscular Disease Group Cochrane Database of Systematic Reviews 2004; 2

35. Rothstein JD, Kuncl RW. Neuroprotective strategies in a model of chronic glutamate-mediated motor neuron toxicity. J Neurochem 1995; 65: 643–51

36. Miller R, Moore DH, Young L, Group WS. Placebo-controlled trial of gabapentin in patients with amyotrophic lateral sclerosis. Neurology 1996; 47: 1383–8

37. Miller RG, Moore DH, Gelinas DF, et al. Phase III randomized trial of gabapentin in patients with amyotrophic lateral sclerosis. Neurology 2001; 56: 843–8

38. Skradski S, White H. Topiramate blocks kainate-evoked cobalt influx into cultured neurons. Epilepsia 2000; 41 (Suppl 1): S45–7

39. Maragakis N, Jackson M, Ganel R, Rothstein J. Topiramate protects against motor neuron degeneration in organotypic spinal cord cultures but not in G93A SOD1 transgenic mice. Neurosci Lett 2003; I338: 107–10

40. Cudkowicz M, Shefner J, Schoenfeld D, et al. A randomized, placebo-controlled trial of topiramate in amyotrophic lateral sclerosis. Neurology 2003; 61: 456–64

41. Askmark H, Aquilonius S, Gillberg P, et al. A pilot trial of dextromethorphan in amyotrophic lateral sclerosis. J Neurol Neurosurg Psychiatry 1993; 56: 197–200

42. Blin O, Azulay JP, Desnuelle C, et al. A controlled one-year trial of dextromethorphan in amyotrophic lateral sclerosis. Clin Neuropharmacol 1996; 19: 189–92

43. Eisen A, Stewart H, Schulzer M, Cameron D. Anti-glutamate therapy in amyotrophic lateral sclerosis: A trial using lamotrigine. Can J Neurol Sci 1993; 20: 297–301

44. Miller RG, Smith SA, Murphy JR, et al. A clinical trial of verapamil in amyotrophic lateral sclerosis. Muscle Nerve 1996; 19: 511–15

45. Sendtner M, Schmalbruch H, Stockli KA, et al. Ciliary neurotrophic factor prevents degeneration of motor neurons in mouse mutant progressive motor neuronopathy. Nature 1992; 358: 502–4

46. Mitsumoto H, Ikeda K, Klinkosz B, et al. Arrest of motor neuron disease in wobbler mice cotreated with CNTF and BDNF. Science 1994; 265: 1107–10

47. Sendtner M, Holtmann B, Kolbeck R, et al. Brain-derived neurotrophic factor prevents the death of motoneurons in newborn rats after nerve section. Nature 1992; 360: 757–9

48. Novikov L, Novikova L, Kellerth JO. Brain-derived neurotrophic factor promotes survival and blocks nitric oxide synthase expression in adult rat spinal motoneurons after ventral root avulsion. Neurosci Lett 1995; 200: 45–8

49. A controlled trial of recombinant methionyl human BDNF in ALS: The BDNF Study Group (Phase III). Neurology 1999; 52: 1427–33

50. Martinou JC, Martinou I, Kato AC. Cholinergic differentiation factor (CDF/LIF) promotes survival of isolated rat embryonic motoneurons in vitro. Neuron 1992; 8: 737–44

51. Mitsumoto H, Ikeda K, Holmund T, et al. The effects of ciliary neurotrophic factor on motor dysfunction in wobbler mouse motor neuron disease. Ann Neurol 1994; 36: 142–8

52. Miller R, Petajan J, Bryan W, et al. A placebo-controlled trial of recombinant human ciliary neurotrophic (rhCNTF) factor in amyotrophic lateral sclerosis. Ann Neurol 1996; 39: 256–60

53. Group ACTS. A double-blind placebo-controlled clinical trial of subcutaneous recombinant human ciliary neurotrophic factor (rhCNTF) in amyotrophic lateral sclerosis. Neurology 1996; 46: 1244–9

54. Barinaga M. Neurotrophic factors enter the clinic. Science 1994; 264: 772–4

55. Penn RD, Kroin JS, York MM, Cedarbaum JM. Intrathecal ciliary neurotrophic factor delivery for treatment of amyotrophic lateral sclerosis (phase I trial). Neurosurgery 1997; 40: 94–9; discussion 99–100

56. Lewis ME, Vaught JL, Neff NT, et al. The potential of insulin-like growth factor-I as a therapeutic for the treatment of neuromuscular disorders. Ann NY Acad Sci 1993; 692: 201–8

57. Lai E, Felice K, Festoff B, et al. Effect of recombinant human insulin-like growth factor-I on progression of ALS. A placebo controlled study. The North

America ALS/IGF-1 Study Group. Neurology 1997; 49: 1621–30

58. Borasio GD, Robberecht W, Leigh PN, et al. A placebo-controlled trial of insulin-like growth factor-I in amyotrophic lateral sclerosis. European ALS/IGF-I Study Group. Neurology 1998; 51: 583–6

59. Mitchell JD, Wokke JH, Borasio GD. Recombinant human insulin-like growth factor I (rhIGF-I) for amyotrophic lateral sclerosis/motor neuron disease. Cochrane Database Syst Rev 2002: CD002064

60. Fournier J, Steinberg R, Gauthier T, et al. Protective effects of SR 57746A in central and peripheral models of neurodegenerative disorders in rodents and primates. Neuroscience 1993; 55: 629–41

61. Lacomblez L, Bensimon G, Douillet P, et al. Xaliproden in amyotrophic lateral sclerosis: Early clinical trials. Amyotroph Lateral Scler Other Motor Neuron Disord 2004; 5: 99–106

62. Meininger V, Bensimon G, Bradley W, et al. Efficacy and safety of xaliproden in amyotrophic lateral sclerosis: Results of two phase III trials. Amyotroph Lateral Scler Other Motor Neuron Disord 2004; 5: 107–17

63. Butterfield DA, Castegna A, Drake J, et al. Vitamin E and neurodegenerative disorders associated with oxidative stress. Nutr Neurosci 2002; 5: 229–39

64. Gurney M, Cutting F, Zhai P, et al. Benefit of vitamin E, riluzole and gabapentin in a transgenic model of familial ALS. Ann Neurol 1996; 39: 147–57

65. Norris FH, Denys EH. Nutritional supplements in amyotrophic lateral sclerosis. Adv Exp Med Biol 1987; 209: 183–9

66. Desnuelle C, Dib M, Garrel C, Favier A. A double-blind, placebo-controlled randomized clinical trial of alpha-tocopherol (vitamin E) in the treatment of amyotrophic lateral sclerosis. ALS riluzole–tocopherol Study Group. Amyotroph Lateral Scler Other Motor Neuron Disord 2001; 2: 9–18

67. Andreassen OA, Dedeoglu A, Klivenyi P, et al. N-Acetyl-L-cysteine improves survival and preserves motor performance in an animal model of familial amyotrophic lateral sclerosis. Neuroreport 2000; 11: 2491–3

68. Louwerse ES, Weverling GJ, Bossuyt PMM, et al. Randomized, double-blind, controlled trial of acetylcysteine in amyotrophic lateral sclerosis. Arch Neurol 1995; 52: 559–64

69. Masui Y, Mozai T, Kakehi K. Functional and morphometric study of the liver in motor neuron disease. J Neurol 1985; 232: 15–19

70. Nakano K, Hirayama K, Terai K. Hepatic ultrastructural changes and liver dysfunction in amyotrophic lateral sclerosis. Arch Neurol 1987; 44: 103–6

71. Sasaki S, Iwata M. Ultrastructural change of synapses of Betz cells in patients with amyotrophic lateral sclerosis. Neurosci Lett 1999; 268: 29–32

72. Hirano A. Cytopathology in amyotrophic lateral sclerosis. Adv Neurol 1991; 56: 91–101

73. Bruijn L, Beal M, Becher M, et al. Elevated free nitrotyrosine levels, but not protein-bound nitrotyrosine or hydroxyl radicals, throughout amyotrophic lateral sclerosis (ALS)-like disease implicate tyrosine nitration as an aberrant in vivo property of one familial ALS-linked superoxide dismutase 1 mutant. Proc Natl Acad Sci USA 1997; 94: 7606–11

74. Dal Canto MC, Gurney ME. The development of central nervous system pathology in a murine transgenic model of human amyotrophic lateral sclerosis. Am J Pathol 1994; 145: 1271–9

75. Pasinelli P, Belford M, Lennon N, et al. Amyotrophic lateral sclerosis-associated SOD1 mutant proteins bind and aggregate with Bcl-2 in spinal cord mitochondria. Neuron 2004; 43: 19–30

76. Liu J, Lillo C, Jonsson PA, et al. Toxicity of familial ALS-Inked SOD1 mutants from selective recruitment to spinal mitochondria. Neuron 2004; 43: 5–17

77. Hemmer W, Wallimann T. Functional aspects of creatine kinase in brain. Dev Neurosci 1993; 15: 249–60

78. Klivenyi P, Ferrante R, Matthews R. Neuroprotective effects of creatine in a transgenic animal model of amyotrophic lateral sclerosis. Mat Med 1999; 5: 347–50

79. Groenveld G, Veldink J, van der Tweel I, et al. A randomized sequential trial of creatine in amyotrophic lateral sclerosis. Ann Neurol 2003; 53: 437–45

80. Slutsky A, Lavery J. Data Safety and Monitoring Boards. N Engl J Med 2004; 350: 1143–7

81. Shefner J, Cudkowicz M, Schoenfeld D, et al. A clinical trial of creatine in amyotrophic lateral sclerosis. Neurology 2004; 63: 1933–5

82. Bezzi P, Carmignoto G, Pasti L, et al. Prostaglandins stimulate calcium-dependent glutamate release in astrocytes. Nature 1998; 391: 281–5

83. Almer G, Romero N, Przedborski S. Upregulation of cyclooxygenase-2 in an animal model of familial amyotrophic lateral sclerosis. Neurology 2000; 54 (Suppl 3): A304

84. Almer G, Teismann P, Stevic Z. Increased levels of the pro-inflammatory prostaglandin PGE2 from ALS patients. Neurology 2002; 58: 1277–9

85. Drachman D, Rothstein J. Inhibition of cyclooxygenase-2 protects motor neurons in an organotypic model of amyotrophic lateral sclerosis. Ann Neurol 2000; 48: 792–5

86. Pompl PN, Ho L, Bianchi M, et al. A therapeutic role for cyclooxygenase-2 inhibitors in a transgenic mouse model of amyotrophic lateral sclerosis. FASEB J 2003; 17: 725–7

87. Klivenyi P, Kiaei M, Gardian G, et al. Additive neuroprotective effects of creatine and cyclooxygenase 2 inhibitors in a transgenic mouse model of amyotrophic lateral sclerosis. J Neurochem 2004; 88: 576–82

88. Tikka T, Usenius T, Tenhunen M, et al. Tetracycline derivatives and ceftriaxone, a cephalosporin antibiotic, protect neurons against apoptosis induced by ionizing radiation. J Neurochem 2001; 78: 1409–14

89. Spector R. Ceftriaxone transport through the blood brain barrier. J Infect Dis 1987; 156: 209–11

90. Kaspar BK, Llado J, Sherkat N, et al. Retrograde viral delivery of IGF-1 prolongs survival in a mouse ALS model. Science 2003; 301: 839–42

91. Jin KL, Mao XO, Greenberg DA. Vascular endothelial growth factor: Direct neuroprotective effect in in vitro ischemia. Proc Natl Acad Sci USA 2000; 97: 10242–7

92. Carmeliet P. Blood vessels and nerves: Common signals, pathways and diseases. Nat Rev Genet 2003; 4: 710–20

93. Oosthuyse B, Moons L, Storkebaum E, et al. Deletion of the hypoxia-response element in the vascular endothelial growth factor promoter causes motor neuron degeneration. Nat Genet 2001; 28: 131–8

94. Lambrechts D, Storkebaum E, Morimoto M, et al. VEGF is a modifier of amyotrophic lateral sclerosis in mice and humans and protects motoneurons against ischemic death. Nat Genet 2003; 34: 383–94

95. Azzouz M, Ralph GS, Storkebaum E, et al. VEGF delivery with retrogradely transported lentivector prolongs survival in a mouse ALS model. Nature 2004; 429: 413–17

96. Miller TM, Cleveland DW. Has gene therapy for ALS arrived? Nat Med 2003; 9: 1256–7

97. Crow J. Treatment with AEOL 10150 results in 2.5 times survival period compared with control in ALS mouse model [online]. Available from the World Wide Web (2004): http://www.incara.com/ALS_Crow_experiments.htm

98. Matthews R, Yang S, Browne S, et al. Coenzyme Q10 administration increases brain mitochondrial concentrations and exerts neuroprotective effects. Proc Natl Acad Sci USA 1998; 95: 8892–7

99. Beal MF. Coenzyme Q10 as a possible treatment for neurodegenerative diseases. Free Radic Res 2002; 36: 455–60

100. Huntington Study Group. A randomized, placebo-controlled trial of coenzyme Q10 and remacemide in Huntington's disease. Neurology 2001; 57: 397–404

101. Shults C, Oakes D, Kieburtz K, et al. Effects of coenzyme Q10 in early Parkinson's disease and evidence for slowing of the functional decline. Arch Neurol 2002; 59: 1541–50

102. Ferrante K, Shefner J, Zang H, et al. Coenzyme Q10 up to 3000 mg per day is well tolerated in amyotrophic lateral sclerosis. Neurology 2005; 65: 1834–6

103. Gordon PH, Moore DH, Gelinas DF, et al. Placebo-controlled phase I/II studies of minocycline in amyotrophic lateral sclerosis. Neurology 2004; 62: 1845–7

104. Meininger V, Asselain B, Guillet P, et al., for the Pentoxifylline European Group. Pentoxifylline in ALS: a double-blind, randomized, multicenter, placebo-controlled trial. Neurology 2006; 66: 88–92

105. Klivenyi P, Ferrante R, Matthew R, et al. Neuroprotective effects of creatine in a transgenic animal model of ALS. Nat Med 1999; 5: 347–50

106. Shefner JM, Cudkowicz ME, Schoenfeld D, et al. A clinical trial of creatine in patients with amyotrophic lateral sclerosis. Amyotroph Lateral Scler Other Motor Neuron Disord 2003; 4 (Suppl 1): 28–9

107. Henderson CE, Camu W, Mettling C, et al. Neurotrophins promote motor neuron survival and are present in embryonic limb bud. Nature 1993; 363: 266–70

108. Ikeda K, Klinkosz B, Greene T, et al. Effects of brain-derived neurotrophic factor on motor dysfunction in wobbler mouse motor neuron disease. Ann Neurol 1995; 37: 505–11

109. Arakawa Y, Sendtner M, Thoenen H. Survival effect of ciliary neurotrophic factor (CNTF) on chick embryonic motoneurons in culture: Comparison

with other neurotrophic factors and cytokines. J Neurosci 1990; 10: 3507–15

110. Vaught JL, Contreras PC, Glicksman MA, Neff NT. Potential utility of rhIGF-1 in neuromuscular and/or degenerative disease. Ciba Found Symp 1996; 196: 18–27; discussion 27–38

111. Hantai D, Akaaboune M, Lagord C, et al. Beneficial effects of insulin-like growth factor-I on wobbler mouse motoneuron disease. J Neurol Sci 1995; 129 (Suppl):122–6

112. Pradines A, Magazin M, Schiltz P, et al. Evidence for nerve growth factor-potentiating activities of the nonpeptidic compound SR 57746A in PC12 cells. J Neurochem 1995; 64: 1954–64

113. Duong FH, Warter JM, Poindron P, Passilly P. Effect of the nonpeptide neurotrophic compound SR 57746A on the phenotypic survival of purified mouse motoneurons. Br J Pharmacol 1999; 128: 1385–92

114. Behl C. Vitamin E protects neurons against oxidative cell death in vitro more effectively than 17-beta estradiol and induces the activity of the transcription factor NF-kappaB. J Neural Transm 2000; 107: 393–407

115. Brewer GJ, Wallimann TW. Protective effect of the energy precursor creatine against toxicity of glutamate and beta-amyloid in rat hippocampal neurons. J Neurochem 2000; 74: 1968–78

116. Brustovetsky N, Brustovetsky T, Dubinsky JM. On the mechanisms of neuroprotection by creatine and phosphocreatine. J Neurochem 2001; 76: 425–34

117. Ikeda K, Iwasaki Y, Kinoshita M. Oral administration of creatine monohydrate retards progression of motor neuron disease in the wobbler mouse. Amyotroph Lateral Scler Other Motor Neuron Disord 2000; 1: 207–12

118. Andreassen O, Jenkins B, Dedeoglu A, et al. Increases in cortical glutamate concentrations in transgenic amyotrophic lateral sclerosis mice are attenuated by creatine supplementation. J Neurochem 2001; 77: 383–90

119. Drachman DB, Frank K, Dykes-Hoberg M, et al. Cyclooxygenase 2 inhibition protects motor neurons and prolongs survival in a transgenic mouse model of ALS. Ann Neurol 2002; 52: 771–8

120. Bruijn LT, Kristal BS, Leahy C, et al. Pre-clinical trials of three FDA-approved compounds in a mouse model of ALS. Amyotroph Lateral Scler Other Motor Neuron Disord 2003; 4 (Suppl 1): 76

121. Heemskerk J, Tobin A, Bain L. Teaching old drugs new tricks. Trends Neurosci 2002; 25: 494–6

122. Favit A, Nicoletti F, Scapagnini U, Canonico PL. Ubiquinone protects cultured neurons against spontaneous and excitotoxin-induced degeneration. J Cereb Blood Flow Metab 1992; 12: 638–45

123. Tikka T, Fiebich B, Goldsteins G, et al. Minocycline, a tetracycline derivative, is neuroprotective against excitotoxicity by inhibiting activation and proliferation of microglia. J Neurosci 2001; 21: 2580–8

124. Zhu S, Stavrovskiaya I, Drozda M, et al. Minocycline inhibits cytochrome c release and delays progression of amyotrophic lateral sclerosis in mice. Nature 2002; 417: 74–78

125. Kriz J, Nguyen MD, Julien JP. Minocycline slows disease progression in a mouse model of amyotrophic lateral sclerosis. Neurobiol Dis 2002; 10: 268–78

126. Carlile GW, Chalmers-Redman RM, Tatton NA, et al. Reduced apoptosis after nerve growth factor and serum withdrawal: Conversion of tetrameric glyceraldehyde-3-phosphate dehydrogenase to a dimer. Mol Pharmacol 2000; 57: 2–12

127. Andreassen OA, Dedeoglu A, Friedlich A, et al. Effects of an inhibitor of poly(ADP-ribose) polymerase, desmethylselegiline, trientine, and lipoic acid in transgenic ALS mice. Exp Neurol 2001; 168: 419–24

128. Katz R. FDA: Evidentiary Standards for Drug Development and Approval. NeuroRx 2004; 1: 307–316

129. Armon C, Moses D. Linear estimates of rates of disease progression as predictors of survival in patients with ALS entering clinical trials. J Neurol Sci 1998; 160 (Suppl 1): S37–41

130. Cedarbaum J, Stambler N, Malta E, et al. The ALSFRS-R: a revised ALS functional rating scale that incorporated assessments of respiratory function. J Neurol Sci 1999; 169: 13–21

131. Cedarbaum JM, Stambler N. Performance of the Amyotrophic Lateral Sclerosis Functional Rating Scale (ALSFRS) in multicenter clinical trials. J Neurol Sci 1997; 152 (Suppl 1): S1–9

132. Andres PL, Finison L, Thibodeau LM, Munsat TL. Use of composite scores (megascores) to measure deficit in amyotrophic lateral sclerosis. Neurol 1988; 38: 405–8

133. Bryan WW, Hoagland RJ, Murphy J, et al. Can we eliminate placebo in ALS clinical trials? Amyotroph Lateral Scler Other Motor Neuron Disord 2003; 4: 11–15

19

Palliative care and quality of life in amyotrophic lateral sclerosis

David Oliver, Gian Domenico Borasio

INTRODUCTION

The World Health Organization's definition of palliative care states that it is:

'An approach that improves the quality of life of patients and their families facing problems associated with life-threatening illness, through the prevention and relief of suffering, early identification and impeccable assessment and treatment of pain and other problems, physical, psychosocial and spiritual'[1].

Thus, as there is no curative treatment for amyotrophic lateral sclerosis (ALS), palliative care is appropriate from the time of diagnosis. Moreover, there is often a delay from the time the person experienced the first symptom to diagnosis – often 10 to 12 months – and the person may have progressive disease at the time of diagnosis, with a relatively short prognosis.

There is a need to ensure a multidisciplinary team approach to the care of the person and their family. The team usually includes members of several professions (Table 19.1).

This team approach can be very helpful in enabling the patient to remain as active and independent as possible, living their lives to the full[2]. The roles of different members of the team will vary as the disease progresses – and the problems faced by the person and their family changes.

Table 19.1 Palliative care in amyotrophic lateral sclerosis those involved

Chaplain	Physiotherapist
Dietitian	Physician
Family and close carers	Psychologist
Hospice worker	Social worker
Lay associations	Speech and language therapist
Nurse	
Occupational therapist	Swallowing therapist

AT THE TIME OF DIAGNOSIS

As the symptoms of ALS are often subtle and may be unrecognized for some time, patients may present with advanced disease, and many symptoms. These are discussed below.

The diagnosis of ALS is often a shock to both patient and family. It may be unknown to them all, and may lead to particular fears and concerns. The recent interest and high-profile court cases, regarding euthanasia and physician-assisted suicide, have engendered increased fears about ALS, as there is discussion of the 'distress' of the disease and its progression. Information regarding the disease and involvement of the wider team can be helpful, to allow the fears to be addressed. It is important to encourage communication within the family, so that the concerns of all can be shared, and not hidden.

AS THE DISEASE PROGRESSES

With disease progression the patient faces increasing symptoms (Table 19.2) due to neuronal degeneration. There is a need for multidisciplinary team assessment of these symptoms so that management can be optimized. Particular symptom areas that should be considered are given below.

Weakness

As patients become weaker, the increased involvement of the physiotherapist and occupational therapist will allow mobility to be maintained as much as possible. Early discussion of aids, such as sticks, frames and wheelchairs, is helpful so that the person and their family can adjust to these new losses of independence.

Dysphagia

As the disease progresses, up to 87% of people will develop difficulties in swallowing, due to weakness of the muscles in the mouth, pharynx and oesophagus. Careful feeding is essential, and alteration of the consistency to soft solid foods can be helpful[3]. The insertion of a feeding tube – either a percutaneous endoscopic gastrostomy or a radiologically inserted gastrostomy – should be considered early and insertion arranged before respiratory function has deteriorated too much, as there is increased risk if the forced vital capacity is less than 50% of expected[4]. In advanced stages, insertion of a feeding tube – if warranted – can be safely performed in combination with non-invasive ventilation[5].

As swallowing deteriorates, drooling of saliva may occur. Anticholinergic medication, such as scopolamine (hyoscine orally or as a transdermal patch) or amitriptyline may be helpful. Injection of botulinum B toxin into the salivary glands may be considered for severe problems.

Table 19.2   Symptoms of amyotrophic lateral sclerosis
Direct
Weakness and atrophy
Fasciculations and muscle cramps
Spasticity
Dysarthria
Dysphagia
Dyspnea
Pathologic laughing/crying
Indirect
Psychological disturbances
Sleep disturbances
Constipation
Drooling
Thick mucous secretions
Symptoms of chronic hypoventilation
Pain

Speech problems

Of affected individuals, 71% may develop problems with communication[6]. The early involvement of the speech and language therapist can allow the timely provision of appropriate communication aids[7].

Dyspnea

Dyspnea is a problem faced by up to 85% of those with ALS[6] and may be helped by opioids (starting at a dose of 2.5–5 mg every 4 hours). If anxiety is prominent, benzodiazepines may be started. Chronic hypoventilation may cause poor and disturbed sleep, anorexia, morning headache, nightmares and lethargy. Non-invasive ventilation (NIV) can be helpful in relieving these symptoms, but careful discussion is needed before starting[8]. As the respiratory muscles and diaphragm weaken further, the symptoms will recur, and it is important to have made plans as to how this will be managed. If not, there is the risk of a sudden deterioration and invasive ventilation via tracheostomy being started without time for full consideration of the consequences. These include progressive weakness and dependency and, in about 15–20%, the patient becoming totally 'locked-in' with no form of communication. It is important to reassure the patients that, whenever they may decide to stop NIV, all necessary care and appropriate medication will be available to ensure a peaceful death.

Pathologic laughing/crying

This symptom, which occurs in around 25% of patients[6], can be socially distressing and responds well to treatment with **amitriptyline** or **fluvoxamine**.

Pain

Up to 73% of people with ALS/MND complain of pain[6], even though the sensory nerves are unaffected. Pain needs to be assessed and appropriately treated:

- Musculoskeletal pain, due to atrophy and the altered tone around joints, may benefit from physiotherapy and non-steroidal anti-inflammatory medication

- Muscle spasm, from spastic muscles, may be helped by passive movements and muscle relaxants, such as baclofen. Muscle cramps can be relieved by quinine sulfate

- Skin pressure pain can be relieved by the use of regular opioids, such as morphine[9]

A list of medications and dosages commonly used for symptomatic treatment in ALS is shown in Table 19.3.

QUALITY OF LIFE ISSUES

The quality of life (QoL) of patients with severe illness is affected by several factors outside the physical domain. The natural history of ALS is one of a continuous series of losses, both physical and psychosocial/spiritual (Table 19.4), the latter

Table 19.3 Symptomatic medication in amyotrophic lateral sclerosis

Fasciculations and muscle cramps	Dosage*
If mild	
Magnesium	5 mmol qd-tid
If severe	
Quinine sulfate	200 mg bid
Carbamazepine	200 mg bid
Phenytoin	100 mg qd-tid
Spasticity	
Baclofen	10–80 mg
Tizanidine	6–24 mg
Memantine	10–60 mg
Tetrazepam	100–200 mg
Drooling	
Glycopyrrolate	0.1–0.2 mg sc/im tid
Transdermal hyoscine patches	1–2 patches
Amitriptyline	10–150 mg
Atropine/benztropine	0.25–0.75 mg/1–2 mg
Pathologic laughing/crying	
Amitriptyline	10–150 mg
Fluvoxamine	100–200 mg
Sedatives	*Dosage nocté*
Chloral hydrate	250–1000 mg
Diphenhydramine	50–100 mg
Diazepam (beware of respiratory depression)	5–10 mg

*Usual range of adult daily dosage; some patients may require higher dosages, e.g. of antispastic medication

playing the major role for the patients' QoL. Accordingly, several studies have shown that QoL in patients with ALS is not primarily dependent on physical function, but relies mainly on psychological, social and spiritual aspects[10,11].

Psychological aspects

As the person with ALS faces the progressive deterioration with the disease, they may experience a

---

Table 19.4   Amyotrophic lateral sclerosis: a series of losses

Physical
Loss of ambulation
Loss of manual dexterity
Loss of writing ability
Loss of driving ability
Loss of working ability
Loss of self-care ability
Loss of ability to swallow
Loss of speech
Loss of breathing ability
Loss of all communication (locked-in)

Psychosocial/spiritual
Loss of emotional control
Loss of independence
Loss of social role
Loss of family role
Loss of intimacy
Loss of dignity
Loss of hope
Loss of faith
Loss of meaning in life

---

wide range of emotions – fears of the disease, of deterioration, of dependency, of disability, and of dying and death. There is a need to be open to the person and their family and to allow discussion of these issues, particularly while the person can still speak – as discussion with a communication aid can become increasingly difficult and distressing for all concerned.

Social aspects

Most people with ALS are part of wider relationships or families. The others in these relationships may have similar concerns: of the disease, deterioration, finances, dying and death, and communication with children[12]. Sexuality is an important issue for many patients and couples, and is often unrecognized[13]. These concerns need to be discussed, and a social worker or counselor may be helpful in encouraging the wider discussion of the difficult issues.

Spiritual aspects

The issues regarding the deeper meaning of life often come to the fore when facing a progressive, life-threatening disease[13]. Opportunities should be provided for the person with ALS, and their family and carers, to look at these aspects of care – which may not necessarily be religious. Cultural aspects of care are also important and need to be addressed.

THE FINAL STAGES

Many people with ALS fear the final stages of the disease progression, and there are particular fears of choking, dyspnea and pain. However, research has shown that, with good palliative care, over 90% of people die peacefully and choking is very rare[14,15]. Often the terminal stage occurs when the person develops a respiratory tract infection and the changes occur over only a few days; 48–72% of patients deteriorate rapidly and die within 24 hours[14,15].

It is important to anticipate the sudden deterioration. Discussion between the person with ALS, their family and the professional carers is essential, so that all are aware of the plans if a deterioration occurs. Medication may be provided: injections of morphine, for pain and dyspnea[9,14]; midazolam, to provide relaxation and sedation; glycopyrronium bromide, for chest secretions; and buccal lorazepam, to be given by family carers, to reduce distress while awaiting help

In the UK the Motor Neurone Disease Association has developed the Breathing Space Programme[6]. This has leaflets for the person with ALS and their family and for health-care professionals to encourage discussion of these issues at the end of life. There is also a box for the medication, so that it can be stored easily in the person's house and is readily available for any health-care professional to use if there is a sudden deterioration. The presence of the medication, together with the ongoing discussion and support of the professional carers, can be reassuring for both patient and family.

The majority of people with ALS wish to remain at home and, with good support, anticipation and the involvement of a co-ordinated team approach, this is often possible[14,15]. A multidisciplinary team approach is essential and regular meetings, to co-ordinate care and support all those involved, are helpful. There is a need for ongoing support from the time of diagnosis, but the team member involved most closely may vary over time. In the earlier stages of the disease the physiotherapist may be most involved, but later in the terminal stages the medical and nursing team may take the lead.

BEREAVEMENT

After the death, the family may need bereavement support. They have faced a progressive loss of the person with ALS, as the disease has progressed. There may be mixed emotions – of relief and then guilt. Support can be helpful, in allowing all these emotions to be expressed[16].

CONCLUSION

During the disease progression of ALS, the patient and their family face many losses – of mobility, speech, swallowing, breathing – and for the majority of patients the mind remains clear and aware. Palliative care has much to offer in allowing those with ALS to retain the capabilities they do have and to make the most of the activities that remain possible for them. With good palliative care from the multidisciplinary team, patients with ALS can die peacefully, and in control of their lives.

ACKNOWLEDGMENT

This chapter is based in part on material from reference 17. We thank the editor and publishers of the *European Journal of Palliative Care* for their permission to use the material.

REFERENCES

1. World Health Organization. National Cancer Control Programmes: Policies and Managerial Guidelines, 2nd edn, Geneva: WHO, 2002: 83–91
2. Oliver D. Palliative care. In: Oliver D, Borasio GD, Walsh D, eds. Palliative Care in Amyotrophic Lateral Sclerosis. Oxford: Oxford University Press, 2000; 23–8
3. Wagner-Sonntag E, Allison S, Oliver D, et al. Dysphagia. In: Oliver D, Borasio GD, Walsh D, eds. Palliative Care in Amyotrophic Lateral Sclerosis. Oxford: Oxford University Press, 2000: 62–72
4. Miller RG, Rosenberg JA, Gelinas DF, et al., and the ALS Practice Parameters Task Force: Practice Parameter. The care of the patient with amyotrophic lateral sclerosis (an evidence-based review): Report of the Quality Standards Subcommittee of the American Academy of Neurology: ALS Practice Parameters Task Force. Neurology 1999; 52: 1311–23
5. Gregory S, Siderowf A, Golaszewski AL, McCluskey L. Gastrostomy insertion in ALS patients with low vital capacity: Respiratory support and survival. Neurology 2002; 58: 485–7
6. Oliver D. The quality of care and symptom control – The effects on the terminal phase of ALS/MND. J Neurol Sci 1996; 139 (Suppl): 134–6
7. Scott A. Foulsom M. Speech and language therapy. In: Oliver D, Borasio GD, Walsh D, eds. Palliative Care in Amyotrophic Lateral Sclerosis. Oxford: Oxford University Press, 2000: 117–25
8. Lyall R, Moxham J, Leigh N. Dyspnoea. In: Oliver D, Borasio GD, Walsh D, eds. Palliative Care in Amyotrophic Lateral Sclerosis. Oxford: Oxford University Press, 2000: 43–56
9. Oliver D. Opioid medication in the palliative care of motor neurone disease. Palliat Med 1998; 12: 113–15
10. Murphy PL, Albert SM, Weber CM, et al. Impact of spirituality and religiousness on outcomes in patients with ALS. Neurology 2000; 55: 1581–4
11. Neudert C, Wasner M, Borasio GD. Individual quality of life is not correlated with health-related quality of life or physical function in patients with amyotrophic lateral sclerosis. J Palliat Med 2004; 7: 551–7

12. Gallagher D, Monroe B. Psychosocial care. In: Oliver D, Borasio GD, Walsh D, eds. Palliative Care in Amyotrophic Lateral Sclerosis. Oxford: Oxford University Press, 2000: 92–103

13. Wasner M, Bold U, Vollmer TC, Borasio GD. Sexuality in patients with amyotrophic lateral sclerosis and their partners. J Neurol 2004; 251: 445–8

14. O'Brien T, Kelly M, Saunders C. Motor neuron disease: A hospice perspective. Br Med J 1992; 304: 471–3

15. Neudert C, Oliver D, Wasner M, Borasio GD. The course of the terminal phase in patients with amyotrophic lateral sclerosis. J Neurol 2001; 248: 612–16

16. McMurray A. Bereavement. In: Oliver D, Borasio GD, Walsh D, eds. Palliative Care in Amyotrophic Lateral Sclerosis. Oxford: Oxford University Press, 2000: 169–181

17. Oliver D, Borasio GD. Palliative care for sufferers of ALS (MND). Eur J Palliat Care 2004; 11: 185–7

Index

T - #0488 - 071024 - C8 - 246/189/17 - PB - 9780367390631 - Gloss Lamination